Neurobiology of Nociceptors

Neurobiology of Nociceptors

Edited by

CARLOS BELMONTE

Instituto de Neurociencias
Universidad de Alicante
Alicante

and

FERNANDO CERVERO

Departamento de Fisiología y Farmacología
Universidad de Alcalá de Henares
Madrid

OXFORD NEW YORK TOKYO

OXFORD UNIVERSITY PRESS

1996

Oxford University Press, Walton Street, Oxford OX2 6DP
Oxford New York
Athens Auckland Bangkok Bombay
Calcutta Cape Town Dar es Salaam Delhi
Florence Hong Kong Istanbul Karachi
Kuala Lumpur Madras Madrid Melbourne
Mexico City Nairobi Paris Singapore
Taipei Tokyo Toronto
and associated companies in
Berlin Ibadan

Oxford is a trade mark of Oxford Unversity Press

Published in the United States
by Oxford University Press Inc., New York

A catalogue record for this book is available from the British Library

Library of Congress Cataloging in Publication Data
Neurobiology of nociceptors / edited by Carlos Belmonte and Fernando Cervero. – 1st ed.

Includes bibliographical references and index.
1. Nociceptors. I. Belmonte, C. II. Cervero, Fernando.
[DNLM: 1. Nociceptors – physiology. WL 102.9 N4934 1996]
QP451.4.N49 1996   612.8'8 – dc20   96–4636

ISBN 0 19 852334 3

Typeset by Hewer Text Composition Services, Edinburgh
Printed in Great Britain by Bookcraft (Bath) Ltd, Midsomer Norton, Avon

Preface

It is almost 100 years since Sherrington introduced the concept of 'Nociceptor' as a hypothetical category of sensory receptor concerned with the signalling and encoding of harmful and potentially harmful events. This proved to be a seminal idea that led to a large number of investigations and eventually to the identification and characterization of this kind of sensory receptor. In the intervening century, and particularly in the last 30 years, there have been numerous studies on the physiology, anatomy, and neurochemistry of these sensory afferents and a good deal has been learned about the functional roles of nociceptors in animals and in man.

It is therefore surprising that this is the first attempt at producing a book specifically dedicated to the neurobiology of nociceptors. If we consider the large number of volumes on the physiology of photoreceptors and of receptors concerned with hearing, olfaction, or taste, then it is clear that a monograph such as the present one is much needed.

The starting point of this book was a symposium that we organized in Madrid with the title 'What do nociceptors tell the brain?' This meeting, sponsored by the Juan March Foundation, was attended by many of the authors that have contributed chapters to this book. At the time of the meeting we realized the need for a book such as the present one and, although it has taken a few years, we have finally achieved our aim. We wanted to produce a comprehensive book rather than the often patchy and incomplete proceedings report of a specialized symposium. Therefore we started from scratch and planned a multi-author book covering all aspects of nociceptor function.

The aim of this book is to offer the reader a set of papers that will provide the experimental evidence for most of our current knowledge about nociceptors. A central issue is the analysis of the role of nociceptors in pain sensation and, therefore, most chapters address this question directly or indirectly. We have included chapters on the structure of nociceptive endings, on the neurochemistry of these afferents, and on evolutionary aspects of nociceptor function. There are reviews of the functional properties of nociceptors innervating somatic and visceral organs and of the biophysical mechanisms that underlie the transduction process in nociceptors. The functions of nociceptors are reviewed in detail, particularly their role in normal and abnormal pain sensations, including their contribution and that of other cutaneous receptors to hyperalgesic states. Finally, there are also sections on the plastic changes expressed by nociceptors, on the alterations induced in their transduction properties by nerve injury and regeneration, and on the physiopathology of nociceptor function.

In order to produce an informative and authoritative book we have asked a group of experts in this field of research to produce the individual chapters. They have had complete freedom to express their ideas and have been encouraged to produce papers containing not only experimental observations but also their opinions and working hypotheses. The authors of this monograph are scientists with considerable experience in this field that have contributed a great deal to current knowledge of the neurobiology of nociceptors. We believe that the readers will appreciate having their personal opinions and not just a set of dry facts. The small amount of intentional overlap between chapters is, in fact, beneficial to the book as it allows the expression of several views, not necessarily unanimous, on a particular topic.

We are aware that there are some aspects that have not been covered in great depth and that others have been approached by several authors. This is only a reflection of current interest in the field with certain topics being more fashionable than others. We take full responsibility for this and offer apologies to those readers that may be disappointed. We would, of course, be very happy if any shortcomings of this book would spur others to produce alternative publications. After all, this topic deserves more than one book every 100 years!

We wish to express our appreciation to all the authors for taking time to write these chapters and for all the hard work that they have put into this project. It is absolutely obvious that without their contribution this book would not have been produced. We are also indebted to Dr Jenny Laird for her considerable help with the editing, both scientific and linguistic, and for agreeing to become a test reader. Finally, we are very grateful to Oxford University Press for offering us an ideal publishing channel for the book and in particular to Vanessa Whitting for her help and encouragement with the management of this project. To all of them our thanks.

Alicante and   C.B.
Alcalá de Henares   F.C.
August, 1995

Contents

Contributors

Carlos Belmonte, Instituto de Neurociencias, Universidad de Alicante, 03080 Alicante Spain.

Stuart Bevan, Sandoz Institute for Medical Research, London, WC1E 6BN, UK

James N. Campbell, Department of Neurosurgery, Johns Hopkins Medical School, Baltimore, MD 21287, USA.

Mario Campero, Department of Neurology, Neuromuscular Division, Neurological Sciences Center, Portland, OR 97210, USA.

Fernando Cervero, Departamento de Fisiologia y Farmacologia, Universidad de Alcalá de Henares, Facultad de Medicina, 28871 Madrid, Spain.

Juana Gallar, Instituto de Neurociencias, Universidad de Alicante, 03080 Alicante Spain.

Zdenek Halata, Anatomisches Institut, Universitäts-Krankenhaus Eppendorf, 20246 Hamburg, Germany.

Hermann O. Handwerker, Physiologisches Institut I, Universität Erlangen-Nürnberg, 91054 Erlangen, Germany.

Michaela Kress, Physiologisches Institut I, Universität Erlangen-Nürnberg, 91054 Erlangen, Germany.

Lawrence Kruger, Department of Neurobiology, UCLA Medical Center, Los Angeles, CA 90095, USA.

Takao Kumazawa, Department of Neural Regulation, Research Institute of Environmental Medicine, Nagoya University, Nagoya 464-01, Japan.

Robert H. Lamotte, Department of Anaesthesiology, Yale University School of Medicine, New Haven, CT 06510, USA.

Sally N. Lawson, Department of Physiology, University of Bristol Medical School, Bristol BS8 1TD, UK.

Stephen J. W. Lisney, Department of Physiology, University of Bristol Medical School, Bristol BS8 1TD, UK.

Bruce Lynn, Department of Physiology, University College London, London WC1E 6BT, UK.

Lorne M. Mendell, Department of Neurobiology and Behavior, State University of New York, Stony Brook, NY 11794, USA.

Siegfried Mense, Institut für Anatomie und Zellbiologie, Universität Heidelberg, 69120 Heidelberg, Germany.

Richard A. Meyer, Applied Physics Laboratory, Johns Hopkins University, Laurel, MD 20723, USA.

José L. Ochoa, Department of Neurology, Neuromuscular Division, Neurological Sciences Center, Portland, OR 97210, USA.

Edward R. Perl, Department of Physiology, University of North Carolina School of Medicine, Chapel Hill, NC 27599, USA.

Srinivasa N. Raja, Department of Anesthesiology and Critical Care, Johns Hopkins Medical School, Baltimore MD 21287, USA.

Peter W. Reeh, Physiologisches Institut I, Universität Erlangen-Nürnberg, 91054 Erlangen, Germany.

Hans-Georg Schaible, Physiologisches Institut, Universität Würzburg, 97070 Würzburg, Germany.

Martin Schmelz, Physiologisches Institut I, Universität Erlangen-Nürnberg, 91054 Erlangen, Germany.

Robert F. Schmidt, Physiologisches Institut, Universität Würzburg, 97070 Würzburg, Germany.

Jordi Serra, Department of Neurology, Neuromuscular Division, Neurological Sciences Center, Portland, OR 97210, USA.

Christoph Stein, Department of Anaesthesiology and Critical Care Medicine, Johns Hopkins Medical School, Baltimore, MD 21287–8711, USA.

H. Erik Torebjörk, Department of Clinical Neurophysiology, University Hospital, Uppsala, Sweden.

Edgar T. Walters, Department of Integrative Biology, University of Texas, Houston Medical School, Houston, TX 77030, USA.

Principles of classification and nomenclature relevant to studies of nociceptive neurones

BRUCE LYNN

Many classifications of neurones will be used in this book. How are we to evaluate them? Why do different authors sometimes use apparently quite dissimilar classifications? This brief article offers some views on these and related matters. The emphasis is on basic ideas and specific citations are not given. A list of sources is given at the end.

Let us first consider why making classifications is so useful. Principally, classification gives us a way of handling the number problem. In simple organisms such as *Caenorhabditis elegans* or the leech there are only small numbers of neurones and it is possible to treat each one as an individual. In the vertebrates, however, this is not possible and we have to deal with populations of neurones. Clearly, finding the appropriate functional groupings is crucial to developing sensible hypotheses about how the system operates. This is really the key to good classifications. They lead to new insights into how the system functions and provide an efficient terminology for describing system function. For example, the discovery of the X, Y, and W classes of retinal ganglion cells led to major developments in our understanding of visual processing, particularly the importance of parallel processing by functionally distinct groups of neurones. A good classification should also lead to insights into how adult neurones develop. Consider the parallel with taxonomy. The classification of plants and animals suggested interrelationships between groups and stimulated thinking about how such groups were formed, eventually playing a major part in the development of the theory of evolution.

How can we tell a good classification from a bad one? A good classification will utilize many variables, probably including both functional and morphological measures. Classifications depending on just one or two 'essential' features are liable to be superseded if just one significant new factor is discovered. Numerical methods can help in assessing multiple variables. Once there are more than four variables to consider, visualizing the *n*-dimensional space in which the data needs to be placed becomes a serious challenge to the imagination! But be warned, numerical methods such as the various forms of cluster analysis do not in themselves tell you how many groups are present. They can only indicate the probable groupings and should be used as part of the hypothesis-building process. Obvious limitations of numerical methods are how they can handle different tyes of variable (nominal, numerical, etc.), whether all variables should be weighted equally, and how to handle conditional variables (for example, response to hair movement is only a variable for units from hairy skin, so a study covering hairy and glabrous skin has to deal with the fact that this parameter is only present for a subset of the sample).

A not uncommon problem occurs with classifications that are really only subdivisions. In science, as in other activities there are 'lumpers' and 'splitters'. A group of neurones with a wide range of properties will commonly be split into subgroups, without any consideration of whether the subdivisions represent separate classes. To be a class, a group of neurones must show a distinct set of properties not shared by other members of the sample. It may occasionally be useful to subdivide a population into arbitrary groups in this way, but this process is not classification, merely dissection.

The importance of basing classifications on several variables has been stressed, but in real life the identification of the class of a neurone needs to be based on a small number of easily measured variables. It is important to distinguish the process of identification from the process of classification. Identifiers will be a subset of the classifiers that give a high probability of correct classification, and are also easy to measure. They may not be particularly important parameters for the main function of the neurone. For example, conduction velocity is an important identifier for many afferent neurones, but is often of much less importance for their function than measures such as receptive field properties or thresholds for adequate stimulation.

A final important distinction to maintain is between nomenclature and classification. Choosing names for classes is good fun, but, compared with defining the classes themselves, is essentially trivial. As an example, consider the large population of C-fibre cutaneous afferents that respond to pressure, heat, and irritant chemicals. These are called either polymodal or mechanoheat. I have argued that the polymodal designation is preferable, but in practice the important thing is to recognize this distinct class of neurones. The question of which term is the best name is quite secondary. Good class names are helpful, however, and a profusion of parallel terminology can be confusing. It has been argued that class names such as polymodal nociceptor are dangerous, since they presuppose the function. More neutral terminology (e.g. type I and type II mechano-receptor) is supposedly less prone to embarrassing error. The literature is full of examples of inappropriate names. Vasopressin, rather than antidiuretic hormone, is one of my favourites. However, where function is well established it does have the advantage of conveying information and, often, of being easier to remember. Where would we be without our nociceptors, mechanoreceptors, and thermoreceptors! In the end, though, nomenclature is secondary to classification. To quote: 'What's in a name? That which we call a rose by any other name would smell as sweet' (Shakespeare, *Romeo and Juliet*).

References

This brief account has borrowed heavily from the following sources.

Gordon, A.D. (1981). *Classification. Methods for the exploratory analysis of multivariate data.* Chapman & Hall, London.

Hughes, A. (1979). A rose by any other name . . . On 'Naming of neurones' by Rowe and Stone. *Brain Behav. Evol.* **16**, 52–64.

Lynn, B. (1994). The fibre composition of cutaneous nerves and the classification and properties of cutaneous afferents with particular reference to nociception. *Pain Rev.* **1**, 172–83.

Rowe, M.H. and Stone, J. (1977). Naming of neurones. Classification and naming of cat retinal ganglion cells. *Brain Behav. Evol.* **14**, 185–216.

Rowe, M.H. and Stone, J. (1979). The importance of knowing our own presuppositions. *Brain Behav. Evol.* **16**, 65–80.

Tyner, C.F. (1975). The naming of neurones: applications of taxonomic theory to the study of cellular populations. *Brain Behav. Evol.* **12**, 75–96.

PART 1
Basic aspects of nociceptor function

1 Pain and the discovery of nociceptors

EDWARD R. PERL

Nociceptors are primary afferent neurones signalling the presence of tissue-damaging stimuli or the existence of tissue damage. Their activity produces adversive and protective reactions including the sensation of pain. The evolution of ideas about such sense organs and the eventual documentation of their existence traces a history of concepts about pain and pain mechanisms. That chronicle is as convoluted as most annals of human thought about complex phenomena. The issues have been several. One concerns the organ of the mind, of consciousness and perception. Another is the nature of pain. Does pain belong to one of the senses or is it akin to an emotion, such as anger, despair, fear? The ancient Greek philosophers touched on these points and left an enduring legacy. In this, Aristotle's (384–322 BC) view that pain is an affect and that the heart is the seat of the mind had a most profound influence upon subsequent Western thinking. After him, the crystallization of ideas proved slow and tortuous. But Aristotle and other early Western philosophers were not alone in perpetuating conceptions eventually shown to be erroneous. The Chinese Canon of Medicine, the *Nei Ching* (2000–250 BC), also left legacies of myth for Eastern thinking about sensation and the functions of the nervous system that persist to the present.

The heart as the seat of feeling

Greek philosophers such as Aristotle were handicapped in their considerations of the structures responsible for feeling and intelligence by the lack of first-hand knowledge about human anatomy. For Aristotle the heart was the dominant organ of the body and the source of sensibility and emotion. He argued for differences in sensibility among different creatures and different individuals. He linked the heart in particular to the sense of touch, viewing it as the most basic sensation. In Aristotle's construction, a person of low sensibility had a small, firm heart while individuals with greater sensibility and more generous reactions had softer hearts (Aristotle: *De partibus animalium*). These ideas probably represent the origin of the terms 'hard-hearted' or 'soft-hearted' (Keele 1957).

Aristotle, as others before him, recognized five senses: sight; hearing; smell; taste; and touch. Each of these had obvious tissue organs associated with the sense. In Aristotle's view, sense organs were intimately related to the media by which they were excited. To him, pain was not a separate sense but rather a variety of touch and of other senses. All senses could lead to either pain or pleasure. Pain would be produced when a medium was in excess and destructive (Aristotle 1951, De Anima, Book II, Chapter 6). By the latter, he implied a relationship between excessive stimulation and tissue damage, a connection that in modern times helped define the common ground for sense organs responsible for pain. Thus, Aristotle made monumental contributions to philosophical thought and to the understanding of nature and provided insights about a possible significance of pain;

however, he failed to appreciate the importance of the brain for sensory experience and classified pain as an emotion rather than a separate sense.

It is not surprising that Aristotle and many after him considered pain to be different from vision, hearing, taste, and smell. Pain is usually associated with discomfort and, if severe, with anguish and suffering. While such affects can arise from other sensations, the connection is not as consistent. What we perceive through vision can be unpleasant or cause fear or despair, but often visual perception is dispassionate or pleasurable. Ordinary experience illustrates that the same variety of emotions follows auditory, gustatory, olfactory, and tactile stimuli. The perception that a circumstance or stimulus is painful and the associated emotional impact appears to differ from other sensations by its common linkage to a negative reaction.

While disagreement with Aristotle's concept of the sensory nature of the heart emerged relatively soon after his time, his views proved hard to overcome. Galen of Alexandria (AD 130–201), five centuries later, provided strong arguments in favour of the brain as the master organ of sensation, thought, and intelligence, supporting similar ideas by earlier commentators from Alexandria. He, in contrast to the Greek philosophers, had a substantial understanding of anatomy and, as a physician, of disease. Galen did experiments that established the functional importance of the brain and its appendages. He described the effects of lesions in animals demonstrating the essential role of the spinal cord in movement and sensation from the body. Galen implicated peripheral nerves as passageways to the brain related to sensation; however, he conceived the transfer as movement of particles or substances extracted from the environment, an Aristotelian view that was not to be dispelled for many centuries. Galen was interested in pain and recognized its value in warning of damage or disturbance but apparently did not comment on whether pain was independent of other senses. Galen's ideas lost favour during the dark and middle ages, in spite of their clarity and support from anatomical observations, perhaps because his heretical views on the mortality of the soul offended Christian beliefs (Keele 1957). As a consequence, Galen did not dissuade subsequent thought from the notion of the sensory heart. Whatever else, he clearly put pain into the class of sensory experiences rather than that of emotions and recognized unambiguously that pain was dependent upon the continuity of the peripheral nerves. Unfortunately for the progress of ideas, these insights remained largely submerged for over a thousand years. A late medieval illustration diagramming a mixture of Aristotle's idea of the heart as the organ for sensation and Galen's views that sensation involved peripheral nerves and the brain appears in Fig. 1.1.

Challenges to the idea of pain as a purely affective phenomenon after Galen came from other physicians. The renowned Muslim physician and philosopher, Avicenna (AD 980–1038), suggested not only that touch was composed of several subvarieties of sensation but also that pain, particularly as produced by injury, was a separate sense (Avicenna: *The canon of medicine* quoted in Gruner 1930). Avicenna's views on medicine had wide influence; however, those about pain did not lessen the general acceptance of Aristotle's ideas. An upheaval in concepts awaited the progressive development of an understanding of how neurones and nerves functioned, a more scientific aproach to questions of natural history, and both clinical and experimental evidence on the dissociation of sensation produced by lesions of nerve or of the central nervous system.

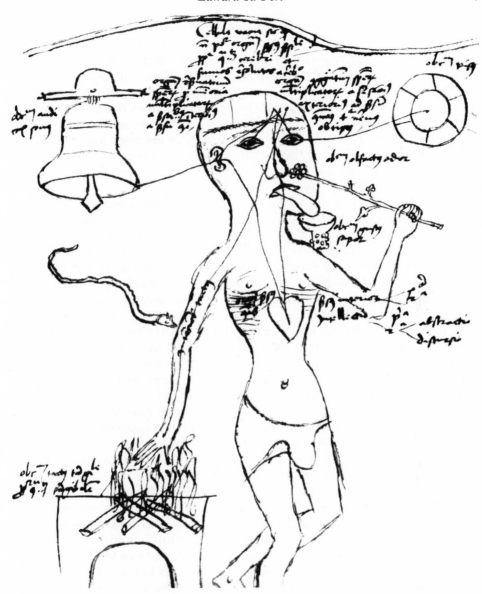

Fig. 1.1 A late fifteenth-century drawing combining the Aristotelian view of the heart as the seat of sensation and the concepts of Galen and Avicenna about the brain and nerves. It shows various senses—audition, vision, smell, and taste—and pain from heat and snake bite impinging upon a 'cell' in brain and being sent to the heart. The heart is labelled as 'sensus communis'. From an incunable in the Wellcome Institute for the History of Medicine, with permission (1954, p. 283). Also reproduced in Keele (1957, Plate 11) and in Clarke and Dewherst (1972, fig. 14).

The light from anatomy

From Galen on through the Middle Ages, little progress was evident in Western thought about pain mechanisms but, with the Renaissance, new views emerged with a revival of interest in anatomy. Knowledge of anatomy, particularly that of the central nervous system, progressed considerably in the years after AD 1400, although not all accepted what was uncovered. The man of all seasons, Leonardo da Vinci (1452–1519), recognized the importance of the nervous system for pain and added to the understanding of the structure of both. Leonardo noted variability in pain responsiveness in different parts of the body and proposed that pain was a sensory experience mediated by the same nerves as those responsible for touch. He had put aside the Aristotelian view of the heart as the source of sensation and control of the body; however, William Harvey, although of the same period and the discoverer of the circulation of blood, still clung to the notion that in some way the heart had to do with conscious experience. René Descartes (1596–1650), famous for his mechanistic approach to human function, still conceived of a physical aspect of the external world as being carried to the brain to produce sensation; however, he, as Galen, proposed the peripheral nerves as the means of this transport. Descartes' idea of man as a machine did recognize pain as a sensation associated with touch. On the other hand, while considering sensation as the work of a part of the brain (the pineal gland), Descartes still had emotion arising from the heart. Thomas Willis (1622–75), a contemporary of Descartes, made many notable observations on central nervous system structures and, in particular, proposed the existence of specific pathways within the nervous system. Willis anticipated the discovery of nerve impulses by presuming that nerves carried something intrinsic along their pathways rather than transmitting an agent from the material world.

As the result of animal vivisection, the seventeenth century saw strides forward in understanding not only the anatomy of the brain, but also its function. For example, Willis found that the meninges gave rise to responses, which led him to attribute to them sensory capacity, a knowledge that could only have come from exploring the brain of a living creature. The intellectual ferment of the Renaissance produced many advances in the understanding of nature and some carried over to the question of pain. Isaac Newton (1642–1727) argued for a propagation along nerves from the organs of sense to the brain as movement of 'a very subtle spirit' integral to the nerve. By the middle of the sevententh century, many of the minds that had considered the issue of pain categorized it as a sensation; however, whether it was a special sense in its own right was far from settled. In that era, pain commonly was still set as the Aristotelian opposite of pleasure and, thereby, if pain was a sensation so was pleasure.

The spinal roots and sensory specificity

A great advance in understanding the mechanisms of sensation came about as a consequence of the insight and evidence showing that the dorsal and ventral spinal roots differed in function, the dorsal roots being sensory and ventral roots motor. Explicit hypotheses about sensory nerve function were other seminal steps. The major seventeenth and eighteenth century discoveries about the natural world, insights into the nature of many chemical substances and of light and sound, were the background for these advances. Charles Bell (1774–1842) contributed to enlightenment about both the spinal roots and the function of sensory neurones. While principally an anatomist, Bell thought in physiological terms and experimented on living animals to confirm his ideas. He was the first to recognize correctly the distinction between dorsal and ventral spinal roots, pointing out that the ventral roots were motor. Moreover, in an 1811 monograph Bell unequivocally proposed that each kind of sense organ was specialized to respond to a particular kind of circumstance or event. Bell later postulated pain to be a distinct sensory experience, which varied with the part of the body, and argued it to have protective value. Across the English Channel, Bell's observations and ideas inspired Francois Magendie to do experiments that led to the formal proposal that dorsal roots were sensory in function, a point that Bell apparently recognized but never explicitly stated.

This early nineteenth century work and the 'Bell and Magendie law' about the spinal roots were the background for Johannes Müller's (1842) codification of the specificity of sensory nerves. Müller argued that each type of sensory nerve has characteristics that make it susceptible to a particular form of stimulation. He also pointed out that the central connections of the nerves of sense were related to specific sensory functions. Furthermore, Müller joined Willis and Newton in anticipating the discovery of the nerve impulse by proposing that a property of the nerve is the factor conveyed to central structures. Müller put pain into the category of sensation, although his attention was largely directed at the special senses of the head. He did not distinguish between various aspects of what was called 'common sensibility' related to the nerves of feeling (*gefühlsnerven*). Müller's formalization of ideas about conveyance of messages to the central nervous system by nerves and the concept that different nerves carry different types of information according to their own peculiar properties probably represented an intellectual turning point (Dallenbach 1939; Keele 1957). Along with the knowledge of separation of sensory and motor function by the spinal roots, these ideas provided a basis for further experimentation and analyses. Now the question could be legitimately asked: if pain is a sensation and there are special nerves for different sensations, are there special nerves for pain?

Dissociation, specificity, and intensity

Once a sensory function for the dorsal roots had been established and an explicit concept about sensory neurones put forth in an era of a burgeoning scientific exploration, the development of information and ideas about pain accelerated. A few years after Müller's concepts, Moritz Schiff, a student of Magendie, described the dissociation of tactile and pain-related responses by experimental lesions of the spinal cord. Schiff (1858) found that lesions of the spinal cord white matter in young canines abolished tactile-evoked reactions while leaving intact responses to pain-causing stimuli. On the other hand, damage of the spinal grey matter caused the converse; reactions to tactile stimuli remained but those evoked by usually painful stimuli disappeared. This dissociation led Schiff in 1858, referring to these observations of some years previous, to postulate explicitly that pain was a separate and particular sensation, independent of touch. While others had argued for pain as a distinct sense, Schiff's evidence and hypothesis were more concrete and it probably is fair to attribute to him the concept of a specific sense of pain.

Although Schiff may have been the first to repeat Galen's experiments showing the spinal cord to be crucial in transmission of information, Brown-Séquard's name is usually attached to the dissociation of sensation as a consequence of lesions of the spinal cord. For generations medical students have learned that hemisection of the spinal cord produces the Brown-Séquard syndrome, characterized by ipsilateral loss of vibration and position sense and contralateral loss of pain and temperature sensibility (Brown-Séquard 1860; 1868). The dissociation of sensation as a result of lesions or manipulation of nervous tissue proved to be a powerful tool in the eventual establishment of the sensory nature of pain; however, the legacy of past concepts was hard to overcome even though the clinicians of the latter part of the nineteenth century seized upon the insights provided by the new evidence. Famous names of nineteenth century neurology (for example, Charcot, Gowers) provided clinical corroboration of Schiff's and Brown-Séquard's experiments.

While pain may be a sensory experience in its own right, this conclusion does not prove that it begins from special sense organs. That point was emphasized by W. Erb (1874) of Heidelberg who used analyses of diseases of peripheral nerve as the basis of a proposal that pain represents a quantitative rather than a qualitative variation of sensation. Erb argued that every kind of stimulus capable of evoking a sensory experience would initiate pain if intense enough; by this formulation he enunciated the 'intensive theory of pain', although again this idea had ancient roots.

The latter quarter of the nineteenth century saw a vigorous and heated debate about the nature of pain among proponents of the then three major viewpoints: pain as an emotion; pain as an intensive concomitant of other sensation; and a pain as a particular sensation (Dallenbach 1939). Only the latter demanded specialized sense organs. In this fray, the physicians were largely on the side of a specific sense. The philosophers tended to hold the traditional (Aristotelian) view and favoured affect. A new class of experimentalists, the human psychophysicists, stepped into the dispute. M. Blix (1884) discovered that the skin was not uniform for the sensory experiences evokable by punctate stimuli. He reported that needle pressure initiated pain from some spots of the skin but a pressure-tactile sense from others, an observation soon confirmed by A. Goldscheider (1885). While Blix and Goldscheider both changed opinions about the existence of cutaneous pain spots, another psychophysicist, Max von Frey (1894, 1922) did not. von Frey's clearly described experiments on skin sensibility and his quantitative approach convinced many, particularly the physiologists and clinicians of the time; the latter were otherwise prepared to be counted in the camp espousing pain as a specific sensation on the basis of the observations on sensory dissociation. von Frey reported a remarkable mosaic of cutaneous sensibility. He described pressure, cold, warm, and pain spots, each separated from each other, and quantitated the relative frequency of each kind in different parts of the body. This frequency of occurrence of each category of spot was compared to the reported density of different types of nerve terminations in equivalent skin regions from histological studies. From this, von Frey (1894, 1897) deduced the morphological type of afferent terminal related to each kind of skin spot and, therefore, to a particular form of cutaneous sensations. He attributed pain to the many fine nerve terminals without capsules or other specialized associated cells on the basis of this circumstantial linkage. The picture his experiments and concepts painted was that of a highly organized system linking a particular type of sense organ in the skin to its own class of sensation. Pain was included in this specificity as proposed by Schiff and predecessors going back at least to Avicenna.

von Frey's views fell on fertile soil, the observations indicative of a particular pathway within the spinal cord for pain and temperature resulting from Schiff's and Brown-Séquard's studies along with corroborating clinical cases. The idea that pain was a sensation with its own neural apparatus was widely accepted by the beginning of the twentieth century; however, the vexing problem of its stimulus remained. Pain is caused by mechanical stimuli when they are strong enough, by heat when the temperature is high enough, cold when the temperature is low enough, and by a variety of chemical agents. This spectrum of stimuli does not fit what was known about the accepted classical sensations. Vision was understood to be the product of waves of energy with clearly defined dimensions. Hearing was believed to result from limited frequencies of pressure changes in the atmosphere. Smell and taste had their own respective effective stimuli. Touch and pressure came from definable mechanical deformations of skin and subcutaneous tissues.

Tissue damage and nociception

A solution to the dilemma of pain stimuli came from the famed neurophysiologist of the turn of the twentieth century, Charles Sherrington. Sherrington had performed a remarkable set of analyses of mammalian neural function, which he summarized in a 1906 volume titled, *The integrative action of the nervous system*. That book, to a substantial degree, refashioned thinking about nervous function. Sherrington's studies had defined withdrawal reflexes in which a decerebrate or spinal animal removes a limb from contact with a source of strong stimulation by the activation of muscles flexing joints and bringing the limb closer to the body. These flexor withdrawal reflexes were interpreted as protective in part because they were most powerfully evoked by natural stimuli that were of such intensity to be pain-causing. Such protective withdrawal reflexes were linked to pain, and Sherrington proposed pain to be their sensory concomitant. This notion, of course, built upon recognition of the protective value of pain by Galen, Charles Bell, and others. Sherrington added the insight that pain was ordinarily produced when tissue was damaged and argued that the receptors for pain could be considered detectors of tissue damage or of the physical threat of such damage. Tissue-damaging or noxious stimuli could be any of several types: mechanical; thermal; or chemical. Therefore, in Sherrington's construct, receptors for noxious stimuli, 'noci-receptors', were detectors of impending or actual tissue damage. The concept of 'noci-reception' and the term 'nociceptors' originated from his insights; however, the documentation and definition of such sense organs waited more than another half century.

Specificity versus pattern

The studies on dissociation of sensation by experimental lesions of the spinal cord suggested that a crossed pathway was important for the preservation of pain or pain-associated reactions. The crossed sensory pathway was further localized to the ventrolateral white matter by clinical findings (Charcot 1888). By the end of the nineteenth century it was recognized that a crossed sensory pathway originated from the opposite grey matter of the dorsal horn of the spinal cord (Edinger 1890; Bechterev 1899). The final connection between the crossed afferent pathway and pain was made by clinicians who showed, through the accidents of nature and disease, a relationship between the crossed pathways of the lateral and ventrolateral portions of the spinal cord and the capacity of human patients to feel painful stimuli (Gowers 1892, 1899; Spiller 1905).

Other studies of the epoch, in describing a differential return of sensation after experimental division of a human peripheral nerve, suggested that somatic sensation was comprised of two distinctive forms—a crude, protopathic variety and a finely discriminative, epicritic version (Head *et al.* 1905). Pain and rough temperature appreciation were classified as protopathic, while fine spatial discrimination, recognition of texture and vibration, and fine temperature discrimination made up the epicritic forms. Such a division among the senses of the body implied differences in the peripheral and central organization.

The establishment of an ascending pathway as necessary for pain proved important in eventually uncovering the relevant sense organs, partially as a result of observations on how the primary afferent fibres from the dorsal roots enter the spinal cord. Edinger (1892) and other anatomists had observed dorsal roots to separate into medial, thick-fibred and lateral, thin-fibred divisions. These observations were amplified by Ranson (1913, 1915) who found that the lateral division of the dorsal roots with its fine fibres entered into a dorsolateral tract and terminated in the most superficial portions of the spinal dorsal grey matter. Preceding anatomical studies had suggested that the origin of the crossed ascending spinal pathway was in the dorsal part of the dorsal grey matter. Ranson (1915) proposed that fibres of the lateral division were responsible for pain and other protopathic sensations. This idea was supported by subsequent observations demonstrating that interruption of the lateral but not the medial division of the dorsal root blocked reflex reactions typically associated with pain (Ranson and Billingsly 1918). Thus, early in the twentieth century, before direct studies of the functional properties of sense organs were available, indications and proposals had come forth that thin afferent fibres from the periphery carried messages essential for pain and pain-related reactions.

At this juncture, the pieces necesssary for a comprehensive theory about pain as a sensation in its own right seemed in place. Different central pathways for pain and a number of non-painful sensations from the body had been shown to exist. In the skin, particular spots from which pain could be evoked had been described. A rationale for the effective stimulus for pain had been given and the term 'nociception' had been coined. However, the sense organ part was far from solved. For instance, Goldscheider (1891), who had originally reported particular pain spots in the skin, abandoned that view and argued instead that it was excessive stimulation of the tactile nerves that caused pain (Goldscheider 1920, 1926). von Frey maintained his conviction on the existence of specific pain spots in the skin (1922); however, several authoritative investigators found problems with the linkage of cutaneous pain spots to anatomically definable nerve terminations, calling into question the stability of such spots (MacKenzie 1918; Head 1920; Dallenbach 1927, 1929).

Early electrophysiology

The dawn of studies recording electrical signals from nerve sent equivocal messages about specific primary afferent neurones for pain. The recordings of compound action potential by Gasser and Erlanger showed peripheral nerve to be composed of groups of fibres conducting action potentials at different velocities related to their cross-sectional diameter. The fibre groups and the corresponding deflection in the compound potential were labelled alphabetically according to the sequence in which they appeared after a single, brief electrical stimulus; the A-deflection and the fibres producing it were the product of the most rapidly conducting fibres and the C-deflection that of those most slowly conducting fibres. Differential actions by pressure on the nerve, by the effects of local anaesthetic, and by the strength of electrical stimuli were used to determine the sensory effects related to the various fibre groups. Pressure blocked conduction in the rapidly conducting fibres before it affected the more slowly conducting ones; local anaesthetics blocked the thinnest, slowest fibres before the thicker, faster fibres; thicker, more rapidly conducting fibres had lower electrical thresholds than thinner, slower fibres. These correlations permitted comparison of the effects of each category in the reactions of lower animals or for sensation in people (Gasser and Erlanger 1927; Lewis *et al.* 1931; Heinbecker *et al.* 1932, 1933; Zotterman 1933; Clark *et al.* 1935). The studies generally agreed that the sensory or behavioural reactions evoked by activity in the more rapidly conducting, larger-diameter afferent fibres were tactile or proprioceptive. In contrast, activity in the thinner, more slowly conducting fibres appeared essential for pain, adversive reactions, and temperature sense. While the selective block or initiation of conduction of populations of fibres in nerve indicated the importance of slowly conducting primary afferent fibres for the production of pain and related reactions, they did not establish a specific subset of sense organs for these effects.

Ambiguous results emerged from the early recordings of unitary activity in primary afferent fibres of peripheral nerve by Adrian (1926, 1928) and Adrian and Zotterman (1926*a*, *b*). These workers interpreted their observations as indicating specific characteristics for different types of receptive units, but this interpretation was not universally accepted. The first electrophysiological recordings of unitary activity from peripheral nerve contained the activity of more than one fibre. As a consequence, in the view of at least one articulate commentator, Nafe (1929, 1934), the data were equivocal. Nafe (1929) counterproposed that the published records showed different patterns of activity for different kinds of stimuli. This alternative interpretation was fuelled by Nafe's objection to the specificity of cutaneous sense as formulated by von Frey, which we have seen was based on a mosaic of cutaneous sensitive spots and the correlation of these points of sensibility to morphological terminations. Nafe offered in place of specificity a theory for cutaneous sense including pain that postulated patterns of activity from a single class of receptive fibres as representing the signals that produced different somatic sensations.

The early unitary discharge records from mammals did not display elements specifically excited by stimuli expected to cause pain (Adrian 1926); however, an ingenious experiment soon afterwards addressed the intensive theory. Erb (1874) suggested that all sensory experiences, when intense enough, were transformed to pain. In the hands of Goldscheider (1891) and others, this concept was translated into one wherein activity from mechanoreceptors producing tactile-pressure sensations, when quantitatively large enough, initiates pain and its associated reactions. To test the intensive idea, Adrian, Cattell and Hoagland (1931) made use of a tactile stimulator consisting of a source of air under pressure blowing across a rotating disk with small holes spaced around its circumference. This device permitted puffs of air to be delivered at a wide range of repetitions. Each puff of air evoked a burst of impulses from single tactile receptors of the frog skin in recordings from the dorsal cutaneous nerves. Puffs repeating at 100 or more per second evoked maximal discharges from these tactile receptors. When the same rapidly repeating air puffs were applied to intact frogs, the animals did not evidence discomfort or avoidance. In contrast, pinprick to the skin of a frog that had ignored the air puffs promptly initiated adversive movements and reactions. Thus, maximal discharge by a tactile sense organ did not evoke reactions associated with pain. At the time these observations were taken to indicate that the quantity of nerve activity by itself was insufficient to initiate reactions typical of pain.

Electrophysiology: 1930–50

In 1932, Adrian, again working with the fine dorsal cutaneous nerves of the frog, reported that tactile stimuli evoked large action potentials, while under comparable conditions sympathetic discharges were represented by only very small action potentials. He found that small-amplitude action potentials similar to those of sympathetic discharges were uniquely initiated from the frog skin by acid solutions, solutions that routinely evoked protective reactions from intact animals. The deduction that the small action potentials induced by acid came from fibres as thin as those contributing to sympathetic discharges was, of course, circumstantial, too much so for some critics of electrophysiological observations and presumptions. A few years later Adrian's former colleague, Yngve Zotterman (1936), illustrated action potentials he presumed to originate from the most slowly conducting (C) fibres of the cat lingual nerve. By demonstrating discharges from the most slowly conducting peripheral fibres in a mammal he apparently succeeded where his mentor had failed. Consistent with Adrian's observations on nerves supplying frog skin, Zotterman reported that light pressure on the tongue evoked large action potentials in the lingual nerve (Fig. 1.2 (D)) which he suggested originated in large-diameter fibres. In contrast, hot water initiated activity in fibres producing very small action potentials (Fig. 1.2 (E)).

On the other hand, a 1939 report by Zotterman clouded the issue of the relationship between sense organs and pain. Zotterman estimated the conduction velocity of peripheral afferent fibres from the relative amplitude of action potentials in extracellular recordings of discharges. In the cat lingual nerve, small action potentials, which according to his calculations originated from fibres conducting at the speed of the Aδ group, were activated by light touch and by locally applied heat. He also reported that action potentials from fibres judged to be those producing the C-deflection and, therefore, unmyelinated were also initiated by the lightest of skin contact and by localized damaging heat. While his interpretation of these observations implied that different sets of fibres might be involved in the various responses, the evidence again was circumstantial and seemed to compromise the idea that slowly conducting fibres signalled the presence of pain-causing stimuli.

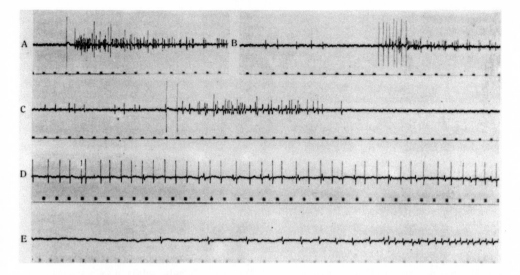

Fig. 1.2 Recordings made from a filament of the lingual nerve of cat. Trace E is of particular interest in its documentation of small-amplitude action potentials evoked by hot water (60°C) applied to the tongue. This appears to be the first published recording of activity by a single mammalian C-fibre that was evoked by noxious stimuli (see text). Trace A, Record from a lingual nerve preparation showing the activity evoked by a drop of water at 14°C on the tongue. Contact with the tongue is indicated by the first large-amplitude action potential. Trace B, Same preparation as in A showing the effect of blowing cool air across the tongue followed by the effect of a stronger blast of air. Trace C, Same preparation as in A. Activity generated by cool air in the background followed by (two large action potentials) the activity evoked by a drop of 80°C water placed on the tongue. Trace D, Recording from another lingual nerve preparation showing the effects of moderate to strong pressure on the tongue produced by a wooden stimulator 1 mm in diameter. Trace E, Same preparation as in D (see above). Reproduced with permission from Zotterman (1936, plate 2).

Post World War II and the challenge from Oxford

The expanding electrophysiological analyses of nervous function in the 1930s were substantially slowed by World War II, but after its end they were renewed with vigour. The resurgence was helped by the postwar explosion of available electronic technology; much improved analogue electronic amplifiers, oscilloscopes, and recording techniques made sampling activity from single neurones or fibres more readily accessible. The decade of the 1950s produced a number of publications dealing with the sense organs responsible for pain and the mechanisms underlying it as a sensation. Once again, however, the quality of the evidence and the interpretations were mixed.

In 1953 Landau and Bishop described analyses of pain produced by electrical, mechanical, and chemical agents. After selective block of myelinated or unmyelinated fibres in human subjects, they suggested distinct differences in the experience associated with activity of each category, broadening earlier analyses by Lewis, Pickering, and Rothschild (1931) and Zotterman (1933). Landau and Bishop concurred with previous studies that slowly conducting myelinated fibres were related to the initial pain felt after a sudden stimulus, which had a pricking or sharp quality. In contrast, the pain initiated from unmyelinated fibres (C) had a diffuse, burning characteristic and a notable conduction delay. Double pain from abrupt stimulation of the skin had been reported previously by Lewis and Pochin (1937); the delay between the two pains was noted to be prolonged with the increasing distance of the stimulated sites from the spinal cord. Landau and Bishop's observations presented more direct evidence than had been obtained before that the two pains were the product of separate groups of fibres from cutaneous and subcutaneous tissues. They interpreted their results in accordance with the concept of particular sense organs for particular sensory experiences. Quite different interpretations were accorded to other studies of the same era.

Until this point there had been few reports of unambiguous recording from single peripheral nerve fibres conducting at C-fibre velocity. Like Zotterman's recordings, these reports detailed the activity presumed to be generated by one fibre in nerve bundles containing several to many active fibres, usually through selective stimulation of the peripheral receptive tissues. An exception was a largely unheralded description from Tasaki's laboratory (Maruhashi et al. 1952) of recordings made after microdissection of peripheral nerve into filaments in which only a single fibre was visible. Fibre diameter in toad and cat nerves was measured using a compound microscope and then related to conduction velocity and the nature of effective stimuli. In both species Maruhashi et al. (1952) reported the existence of myelinated fibres described as nociceptive because they were excited more effectively by strong stimuli such as pinprick, heat, or pulling of hairs than by gentle skin contact. In the toad they reported the successful recording of discharges from single unmyelinated fibres. While they gave no details, their paper mentioned that it was difficult to excite such fibres using light tactile stimuli but that cold, heat, and acid activated them.

A spirited disagreement with the concept of specificity in somatosensory arrangements came from G. Weddell and associates from Oxford. The latter's studies began as attempts to correlate skin spots from which specific cutaneous experiences were elicited with underlying histologically defined nerve structures. The initial aims of work with Woollard and Harpman (Woollard et al. 1940) were to test von Frey's correlations and hypotheses and to examine Thomas Lewis' (1937a, b, 1938, 1942) ideas about a 'nocifensor' system of special nerves subserving efferent effects from cutaneous fibres (Woollard et al. 1940). Lewis presumed that the nocifensor system represented an interconnected network of peripheral fibres independent of connections to the central nervous system and not necessarily responsible for the sensory aspects of pain. In the examination of skin innervation from human subjects, Woollard et al. (1940) found no morphological evidence of the network that Lewis envisioned for his nocifensor apparatus; they concluded 'that all varieties of cutaneous pain are subserved by the same nerve apparatus'. In spite of differences with von Frey's attribution of different cutaneous sensations to particular morphologically defined entities, they interpreted their findings as 'establishing that cutaneous pain behaves in accordance with the doctrine of specific nervous activity'.

Some 12 years later, Sinclair, Weddell, and Zander (1952) described only two types of peripheral afferent termination in histological examination of the skin of the human ear, while noting that this skin gives rise to 'the four customarily recognized sensory modalities', namely, touch, pinprick, cold, and warm. In a dramatic change from the earlier position, the conclusions stated 'the current theory of cutaneous sensation, which demands specific receptors for each modality or sensation, cannot be of universal application to the human body, and thus its standing must be seriously called in question'. Other volleys of the same genre were soon fired from their pens. Lele and Weddell (1956) reported that the sensory experiences evokable from the human cornea included touch, warmth, cold, and pain. On the other hand, these workers' light-level histology of the cornea suggested no specialization in the pattern of neural termination. This and the earlier histological studies led to a challenge to the notion of 'the doctrine of specific energy' and agreement by Weddell (1955) and Sinclair (1955) in favouring the pattern concept proposed nearly three decades before by Nafe.

A second, less frontal challenge to the idea of selective signalling of pain-causing stimuli by thin fibres came as the result of experiments by Douglas and Ritchie (1957*a*, *b*) that utilized the refractory period of peripheral fibres to modify compound action potentials. Compound action potentials recorded near the peripheral distribution of an intact cutaneous nerve were initiated by single brief electrical pulses applied centrally. Orthodromic impulses generated by 'natural' stimulation of the skin were used to collide with the electrically initiated compound activity; refractoriness of the fibres activated by skin stimulation suppressed components of the compound potential. Douglas and Ritchie found light skin contact and cooling stimuli to occlude a large fraction of the C and Aδ reflections and concluded that the majority of the more slowly conducting afferent fibres from a skin nerve were involved in transmitting tactile information. They also noted that the touch-evoked responses appeared to adapt slowly and persist beyond duration of the stimulation. This ingenious approach appeared to confirm Zotterman's earlier conclusions from unitary recordings and had considerable influence on ideas about pain at the time. The evidence that innocuous stimuli excited precisely the subset of fibres linked to pain by much previous work again appeared to bring into question the idea of the existence of sensory neurones that selectively signalled the presence of painful stimuli.

The strong and articulate attacks on what represented the 'specificity theory' of pain mechanisms were the environment for Ainsley Iggo's observations in mammals on the discharges of single unmyelinated primary afferent fibres. Iggo succeeded in the late 1950s at what had largely escaped others before him, namely, recording from identified, single C-fibres by dividing peripheral nerve into the fine filaments under microscopic vision. The novel utilization of small bits broken from razor blades allowed him to prepare very fine filaments by cutting the connective tissue binding together bundles of fibres, in a bath of mineral oil to prevent drying. To confine activity in the dissected fine filaments to that from a single fibre and confirm its origin, Iggo restricted stimulation to the receptive field of a given fibre, confirming Adrian's and Zotterman's findings that the fibres in a fine nerve or filament usually had distinctive small regions from which they could be excited without generating activity in other fibres. In addition, Iggo used the suppression of a discharge due to the refractoriness of a fibre excited by both electrical stimulation of the parent nerve, and simultaneously to adequate stimulation of the receptive field to prove their common origin. Iggo (1959*a*) reported on 17 cutaneous afferent fibres from a cat conducting at C velocities that responded to large temperature changes. Most of these units were excited by raising the temperature of the skin and had thresholds well above normal physiological ranges. Other units were activated by cold, again below the normal physiological range. All fibres tested by mechanical stimuli were described as having thresholds higher than those for other mechanoreceptors in the same nerves. His paper reporting these observations appears to make a firm link neither to pain or to the concept of nociception, although an article published in a symposium volume (Iggo 1959*b*) made a stronger case for connecting the same data to pain. One year later, Iggo (1960) provided further observations from 58 C-fibre recordings that proved to make the relationship of C fibres to pain more tortuous by describing an apparent continuum of mechanical responsiveness in the C-fibre population. Responses in different fibres were stated to range from those initiated by mechanical stimuli that were subthreshold for human experience to ones evoked by mechanical stimuli sufficient to elicit pricking pain. These mechanically excitable elements were unresponsive to heat, although a number gave a brief discharge to skin cooling. This report did not directly connect even those C fibres with elevated thresholds for mechanical stimuli to a special signalling task related to pain. On the contrary, one conclusion was that 'the non-myelinated cutaneous fibers can no longer be regarded as exclusively nociceptive in function, since the most sensitive C-mechanoreceptors and C-thermoreceptors are comparable in sensitivity with touch and temperature sense in man'. On balance, the latter was taken as support for those opposed to the notion of specific neural systems for pain.

While Iggo's published interpretation of his results was equivocal and, in part, begged the question of selective responsiveness by sense organs with thin fibres, other contemporary accounts were less tentative. Iriuchijima and Zotterman (1960) described recordings from single C afferent fibres in cutaneous nerve of mammals with particular focus on those that were consistently excited by either increases or decreases of temperature by a contact thermode of 1°C or less. In addition to these 'warm' or 'cold' fibres, they mentioned observations on fibres 'found fairly often' that were activated by extremes of temperature and by strong mechanical stimuli, confirming the observations published by Iggo the previous year.

Until the late 1950s, the attempts to record action potentials from thin primary afferent fibres had focused on skin nerves. At the beginning of the 1960s, two studies significant in this history dealt with thinly myelinated afferent fibres of muscle nerve. Such afferent fibres, with conduction velocities generally corresponding to the Aδ group, were also called the group III fibres of the limb muscle nerves (Lloyd and Chang 1948). It had been established that activity in group III fibre muscle nerve evoked particularly potent withdrawal reflexes along with contralateral extension, a pattern different from that seen with activation of the more rapidly conducting afferent elements of the same nerve (Perl 1958). Paintal (1960) appeared to provide an explanation for special reflex effects by characterizing the thinly myelinated afferent fibres comprising muscle nerve's group III as 'pressure-pain' receptors. Group III fibres were reported to respond to strong mechanical pressure on the muscle and also to be excited by intramuscular injections of hypertonic saline. While agreeing with this characterization for some of the group III fibres, Bessou and LaPorte (1961) noted that a number of group III fibres were excited by innocuous elongation of the muscle, including some that had characteristics similar to those that had been establisheld as associated with the length-detecting muscle spindle. Thus, nerves supplying muscle, such as those of skin, include a number of thin primary afferents that are activated by less than harmful stimuli.

The early 1960s served up other cross-currents. Hunt and McIntyre (1960*a–c*) produced a major analysis of the afferent characteristics of myelinated afferent fibres from skin and subcutaneous distributions. Their sample of fibres conducting over the entire Aαβδ ranges confirmed that the majority of these sensory units were responsive to innocuous mechanical disturbances of the skin. However, seven of the 421 fibres they described were responsive only to strong mechanical stimulation of the skin, a number that was soon to be used in an argument countering the existence of specific sense organs for pain.

In this same period, Witt (1962; Witt and Griffin 1962) also clouded the issue about the nature of sensory units with C fibres from the skin but at the same time brought to attention the sensitization of mammalian sense organs. Witt had worked with Hensel and Iggo (Hensel *et al.* 1960) on sensitive cutaneous thermoreceptors reported on concurrently by Iriuchigima and Zottermman (1960). She focused independently on 'non-specific' receptors found to respond to mechanical and thermal stimuli and irritant chemicals. She mentions in her description that many of these 'non-specific' afferent fibres were excited by innocuous mechanical stimuli although they gave their largest responses to temperature extremes, particularly heat. Shortly thereafter, Witt and Griffin (1962) described an enhancement of response and apparent lowering of threshold of presumably similar fibres after exposure to noxious heat and irritant chemicals. An enhanced response of amphibian C-fibre receptors had been observed some years earlier (Hogg 1935; Echlin and Propper 1937; Habgood 1950). In the frog it was manifested by increased responses to mechanical stimuli after scraping of the skin or antidromic stimulation of cutaneous nerves. Habgood (1950) suggested that the sensitization involved the release of a substance at the nerve endings. Both in the frog and in the cat, spontaneous activity was found to follow injurious stimuli. These several reports did not make clear the type of sensory unit concerned or whether all types participated in the enhanced responsiveness and ongoing discharge, although Witt's article indicated that some units particularly effectively excited by high temperatures were involved. Unfortunately, the clear impression from Witt's studies was that C-fibre units were variable in their response with a major feature being persistence of activity (after discharge) following an adequate stimulus.

The gate theory

This mixture of observations and concepts was the setting for a review by R. Melzack and P. Wall (1962) that again challenged the concept of specificity in neural arrangements for the various modalities of cutaneous sensation. Their analysis was based, in part, on reports from the Oxford workers a few years previously. Melzack and Wall concluded that, while differences among peripheral sensory receptors exist, 'there can no longer be any doubt that temporal and spatial patterns of nerve impulses provide the basis of our sensory perceptions'. Consequently, they attributed many of the essential mechanisms for differentiation of characteristics of stimuli to neurones of the central nervous system. While it was apparent that Melzack and Wall had chosen to emphasize observations questioning specificity more than those supportive of that concept, their ideas did reflect doubts in many minds about the nature of neural mechanisms for somesthesis.

Three years later Melzack and Wall (1965) crowned their thesis by an explicit theory about pain. In their presentation of 'the gate control theory', they leaned heavily on the relative paucity of descriptions of sensory units that 'respond exclusively to high-intensity stimulation'. In particular, several of the studies mentioned above were cited, singling out those by Maruhalshi *et al.* (1952), Douglas and Ritchie (1957*a*, *b*), Iggo (1959*a*, *b*, 1960), and Hunt and McIntyre (1960*a–c*). The conclusion from their review of the existing evidence was that sensory units with myelinated or unmyelinated fibres that responded to intense stimulation probably only represented 'the extreme of a continuous distribution of receptor-fibre thresholds'. They also criticized the evidence for specific groups of central cells responsive only to intense stimulation and aired circumstances from the clinic that seemed hard to square with central neural arrangements fully dedicated to conveying pain-related activity. Their concept was of a neural gate in the substantial gelatinosa of the dorsal horn of the spinal cord operated by the balance of activity between large-diameter and small-diameter primary afferent fibres. Activity in the small fibres was presumed to open the 'gate' in the spinal substantia gelatinosa closed by impulses in large fibres, because the former adapted more slowly to strong stimuli. The latter notion took its premise partially from a paper by Wall (1960) that concluded that, of cutaneous afferent A fibres, the more rapidly conducting adapted more quickly than the slowly conducting. The theory also brought in the concept of descending (from the brain) control of somatosensory afferent transmission, an arrangement established to exist a decade previously by Hagbarth and Kerr (1954). The idea of neural gating also was not new; the classical reflex studies by Sherrington had established the principle of integrative control or modulation, a concept that incorporated changing one reaction to accommodate another. Prior to the gate theory proposal, two laboratories independently had demonstrated neural switching (gating) in the spinal cord by descending modulation of reflexes, resulting in the suppression of withdrawal reactions in decerebrate rigidity (Eccles and Lundberg 1959; Kuno and Perl 1960).

The gate theory caught the imagination of many psychologists and clinicians partially because its basic concept utilized a process and a term in the language of the emerging and exciting fields of digital electronics and computer processing. It also introduced a flexibility of arrangement necessary to account for variations in symptoms observed under pathological circumstances. One fundamental assumption of the theory was that neither peripheral nor central neurones selectively (specifically) responding to strong stimuli exist, although it was admitted that the integrity of certain subsets of fibres (for example, the thin fibres) and certain central pathways (the crossed spinothalamic system) were essential for a normal pain reception. As outlined below, this underlying assumption of the theory was soon shown to be incorrect.

Whatever else, the Melzack and Wall theory created controversy. It also sparked my concern about the nature and range of peripheral afferent features. Our previous work had largely focused on central neural mechanisms, establishing projection and reflex mechanisms uniquely associated with thin myelinated fibres (Perl 1957, 1968; Perl and Whitlock 1961; Beacham and Perl 1964*a*, *b*). My opinion at the time was that Melzack and Wall's account of work on sense organs was unbalanced. Among challengable points, it ignored the technical problems in recording from thin afferent fibres, which, given the techniques used, would hamper random sampling. Their argument that the paucity of sensory units described as having high thresholds and the lack of consistency in the observations indicated the absence of specific subgroups of sensory units selective for strong stimuli was valid only if the numbers came from random and adequate samples. Samples biased against thin fibres might easily account for imperfect surveys of sensory fibres with a tilt towards the more easily recorded or identified units.

Nociceptors as distinctive primary afferent neurones

Until the mid-1960s, recordings from single afferent fibres of peripheral nerve had, with few exceptions, been obtained by teasing the nerve with needles or other fine instruments into fine filaments. Such microdissection was continued until the electrical activity of single fibres could be identified when leading potentials from a filament. Ordinarily, after each division of the nerve fibre bundles, the tissue of the nerve's distribution was tested by various mechanical or thermal manipulations. These stimuli generally were moderate in intensity to minimize damage to the peripheral tissues. The dissection process typically is delicate and tedious; irreversible damage of the receptive tissue could render valueless much dissection effort. Thus, there was an understandable tendency by investigators to focus upon the many afferent units activated by weak or moderate stimuli. To test the assumptions of the gate or other theories about the peripheral afferent bases of sensation, it appeared essential to make an extensive survey of slowly conducting fibres using a search for afferent units unbiased in selection. As an alternative to the tedious and time-consuming nature of the teased-filament method, I chose to try glass micropipette electrodes inserted into the peripheral nerve. After Ling and Gerard (1949) had proposed such electrodes for recording from neural tissue, they had become the method of choice for intracellular recording from nerve cell bodies. Moreover, Tasaki (1953) had shown that electrodes of this type could record from peripheral nerve fibres. Trials made on sympathetic nerves suggested that this procedure was promising for recordings from thin fibres.

In the summer of 1965, P.R. Burgess and I evolved an experimental arrangement wherein a peripheral nerve intact to the periphery was placed upon a small plastic support to allow fine glass micropipettes (< 0.1 µm) to be slowly driven into a mechanically stabilized region of a cutaneous nerve. Movement of the fine tip of the electrode through the packed fibres of a peripheral nerve seemingly should allow the experimenter to record the electrical signs of activity from numerous fibres, one at a time. The technique appeared appropriate to establish the nature and range of characteristics of the population of fibres making up the afferent component of typical peripheral nerves. Importantly, the primary search stimulus was electrical excitation of the nerve at intensities adequate to activate all afferent fibres. Thus, the selection of a fibre for study was based upon the chance of the microelectrode encountering a favourable recording position relative to a fibre.

It was hoped that this method would permit the sampling of the receptive characteristics of unmyelinated fibres; the greatest uncertainty existed about their range of signalling characteristics. Use of cutaneous nerve with a relatively thin epineurium aided penetration by the microelectrode and permitted ready exploration of the receptive field. Recording from myelinated fibres with this technique proved easy; on the other hand, activity from fibres conducting at the C-fibre velocity was encountered rarely and fleetingly. During one experiment after many months of such trials, many fibres of the

myelinated range were found to be excited as usual by innocuous mechanical manipulations of the skin in confirmation of previous descriptions. One relatively slowly
conducting myelinated fibre, however, proved unresponsive to these manipulations.
After considerable exploration of the area of skin served by the nerve and confirmation
of the continued presence of the response to electrical stimulation of the nerve, the skin
was pinched with a tissue forceps. This promptly evoked a repeatable discharge from a
particular area of skin. The fibre in question had a mechanical threshold many times that
of the ordinary mechanoreceptors in the same nerve, including those with similar
conduction velocities. From that observation on, our search efforts concentrated on
myelinated fibres conducting under 30 m/s. In subsequent experiments, single afferent
fibres with notably high mechanical thresholds and other features setting them apart
from other myelinated fibres were regularly found. Rubbing the skin with a blunt object,
even when exerting sufficient force to visibly deform the skin or soft subcutaneous
tissues, was ineffectual in exciting a response. The responses of one of these high-
threshold mechanoreceptors are shown in Fig. 1.3. These sensory units had receptive
fields differing from those of other myelinated fibre units in that they regularly consisted
of multiple (5 to > 20) punctate areas from which responses were evokable by prodding
with a needle or a stiff filament separated by regions in which equivalent stimuli were
ineffective (see below).

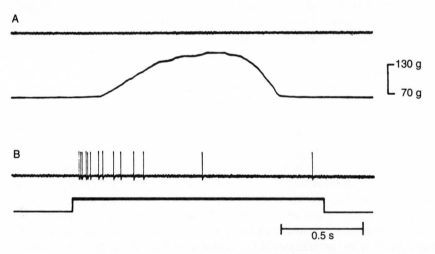

Fig. 1.3 Activity of a myelinated mechanical nociceptor of mammalian skin evoked by mechanical stimuli.
Trace A is a recording obtained from a micropipette in the posterior femoral cutaneous nerve. The conduction
velocity of the afferent fibre was 25 m/s. Trace A, Pinch of a fold of skin containing the receptive field. The force
was applied with blunt forceps with tips approximately 3 mm across as indicated by a calibrated strain gauge.
The scale is in grams. Trace B indicates the time of application of a pinch to the same fold of skin used in trace
A, this time with a serrated (with teeth) tissue forceps. Reproduced with permission from Burgess and
Perl (1967).

Many slowly conducting myelinated fibres did not have these characteristics. In
confirmation of earlier studies by Zotterman (1939), Maruhashi *et al.* (1952), and Hunt
and McIntyre (1960*a–c*), in cat cutaneous nerves the majority of myelinated fibres
conducting at the Aδ velocity were excited by the most gentle manipulations of hair or

light contact with the skin. The results in our survey made it evident that the population of slowly conducting myelinated fibres was made up of distinct subsets, one of which had a high threshold to all forms of mechanical distortion.

The threshold mechanical distortion for activation of a punctate receptive region of these myelinated high-threshold mechanoreceptors varied substantially from one fibre to another. Some responded to moderate pressure with a blunt object, while others needed overtly tissue-damaging mechanical stimuli for excitation. None gave prompt responses to noxious skin heating (> 42°C) or cooling of the skin surface to 10°C. Regardless of differences in sensitivity, the high-threshold myelinated afferent units all produced more action potentials and higher discharge frequencies in response to frankly damaging stimuli than to any form of innocuous mechanical manipulation. In describing the results, we turned to Sherrington's (1906) argument about the relationship of pain and tissue damage and embraced his term, noci-receptive. The very highest threshold of these mechanical receptors were named 'nociceptors', for the first time using Sherrington's suggested label for a functionally defined set of sense organs (Burgess and Perl 1967).

Despite the prevailing uncertainty about the existence of specific pain receptors, these findings and their interpretations as demonstrating the existence of cutaneous myelinated fibre nociceptors encountered relatively little objection. One reason was the novel recording technique that yielded a sample of over 500 fibres for the initial description, 74 of which were categorized as nociceptors. Moreover, contrary to previous descriptions of fibres with elevated thresholds for one or another type of stimulation, our study established a coherent set of characteristics for the presumed nociceptors. The first observations were made on cat, the then pre-eminent experimental animal for *in vivo* investigation of the nervous system. The question of species specificity was soon settled by showing, using a similar microelectrode recording technique, that cutaneous afferent fibres with almost identical characteristics existed in monkey (Perl 1968). Figure 1.4 reproduces diagrams illustrating the receptive field organization for several high-threshold myelinated mechanical receptors in a primate. The primate work also specifically addressed the question of the ability of low-threshold mechanoreceptors to signal differences between strong innocuous stimuli and stimuli producing damage to the skin. In mechanoreceptors of the low-threshold variety, skin-damaging stimuli did not evoke a response uniquely different from that provoked by moderate non-damaging stimuli. Neither the frequency nor the pattern of discharges from low-threshold sense organs provided a distinctive coding for noxious stimuli. This contrasted with the unequivocal graded signalling of tissue-damaging stimuli provided by the high-threshold mechanoreceptors.

The die was cast. At least one particular type of nociceptor had been shown to have a clearly definable set of features, but the uncertainties about the unmyelinated fibres remained. Unhappily, our hopes of using microelectrode recordings to survey the C fibres in peripheral nerve proved in vain. In spite of efforts to improve recording stability, recordings from fibres with C-conduction velocities remained so rare and unstable that an adequate determination of their receptive properties could not be made.

A survey similar to that done for the slowly conducting myelinated fibres was needed for the unmyelinated population. The failure of the microelectrode approach to record C fibres in nerve prompted a decision to turn to the dissected-filament method with the intent to sample randomly and extensively. We (Bessou and Perl 1969) began such a

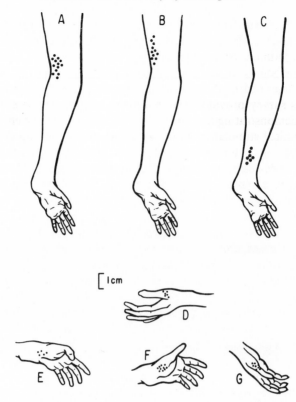

Fig. 1.4 Sketches of the monkey hindlimb and hand showing on each drawing the receptive field of the single myelinated cutaneous mechanical nociceptor. Each sensory unit was excited from locations indicated by dots and was unresponsive to stimuli between dots or alongside them. The nociceptors whose receptive fields are shown in B, C, and G had lower thresholds than the others, although they also gave progressively graded responses to progressively stronger overtly noxious stimuli. Reproduced with permission from Perl (1968).

survey in 1968 on the cutaneous hindlimb nerve of cat. Using the search paradigm that had proved successful for the myelinated fibres, nerve filaments were subdivided centrally along the course of the nerve with their activity tested by stimulating the nerve peripherally at intensities sufficient to excite all C fibres. Prior to the isolation of the discharge of a C fibre from the other activity in the nerve to the point that its action potentials were unequivocally recognizable, the peripheral receptive field was not stimulated. Thus, the elements studied were selected by the chance of the dissection process. In the course of a year, over 100 cutaneous afferent C fibres were characterized, chosen solely on the basis of conduction at C velocity. The population of afferent units fell into five categories based upon a range of stimuli relevant to the natural history of a free-ranging animal. At least two categories were clearly noci-receptive and appeared properly classifiable as nociceptors. The most common nociceptors in our C-fibre sample (40 per cent) were named polymodal because they were excited by strong mechanical stimulation, by noxious heat, and by irritant chemicals (Figs 1.5–1.7). These probably were the type of units noted previously by Iggo (1959a, b) and Witt (1962). About 10 per cent of the C fibres did not respond either to strongly noxious heat (60°C) or to cooling to clearly abnormal skin temperatures (10°C) but could be activated by intense mechanical stimulation. Roughly one-half of the sample were excited by the most gentle mechanical stimuli, explaining the very sensitive units reported before. A rare (2 per cent) unit responded to small temperature changes in the innocuous range as had been previously described (Zotterman 1936; Iriuchijima and Zotterman 1960; Hensel *et al.* 1960). This survey provided reasonable explanation of the earlier confounding observations by demonstrating that the C-fibre afferent units most effectively excited by innocuous mechanical stimulation in the cat represented a group distinct from those with high thresholds to all forms of stimuli. The convincing evidence for special sets of noci-receptive C fibres came from a systematic comparison of the characteristics of different elements in a sample large enough to bear a relationship to the population existing in a typical nerve.

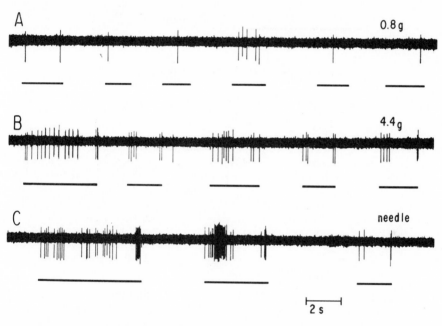

Fig. 1.5 Activity evoked in the afferent fibre of a mammalian C-fibre polymodal nociceptor by punctate mechanical stimuli. The recording was obtained from a fine filament teased from the posterior femoral cutaneous nerve of cat. The conduction velocity of the afferent fibre was 1 m/s. The lines under each trace mark the time of skin contact. Force A, Stimulation by a flexible hair bending at 0.8 g. Trace B, Stimulation by a flexible hair bending at 4.4 g. Trace C, Pressure with a sewing needle sufficient to penetrate the cutaneous surface. Reproduced with permission from Bessou and Perl (1969).

P.R. Burgess persisted in trying to record from the unmyelinated fibres with microelectrodes. Acting on a suggestion by W.S. Beacham, he turned to recording from the dorsal ganglia (DRG) that harboured the somata of the primary afferent fibres. By judicious choice of ganglia, reasonably stable intracellular recordings were obtained from DRG neurones *in vivo*. By working in the segments supplying the cat's tail, a sample of unmyelinated fibres cells innervating hairy skin was obtained. Efforts from the two techniques were combined and soon a substantial population of C fibres obtained by

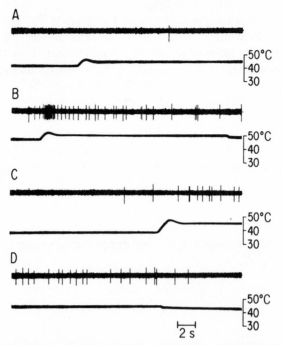

Fig. 1.6 Activity recorded from a C-fibre polymodal nociceptor in response to cutaneous heating. Same unit as shown in Fig. 1.5. Records A and B are separated by 10 s; B and C are separated by 80 s during which the thermode had passively cooled. Contact thermode temperatures are indicated by the trace below each electrophysiological reading. The approximately 2 mm^2 thermode contact area was centred upon the mechanically excitable receptive field. Reproduced with permission from Bessou and Perl (1969).

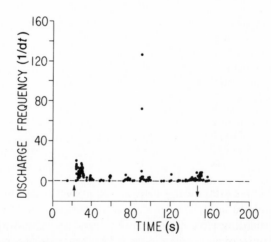

Fig. 1.7 Activity evoked in a C-fibre polymodal nociceptor in response to dilute acid placed upon intact skin covering the mechanically defined receptive field. The recording was obtained from a fine filament dissected from a posterior femoral cutaneous nerve of cat. Each impulse is plotted as a dot located on the horizontal axis at the time of the occurrence (relative to the beginning of the plot) and on the vertical axis at 1/time (1/dt) from the previous impulse ('instantaneous frequency'). The conduction velocity of the afferent fibre was 0.8 m/s. Reproduced with permission from Bessou and Perl (1969).

the two methods were shown to be congruent and supportive of the initial classifications (Bessou *et al.* 1971). The latter work also demonstrated that the low-threshold C mechanoreceptors do not provide signals that by pattern or frequency of discharge distinguish strong, undamaging stimuli from those causing unambiguous tissue injury (Fig. 1.8).

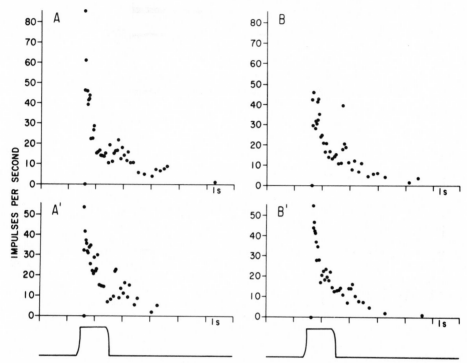

Fig. 1.8 Responses of a cat C-fibre mechanoreceptor (low-threshold) to innocuous and to noxious mechanical stimuli. The responses in A and B were evoked by a 1-mm diameter probe deflecting the skin 1.2 mm and causing no visible injury. The stimulation was not painful to human subjects. In A′ and B′, the responses were initiated by the same deflection of a needle tip centred on the identical receptive field. The stimuli in A′ and B′ produced visible holes in the skin. A and A′ were the first in a series of identical stimuli repeated at 100-s intervals, B and B′ were the third such stimuli. The traces below the graphs show the movement of the electromechanical stimulator. The plots were formed as described for Fig. 1.7. Note the lack of distinction between the responses evoked by the innocuous (A and B) and noxious (A′ and B′) stimuli. Reproduced with permission from Bessou *et al.* (1971).

The surveys of C fibres establishing distinct subsets with appropriate characteristics for nociceptors brought to light other aspects of the peripheral afferent innervation that helped clarify long-standing issues. A given cutaneous nerve was shown to contain at least two distinctive types of nociceptors differing in functional characteristics other than the velocity of conduction of the peripheral fibre. Some nociceptors were excited, at least initially, only by intense mechanical deformation, while another subset responded to a variety of stimuli threatening the physical integrity of the skin. If central mechanisms maintained these distinctions, this offered an explanation of the differences in sensory experiences attributed to the pain associated with A and C fibres (Landau and Bishop

1953). Sensitization, a phenomenon that had been recognized previously (see above) but indifferently documented for mammals, was another aspect. In particular, the C polymodal nociceptors were shown to become more responsive after once being excited by heat. Enhanced responsiveness after stimulation was not a general property of C-fibre afferent units since the low-threshold C mechanoreceptors do not exhibit it. Lowering of threshold, increased response, and development of background discharge appear prominently in C polymodal fibres after their receptive fields are stimulated sufficiently to evoke a response. The manner in which the activity of a C polymodal type of nociceptor to heat stimuli can be altered by sensitization is illustrated in Fig. 1.9. Sensitization of nociceptors has an evident link to some forms of hyperalgesia, the increased pain experienced by human beings in the manipulation of injured or inflamed tissue—phenomena that have long interested clinicians and experimentalists (see, for example, Lewis 1942).

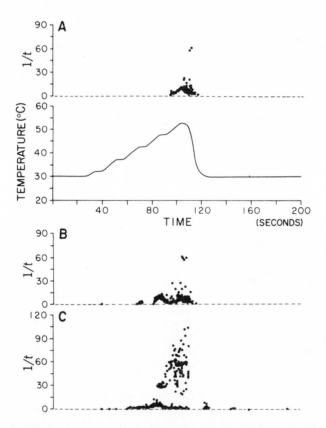

Fig. 1.9 Activity evoked from a primate C-fibre polymodal nociceptor by repeated heating of the mechanically excitable receptive field by a small contact thermode. Recording of single unit activity from a fine filament dissected from peripheral nerve. The graphs with dots were constructed as described for Fig. 1.7 and represent the 'instantaneous frequency' of discharge. Identical heat trials as shown in the lower part of A were produced every 200 s. (A) First heat test; (B) third heat test; (C) fifth heat test. Graphs B and C were aligned to A by superimposition of a temperature record from the thermode for each trial. Reproduced with permission from Kumazawa and Perl (1977).

The importance of the input from nociceptors in central nervous organization was promptly established thereafter. Christensen and Perl (1970) found that certain neurones of the superficial portion of the spinal dorsal horn were excited only by noxious stimulation of the skin from a peripiheral pathway involving either thinly myelinated fibres and/or unmyelinated fibres. This evidence for a selective noci-receptive input hinged on firm knowledge of the receptive characteristics of both noci-receptive and low-threshold primary afferent fibres. Subsequently, the central termination pattern of nociceptor fibres was shown to be distinctive from that of low-threshold fibres by intracellular labelling of identified myelinated (Light and Perl 1979) and unmyelinated (Sugiura *et al.* 1986) nociceptors. An example of the central termination of a cutaneous myelinated nociceptor, intracellularly labelled with horseradish peroxidase, is shown in Fig. 1.10 and that of an unmyelinated nociceptor labelled with a plant lectin (*Phaseolus vulgaris* leucoagglutinin) in Fig. 1.11. The concentration of central terminations from

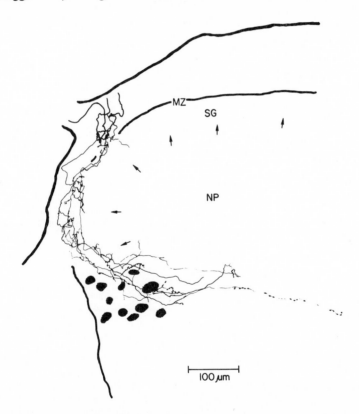

Fig. 1.10 Central terminations of a cutaneous mechanical nociceptor of the cat. Camera lucida drawing of the fibre trajectory as visualized by intracellular application of horseradish peroxidase at the dorsal root spinal cord junction after functional identification of receptive characteristics. Drawn from nine serial 80 μm thick transverse sections. The conduction velocity of the afferent fibre was 15 m/s. MZ, Marginal zone (lamina I); SG, substantia gelatinosa (lamina II); NP, nucleus proprius. Arrows mark the approximate junction of the SG and the NP. This termination pattern is typical for such primary afferent units in both cat and monkey. The dark ovals at the lower left of the drawing indicate longitudinal bundles of myelinated fibres that reticulate the lateral portion of lamina V. Reproduced with permission from Light and Perl (1979).

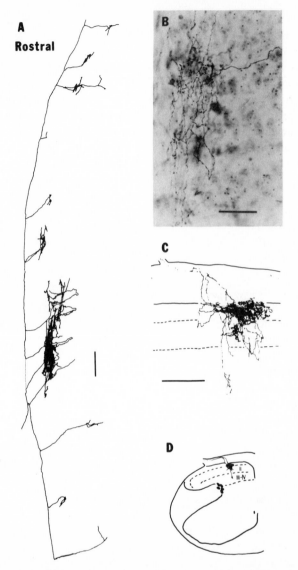

Fig. 1.11 Central termination of a C-fibre polymodal nociceptor in the lumbar segment of the spinal cord of a guinea-pig. The primary afferent neurone was labelled intracellularly in the L-6 dorsal root ganglion with *Phaseolus vulgaris* leucoagglutinin (PHA-L) after functional determination of receptive characteristics. (A) Sagittal rendering of the termination pattern of the fibre that bifurcated into an ascending and descending branch from the point of entry (lower left). (B) Photomicrograph showing the labelled fibre and terminal swellings at one of the regions of concentration of terminals. (C) Transverse view of the terminal pattern at a region of concentration. (D) Transverse drawing locating the C-fibre terminals relative to various laminae of the spinal dorsal horn. Rearranged with permission from Sugiura *et al.* (1986).

nociceptors in the marginal layer and outer substantia gelatinosa (laminae I and II) of the spinal dorsal horn suggests that at least certain connections to neurones of these regions selectively excited by noxious stimuli are direct, that is monosynaptic. Essential points from the early observations on afferent fibres from nociceptors are: (1) that nociceptors provide distinctive signals to the central nervous system about events threatening the physical integrity of peripheral tissue; (2) that nociceptors deliver this information to specific central regions by means of a unique termination pattern; and (3) that at least some central connections functionally segregate information from nociceptors and that provided by other sense organs.

Once reasonable sets of functional characteristics for nociceptors were established, evidence about their properties and central connections quickly accumulated. Other chapters of this volume document much that has been learned about them and the mechanisms of their sensitization.

The link to pain

The story has come full circle. The question of the nature of the receptors for the experience of pain was posed once the sensory nature of the experience was understood. After a set of primary afferent neurones had been identified as nociceptors, the relationship of the characteristics of such receptive elements could be compared to the features of pain in normal and abnormal circumstances. This volume deals with these issues at length. The present evidence makes clear that different subgroups of nociceptors have distinctive characteristics, which in some cases are altered by past history and the circumstances of the moment. In other words, past stimuli, post-injury effects, or inflammation can profoundly change the manner in which nociceptors signal the central nervous system about events in the periphery.

As a final point, observations from the technique of percutaneous neurography pioneered by Hagbarth and Vallbo (1968) are pertinent. In this procedure, fine metal electrodes inserted through the skin into the peripheral nerve of human beings are manipulated by a skilful operator to permit electrical recording from individual myelinated or unmyelinated fibres. While the technique rarely allows the total isolation of the activity of a fibre from that of other fibres, as is possible with the much finer glass pipette electrodes, it does permit the recording of the identifiable activity of an individual element. With persistence, the amplitude of one unit can often be made substantially greater than that of other discharges recordable at the same locus. When a large unitary potential is present under such circumstances and the electrode is converted from recording to a source of electrical stimulation, there is a remarkable concurrence between the receptive field for the largest action potential evoked by tissue stimulation and the human subject's location of the sensory experience evoked by threshold electrical stimulation through the electrode. In recordings in which the largest unitary potential was generated by a nociceptor, as established by cutaneous stimuli, threshold electrical stimuli through the electrode (for sensation) evoke an experience reported by the subject to be a pricking or sharp 'pain-like' feeling referred to the afferent unit's receptive field (Torebjörk and Ochoa 1980; Konietsky *et al.* 1981; Ochoa and Torebjörk 1983, 1989). Non-painful sensations are provoked when stimulating with the recording electrode if discharges from low-threshold mechanoreceptors in the same nerve are the most prominent in the record. While the method of intraneural stimulation has been criticized (Wall and McMahon 1985), its assumptions have been validated by crucial tests (Torebjörk 1987). In addition, psychophysical comparisons between the experiences or effects evoked by particular stimuli in human beings and animals and the responses of nociceptors to equivalent stimuli have strongly supported a close link between nociceptor activity and pain in normal individuals (Dubner *et al.* 1977; LaMotte and Campbell 1978; Yarnitsky *et al.* 1992).

In summary, the present evidence argues that the neural organization associated with pain follows that of other sensations in terms of having particular afferent units that provide the essential information to the central nervous system about the nature of peripheral events important for the sensory experience. The central nervous system deciphers peripheral signals leading to pain with the clues of threshold that are an inherent property of the spectrum of peripheral afferent units. Thus, theories that presume normal pain to be a unique product of special combinations of activity in sense organs that are also responsible for other experiences through patterns or gates, are contradicted by the present evidence. If and how the responsiveness of nociceptors and the connectivity of peripheral receptors to central mechanisms may alter as a consequence of the malfunctions caused by disease, injury, or abnormal development are other issues.

References

Adrian, E.D. (1926). The impulses produced by sensory nerve-endings. Part 4. Impulses from pain receptors. *J. Physiol., London* **62**, 33–51.

Adrian, E.D. (1928). *The basis of sensation.* Norton, New York.

Adrian, E.D. (1932). *The mechanism of nervous action.* University of Pennsylvania Press, Philadelphia.

Adrian, E.D., Cattell, M., and Hoagland, H. (1931). Sensory discharges in single cutaneous nerve fibres. *J. Physiol.* 72, 377–91.

Adrian, E.D. and Zotterman, Y. (1926*a*). The impulses produced by sensory nerve endings. Part 2. The response of a single end-organ. *J. Physiol., London* **61**, 151–71.

Adrian, E.D. and Zotterman, Y. (1926*b*). The impulses produced by sensory nerve endings. Part 3. Impulses set up by touch and pressure. *J. Physiol., London* **61**, 465–83.

Aristotle. *De anima* (version by William of Muerbeke, trans. K. Foster and S. Humphries (1951). Yale University Press, New Haven.

Beacham, W.S. and Perl, E.R. (1964). Background and reflex discharge of sympathetic preganglionic neurones in the spinal cat. *J. Physiol., London* **172**, 400–16.

Beacham, W.S. and Perl, E.R. (1964). Characteristics of a spinal sympathetic reflex. *J. Physiol., London* **173**, 431–48.

Bechterev, V.M. (1899). *Les voies de conduction du cerveau et de la moelle.* Paris.

Bell, C. (1811). *Idea of a new anatomy of the brain submitted for the observation of his friends.* London.

Bessou, P. and LaPorte, Y. (1961). Étude des récepteurs musculaires innervés par les fibres afférentes du groupe III (fibres myelinisées fines) chez le chat. *Arch. Italiennes Biol.* 99, 293–321.

Bessou, P. and Perl, E.R. (1969). Response of cutaneous sensory units with unmyelinated fibers to noxious stimuli. *J. Neurophysiol.* 32, 1025–43.

Bessou, P., Burgess, P.R., Perl, E.R., and Taylor, C.B. (1971). Dynamic properties of mechanoreceptors with unmyelinated (C) fibers. *J. Neurophysiol.* 34, 116–31.

Blix, M. (1884). Experimentelle Beiträge zur lösung der Frage über die specifische Energie der Hautnerven. *Z. Biol.* **20**, 141–56.

Brown-Séquard, C.E. (1860). *Course of lectures on the physiology and pathology of the central nervous system.* Collins, Philadelphia.

Brown-Séquard, C.E. (1868). Lectures on the physiology and pathology of the nervous system; and on the treatment of organic nervous affections. *Lancet* 2, 593–6, 659–62, 755, 757, 821–3.

Burgess, P.R. and Perl, E.R. (1967). Myelinated afferent fibres responding specifically to noxious stimulation of the skin. *J. Physiol., London* **190**, 541–62.

Charcot, J.-M. (1888). *Localization dans la moelle epiniere.* Paris.

Christensen, B.N. and Perl, E.R. (1970). Spinal neurons specifically excited by noxious or thermal stimuli: marginal zone of the dorsal horn. *J. Neurophysiol.* **33**, 293–307.

Clark, D., Hughes, J., and Gasser, H.S. (1935). Afferent function in the group of nerve fibers of slowest conduction velocity. *Am. J. Physiol.* **114**, 69–76.

Clarke, E. and Dewherst, K. (1972). *Illustrated history of brain function.* University of California Press, Berkeley.

Dallenbach, K.M. (1927). The temperature spots and end-organs. *Am. J. Psychol.* **39**, 402–27.

Dallenbach, K.M. (1929). A bibliography of the attempts to identify the functional end-organs of cold and warmth. *Am. J. Psychol.* **41**, 344.

Dallenbach, K.M. (1939). Pain: history and present status. *Am. J. Psychol.* **52**, 331–47.

Douglas, W.W. and Ritchie, J.M. (1957*a*). A technique for recording functional activity in specific groups of medullated and non-medullated fibres in whole nerve trunks. *J. Physiol.* **138**, 19–30.

Douglas, W.W. and Ritchie, J.M. (1957*b*). Non-medullated fibres in the saphenous nerve which signal touch. *J. Physiol.* **139**, 385–99.

Dubner, R., Price, D.D., Beitel, R.E., and Hu, J.W. (1977). Peripheral neural correlates of behavior in monkey and human related to sensory-discriminative aspects of pain. In *Pain in the trigeminal region* (ed. D.J. Anderson and B. Matthews), pp. 57–66. Elsevier/North-Holland Biomedical Press, Amsterdam.

Eccles, R.M. and Lundberg, A. (19959). Supraspinal control of interneurones mediating spinal reflexes. *J. Physiol.* **147**, 565–84.

Echlin, F. and Propper, N. (1937). 'Sensitization' by injury of the cutaneous nerve endings in the frog. *J. Physiol.* **88**, 388–400.

Edinger, L. (1890). Einigles von Verlauf der Gefühlsbahnen in centralen Nervensysteme. *Deutsche Med. Woch.* **16**, 421–6.

Edinger, L. (1892). *Zwolf Vorlesungen über den Blau der nervosen Centralorgane, 3 Auflage.* Davis, Leipzig.

Erb, W. (1874). *Handbuch der Krankheiten des Nervensystems* II, pp. 1–18. Leipzig.

Gasser, H.S. and Erlanger, J. (1927). The role played by the sizes of the constituent fibers of a nerve trunk in determining the form of its action potential wave. *Am. J. Physiol.* **80**, 522–47.

Goldscheider, A. (1885). Neue Thatsachen über die Hautsinnesnerven. *Arch. J. Physiol., Leipzig,* 1–110.

Goldscheider, A. (1891). Ueber die Summation von Hautreizen. *Arch. J . Physiol.* 164–9.

Goldscheider, A. (1920). *Das Schmerzproblem.* Springer-Verlag, Berlin.

Goldscheider, A. (1926). Beiträge zur Physiologie der Gemeingefühle. *Z. Sinnesphysiol.* **57**, 1–14.

Gowers, W.R. (1892). *Diseases of the nervous system* (2nd edn). Blakiston, London.

Gowers, W.R. (1899). *Diseases of the nervous system* (3rd edn). Blakiston, London

Gruner, O.C. (1930). *A treatise on 'The canon of medicine of Avicenna'.* Luzac & Co, London.

Hagbarth, K.-E. and Kerr, D.I.B. (1954). Central influences on spinal afferent conduction. *J. Neurophysiol.* **17**, 295–307.

Hagbarth, K.-E. and Vallbo, Å.B. (1968). Discharge characteristics of human muscle afferents during muscle stretch and contraction. *Exp. Neurol.* **22**, 674–94.

Habgood, J.S. (1950). Sensitization of sensory receptors in the frog's skin. *J. Physiol.* **111**, 195–213.

Head, H. (1920). *Studies in neurology.* Oxford University Press, London.

Head, H., Rivers, W.H.R., and Sherren, J. (1905). The afferent nervous system from a new aspect. *Brain* **28**, 99–115.

Heinbecker, P., Bishop, G.H., and O'Leary, J. (1932). Fibers in mixed nerves and their dorsal roots responsible for pain. *Proc. Soc. exp. Biol. Med.* **29**, 928–30.

Heinbecker, P., Bishop, G.H., and O'Leary, J.L. (1933). Pain and touch fibers in peripheral nerves. *Arch. Neurol. Psychiat.* **29**, 771–89.

Hensel, H., Iggo, A., and Witt, I. (1960). A quantitative study of sensitive cutaneous thermo-receptors with C afferent fibres. *J. Physiol., London* **153**, 113–26.

Hogg, B.M. (1935). Slow impulses from the cutaneous nerves of the frog. *J. Physiol.* **84**, 250–8.

Hunt, C.C. and McIntyre, A.K. (1960a). Characteristics of responses from receptors from the flexor longus digitorum muscle and the adjoining interosseous region of the cat. *J. Physiol., London* **153**, 74–87.

Hunt, C.C. and McIntyre, A.K. (1960b). Properties of cutaneous touch receptors in cat. *J. Physiol., London* **153**, 88–98.

Hunt, C.C. and McIntyre, A.K. (1960c). An analysis of fibre diameter and receptor characteristics of myelinated cutaneous afferent fibres in cat. *J. Physiol., London* **153**, 99–112.

Iggo, A. (1959a). Cutaneous heat and cold receptors with slowly conducting (C) afferent fibres. *Quart. J. exp. Physiol.* **44**, 362–70.

Iggo, A. (1959b). A single unit analysis of cutaneous receptors with C afferent fibres. In *Pain and itch*, Ciba Foundation Study Group No. 1 (ed. C.E. Wolstenholme and M. O'Conner), pp. 41–59. Little, Brown & Co, Boston.

Iggo, A. (1960). Cutaneous mechanoreceptors with afferent C fibres. *J. Physiol., London* **152**, 337–53.

Iriuchijima, J. and Zotterman, Y. (1960). The specificity of afferent cutaneous C fibres in mammals. *Acta physiol. scand.* **49**, 267–78.

Keele, K.D. (1957). *Anatomies of pain*. Blackwell, Oxford.

Konietsky, F., Perl, E.R., Trevino, D., Light, A., and Hensel, H. (1981). Sensory experiences in man evoked by intraneural electrical stimulation of intact cutaneous afferent fibers. *Exp. Brain Res.* **42**, 219–22.

Kumazawa, T. and Perl, E.R. (1977). Primate cutaneous sensory units with unmyelinated (C) afferent fibres. *J. Neurophysiol.* **40**, 1325–38.

Kuno, M. and Perl, E.R. (1960). Alteration of spinal reflexes by interaction with suprasegmental and dorsal root activity. *J. Physiol., London* **151**, 103–22.

LaMotte, R.H. and Campbell, J.N. (1978). Comparison of responses of warm and nociceptive C-fiber afferents in monkey with human judgements of thermal pain. *J. Neurophysiol.* **41**, 509–28.

Landau, W. and Bishop, G.H. (1953). Pain from dermal, periosteal, and facial endings and from inflammation. *Arch. Neurol. Psychiat.* **69**, 490–504.

Lele, P.P. and Weddell, G. (1956). The relationship between neurohistology and corneal sensibility. *Brain* **79**, 119–54.

Lewis, T. (1937a). The nocifensor system of nerves and its reactions. Part 1. *Br. med. J.* **1**, 431–5.

Lewis, T. (1937b). The nocifensor system of nerves and its reactions. Part 2. *Br. med. J.* **1**, 491–4.

Lewis, T. (1938). Suggestions relating to the study of somatic pain. *Br. med. J.* **1**, 321–5.

Lewis, T. (1942). *Pain*. Macmillan, New York.

Lewis, T. and Pochin, E.E. (1937). The double pain response of the human skin to a single stimulus. *Clin. Sci.* **3**, 67–76.

Lewis, T., Pickering, G.W., and Rothschild, P. (1931). Centripetal paralysis arising out of arrested bloodflow to the limb, including notes on a form of tingling. *Heart* **16**, 1–32.

Light, A.R. and Perl, E.R. (1979). Spinal termination of functionally identified primary afferent neurons with slowly conducting myelinated fibers. *J. comp. Neurol.* **186**, 133–50. Copyright 1979 Wiley-Liss, Inc.

Ling, G. and Gerard, R.W. (1949). The normal membrane potential of frog sartorious fibers. *J. cell. comp. Physiol.* **34**, 383–96.

Lloyd, D.P.C. and Chang, H.T. (1948). Afferent fibers in muscle nerves. *J. Neurophysiol.* **11**, 199–208.

Mackenzie, J. (1918). *Symptoms and their interpretation* (3rd edn). London.

Maruhashi, J., Mizuguchi, K., and Tasaki, I. (1952). Action currents in single afferent nerve fibres elicited by stimulation of the skin of the toad and the cat. *J. Physiol., London* **117**, 129–51.

Melzack, R. and Wall, P.D. (1962). On the nature of cutaneous sensory mechanisms. *Brain* **85**, 331–56.

Melzack, R. and Wall, P.D. (1965). Pain mechanisms: a new theory. *Science* **150**, 971–9.

Müller, J. (1842). *Elements of physiology*, Vol. 2. Taylor and Walton, London.

Nafe, J.P. (1929). A quantitative theory of feeling. *J. gen. Psychol.* **2**, 199–211.

Nafe, J.P. (1934). The pressure, pain, and temperature senses. In *Handbook of general experimental psychology* (ed. C. Murchison), pp. 1037–87. Clark University Press, Worcester, Massachusetts.

Ochoa, J. and Torebjörk, E. (1983). Sensations evoked by intraneural microstimulation of single mechanoreceptor units innervating the human hand. *J. Physiol., London* **342**, 633–45.

Ochoa, J. and Torebjörk, E. (1989). Sensations evoked by intraneural microstimulation of C nociceptor fibres in human skin nerves. *J. Physiol., London* **415**, 583–99.

Paintal, A.S. (1960). Functional analysis of group III afferent fibres of mammalian muscles. *J. Physiol., London* **152**, 250–70.

Perl, E.R. (1957). Crossed reflexes of cutaneous origin. *Am. J. Physiol.* **188**, 609–15.

Perl, E.R. (1958). Crossed reflex effects evoked by activity in myelinated afferent fibers of muscle. *J. Neurophysiol.* **21**, 101–12.

Perl, E.R. (1968). Myelinated afferent fibres innervating the primate skin and their response to noxious stimuli. *J. Physiol., London* **197**, 593–615.

Perl, E.R. and Whitlock, D.G. (1961). Somatic stimuli exciting spinothalamic projections to thalamic neurons in cat and monkey. *Exp. Neurol.* **3**, 256–96.

Ranson, S.W. (1913). The course within the spinal cord of the non-medullated fibers of the dorsal roots: a study of Lissauer's tract in the cat. *J. comp. Neurol.* **23**, 259–81.

Ranson, S.W. (1915). Unmyelinated nerve-fibres as conductors of protopathic sensation. *Brain* **38**, 381–9.

Ranson, S.W. and Billingsley, P.R. (1918). The conduction of painful afferent impulses in the spinal nerves. *Am. J. Physiol.* **340**, 571–84.

Schiff, J.M. (1858). *Lehrbuch der Physiologie des Menschen. Muskel und Nervenphysiologie*, Vol. 1. Lahr, Schauenburg.

Sherrington, C.S. (1906). *The integrative action of the nervous system*. Scribner, New York.

Sinclair, D.C. (1955). Cutaneous sensation and the doctrine of specific energy. *Brain* **78**, 584–614.

Sinclair, D.C., Weddell, G., and Zander, E. (1952). The relationship of cutaneous sensibility to neurohistology in the human pinna. *J. Anat.* **86**, 402–11.

Spiller, W.G. (1905). The occasional clinical resemblance between caries of the vertebrae and lumbothoracic syringomyelia, and the location within the spinal cord of the fibres for the sensations of pain and temperature. *Univ. Pa. med. Bull.* **18**, 147–54.

Sugiura, Y., Lee, C.L., and Perl, E.R. (1986) Central projections of identified unmyelinated (C) afferent fibers innervating mammalian skin. *Science* **234**, 358–61. Copyright 1986 American Association for the Advancement of Science.

Tasaki, I. (1953). Properties of myelinated fibers in frog nerve and in spinal cord as examined with micro-electrodes. *Jap. J. Physiol.* **3**, 73–94.

Torebjörk, E. and Ochoa, J. (1980). Specific sensations evoked by activity in single identified sensory units in man. *Acta physiol. scand.* **110**, 445–7.

Torebjörk, E., Allbo, Å.B., and Ochoa, J.L. (1987). Intraneural microstimulation in man. Its relation to specificity of tactile sensations. *Brain* **110**, 1509–29.

von Frey, M. (1894). Beiträge zur Physiologie des Schmerzsinns. *Koenigl. Saechs. Ges. Wiss., Math.-Phys. Klasse* **46**, 185–96.

von Frey, M. (1897). Beiträge zur Sinnesphysiologie der Haut. Part Iv. *Koenigl. Saechs. Ges. Wiss., Math.-Phys. Klasse* **49**, 462–8.

von Frey, M. (1922). Versuche über schmerzerregende Reize. *Z. Biol.* **76**, 1–24.

Wall, P.D. (1960). Cord cells responding to touch, damage, and temperature of skin. *J. Neurophysiol.* **23**, 197–10.

Wall, P.D. and McMahon, S.B. (1985). Microneurography and its relation to perceived sensation: a critical review. *Pain* **21**, 209–29.

Weddell, G. (1955). Somesthesis and the chemical senses. *Ann. Rev. Psychol.* **6**, 119–36.

Wellcome Trust (1954). *Catalog of incunabula in the Wellcome historical medical library.* Oxford University Press, London.

Witt, I. (1962). Aktivtät einzelner C-Fasern bei schmerzhaften und nicht schmerzhaften Hautreizen. *Acta neuroveg.* **24**, 208–19.

Witt, I. and Griffin, J.P. (1962). Afferent cutaneous C-fibre reactivity to repeated thermal stimuli. *Nature* **194**, 776–7.

Woollard, H.H., Weddell, G., and Harpman, J.A. (1940). Observations on the neurohistological basis of cutaneous pain. *J. Anat.* **74**, 413–40.

Yarnitsky, D., Simone, D.A., Dotson, R.M., Cline, M.A., and Ochoa, J.L. (1922). Single C nociceptor responses and psychophysical parameters of evoked pain: effect of rate of rise of heat stimuli in humans. *J. Physiol.* **450**, 581–92.

Zotterman, Y. (1933). Studies in the peripheral nervous mechanism of pain. *Acta med. scand.* **80**, 185–242.

Zotterman, Y. (1936). Specific action potentials in the lingual nerve of cat. *Skand. Arch. Physiol.* **75**, 105–20.

Zotterman, Y. (1939). The nervous mechanism of touch and pain. *Acta psychiat. neurol.* **XIV**, 91–7.

2 Structure of nociceptor 'endings'

LAWRENCE KRUGER AND ZDENEK HALATA

Introduction: The identification of nociceptors

Determining the association of specific sense organs with a specific sensory 'quality' or 'modality' has been a long and controversial quest, largely successful in relating the variety of elaborate sensitive mechanoreceptors to the complex events constituting tactile and kinaesthetic sensations. The evidence inferred for assigning the large corpuscular elements supplied by large, myelinated, fast-conducting afferent axons has been secured by combined electrophysiological and morphological observations and thus about one-half of afferent axons, derived from approximately one million large sensory ganglion cells in humans, can be accounted for in terms of both sensory function and an associated complex end-organ. The other half, constituting the thin, unmyelinated, slowly conducting axons originating principally in small sensory ganglion cells, remains elusive, although it is generally conceded that the vast majority probably constitute the nociceptive sense organs underlying the variety of sensory qualities usually described as 'pain'. No other sensation has eluded the designation of a specific structure as successfully as the nociceptor, and indeed it should be noted that some modern, seminal reviews, including the widely studied 'gate control theory' of pain (Melzack and Wall 1965), denied the very existence of nociceptors until the electrophysiological studies of Iggo and of Perl and their collaborators confirmed the widely held nineteenth century belief that cutaneous sensation was punctate and that each quality was associated with a discrete morphological arrangement serving as a sense organ, a view championed by Max von Frey (see Perl, Chapter 1, this volume). By the end of the nineteenth century, it was generally believed that 'free nerve endings' associated with thin, largely unmyelinated axons provided the morphological substrate for pain, and Sherrington (1900) noted that those sructures that he believed to be innervated solely by unmyelinated axons were zones from which only a sensation of pain could be elicited; these were the cornea, the dental pulp, and the internal surface of the tympanic membrane. Although the sensory quality attributable to stimulating these regions may be argued and the fibre spectrum innervating them extends into the thinly myelinated range in some species, the intuitive correlation between free endings, thin axons, and pain seemed basically sound.

An exclusionary principle proved more elusive, and the association of thin, largely unmyelinated axons with thermal sensations and the poorly understood qualities of tickle and itch at the other end of the hedonic spectrum presents a problem that remains unresolved. Aside from the uncertainty concerning the several sensory qualities associated with thin, unmyelinated, slowly conducting axons possessing a relatively simple terminal structure, it has been argued that many afferent axons are rarely, if ever, likely to be associated with any 'sensation' and that these axons primarily subserve an efferent or effector role, playing a role in the body's defence system as 'noceffectors' (Kruger 1987; Kruger et al. 1989). The electrophysiological observation of thin axons conducting in the C-fibre range that are apparently unexcitable by natural stimuli (Meyer et al. 1991) also renders fallible any exclusionary principle for attributing a specific morphology to nociception. Indeed, there are remarkably few examples of electrophysiologically identified receptive field 'spots' that have been studied in detail and, even in those studied in serial sections by electron microscopy, there can be no guarantee that there is only a single axon terminal in the marked zone. The only *direct* evidence that a single C fibre may merit a 'pain' designation derives from microstimulation of a presumed *single* fibre where the character and locus of the receptive field can be matched with the human subect's sensory report (Ochoa and Torebjörk 1989). The anatomical isolation of solitary axons in man (Fig. 2.1) provides one of the notable criteria in establishing a specific 'labelled line' serving pain. In the following account, the description of the characteristics of axon terminals *probably* associated with nociception and perhaps pain, is tempered by the caveats mentioned above and the certainty that there are other alternatives (including at least thermoreceptors and sensitive C mechanoreceptors) for the sensory modalities associated with 'free nerve endings'. Fortunately, popular beliefs cannot substitute for objective scientific evidence and the prevailing curent opinion that 'free' nerve endings constitute nociceptors should be considered an inference quite susceptible to other interpretations.

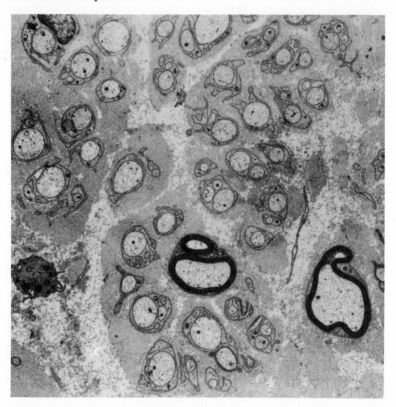

Fig. 2.1 Electron micrograph of human sural nerve. Many *solitary* unmyelinated axons can be found within each Schwann cell, a significant feature in interpreting reports of pain in human subjects (Ochoa and Torebjörk 1989). Micrograph courtesy of Professor José L. Ochoa.

'Silent nociceptors'

The number and proportion of thin afferent fibres that might be difficult or unlikely to be detected by means of conventional electrophysiological exploration could logically constitute a very substantial population. Although some experienced investigators indicate that they are rather rare in cutaneous nerves (Kress *et al.* 1992), if a sufficient range of mechanical and thermal stimuli is applied, the proportion of 'inexcitable' units ranges from 10 per cent (Bessou and Perl 1969), up to 28 per cent or about half of the C fibres (Handwerker *et al.* 1991b) in rat skin nerves (Lynn and Carpenter 1982; Pini *et al.* 1990) and 48 per cent of Aδ fibres and 30 per cent of C fibres in monkey skin (Meyer *et al.* 1991b). The proportions can be considerably higher in deep joint and muscle nerves (Kniffki *et al.* 1976; Schaible and Schmidt 1983, 1985, 1988a; Grigg *et al.* 1986), but many of them can be sensitized by inflammation and can be excited by hypertonic KCl, leading Schaible and Schmidt (1988b) to call them 'sleeping' rather than 'silent' units. It can be argued that it is dangerous to infer inexcitability from negative observations (Lynn 1991), but the large proportion of apparently unresponsive fibres in visceral nerves (Jänig and Koltzenburg 1990) that can be rendered active by inflammation has led to the proposal that there is a large class of visceral receptor fibres that are mainly concerned with signalling tissue injury; they become active only after inflammation of a peripheral organ (McMahon and Koltzenburg 1990a, b), for example, as demonstrated in urinary bladder thin fibres (Habler 1990, 1993).

Chemical stimuli, especially those that might be released consequent to inflammation (such as bradykinin, histamine, serotonin, prostaglandins, and leukotrienes), can sensitize high-threshold mechanoreceptors (for example, Perl *et al.* 1976; Martin *et al.* 1987, 1988; Cohen and Perl 1990; Dray *et al.* 1992), but it is likely that there is a novel class of thin afferent fibres that are chemoreceptive mediating chemogenic pain (Lang *et al.* 1990; LaMotte *et al.* 1991, 1992) and there are suggestive data for C-fibre chemoreceptors signalling itch (for example, Torebjörk and Ochoa 1981; Tuckett and Wei 1987; Wei and Tuckett 1991) as well as evidence of a 'sensitive' C mechanoreceptor class (Kumazawa and Perl 1977; Shea and Perl 1985a and b) that discharge when excited by gentle, moving tactile stimuli that might conceivably elicit a human sensory report of 'tickle'. It also should be noted that a substantial portion of the unmyelinated population includes sympathetic postganglionic efferents (Baron and Jänig 1988), but the 'insensitive' (silent or sleeping) class of C-fibres is amply demonstrable after surgical sympathectomy (Meyer *et al.* 1991a; Davis *et al.* 1993).

Sensitive C mechanoreceptors

A substantial number of unmyelinated afferents can be excited by innocuous mechanical stimuli (Douglas and Ritchie 1957; Iggo 1960; Bessou *et al.* 1971), and, as noted, it has been suggested that their discharge may be related to itch (Handwerker *et al.* 1991a; McMahon and Koltzenburg 1992). In human neuronography, C units appear to be almost exclusively activated by noxious or by thermal stimuli (Torebjörk and Hallin 11974) and perhaps gentle tactile stimuli in trigeminal neuralgia (Nordin 1990), but this may be a consequence of conspicuous regional differences, wherein sensitive C mechanoreceptors are evident in forelimb hairy skin but absent in distal glabrous skin in monkeys (Kumazawa and Perl 1977), a finding recently corroborated in humans (Vallbo *et al.* 1993).

Thermoreceptive endings

Extensive electrophysiological evidence for both 'cold' and 'warm' fibres conducting at velocities consistent with unmyelinated axons (reviewed by Spray 1986) supports the view championed by Weddell *et al.* (1955) that both types of thermoreceptors are subserved by 'free' nerve endings. The early opinions purporting to associate Krause end bulbs with cold receptors and Ruffini endings with warm receptors is still represented in some textbooks, although the *mechanoreceptive* properties of these elaborate 'corpuscular' endings are firmly established. The sequential dissociation of cold and warm sensations with local anaesthetic block (Fruhstorfer *et al.* 1974) is consistent with electrophysiological evidence of a smaller proportion of 'cold' than 'warm' C fibres. There is only limited evidence of a distinctive terminal morphology in a cold receptor (Hensel 1974) and there is virtually nothing known about warm receptors, but findings obtained in the free nerve endings in the pit organs of crotaline snakes (Bleichmar and De Robertis 1962; Terashima *et al.* 1970), known to be infrared thermoreceptors (Bullock and Fox 1957), may provide some insights into the characteristics of the vesicles found in afferent axon terminals (see below).

Finally, it has been argued that there may be a class of thin afferent axons that lack a sensory role, largely subserving efferent influences (Kenins 1981), possibly of a 'trophic' nature (Kruger 1988; McMahon and Koltzenburg 1990*a,b*). There is an extensive literature dating from the beginning of the century (Bayliss 1901) for an 'axon reflex' in which vasodilatation and plasma extravasation can be elicited in sympathectomized, cutaneous nerves, specifically in the slowly conducting fibres (Hinsey and Gasser 1930, Kenins 1981), and largely comprising a neuropeptide-dependent 'effector' action of 'sensory' nerves (Gamse *et al.* 1980; Lembeck and Gamse 1982; Maggi and Meli 1988).

The classification of small sensory ganglion cells

The main thrust of this review deals with the fine structural characterization of the terminals derived from thin axons, but it is becoming increasingly evident that the smaller-diameter dorsal root and trigeminal ganglion cells express extraordinary biochemical diversity compared with their larger counterparts that give rise to the thick, myelinated axons associated with a variety of specific, sensitive mechanoreceptors. Chapter 3 in this volume, by Lawson, expands upon this subject in detail, but a few broad features may prove relevant for solving the problem of modality assignment—a crucial issue for inferring nociceptive function in unmyelinated afferent axons.

Peptidergic markers

A convenient and widely used means of identifying thin sensory axons, is based on the presumption that sensory ganglion neurones manufacture molecules unique to that population. The discovery of substance P and other neuropeptides in a restricted population of sensory neurones and their axons proved of special interest and value, because peptides are found predominantly in numerous small cells and their thin axons, which, by inference, probably include a substantial proportion of nociceptors. The tissues innervated by peptidergic axons are largely sites from which pain can be elicited and, since a vast number of unmyelinated and thinly myelinated axons possess nociceptive properties that have enabled them to be identified electrophysiologically, it has been inferred that 'sensory' neuropeptides are selectively limited to nociceptive neurones. Selectivity is a key issue, but it also must be established that a 'sensory' neuropeptide is not expressed by other neurones. Fortunately, the most prevalent peptides found in small sensory ganglion cells, calcitonin gene-related peptide (CGRP) and galanin (Ju *et al.* 1987; Klein *et al.* 1990) are apparently absent from sympathetic postganglionic neurones. Although many sympathetic neurones are surounded by peptidergic axon terminals, especially those containing tachykinins and CGRP, these are presynaptic (Silverman and Kruger 1989), and evidence for perikaryal labelling in sympathetics is weak. On the other hand, there are numerous parasympathetic postganglionic neurones in the several ganglia examined in detail (Silverman and Kruger 1989) that have been shown to express substantial quantities of the prevalent 'sensory' neuropeptides. Thus, some proportion of peptide-labelled unmyelinated axons is probably autonomic, although numerically they constitute only a minor population.

A relatively unexplored feature of the ganglion cell bodies giving rise to the thin axons purported to be nociceptors is the variety of axon morphology. Figure 2.2 illustrates some peptidergic (CGRP-immunoreactive) cells with a variety of axon diameters and, interestingly, some axons display a variety of beaded appearances near the soma. Peripheral (distal) axons with varicosities have been recognized since the nineteenth century, but it remains to be determined whether axonal form constitutes a specific class, a functional variant of all classes or an artefact (Ochs and Jersild 1990), although the latter would not readily explain the axonal varieties exhibited within the ganglion itself (Fig. 2.2).

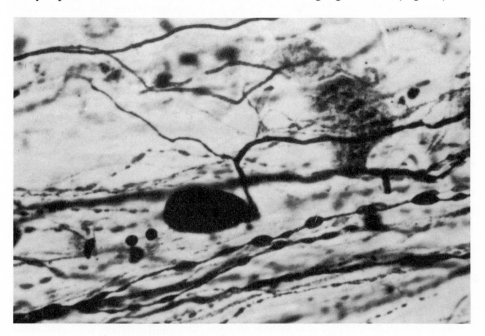

Fig. 2.2 A rat peptidergic (CGRP-immunoreactive) sensory (trigeminal) ganglion cell exhibiting the bifurcation of its thick (distal) and thin (central) branch. Note the range of axonal morphologies varying in thickness, beading, varicosities, etc. in individual axons.

The literature on peptidergic sensory neurones is beyond the scope of this survey (see Lawson, Chapter 3, this volume), but several features relevant to the classification of nociceptors derive from the selective distribution of neuropeptides and their receptors. A prominent feature of the 'sensory' peptidergic endings is their relation to autonomic targets containing smooth muscle and glands, especially blood vessels and sphincters (Kruger *et al*. 1989; Silverman and Kruger 1989). This contrasts with a largely non-peptidergic unmyelinated fibre population, characterized by specific glycoconjugates and traceable with specific lectins (Silverman and Kruger 1990*a*). The latter population constitutes the fluoride-resistant acid phosphatase (FRAP)-positive small sensory ganglion cells, once thought to prevail only in rodents (Silverman and Kruger 1988*a*). This subset of small, 'type B', sensory ganglion cells has been shown to express α 1,3-galactosyl-extended lactoseries carbohydrate epitopes that can be labelled by specific monoclonal antibodies (Dodd and Jessell 1985; Lawson *et al*. 1985). The cell-surface glycoconjugates expressed by these cells render them readily labelled by galactose and *N*-acetylgalactosamine-binding lectins. The lectin-reactive cell surface carbohydrate expression enables the labelling of axonal processes of a substantial proportion of the unmyelinated fibre population (Streit *et al*. 1986) which is largely distinct from the peptidergic population of dorsal root ganglia (DRG) neurones (Nagy and Hunt 1982; Silverman and Kruger 1990) and most prominently in their peripheral terminal distribution, for example in whole mounts where lectin-reactive axons appear to be unrelated to the small blood vessel distribution, which is contrastingly heavily decorated with peptidergic endings (see below and Fig. 2.11). The implication of the differential distribution is that those peptidergic axons containing the potent vasodilator, CGRP, are predominantly involved in vascular regulation and may more readily serve an effector role than the lectin-reactive axon terminals that appear to distribute in a 'free' fashion lacking any obvious target cells and corresponding receptor binding sites. The possibility that the non-peptidergic, lectin-positive neurones might be strictly nociceptive and may constitute a distinctive sensory class has not been supported by electrophysiological studies (see Lawson, Chapter 3, this volume). It should also be noted that peptidergic sensory axons are abundantly distributed in the avascular cornea (Silverman and Kruger 1989) and that CGRP-immunoreactive axons include *sensitive* mechanoreceptors (for example, Hoheisel *et al*. 1994) and thus also are unlikely to constitute a single functional class in either afferent or efferent terms.

The 'noceffector' concept

This concept arose from the need to account for the distribution of peptidergic thin 'sensory' axons whose efferent roles are not likely to be in the form of vascular effector actions or 'axon reflexes' and are more probably of a trophic nature (Kruger 1988). The argument derived originally from observation of the extraordinarily rich innervation of the dentinal tubules of molar teeth by CGRP-immunoreactive afferent fibres (Silverman and Kruger 1987) where only a small number of fibres might be required for 'nociceptive' function in the exceedingly rare instance of injury and pain from this location. This and other examples of innervation that presumably are not nociceptive are discussed below. The putative 'effector' roles in terms of some 'trophic' influences have been widespread for peptidergic afferents (Micevych and Kruger 1992), but there is no direct evidence that these constitute the 'silent' or 'sleeping' nociceptor afferent class.

Selective degeneration of nociceptive axons has been deduced from experiments based on systemic administration of capsaicin to rodents (Jancsó *et al.* 1977). In newborn animals, use of this agent results in extensive elimination of unmyelinated axons and small sensory ganglion cells accompanied by a behavioural deficit consisting of reduced responsiveness to thermal and noxious mechanical stimuli (reviewed by Buck and Burks 1986; Fitzgerald 1983). Fine structural examination reveals severe depletion of peri-vascular fibres (Papka *et al.* 1984) and of intraepithelial endings in the ear drum (Yeh and Kruger 1984) and epidermis (Kruger *et al.* 1985) following neonatal capsaicin treatment; there is no evident loss following chemical sympathectomy (Kruger *et al.* 1985), although the capsaicin-induced loss of peptidergic fibres has been questioned by other workers (Kashiba *et al.* 1990). In adult rats, following capsaicin treatment the sensory defect is evident without obvious loss of sensory ganglion cells or in dorsal root fibre counts (Chung *et al.* 1985) despite obvious degeneration of distal axons (Hoyes and Barber 1981), but quantitative analysis of subepidermal axon bundles suggests severe loss of the distal portions of unmyelinated nerves without detectable loss in their supplying cutaneous (sural) nerve (Chung *et al.* 1990). These authors also suggest that these intact axons do not regenerate (at least within 112 days) consistent with the prolonged selective action of this toxin (Lynn *et al.* 1987). Joo *et al.* (1969) claim that there is long-term mitochondrial damage in the small sensory ganglion cells associated with the sensory disturbance induced by capsaicin.

Regional variation

The distribution of thin afferent axons does not appear to obey any simple rule based on sensory requirements, probable exposure to noxious stimuli, or putative effector roles, but nineteenth century histologists had already established that the innervation of the skin differed considerably in different locations and surmised that these variants should relate to features of sensory discrimination. It is beyond the scope of this brief survey to review systematically the broad range of regional variation for which some general articles are available; we select here observations relevant to a few specialized regions of the body whose examination provides some insight into the problem of identifying nociceptors.

Glabrous skin

The principal emphasis has generally been placed on the structure of sense organs in glabrous digital skin because of its prominent role in exploratory behaviour. The descrip-tion by Cauna (1980) of thin axonal endings in human digital skin opened the modern period in which a range of variants were sought, following his description of three types of 'free' nerve endings — open; beaded; and plain. Their thin axons distribute vertically in a 'punctate pattern', some apparently terminating in the dermis and others penetrating the epidermal basal lamina, invaginating the basal layer. Cauna (1973, 1980) also noted a branched 'penicillate' distribution, more common in hairy human skin. An example of the branching pattern from a thinly myelinated axon from the lip of a marsupial is illustrated in Fig. 2.6. The meaning of such distinctions in functional terms (that is, modality) is largely unknown, and the few morphological studies of electrophysiologically characterized endings generally exploited the idiosyncratic features of specific tissues.

Intraepidermal axons

The existence of thin axons penetrating far up into the epidermis was illustrated in the mid-nineteenth century in a drawing by Langerhans (1868) and confirmed by numerous histologists using silver impregnation methods, but tracing their vertical course proved more elusive by electron microscopy (Breathnach 1971; Cauna 1959, 1980; Kadaroff 1971). The sensory nature of intraepithelial axons was demonstrated by electron microscopic autoradiography in the palatal epithelium employing a radioactive axonal transport label (Yeh and Byers 1983). Numerous studies have revealed peptidergic intraepidermal axons distributed in a manner resembling that of the more general axonal marker, protein gene product 9.5 (PGP9.5), suggesting that a large proportion of intraepidermal fibres are peptidergic (see, for example, Gibbins *et al.* 1985; Kruger *et al.* 1985, 1989; Dalsgaard *et al.* 1989; Karanth *et al.* 1991; Ribeiro da Silva *et al.* 1991; Hosoi *et al.* 1993; Kennedy and Wendelschafer-Crabb 1993; Rice *et al.* 1993). It should be emphasized that these axons do not penetrate above the stratum spinosum and that their sensory function has not been established. The peptidergic axons have been implicated in effector functions in regulating Langerhans ('dendritic') cell phenotypic expression (Hosoi *et al.* 1993; Hsieh *et al.* in press) and keratinocyte proliferation (Kjartansson and Dalsgaard 1987).

Among the puzzles in interpreting the functional significance of intraepidermal unmyelinated axons are findings concerning calcium-binding proteins. Immunoreactivity for calbindin (CB) and calretinin (CR) appears to be associated with rapidly adapting sensitive mechanoreceptors in both cutaneous and deep avian tissues and these proteins are apparently absent in slowly adapting axons (Duc *et al.* 1993). The identification of CR-immunoreactive intraepidermal axons in rat digital skin by Duc *et al.* (1994) presents a special problem as these workers have now established the general principle of calcium-binding proteins in mammalian rapidly adapting mechanoreceptive axons. The high affinity of these proteins for calcium could signify a role in controlling intracellular Ca^{2+} levels and thereby modulate impulse generation properties, but comparison of CB and CR amino acid sequences in diverse species indicates that calcium-binding sites are not the most conserved regions of these proteins, and it has been suggested that the interspersed segments actually may be crucial in interacting with intracellular macromolecules, independently of the role of calcium ions in transduction (Parmentier 1990). Whether these proteins are singularly associated with rapidly adapting mechanoreceptors remains uncertain because it has often been inferred that intraepidermal axons extending deep into the stratum spinosum of glabrous skin derive from unmyelinated parent axons and thus probably constitute 'nociceptors', unlike the thinly myelinated 'delta' mechano-nociceptors terminating in or near the basal stratum (Kruger *et al.* 1981) in cat hairy skin. The nature of deep epidermal 'free' nerve endings enveloped by keratinocytes and terminating below the stratum corneum merits inquiry concerning a possible role as sensitive mechanoreceptors with axons conducting at C-fibre velocities. In this context, it should be noted that the intrapithelial axons that penetrate almost to the surface of the cornea (see Fig. 2.7) identified by MacIver and Tanelian (1993) include C 'nociceptors' that respond to delicate mechanical stimuli, although in this location their excitation usually results in sensory reports of discomfort, if not pain, in human subjects (see Belmonte and Gallar, Chapter 6, this volume).

Thinly myelinated (Aδ) endings

The thinly myelinated axons that lose their myelin sheath and penetrate to the basal layer of the epidermis described by Cauna (1980) have been noted in various cutaneous sites, including several electron microscopic studies thereof (Fig. 2.3). In one early study (Hensel *et al.* 1974), a terminal of this type, identified electrophysiologically as a 'cold' spot receptive field, was illustrated by a drawing, but there apparently is no evidence to date that enables morphological distinction between 'cold spots' or the mechanoreceptive 'spots' of nociceptors. In a study of cat hairy skin, Kruger *et al.* (1981) examined a series of units identified as conducting in the myelinated Aδ conduction velocity range, and were able to identify axon terminals in the basal epidermis at identified nociceptive 'spots' that were not found in the intervening insensitive regions of the receptive field (Fig. 2.4). The several electron microscopic studies of epidermal basal layer endings reveal aggregations of vesicles and mitochondria, but little else that might distinguish these 'terminals' as specialized sense organs and, in the absence of serial sections before and after encountering the putative ending, there can be no assurance as to whether or not a branch might continue further into the stratum spinosum since such axons have been observed by many workers and in diferent species. Examples traced from thinly myelinated cutaneous axon to their presumptive terminal containing an accumulation of mitochondria and a few vesicles (Fig. 2.5) and the terminal branching pattern (Fig. 2.6) are illustrated here in marsupial skin.

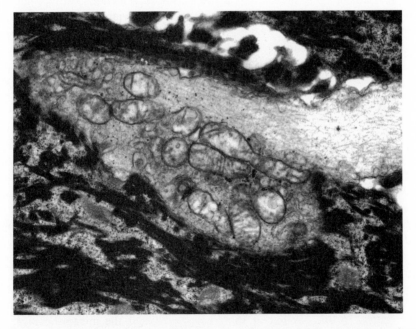

Fig. 2.3 Electron micrograph of an axon terminating in the nasal epidermal stratum spinosum of opossum. The 'free' ending contains numerous mitochondria and dispersed clear vesicles, glycogen granules, and amorphous matrix material. The axon was traced from the dermis and is a thinly myelinated Aδ fibre.

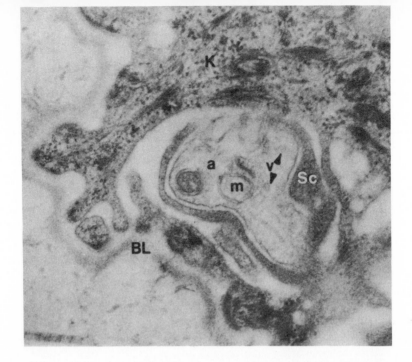

Fig. 2.4 Electron micrograph of an Aδ terminal found in an electrophysiologically identified nociceptive receptive field. The axon (a) containing mitochondria (m) and clear vesicles (v) has penetrated the epidermal basal lamina (BL) emerging from its surrounding Schwann cell processes (Sc) before becoming enveloped by keratinocyte processes (K). Taken with permission from Kruger *et al.* (1981).

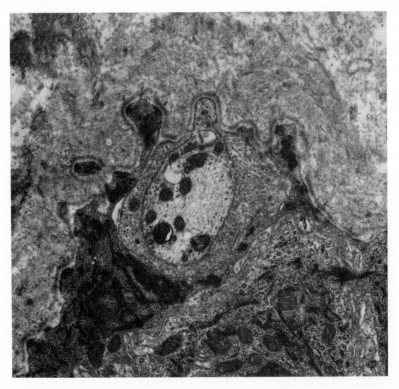

Fig. 2.5 Electron micrograph of an axon terminal traced from an Aδ fibre into the basal epidermal layer of opossum palmar skin. The axon is enveloped by Schwann cell cytoplasm surrounded by keratinocyte processes and contains (on the right side) a cluster of mitochondria and a few clear spherical vesicles.

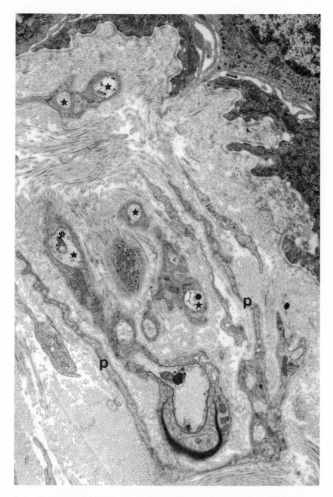

Fig. 2.6 Electron micrograph of the unmyelinated branches (*) of a thinly myelinated parent fibre in the superficial dermis of the lip (marsupial), at the site where myelin and perineurial (p) sheaths end.

Cornea

A recent study by MacIver and Tanelian (1993) in which thin polymodal fibres were studied electrophysiologically, while observed in the living cornea (*in vitro*) using epifluorescence, offers much promise. The mechanical- and heat-sensitive Aδ fibres were associated with horizontally directed processes described as basal epithelial branched 'leashes' that could be distinguished from the 'delicate stranded endings' traced into superficial epithelial layers and which are associated with 'polymodal' C fibres. Although MacIver and Tanelian (1993) present no fine structural data, their findings clearly distinguish separate classes of 'free nerve endings' that can be functionally interpreted in the context of the several accounts of corneal innervation (Zander and Weddell 1951; Matsuda 1968; Hoyes and Barber 1976; Tervo *et al.* 1979; Rozsa and Beuerman 1982; Tanelian and Beuerman 1984; Silverman and Kruger 1988*b*, 1989; Jones and Marfurt 1991; Ogilvy *et al.* 1991). The 'leash-like' arrangement of the basal fibres and endings associated with Aδ fibres (Fig. 2.7) may account for the directional selectivity of these mechano-sensitive units (MacIver and Tanelian 1993), but this is probably not a functionally homogeneous population as it comprises units with high and low mechanical thresholds as well as some with heat sensitivity (Belmonte *et al.* 1991; Belmonte and Gallar, Chapter 6, this volume) and, although some of these fibres are peptidergic (Silverman and Kruger 1989; Jones and Marfurt 1991), there is a lectin-reactive population (Silverman and Kruger 1988*b*) that is predominantly associated with thinner C fibres.

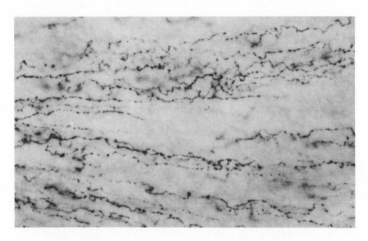

Fig. 2.7 CGRP-immunoreactive axon branches traced into the superficial layers of the epithelium of a rat corneal flat-mount preparation. Taken with permission from Silverman and Kruger (1989).

The corneal C fibres are of particular interest, in that they not only clearly penetrate vertically into the depths of the epithelium close to the surface, but also are the only sensory endings that undergo continuous growth and remodelling, spectacularly observed continuously in the living cornea by Harris and Purves (1989). While it is tempting to assume that these axons are nociceptive and polymodal, often possessing low mechanical threshold, thermal sensitivity and chemosensitivity, this is a complex problem for which the morphological correlates require further detailed examination.

Tooth

The innervation of the interior of teeth is numerically rich and of special interest because the only sensory quality reported on its stimulation in humans is invariably intense pain. The extensive innervation of dental pulp blood vessels is not surprising, although much of it is presumably of sympathetic origin. Peptidergic 'sensory' fibres are also quite numerous, but the unexpected finding is the richness of CGRP-immunoreactive axons within the coronal dentinal tubules (Silverman and Kruger 1987), which in terms of density (that is, number of axons/unit area) is richer than the exposed, superficial cornea and any other tissue we know of (Fig. 2.8). It was largely this finding that led to the proposal of the 'noceffector' concept (Kruger 1988), because afferent activation of these axons would seem unlikely in normal circumstances. It should also be noted that pulpal afferents apparently derive from numerous large ganglion cells with myelinated axons, many of which contain calcium-binding proteins (Ichikawa *et al.* 1994; Sugimoto *et al.*

1988), reducing the likelihood that these proteins might be exclusive mechanoreceptor markers unless the retrograde fluorescent label used in these experiments leaked to periodontal mechanoreceptors—an unlikely occurrence.

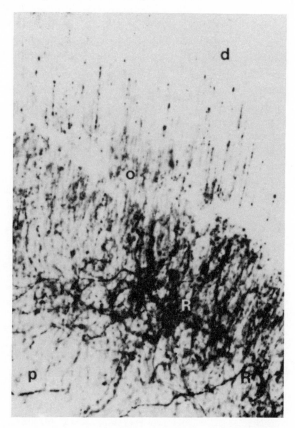

Fig. 2.8 CGRP-immunoreactive axons in the dental pulp (p) of a rat molar can be traced through Raschkow's plexus (R) and the odontoblast layer (o) into numerous dentinal tubules (d). Magnification, 200 ×. Taken with permission from Silverman and Kruger (1987).

Pulpal innervation appears to be especially disconcerting for sustaining some general principles concerning nociceptors. The sensory report by pulpal excitation, even using stimuli that would be innocuous when applied to other tissues, is invariably intense pain in humans, yet it clearly contains some myelinated axons derived from large, light ganglion cells. However, the fibre spectrum of the trigeminal nerve differs from other somatic afferent nerves in possessing a higher ratio of myelinated to unmyelinated fibres. If these fibres serve a nociceptive function, especially encased in a crystalline protective casing of enamel, it is not obvious why numerous axons would be useful as required for signalling 'pain'.

Tympanic membrane

This structure is particularly interesting in possessing an outer surface constituting the thinnest epidermis of the entire body and innervated by thick and thin axons but lacking in specialized corpuscular endings, although it is clearly suitable for tactile function. The inner mucosal surface facing the middle ear cavity is a sparsely innervated thin epithelium innervated solely by unmyelinated axons, and it is generally believed that their excitation can only elicit the sensory quality of slow, prolonged pain. These fibres can be visulized conveniently in whole-mount preparations (Colin and Kruger 1986) and traced to their single ending (Fig. 2.9). Fine structural analysis (Yeh and Kruger 1984) reveals superficial axon terminals lying immediately beneath the mucosal basal lamina, and many of these endings contain granular core vesicles and mitochondria (Fig. 2.10) typical of peptidergic endings (see (Fig. 2.15) and also seen in the intraepidermal terminals in the outer surface (Yeh and Kruger 1984), These peptidergic axons are extensively, but not totally, eliminated by neonatal capsaicin treatment.

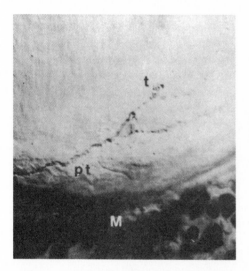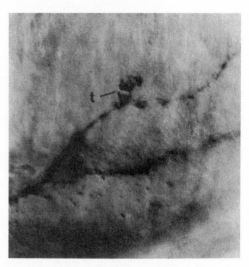

Fig. 2.9 A whole-mount view of the inner surface of the rat tympanic membrane near the attachment of the malleus (M), showing CGRP-immunoreactive axons traversing the pars tensa (pt), with one fibre traced to its terminal (t) enlargement (b). Taken with permission from Colin and Kruger (1986).

In the context of the previous discussion of tooth pulp innervation, it is worth noting that inflammation of the tooth and of the mucosa of the tympanic membrane both result in intense, 'slow' pain but with vast differences in the density of 'free' nerve endings representing the extremes of highest and lowest numerically.

Testis

This organ has been exploited as an optimum region for electrophysiological study of visceral nociceptors largely through the use of an *in vitro* preparation developed by Kumazawa *et al.* (1987). The testes are rarely associated with pain except when elicited by a mechanical insult or an inflammatory process. The sense organs are distributed principally in the tunica vasculosa protected by the collagenous coat of the tunica albuginea, an arrangement that is convenient for identifying the locus of receptive fields in a confined sheet suitable for electron microscopy as well as for whole-mount staining. The whole-mount preparation revealed a propitious vehicle for distinguishing between peptidergic sensory fibres and the large population of generally thinner lectin-reactive

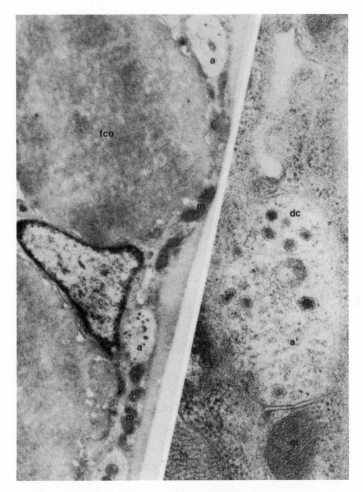

Fig. 2.10 Electron micrograph of the mucosal epithelial surface of the rat tympanic membrane. The thin epithelial cell processes are filled with mitochondria (m) and interspersed are three axon terminals (a), one shown at higher magnification on the right (a') containing several granular 'dense core' (dc) vesicles. Taken with permission from Yeh and Kruger (1984).

unmyelinated sensory organs. The latter are characterized by membrane-associated glycoconjugates with a terminal galactose, are largely non-peptidergic (that is, there is minimal overlap), and co-localize with the FRAP-positive neurone population (Silverman and Kruger 1990). The striking finding using these markers was the predominantly perivascular distribution of the peptidergic axons and their terminals, illustrated by CGRP-immunoreactivity in Fig. 2.11 (a), in contrast to the thin lectin-reactive axons that appear consistently unrelated to blood vessels and in a seemingly random distribution (Fig. 2.11 (b)).

   The distribution of axons in the relatively flat sheet of the tunica vasculosa also facilitated electron microscopic analysis of serial sections through electrophysiologically delimited receptive field 'spots' of characterized 'polymodal' fibres (Fig. 2.12). Kumazawa and his colleagues conservatively avoid commitment to designating these

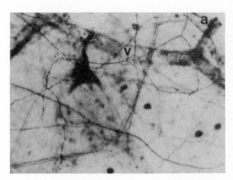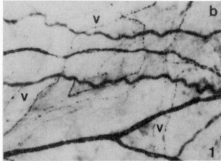

Fig. 2.11   Testicular whole mount of rat tunica vasculosa stained with lectin (GSA-IB₄) in (a) and for CGRP-immunoreactivity in (b). The thin lectin-reactive axonal bundles and terminals are distributed freely with little relation to vasculature (v), the endothelial basal lamina of which is lectin-stained. In contrast, coarse CGRP and bundles and fine granular axon terminals can be traced adjacent to vessel walls (v). Taken with permission from Silverman and Kruger (1988*b*).

nociceptive because the mechanical thresholds are low and, thus, the sensitive zone can be identified with greater precision than with high-threshold mechanoreceptors. The marked receptive fields often contained a nerve bundle and some contained more than one terminal, mostly within the nerve bundle, but those farthest removed from the epididymis and main nerve were occasionally isolated, and serial analysis revealed a terminal swelling, surrounded by a Schwann cell sheath, and containing numerous mitochondria and a small number of dense granules and small, clear spherical vesicles (Fig. 2.13). This terminal was traced serially until its disappearance, almost totally enveloped by a thin rim of Schwann cell cytoplasm and surrounded at a distance of ∼10–50 μm by concentrically arranged smooth muscle.

Nervi vasorum and nervi nervorum

The vascular tree throughout the body was shown to be richly innervated by substance P- and CGRP-immunoreactive sensory axons (Furness *et al.* 1982; Kruger *et al.* 1989), and numerous studies have implicated these fibres with the plasma extravasation and vasodilatation accompanying inflammation (see Holzer 1988; Maggi and Meli 1988 for reviews). There is direct evidence that individual nociceptive axons, when excited electrically, can elicit these peripheral efferent actions (Kenins 1981). These vasoactive fibres are capsaicin-sensitive and their perivascular distribution has been demonstrated using antibodies to several peptides in virtually every tissue examined thus far. Most papers illustrate the rich innervation of large arterial branches, but there are numerouss endings surrounding small vessels entering capillary beds that are distinct, though less numerous, surrounding veins (Kruger *et al.* 1989). In frozen sections, some fibres appear to traverse the mural smooth muscle, but this is probably an artefact and we have never seen a labelled terminal at the electron microscopic level that actually penetrates the adventitia. Thus, it is highly unlikely that there is any direct synaptic action on smooth muscle, but numerous investigators have noted peptidergic axons traceable to the vicinity of mast cells (Fig. 2.14) whose release of histamine when excited to degranulate probably also contributes to 'neurogenic' vascular effects (Coderre *et al.* 1989; Dimitriadou *et al.* 1991).

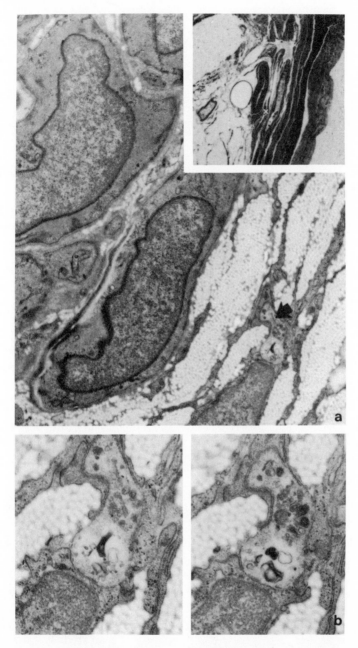

Fig. 2.12 A polymodal receptor terminal in the tunica vasculosa of the dog testis identified electrophysiologically in the laboratory of Professor T. Kumazawa. (a) The receptive field, marked by pinholes, contains an ending indicated in the low-magnification inset by an x next to a blood vessel and indicated by a large arrow. (b) Selected serial electron micrographs through this ending are shown. Note the variety of organelles and the cytoplasmic matrix components of the terminal; although largely enveloped by Schwann cells, one surface is slightly exposed or 'free'.

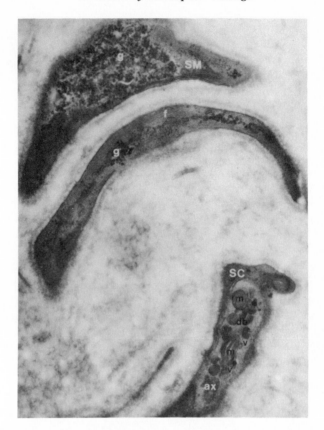

Fig. 2.13 Electron micrograph of an identified polymodal receptor axon terminal (ax) containing mitochondria (m) and clear (v) and dense core (dc) vesicles and surrounded by a thin layer of Schwann cell (SC) cytoplasm. Isolated smooth muscle cells (SM) containing glycogen (g) and filaments (f) loosely envelop the ending. Taken with permission from Kruger *et al.* (1988).

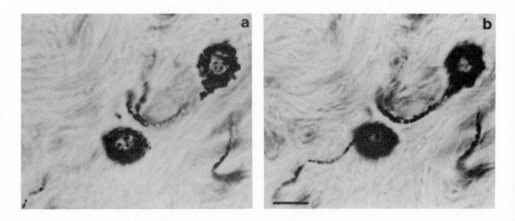

Fig. 2.14 Dermal substance P-immunoreactive axons traced in through-focus photomicrographs to two mast cells. Taken with permission from Kruger *et al.* (1985).

The innervation of nerve bundles resembles that of the vasa nervorum and thus many of the sympathetic as well as of the sensory peptidergic axons surrounding nerves (nervi nervorum) probably exert their effect directly on blood vessels (Hromada 1963; Furness *et al.* 1982; Appenzeller *et al.* 1984; Dhital and Appenzeller 1988). There is suggestive evidence that peptidergic fibres to vessels and nerves might be implicated in pathological conditions associated with chronic pain (Lincoln *et al.* 1993; Zochodne 1993), but the mode of action is poorly understood. Bove and Light (1994) have identified nociceptive fields associated with neurovascular bundles electrophysiologically and suggest that these are related to epineurial CGRP immunoreactivity (Bove and Light 1993), some of which may be non-vascular. A direct effect of nociceptive terminals on or associated with intraneurial axonal bundles is difficult to establish, but putative terminals can be detected with electron microscopy, a striking example of which is illustrated in Fig. 2.15. However, unless the parent axon is traced in its course through the epineural sheath, serial sections showing the disappearance of these rare presumptive 'terminals' should be interpreted with caution, although large clusters of peptidergic vesicles are not generally evident in sagittal sections of axonal varicosities. Unmyelinated axons terminating within small peripheral nerves have been shown in serially reconstructed sections in joint capsules and tendons (Andres *et al.* 1985; Heppelmann *et al.* 1990). The localization of peptides to granular 'dense core' vesicles using colloidal gold immuno-cytochemistry was established earlier by Gulbenkian *et al.* (1986). It should also be noted that small vessels penetrate the nerve sheaths and these presumably might be accompanied by small penetrating axons.

Glands

The peptidergic innervation of glands, especially by CGRP because it is lacking in sympathetic postganglionics, provides some clues to the complex pattern of secretory regulation (see Silverman and Kruger 1989). In general, the acinar portions of exocrine glands receive rather sparse sensory (that is, CGRP-immunoreactive) supply, although there is an abundance of perivascular intraglandular fibres (for example, dermal sweat glands; Kruger *et al.* 1989), and the densest pattern of glandular innervation is associated with excretory ducts and especially their orifices. It should be noted, however, that there are exceptions to such generalizations among the various nasal glands, for example, the Bowman's glands associated with the olfactory epithelium, and the acini of several nasal serous glands are amply supplied with CGRP-immunoreactive fibres, in contrast to the scant innervation of the mucous vomeronasal gland acini. The duct orifices strikingly supplied with sensory peptidergic fibres (for example, Bowman, von Ebner, and vomeronasal glands) imply an efferent role in regulation of secretions, especially in conjunction with chemosensory epithelia, but several exceptions remain unexplained (Silverman and Kruger 1989). In the absence of data suggesting that the efferent axons to glandular acini, ducts, and orifices serve a sensory role, it is tempting to relegate this rich thin-fibre innervation to an effector role, some of which is unrelated to regulation of smooth muscle. Nociceptive protective reflexes may be mediated by some of these fibres, but it would be difficult to account for their number and pattern of distribution strictly on the basis of nociceptive function.

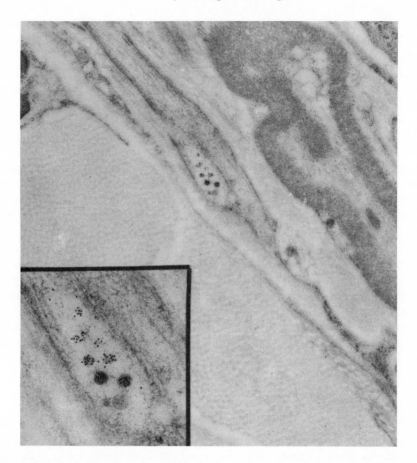

Fig. 2.15 Electron micrograph of an intraneurial presumptive axon terminal in a branch of the rat sural nerve cut longitudinally. The ending contains granular vesicles labelled with colloidal gold (inset) for CGRP-immunoreactivity.

Specialized secretory epithelia

The watery secretions of low protein content, and differing in ionic content substantially from plasma and extracellular fluid, do not appear to be regulated by peptidergic axons; they are conspicuous in their absence from the ocular ciliary processes, the stria vascularis of the inner ear, and the choroid plexuses (Silverman and Kruger 1989). This condition contrasts with the peptidergic innervation of all types of *sensory* epithelia.

Specialized sensory epithelia

The innervation of the renewable chemosensory epithelia—the neural olfactory and vomeronasal mucosae, as well as perigemmal axons surrounding taste buds and their orifices (Silverman and Kruger 1989, 1990*b*)—may be related to the turnover of cells in these renewable epithelia and the putative efferent regulation of mitogenesis by peptide release (Kruger 1987), rather than to joining central somatic nociceptive pathways. Neither of these functional inferences are likely to account for the sensory peptidergic innervation of the non-mitotic vestibular and cochlear hair cells (see Silverman and Kruger 1989). This constitutes another region in which a sensory 'nociceptive' role for these fibres is not evident, and their possible efferent function in regulating the sensitivity of these sense organs has not been elucidated.

Hairs

The vibrissae of those species using their 'whiskers' as exploratory organs (for example, rodents) are among the regions most richly supplied with unmyelinated axons, most prominently to the vibrissal follicle—sinus complex constituting the inner conical body (ICB). Andres (1966) illustrated circumferential 'lanceolate' endings derived from thin myelinated axons and numerous branching unmyelinated axons in the rat—the latter notably sparse in the rabbit and cat. Many of the unmyelinated endings are associated with parallel collagen bundles and are partially encapsulaed by septal cell processes; these are interpreted as Ruffini endings (Munger and Halata 1983; Renehan and Munger 1986). There are three sets of sensitive mechanoreceptors supplied by myelinated axons associated with the ICB including those ending on Merkel cells, small lamellated corpuscles (in monkey), and the lanceolate endings associated with the basal lamina (Halata and Munger (1980), These all obviously possess an unmyelinated terminal portion, but it is unlikely that they serve a nociceptive role.

The ICB of sinus hairs has been studied using high-voltage electron microscopy and serial reconstrucion of the extraordinarily dense array of small bundles of principally unmyelinated axons that terminate in a succession of cytoplasmic expansions resembling a cluster of grapes (Fig. 2.16). The endings are packed with organelles, principally mitochondria, and vesicles of both clear round and dense-core varieties, and they remain surrounded by a thin sheath of Schwann cell and basal lamina such that they are never observed as single 'free' endings (Mosconi et al. 1993). There are two distinct sets of unmyelinated axons: one derived from the deep nervous plexus to the lower third of the blood sinus where they branch and run upwards and the other from the superficial plexus, which are topographically more likely to discharge on pulling or swelling of the blood sinus. The latter are more likely to serve as nociceptors. Both plexuses also contain some thinly myelinated axons.

Other sets of unmyelinated axons surround the mouth of the sinus hair follicle and are deep in the outer root sheath of the hair shaft (Rice 1993; Rice et al. 1993). The location and large number of these branched endings surrounding the ICB would suggest that they are unlikely to serve a purely nociceptive function. Although many of the axons display peptide immunoreactivity (CGRP, galanin, and substance P), there is also a prominent lectin-reactive axonal population, indicating that there is probably a functionally heterogeneous innervation pattern (Mosconi et al. 1991).

Common fur or down hairs are also innervated by circumferential arrays of highly branched unmyelinated axons in their terminal distribution, some of which derive from myelinated parent axons and are arranged in a Ruffini-like pattern (Halata 1988; Halata and Munger 1981). The larger guard hairs are prominently innervated by large myelinated axons that serve as velocity-responsive sensitive mechanoreceptors (see Burgess and Perl 1973). The sensory function of hairs is generally to provide a lever for enhancing mechanosensitivity and it is doubtful that they serve an important role in nociception, although pain can be elicited by pulling on all types of hair. For those hairs most heavily innervated by unmyelinated axons, that is, sinus hairs, it is unlikely that they serve principally as nociceptors. Perhaps these fibres possess an efferent role with respect to altering the dynamic properties of the blood sinus, but the mechanism is unknown.

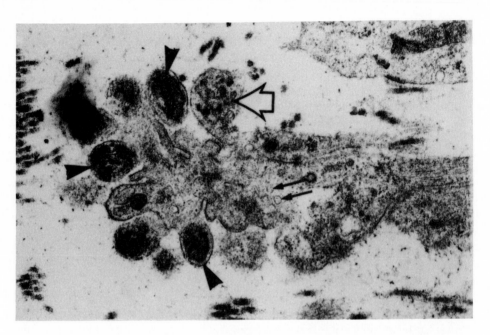

Fig. 2.16   A rat sinus hair terminal traced serially by high-voltage electron microscopy (see fig. 9 of Mosconi *et al.* 1993) revealing a branched 'blebbed' ending containing mitochondria (arrowheads) and clear (small arrows) and granular (large open arrow) vesicles. Taken with permission from Mosconi *et al.* (1993).

Fine structure of axon terminals

Recognition of the terminal *receptive portion* of a distal axon derived from a sensory ganglion cell may be ambiguous for unmyelinated axons unless fully reconstructed in serial sections that extend beyond the terminal in all directions. Most mechanoreceptor afferent fibres end in an encapsulated form, at least in the sense that the perineurial epithelium can be traced to a surrounding corpuscle or sensory apparatus with which it is continuous (Halata 1975), whereas unmyelinated axons often lose their perineurial layer (except perhaps some of its collagen component) before terminal expansion is reached (see Fig. 2.6). It is conceivable that the entire segment of such axons distal to its perineurial epithelial ensheathment constitutes the 'receptive' portion of the axon and there are examples of unensheathed segments along the course of nerves (for example, Yokota 1984). The 'terminal' portion, as defined by the absence of perineurial epithelium, may have multiple sectors of organelle aggregations (cf. vesicles and mitochondria) and there is no direct evidence to preclude the possibility that the entire distal process serves as a 'transducer', especially for C nociceptors that respond to chemical stimuli and possess what appear to be multiple 'endings' for a single axon (Heppelmann *et al.* 1990). The issue is not trivially semantic, for there is a distinction between multiple *branches* of a single axon each with its own terminus and multiple sensor zones along the path of one axon (or branch) each constituting a 'terminal' zone.

Ultimately, most authors have relied on defining the cytoplasmic features of putative endings that distinguish them from other portions of the distal unmyelinated parent axon. There is general agreement, in numerous papers, that mitochondria accumulate in the region of impulse generation in all sensory terminals, although in very thin terminals, a common feature of C fibres, there may be only a few, and similar clusters of mitochondria might be found in the parent nerve trunk. The pattern of cristae and intramitochondrial matrix density differs in individual terminals, often in the same field. Although this may be an irrelevant feature for determining a functional role and is generally ignored in the literature, mitochondrial matrix density is related to functional activity in sensory ganglion cells (Wong-Riley and Kageyama 1986). A number of reports illustrate accumulation of glycogen granules in terminals (see Andres and von Düring 1973; Halata 1975), and it is likely that their apparent absence in many studies is related to the method of tissue preservation and avoidance of anoxia prior to fixation. However, glycogen also is found along the entire axonal length. A feature that has not been noted in any studies is the 'receptor matrix' (Andres 1969; Andres and von Düring 1973), an amorphous, faintly filamentous region located in a focal sector of the terminal often associated with microtubules. Failure to identify this in most reports on unmyelinated axon terminals with nociceptor candidacy also may be related to fixation methodology even when electron micrographs are of obvious high quality, but for the present judgement should be postponed.

The presence of dense bodies (for example, Figs 2.12 and 2.15) is evident in many micrographs from numerous reports and a few also reveal small vacuolar inclusions or organelles, but these are unlikely to serve as diagnostic markers for identifying a 'free' nerve *terminal*. The all-important issue of vesicle accumulation is generally accepted as a particularly reliable criterion for identifying a receptive terminal zone, but there are many micrographs in the literature of putative endings with few or no vesicles. This may be, in part, a sampling problem and we shall deal with the vesicles in some detail below. Finally, there is the issue of identifying a region of bare axolemma lacking envelopment by Schwann cell cytoplasm associated with one or more of the above-mentioned features. A sampling of the growing literature and our own experience indicate that a thin layer of Schwann cell processes and its basal lamina constitute an interface that attenuates the usefulness and accuracy of the term 'free' nerve ending, unless one finds comfort and mitigation in the examples of those small sectors of the axolemma that protrude from one surface of the Schwann cell (Fig. 2.12 (b)). The site of the receptive or transductive surface, the nature of endocytotic and exocytotic processes and especially of peptide release, and the role of the Schwann cell in the interaction between sensory terminals and their surround must be better understood before the concept of a 'free' ending acquires meaning.

Vesicles

The nature of the vesicles found in the peripheral axon terminals of sensory ganglion cells is of special interest because, unlike the central (dorsal root) branch of the same axon, the distal 'sensory' terminal lacks synaptic contact and function and there is clearly no known requirement for neurotransmitter release. The latter statement may not be strictly correct, at least for peptidergic terminals serving an efferent role, especially when the peptide target can be identified by determining the cellular localization of peptide receptor binding sites. A functional role of 'sensory neuropeptides' in impulse generation or even as potent modulators of membrane events in these afferent terminals has not been demonstrated persuasively. It seems most likely that peptides serve a quasi-hormonal role in the various target tissues where receptor-binding sites have been identified. In this context, the role of vesicles containing peptides may be simply to fuse with the axolemma at a locus suitable for release; their effector action is known for smooth muscle but it is probably important in a variety of other cell types expressing sensory neuropeptide receptors. A dramatic example of a receptor-binding site in a lymph node, in addition to those in smooth muscle, where an effector target site might be expected, is illustrated in Fig. 2.17. There also has been some speculation that peptides, for example, CGRP, may play a role in impulse initiation (Beckers *et al.* 1992), but this has not been demonstrated.

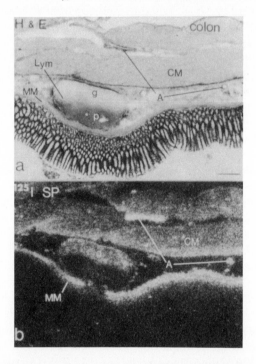

Fig. 2.17 Substance P receptor-binding sites in the canine colon exhibited in a longitudinal section (b) and stained with H & E (a) for orientation. In addition to the expected smooth muscle arterial (A) and muscularis binding sites of the circular (CM) and mucosal (MM) layers, a target effector is shown in the germinal centre (g), but not in the proliferative zone (p) of a lymph nodule (Lym). Scale bar, 0.85 mm. Taken with permission from P.W. Mantyh *et al* (1988).

We shall not attempt to survey the growing body of literature indicating that various peptides can be localized within granular or 'dense-core' vesicles, using colloidal gold immunocytochemistry as illustrated in Fig. 2.15 (see Gulbenkian *et al.* 1986; Ribeiro da Silva *et al.* 1991). The form of these peptide (or protein-precursor)-containing electron-dense vesicles is apparently susceptible to perturbation by various fixation methods such that preservation of the vesicle membrane and the distinct visualization of a halo around a dense interior is not evident in all published micrographs. It should be emphasized that the exclusivity of sequestration of peptides in dense vesicles has not been firmly established in all clases. Furthermore, it is likely that some of the dense-core vesicles are of the catecholaminergic variety (Price and Mudge 1983) and possess distinctly greater electron density. Clear, spherical vesicles are mostly commonly found in sensory axon terminals (Whitear 1974), and it can be inferred reasonably that the same range of excitatory and inhibitory neurotransmitters identified in the *synaptic* terminals of the spinal cord and brainstem are manufactured and apparently indiscriminately transported to both central and peripheral terminals. The nature and variety of these 'transmitters' is reviewed by Lawson (Chapter 3, this volume), but their functional, clearly *non-synaptic* role in peripheral endings is unknown. Some of the most intensively studied synaptic transmitters, popularly known as 'classical', for example acetylcholine and glutamate, are known to act upon non-neural elements. There is also a panoply of substances associated with pain and capable of eliciting impulse discharge in nociceptors, including bradykinins and free radicals. Nitric oxide, a recent 'molecule of the year', implicated in pain (Dawson *et al.* 1992; Meller and Gebhart 1993) is found in a variety of putative nociceptive neurones and their endings (Verge *et al.* 1993; Bscheidl *et al.* 1994). Its actions on a variety of cell types involved in inflammatory reactions obfuscate its neurogenic role and its specificity.

On strictly morphological grounds, it is unlikely that there is a homogeneous population of clear vesicles, for, in addition to some pleomorphic variants, there is a range of sizes, and, in some studies employing methods optimal for preservation of membrane ultrastructure, distinct vesicle coats or cages can be discerned. Recent studies of the 'free' nerve endings of the infra-red sensitive pit organ of crotaline snakes (Terashima and Jiang 1993; Terashima *et al.* 1995) suggest that temperature can alter the size, number, and coats of vesicles in this receptor terminal and Fig. 2.18, taken from Terashima's studies, illustrates the typically larger size of the large spherical coated vesicles. We are unaware of attempts to determine whether the latter are clathrin-coated and exert a distinctive role in endocytosis and exocytosis. The role of the clear, uncoated, vesicles in transmitter cycling, discussed in the extensive literature on synaptic endings (see Heuser and Reese 1973; Basbaum and Heuser 1979; Zimmerman 1979; Tauc 1982; Heuser 1989; Valtorta *et al.* 1990), apparently has not attracted systematic investigation in nociceptive endings, nor has the putative role of neurotransmitters or neuropeptides in impulse generation been examined in a morphological context. Techniques for examining the mechanism of uptake of axonal transport 'markers' can be applied readily to this perplexing question. The absence of terminal transporters for neuropeptides and the lack of information concerning the presence and distribution of vesicle transporters of transmitters have impeded our understanding of vesicle function in *non-synaptic* sensory terminals. Stimulated release of neuropeptides has been established convincingly (Olgart *et al.* 1977; Fujimori *et al.* 1990), and many of their cellular targets have been identified by receptor-binding autoradiography, but the peripheral target cells or hypothetical axon terminal autoreceptors for transmitters involved in rapid depolarization and impulse generation remain remarkably unexplored.

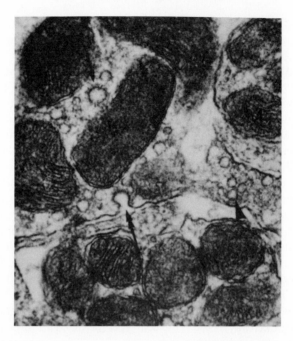

Fig. 2.18   Electron micrograph of a 'free' nerve ending in the infra-red thermoreceptive pit organ of crotaline snakes. Note the high density of mitochondria interspersed between spherical vesicles (arrowhead) and larger coated-vesicles (arrow) one of which opens on to the surface (double-headed arrow). Micrograph courtesy of Professor S. Terashima.

Conclusion

Any survey of morphological studies of putative nociceptor endings reveals that these sense organs have been characterized in very bare detail. A vast literature abounds with non-descriptive constructs implying that nociceptors are 'simple' or 'primitive', an unlikely condition for which evidence is grossly deficient, and, despite a consensus for physiological diversity, we lack a satisfactory taxonomy based on structure. Reluctance to accept the very existence of 'nociceptors' until late in this century may account in part for dilatory progress, but their study has also been hampered by the inherent difficulty of characterizing a structure that requires some degree of damage in order to be identified.

A vast proportion of the thin fibres whose endings might be involved in pain or any sensation related to mechanical, thermal, or chemical stimuli, are arranged in the periphery in a pattern and in numbers suggestive of efferent actions that are independent of nociceptive protective reflexes and instead may be involved in physiological trophic roles in the absence of actual or threatened tissue damage. Peptide-mediated efferent mechanisms, particularly of vascular regulation, may be controlled by impulse generation due to noxious stimuli, although dependence upon afferent activity and peptide release has not been established. The 'noceffector' concept implies that many afferent fibres are *effectors* and that they are rarely, if ever, activated by noxious stimuli (for example, those innervating glands, ducts, sphincters, taste buds, endosteum, dentinal tubules, etc.), and others (such as those innervating cochlear and vestibular hair cells, olfactory epithelium, and sympathetic ganglion cells) may lack any afferent or sensory role whatever.

Another population of apparently non-peptidergic sensory ganglion cells emitting thin, principally unmyelinated axons characterized by specific membrane glycoconjugates and co-localized markers (monoclonal antibodies, lectins, fluoride-resistant acid phosphatase) are not distributed in any identified relation to peripheral target effectors, nor have their electrophysiological correlates been secured. The ostensible 'transmitters' at sensory terminals have been inferred largely from identification of these substances in central (dorsal horn) terminals (acetylcholine, γ-aminobutyric acid (GABA), excitatory amino acids, purines, etc.) and their influence upon events in putative nociceptive endings is obscure. The molecular specificity of neuromodulators found within, or exerting an influence upon, 'nociceptive' endings offers promise in classifying 'nociceptors' as do the many substances that clearly influence or vigorously excite discharge (bradykinins, nitric oxide, and reactive oxygen species). A practical taxonomy of 'nociceptors' based on molecular specificity or on morphological specialization remains elusive, but the popularly held concept of 'free' nerve endings and their identity with nociceptors has probably outlived its usefulness.

Acknowledgements

We are indebted to our colleagues who are too numerous to mention for discussions of the content of this chapter, to Ms Deborah Anderson for preparing the immunogold electron micrograph as well as for assistance in asembling the figures, and to Ramon Colinayo and Lisa Chen for manuscript preparation. The electron micrographs from marsupial skin were obtained from studies in Hamburg supported by the Deutsche Forschungsgemeinschaft Ha 1194/3–1 and the previously unpublished rat electron micrographs were obtained at UCLA supported by a National Institute of Health, grant NS-5685 (a Javits Investigator award).

References

Alvarez, F.J., Rodrigo, J., Jessell, T.M., Dodd, J., and Priestley, J.V. (1989). Ultrastructure of primary afferent fibres and terminals expressing d-galactose extended oligosaccharides in the spinal cord and brainstem of the rat. *J. Neurocytol.* **18**, 631–45.

Andreev, M. and Dray, A. (1994). Opioids suppress activity of polymodal nociceptors in rat paw skin induced by ultraviolet irradiation. *Neuroscience* **58** 793–8.

Andres, K.H. (1966). Uber die Feinstruktur der Rezeptoren an Sinushaaren. *Z. Zellforsch.* **75**, 335–65.

Andres, K.H. (1969). Zur Ultrastruktur verschiedener Mechanorezeptoren von Höheren Wirbeltieren. *Anat. Anz.* **124**, 551–65.

Andres, K.H. and von Düring, M. (1973). Morphology of cutaneous receptors. In *Handbook of sensory physiology*, Vol. II (ed. A. Iggo), pp. 3–28. Springer-Verlag, New York.

Andres, K.H., von Düring, M., and Schmidt, R.F. (1985). Sensory innervation of the Achilles tendon by group III and IV afferent fibers. *Anat. Embryol.* **172**, 145–56.

Appenzeller, D., Dhital, K.K., and Burnstock, G. (1984). The nerves to blood vessels supplying nerves: the innervation of vasa nervorum. *Brain Res.* **304**, 383–6.

Baron, R. and Jänig, W. (1988). Sympathetic and afferent neurons projecting in the splenic nerve of the cat. *Neurosci. Lett.* **94**, 109–13.

Basbaum, C.B. and Heuser, J.E. (1979). Morphological studies of stimulated adrenergic axon varicosities in the mouse vas deferens. *J. Cell Biol.* **80**, 310–25.

Bayliss, W.M. (1901). On the origin of the vaso-dilator fibres of the hind-limb, and on the nature of these fibres. *J. Physiol.* **26**, 173–209.

Beckers, H.J.M., Klooster, J., Vrensen, G.F.J.M., and Lamars, W.P.M.A. (1992). Ultrastructural identification of trigeminal nerve endings in the rat cornea and iris. *Invest. Ophthal. vis. Sci.* **33**, 1979–86.

Belmonte, C., Gallar, J., Pozo, M.A., and Rebollo, I. (1991). Excitation by irritant chemical substances of sensory afferent units in the cat's cornea. *J. Physiol.* **437**, 709–25.

Bessou, P. and Perl, E.R. (1969). Responses of cutaneous sensory units with unmyelinated fibres to noxious stimuli. *J. Neurophysiol.* **32**, 1025–43.

Bessou, P., Burgess, P.R., Perl, E.R., and Taylor, C.B. (1971). Dynamic properties of mechanoreceptors with unmyelinated (C) fibers. *J. Neurophysiol.* **34**, 116–31.

Bleichmar, H. and De Robertis, E. (1962). Submicroscopic morphology of the infrared receptor of pit vipers. *Z. Zell. Forsch. Mikr. Anat.* **45**, 748–61.

Bove, G.M. and Light, A.R. (1993). CGRP-like immunoreactivity of fine afferents innervating peripheral nerve sheaths. *Soc. Neurosci. Abstr.* **19**, 327.

Bove, G.M. and Light, A.R. (1994). Group IV nociceptors of rat paraspinal tissue. *J. Neurophysiol.* **1**, 1–4.

Breathnach, A.S. (1971). *An atlas of the ultrastructure of human skin.* J.A. Churchill, London.

Bscheidl, C., Hanesch, U., and Heppelmann, B. (1994). NADPH-diaphorase reactivity in articular afferents of a normal and inflamed knee joint in the cat. *Brain Res.***668**, 266–70.

Buck, S.H. and Burks, T.F. (1986). The neuropharmacology of capsaicin: review of some recent observations. *Pharmacol. Rev.* **38**, 179–226.

Bullock, T.H. and Fox, W. (1957). The anatomy of the infrared sense organ in the facial pit of pit vipers. *Quart. J. mirosc. Sci.* **98**, 219–234.

Burgess, P.R. and Perl, E.R. (19773). Cutaneous mechanoreceptors and nociceptors. In *Handbook of sensory physiology*, Vol. II (ed. A. Iggo), pp. 29–78. Springer-Verlag, New York.

Cauna, N. (1959). The mode of termination of sensory nerves and its significance. *J. comp. Neurol.* **113**, 169–210.

Cauna, N. (1973). The free penicillate nerve endings of human skin. *J. Anat.* **115**, 227–88.

Cauna, N. (1980). Fine morphological characteristics and microtopography of free nerve endings of the human digital skin. *Anat. Rec.* **198**, 643–56.

Cervero, F., Connell, L.A., and Lawson, S.N. (1984). Somatic and visceral primary afferents in the lower thoracic dorsal root ganglia of the cat. *J. comp. Neurol.* **228**, 422–31.

Chung, K., Schwen, R.J., and Coggeshall, R.E. (1985), Ureteral axon damage following subcutaneous administration of capsaicin in adult rats. *Neurosci. Lett.* **53**, 221–6.

Chung, K., Klein, C.M., and Coggeshall, R.E. (1990). The receptive part of the primary afferent axon is most vulnerable to systemic capsaicin in adult rats. *Brain Res.* **511**, 222–6.

Coderre, T.J., Basbaum, A.I., and Levine, J.D. (1989). Neural control of vascular permeability: interaction between primary afferents, mast cells, and sympathetic efferents. *J. Neurophysiol.* **62**, 48–58.

Cohen, R.H. and Perl, E.R. (1990). Contributions of arachidonic acid derivatives and sustance P to the sensitization of cutaneous nociceptors. *J. Neurophysiol.* **64**, 457–64.

Colin, S. and Kruger, L. (1986). Peptidergic nociceptive axon visualization in whole-mount preparations of cornea and tympanic membrane in rat. *Brain Res.* **398**, 199–203.

Dalsgaard, C.J., Rydh, M., and Haegstrand, A. (1989). Cutaneous innervation in man visualized with protein gene product (PGP9.5) antibodies. *Histochemistry* **92**, 385–9.

Davis, K.D., Meyer, K.A., and Campbell, J.N. (1993).Chemosensitivity and sensitization of nociceptive afferents that innervate the hairy skin of monkey. *J. Neurophysiol.* **69**, 1071–81.

Dawson, T.M., Dawson, V.L., and Snyder, S.H. (1992). A novel neuronal messenger molecule in brain: the free radical, nitric oxide. *Ann. Neurol.* **32**, 297–311.

Devor, M., Jänig, W., and Michaelis, M. (1994). Modulation of activity in dorsal root ganglion neurons by sympathetic activation in nerve-injured rats. *J. Neurophysiol.* **71**, 38–47.

Dhital, K. and Appenzeller, O. (1988). Innervation of vasa nervorum. In *Nonadrenergic innervation of blood vessels*, Vol. II (ed. G. Burnstock and S.G. Griffith), pp. 191–211. CRC Press, Boca Raton, Florida.

Dimitriadou, V., Buzzi, M.G., Moskowitz, M.A., and Theoharrides, T.C. (1991). Trigeminal sensory fibre stimulation induces morphological changes reflecting secretion in rat dura mater mast cells. *Neuroscience* **44**, 97–112.

Dodd, J. and Jessell, T.M. (1985). Lactoseries carbohydrates specify subsets of dorsal root ganglion neurons projecting to the superficial dorsal horn of rat spinal cord. *J. Neurosci.* **5**, 3278–94.

Douglals, W.W. and Ritchie, J.M. (1957). Non-medullated fibres in the saphenous nerve which signal touch. *J. Physiol.***139**, 385–99.

Dray, A. (1992). Neuropharmacological mechanisms of capsaicin and related substances. *Biochem. Pharmacol.* **44**, 611–15.

Dray, A., Patel, I.A., Perkins, M.N., and Rueff, A. (1992). Bradykinin-induced activation of nociceptors: receptor and mechanistic studies on the neonatal rat spinal cord–tail preparation *in vitro. Br. J. Pharmacol.* **107**, 1129–34.

Duc, C., Barakat-Walter, I., and Droz, B. (1993). Peripheral projections of calretinin-immunoreactive primary sensory neurons in chick hindlimbs. *Brain Res.* **632**, 321–4.

Duc, C., Barakat-Walter, I., and Droz, B. (1994). Innervation of putative rapidly adapting mechanoreceptors by calbindin- and calretinin-immunoreactive primary sensory neurons in the rat. *Eur. J. Neurol.* **6**, 264–71.

Fitzgerald, M. (1983). Capsaicin and sensory neurones—a review. *Pain* **15**, 109–30.

Fruhstorfer, H., Zenz, M., Noltle, H., and Hensel, H. (1974). Dissociated loss of cold and warm sensibility during regional anaesthesia. *Pflügers Arch.* **349**, 73–82.

Fujimori, A., Saito, A., Kimura, S., and Goto, K. (1900). Release of calcitonin gene-related peptide (CGRP) from capsaicin-sensitive vasodilator nerves in the rat mesenteric artery. *Neurosci. Lett.* **112**, 173–8.

Furness, J.B., Papka, R.E., Della, N.G., Costa, M., and Eskay, R (1982). Substance P-like immunoreactivity in nerves associated with the vascular system of guinea pigs. *Neuroscience* **7**, 447–59.

Gamse, R.S., Holzer, P., and Lembeck, F. (1980). Decrease of substance P in primary afferent neurons and impairment of neurogenic plasma extravasation by capsaicin. *Br. J. Pharmacol.* **68**, 207–13.

Gibbins, I.L., Furness, J.B., Costa, M., MacIntyre, I., Hillyard, C.J., and Girgis, S. (1985). Co-localization of calcitonin gene-related peptide-like immunoreactivity with substance P in cutaneous, vascular and visceral sensory neurons of guinea pigs. *Neurosci. Lett.* **57**, 125–30.

Grigg. P., Schaible, H.-G., and Schmidt, R.F. (1986). Mechanical sensitivity of group III and IV afferents from posterior articular nerve in normal and inflamed cat knee. *J. Neurophysiol.* **55**, 635–43.

Gulbenkian, S., Merighi, A., Wharton, J., Varndell, I.M., and Polak, J.M. (1986). Ultrastructural evidence for the coexistence of calcitonin glene-related peptide and substance P in secretory vesicles of peripheral nerves in the guinea pig. *J. Neurocytol.* **15**, 535–42.

Habler, H.J., Jänig, W., and Koltzenburg, M. (1990). Activation of unmyelinated afferent fibres by mechanical stimuli and inflammation of the urinary bladder in the cat. *J. Physiol.***425**, 545–62.

Habler, H.J., Jänig, W., and Koltzenburg, M. (1993). Receptive properties of unmyelinated primary afferents innervating the inflamed urinary bladder of the cat. *J. Neurophysiol.* **69**, 395–405.

Halata, Z. (1975). The mechanoreceptors of the mammalian skin: ultrastructure and morphological classification. *Adv. Anat. Embryol. Cell Biol.* **50**, 1–77.

Halata, Z. (1988). Ruffini corpuscle: a stretch receptor in the connective tissue of the skin and locomation apparatus. *Prog. Brain Res.* **74**, 221–9.

Halata, Z. and Munger, B.L. (1980). The sensory innervation of primate eyelid. *Anat. Rec.* **198**, 657–70.

Halata, Z. and Munger, B.L. (1988). Sensory nerve endings in rhesus monkey sinus hairs. *J. comp. Neurol.* **192**, 645–63.

Haley, J.E., Dickinson, A.H., and Schachter, M. (1989). Electrophysiological evidence for a role of bradykinin in chemical nociception. *Neurosci. Lett.* **97**, 198–202.

Handwerker, H.O., Forster, C., and Kirchhoff, C. (1991a). Discharge patterns of human C-fibers induced by itching and burning stimuli. *J. Neurophysiol.* **66**, 307–15.

Handwerker, H.O., Kilo, S., and Reeh, P.W. (1991b). Unresponsive afferent nerve fibres in the sural nerve of the rat. *J. Physiol.* **435**, 229–42.

Harris, L.H. and Purves, D. (1989). Rapid remodeling of sensory endings in the corneas of living mice. *J. Neurosci.* **9**, 2210–14.

Hensel, H., Andres, K.H., and von Düring, M. (1974). Structure and function of cold receptors. *Pflügers Arch.* **352**, 1–10.

Heppelmann, B., Messlinger, K., Neiss, W.F., and Schmidt, R.F. (1990). Ultrastructural three-dimensional reconstruction of group III and IV sensory nerve endings ('free nerve endings') in the knee joint capsule of the cat: evidence for multiple receptive sites. *J. comp. Neurol.* **292**, 103–16.

Heuser, J.E. (1989). The role of coated vesicles in recycling of synaptic vesicle membrane. *Cell Biol. Int. Rep.* **13**, 1063–76.

Heuser, J.E. and Reese, T.S. (1973). Evidence for recycling of synaptic vesicle membrane during transmitter release at the frog neuromuscular junction. *J. Cell. Biol.* **57**, 315–44.

Hinsey, J.C. and Gasser, H.S. (1930). The component of the dorsal root mediating vasodilation and the Sherrington contracture. *Am. J. Physiol.* **92**, 679–89.

Hoheisel, U., Mense, S., and Scherotzke, R. (1994). Calcitonin gene-related peptide-immunor-eactivity in functionally identified primary afferent neurons in the rat. *Anat. Embryol.* **189**, 41–9.

Holzer, P. (1988). Local effector functions of capsaicin-sensitive sensory nerve endings: involvement of tachykinins, calcitonin gene-related peptide, and other neuropeptides. *Neuroscience* **24**, 739–68.

Hosoi, J., Murphy, G.F., Egan, C.L., Lerner, E.A., Grabble, S., Asahina, A., and Granstein, R.D. (1993). Regulation of Langerhans cell function by nerves containing calcitonin gene-related peptide. *Nature* **363**, 159–63.

Hoyes, A.D. and Barber, P. (1976). Ultrastructure of the corneal nerves in the rat. *Cell Tissue Res.* **172**, 133–44.

Hoyes, A.D. and Barber, P. (1981). Degeneration of axons in the ureteric and duodenal nerve plexuses of the adult rat following *in vivo* treatment wih capsaicin. *Neurosci. Lett.* **25**, 19–24.

Hromada, J. (1963). On the nerve supply of the connective tissue of some peripheral nervous tissue components. *Acta anat.* **55**, 343–51.

Hsieh, S-T, Choi, S., Lin, W-M., Chong, Y-C., Mc Arthur, J.C., and Griffin, J-W. Epidermal denervation and its effects on keratinocytes and Langerhans cells. *J. Neurocytol.* (in press).

Ichikawa, H., Deguchi, T.,Mitani, S.H., Nakago, T., Jacobowitz, D.M., and Sugimoto, T. (1944). Neural parvalbumin and calretinin in the tooth pulp. *Brain Res.* **647**, 124–30.

Iggo, A. (1960). Cutaneous mechanoreceptors with afferent C fibers. *J. Physiol.* **1252**, 337–53.

Jancsó, G., Kiraly, E., and Jancsó-Gabor, A. (1977). Pharmacologically induced selective degeneration of chemosensitive primary sensory neurons. *Nature* **270**, 741–3.

Jänig, W. and Koltzenburg, M. (1990). On the function of spinal primary afferent fibres supplying colon and urinary bladder. *J. autonom. nerv. Syst.* **30** (Suppl), S89–S96.

Jessell, T.M. (1985). Cellular interactions at the central and peripheral terminals of primary sensory neurons. *J. Immunol.* **135**, 746S–749S.

Jones, M.A. and Marfurt, C.F. (1991). Calcitonin gene-related peptide and corneal innervation: a developmental study in the rat. *J. comp. Neurol.* **313**, 132–50.

Joo, F., Szolcsányi, J., and Janscó-Gabor, A. (1969). Mitochondrial alterations in spinal ganglion cells of the rat accompanying the long-lasting sensory disturbance induced by capsaicin. *Life Sci.* **8**, 621–6.

Ju, G. Hökfelt, T., Bordin, E., Fahrenkrug, J., Fischer, J.A., Frey, P., Elde, R.P., and Brown, J.C. (1987). Primary sensory neurons of the rat showing calcitonin gene-related peptide immunoreactivity and their relation to substance P-, somatostatin, galanin-, vasoactive intestinal polypeptide-, and cholycystokinin-immunoreactive ganglion cells. *Cell Tissue Res.* **247**, 417–31.

Kadanoff, D. (1971). Die Ultrastruktur und Lage der Nervenfasern und ihrer Endingen in Epithelgewebe. *Z. mikrosk. anat. Forsch.* **84**, 321–2.

Karanth, S.S., Springall, D.R., Kuhn, D.M., Levene, M.M., and Polak, J.M. (1991). An immunocytochemical study of cutaneous innervation and the distribution of neuropeptides and protein gene product 9.5 in man and commonly employed laboratory animals. *Amer. J. Anat.* **191**, 369–83.

Kashiba, H., Senba, E., Ueda, Y., and Tohyama, M. 1990). Relative sparing of calcitonin gene related peptide containing primary sensory neurons following neonatal capsaicin treatment in the rat. *Peptides* **11**, 491–6.

Kenins, P. (1981). Identification of the unmyelinated sensory nerves which evoke plasma extravasation in rsponse to antidromic stimulation. *Neurosci. Lett.* **25**, 137–41.

Kennedy, W.R. and Wendelschafer-Crabb, G. (1993). The innervation of human epidermis. *J. neurol. Sci.* **115**, 184–90.

Kjartansson, J. and Dalsgaard, C.J. (1987). Calcitonin gene-related peptide increases survival of a musculocutaneous critical flap in the rat. *Eur. J. Pharmacol.* **142**, 355–8.

Klein, C.M., Westlund, K.N., and Coggeshall, R.E. (1990). Percentage of dorsal root axons immunoreactive for galanin are higher than those immunoreactive for calcitonin gene-related peptide in the rat. *Brain Res.* **519**, 97–101.

Kniffki, K-D., Mense, S., and Schmidt, R.F. (1976). Response of group IV afferent units from skeletal muscle to stretch, contraction and chemical stimulation. *Exp. Brain Res.* **31**, 511–22.

Kress, M., Koltzenburg, M., Reeh, P.W., and Handwerker, H.O. (1992). Responsiveness and functional attributes of electrically localized terminals of cutaneous C-fibers in vivo and in vitro. *J. Neurophysiol.* **68**, 581–95.

Kruger, L. (1987). Morphological correlates of 'free' nerve endings—a re-appraisal of thin sensory axon classification. In *Fine afferent nerve fibers and pain* (ed. R.F. Schmidt, H.-G. Schaible, and C. Vahle-Hinz), pp. 3–13. VCH Verlagsgesellschaft, Weinheim, Basel.

Kruger, L. (1988). Morphological features of thin sensory afferent fibers: a new interpretation of 'nociceptor' function. In *Prog. Brain Res.* **74**, 253–7.

Kruger, L., Perl, E.R., and Sedivec, M.J. (1981). Fine structure of myelinated mechanical nociceptor endings in cat hairy skin. *J. comp. Neurol.* **198**, 137–54.

Kruger, L., Sampogna, S.L., Rodin, B.E., Clague, J., Brecha, N., and Yeh, Y. (1985). Thin-fiber cutaneous innervation and its intraepidermal contribution studied by labeling methods and neurotoxin treatment in rats. *Somatosens. Res.* **335–56.**

Kruger, L., Kumazawa, T., Mizumura, K., Sato, J., and Yeh, Y. (1988). Observations on electrophysiologically characterized receptive fields of thin testicular afferent axons: a preliminary note on the analysis of fine structural specializations of polymodal receptors. *Somatosens. Mot. Res.* **5**, 373–80.

Kruger, L., Silverman, J.D., Mantyh, P.W., Sternini, C., and Brecha, N.C. (1989). Peripheral patterns of calcitonin gene-related peptide general somatic sensory innervation: cutaneous and deep terminations. *J. comp. Neurol.* **280**, 291–302.

Kumazawa, T. and Perl, E.R. (1977). Primate cutaneous sensory units with unmyelinated (C) afferent fibers. *J. Neurophysiol.* **40**, 1325–38.

Kumazawa, T., Mizumura, K., and Sato, J. (1987). Response properties of polymodal receptors studied using in vitro testis superior spermatic nerve preparations of dogs. *J. Neurophysiol.* **57**, 702–11.

LaMotte, R.H., Lundberg, L.E.R., and Torebjörk, H.E. (1922). Pain, hyperalgesia and activity in nociceptive C units in humans after intradermal injection of capsaicin. *J. Neurophysiol.* **448**, 749–64.

LaMotte, R.H., Schain, C.N., Simone, D.A., and Tsai, E. (1991). Neurogenic hyperalgesia: psychophysical studies on underlying mechanisms. *J. Neurophysiol.* **66**, 190–211.

Lang, E., Novak, A., Reeh, P.W., and Handwerker, H.O. (1990). Chemosensitivity of fine afferents from rat skin in vitro. *J. Neurophysiol.* **63**, 887–901.

Langerhans, P. (1868). Ueber die Nerven der menschlichen Haut. *Virchow Arch.* **44**, 325–38.

Lawson, S.N., Harper, E.I., Harper, A.A., Garson, J.A., Coakham, H.B., and Randle, B.J. (1985). Monoclonal antibody 2C5: a marker for a subpopulation of small neurons in rat dorsal root ganglia. *Neuroscience* **16**, 365–74.

Lembeck, F. and Gamse, R. (1982). Substance P in peripheral sensory process. In *Substance P in the nervous system,* Ciba Foundation Symposium no. 91, pp. 35–49. Pitman, London.

Lincoln, J., Milner, P., Appenzeller, O., Burnstock, G., and Qualls, C. (1993). Innervation of normal human sural and optic nerves by noradrenaline- and peptide-containing nervi vasorum and nervorum: effect of diabetes and alcoholism. *Brain Res.* **632**, 48–56.

Lynn, B. (1991). 'Silent' nociceptors in the skin. *Trends Neurosci.* **14**, 95.

Lynn, B. and Carpenter, S.E. (1982). Primary afferent units from the hairy skin of the rat hind limb. *Brain Res.* **238**, 29–43.

Lynn, B., Pini, A., and Baranowski, R. (1987). Injury of somatosensory afferents by capsaicin: selectivity and failure to regenerate. Effects of injury on trigeminal and spinal somatosensory systems. *Neurol. Neurobiol.* **30**, 115–24.

MacIver, M.B. and Tanelian, D.L. (1993). Structural and functional specialization of Aδ and C fiber free nerve endings innervating rabbit corneal epithelium. *J. Neurosci.* **13**, 4511–24.

McMahon, S.B. and Koltzenburg, M. (1990*a*). Novel classes of nociceptors: beyond Sherrington. *Trends Neurosci.* **13**, 199–201.

McMahon, S.B. and Koltzenburg, M. (1990*b*). The changing role of primary afferent neurons in pain. *Pain* **43**, 269–72.

McMahon, S.B. and Koltzenburg, M. (1992). Itching for an explanation. *Trends Neurosci.* **15**, 497–501.

Maggi, C.A. and Meli, A. (1988). The sensory-efferent function of capsaicin-sensitive sensory neutrons. *Gen. Pharmacol.* **19**, 1–43.

Mantyh, P.W., Mantyh, C.R., Gates, T., Vigna, S.R., and Maggio, J.E. (1988). Receptor binding sites for substance P and substance K in the canine gastrointestinal tract and their possible role in inflammatory bowel disease. *Neuroscience* **43 25**, 817–37.

Martin, H.A., Basbaum, A.I., Kwiat, C., Goetzl, E.J., and Levine, J.D. (1987). Leukotriene and prostaglandin sensitization of cutaneous high-threshold C- and Aδ-mechanoreceptors in the hairy skin of rat hindlimbs. *J. Neurosci.* **22**, 651–9.

Matsuda, H. (1968). Electron microscopic study on the corneal nerve with special reference to its endings. *J. Ophthalmol.* **12**, 163–73.

Meller, S.T. and Gebhart, G.F. (1993). Nitric oxide (NO) and nociceptive processing in the spinal cord. *Pain* **52**, 127–36.

Melzack, R. and Wall, P.D. (1965). Pain mechanisms: a new theory. *Science* **150**, 971–9.

Meyer, R.A., Cohen, R.H., Davis, K.D., Tweede, R.D., and Campbell, J.N. (1991*a*). Evidence for cutaneous afferents that are insensitive to mechanical stimuli. In *Proceedings of the Sixth World Congress of Pain, Adelaide Australia 1990* (ed. M. E. Bond, J.E. Charlton, and C.J. Woolf), pp. 71–5. Elsevier, Amsterdam.

Meyer, R.A., Davis, K.D., Cohen, R.H., Tweede, R.D., and Campbell, J.N. (1991*b*). Mechanically insensitive afferents (MIAS) in cutaneous nerves of monkey. *Brain Res.* **561**, 252–61.

Micevych, P.E. and Kruger, L. (1992). The status of calcitonin gene-related peptide as an effector peptide. *Ann. NY Acad. Sci.* **657**, 379–96.

Mosconi, T.M., Rice, F.L., and Song, M.J. (1991). Sensory endings in the inner conical body of the rat mystacial vibrissa. *Soc. Neurosci. Abstr.* **17**, 106.

Mosconi, T.M., Rice, F.L., and Song, M.J. (1993). Sensory innervation in the inner conical body of the vibrissal follicle-sinus complex of the rat. *J. comp. Neurol.* **328**, 232–51.

Munger, B.L. and Halata, Z. (1983). The sensory innervation of the primate facial skin. *Brain Res. Rev.* **5**, 45–80.

Nagy, J.I. and Hunt, S.P. (1982). Fluoride-resistant acid phosphatase-containing neurons in dorsal root ganglia are separate from those containing substance P or somatostatin. *Neuroscience* **7**, 89–97.

Nordin, M. (1990). Low-threshold mechanoreceptive and nocireceptive units with unmyelinated (C) fibres in the human supraorbital nerve. *J. Physiol.***425**, 229–40.

Ochoa, J. and Torebjörk, E. (1989). Sensations evoked by intraneural microstimulation of C nociceptor fibres in human skin nerves. *J. Physiol.***415**, 583–99.

Ochs, S. and Jersild, R.A. Jr (1990). Myelin intrusions in beaded nerve fibers. *Neuroscience* **36**, 553–67.

Ogilvy, C.S., Silverman, K.R., and Borges, L.F. (1991). Sprouting of corneal sensory fibers in rats treated at birth with capsaicin. *Invest. Ophthalmol. vis. Sci.* **32**, 112–21.

Olgart, L., Gazelius, B., Brodin, E., and Nilsson, G. (1977). Release of substance P-like immunoreactivity from the dental pulp. *Acta physiol. scand.* **101**, 510–12.

Papka, R.E., Furness, J.B., Della, N.G., Murphy, R., and Costa, M. (1984). Time course of effect of capsaicin on ultrastructure and histochemistry of substance P-immunoreactive nerves associated with the cardiovascular system of the guinea pig. *Neuroscience* **12**, 1277–92.

Parmentier, M. (1990). Structure of the human cDNAs and genes coding for calbindin D28k and calretinin. *Ad. exp. Med. Biol.* **269**, 27–34.

Perl, E.R., Kumazawa, T., Lynn, B., and Kenins, P. (1976). Sensitization of high threshold receptors with unmyelinated C) afferent fibers. *Prog. Brain Res.* **43**, 263–77.

Pierau, F.K., Fellmer, G., and Taylor, D.C.M. (1984). Somatovisceral convergence in the cat dorsal root ganglion neurons demonstrated by double-labeling with fluorescent tracers. *Brain Res.* **321**, 63–70.

Pini, A., Baranowski, R., and Lynn, B. (1990). Long-term reduction in the number of C-fibre nociceptors following capsaicin treatment of a cutaneous nerve in adult rats. *Eur. J. Neurosci.* **2**, 89–97.

Price, J. and Mudge, A.W. (1983). A subpopulation of rat dorsal ganglion neurons is catecholaminergic. *Nature* **301**, 241–3.

Renehan, W.E. and Munger, B.L. (1986). Degeneration and regeneration in the rat trigeminal system I: identification and characterization of the multiple afferent innervation of the mystacial vibrissae. *J. comp. Neurol.* **29**, 129–45.

Ribeiro-da Silva, A., Kenigsbery, R.L., and Cuello, A.C. (1991). Light and electron microscopic distribution of nerve growth factor receptor-like immunoreactivity in the skin of the rat lower lip. *Neuroscience* **43**, 631—46.

Rice, F.L. (1993). Structure, vascularization, and innervation of the mystacial pad of the rat as revealed by the lectin Griffonia simplicifolia. *J. comp. Neurol.* **337**, 386–99.

Rice, F.L., Kinnman, E., Aldskogius, H., Johansson, O., and Arvidsson, J. (1993). The innervation of the mystacial pad of the rat as revealed by PGP 9.5 immunofluorescence. *J. comp. Neurol.* **337**, 365–85.

Roozsa, A.J. and Beuerman, R.W. (1982). Density and organization of free nerve endings in the corneal epithelium of the rabbit. *Pain* **14**, 105–20.

Schaible, H.-G. and Schmidt, R.F. (1983). Responses of fine medial articular nerve afferents to passive movements of knee joint. *J. Neurophysiol.* **49**, 1118–26.

Schaible, H.-G. and Schmidt, R.F. (1985). Effects of an experimental arthritis on the sensory properties of fine articular afferent units. *J. Neurophysiol.* **54**, 1109–22.

Schaible, H.-G. and Schmidt, R.F. (1988*a*). Direct observation of the sensitization of articular afferents during an experimental arthritis. In: *Proceedings of the Fifth World Congress of Pain, Hamburg, Germany 1987*, (ed. R. Dubner, G.F. Gebhart, and M.R. Bond), pp. 44–50. Elsevier, Amsterdam.

Schaible, H.-G. and Schmidt, R.F. (1988*b*). Time course of mechanosensitivity changes in articular afferents during a developing experimental arthritis. *J. Neurophysiol.* **60**, 2180–95.

Shea, V.K. and Perl, E.R. (1985*a*). Failure of sympathetic stimulation to affect responsiveness of rabbit polymodal nociceptors. *J. Neurophysiol.* **54**, 513–19.

Shea, V.K. and Perl, E.R. (1985*b*). Sensory receptors with unmyelinated (C) fibers innervating the skin of the rabbit's ear. *J. Neurophysiol.* **54**, 491–501.

Sherrington, C.S. (1900). Cutaneous sensations. In *Textbook of physiology*, Vol. II (ed. E.A. Schafer), pp. 920–1001. Y.J. Pentland, Edinburgh and London.

Silverman, J.D. and Kruger, L. (1987). An interpretation of dental innervation based upon the pattern of calcitonin gene-related peptide (CGRP) immunoreactive thin sensory axons. *Somatosens. Motor Res.* **5**, 157–75.

Silverman, J.D. and Kruger, L. (1988*a*). Acid phosphotase as a selective marker for a class of small sensory ganglion cells in several mammals: spinal cord distribution, histochemical poperties, and relation to fluoride-resistant acid phosphatase (FRAP) of rodents. *Somatosens. Motor Res.* **5**, 219–46.

Silverman, J.D. and Kruger, L. (1988*b*). Lectin and neuropeptide labeling of separate populations of dorsal root ganglion neurons and associated 'nociceptor' thin axons in rat testis and cornea whole-mount preparation. *Somatosens. Motor Res.* **5**, 259–67.

Silverman, J.D. and Kruger, L. (1989). Calcitonin gene-related peptide (CGRP) immunoreactive innervation of the rat head with emphasis on the specialized sensory structures. *J. comp. Neurol.* **280**, 303–30.

Silverman, J.D. and Kruger, L. (1990*a*). Selective neuronal glycoconjugate expression in sensory and autonomic ganglia: relation of lectin reactivity to peptide and enzyme markers. *J. Neurocytol.* **19**, 789–801.

Silverman, V.D. and Kruger, L. (1990*b*). Analysis of taste bud innervation based on glycoconjugate and peptide neuronal markers *J. comp. Neurol.* **292**, 575–84.

Spray, D.C. Cutaneous temperature receptors. *Ann. Rev. Physiol.* **48**, 625–38.

Streit, W.J., Schulte, B.A., Balentine, J.D., and Spicer, S.S. (1986). Evidence for glycoconjugate in nociceptive primary sensory neurons and its origin from the Golgi complex. *Brain Res.* **377**, 1–17.

Sugimoto, R., Takemura, M., and Wakisaka, S. (1988). Cell size analysis of primary neurons innervating the cornea and tooth pulp of the rat. *Pain* **32**, 375–81.

Tanelian, D.L. and Beuerman, R.W. (1984). Responses of rabbit corneal nociceptors to mechanical and thermal stimulation. *Exp. Neurol.* **84**, 165–78.

Tauc, L. (1982). Nonvesicular release of neurotransmitter. *Physiol. Rev.* **62**, 857–93.

Terashima, S. and Jiang, P-J. (1993). The effect of temperature change on the number of vesicles and on the form of mitochondria in free nerve endings. *J. physiol. Soc., Jap.* **55**, 64–5. [In Japanese.]

Terashima, S., Goris, R.C., and Katsuki, Y. (1970). Structure of warm fiber terminals in the pit membrane of fibers. *J. ultrastruct. Res.* **31**, 494–506.

Terashima, S., Jiang, P.J., Mizuhira, V., Hasegowa, H. and Notoya, M. (1995). Temperature-induced changes in the number of vesicles in the free nerve endings of temperature neurons of the snake. *Somatosens. Motor Res.* **12**, 143–50.

Tervo, T., Joo, F., Kuikuri, K.T., Toth, I., and Palkama, A. (1979). Fine structure of sensory nerves in the rat cornea: an experimental nerve degeneration study. *Pain* **6**, 57–70.

Torebjörk, H.E. and Hallin, R.G. (1974). Identification of afferent C units in intact human skin nerves. *Brain Res.* **67**, 387–403.

Torebjörk, H.E. and Ochoa, J.L. (1981). Pain and itch from C-fiber stimulation. *Soc. Neurosci. Abstr.* **7**, 228.

Tuckett, R.P. and Wei, W.Y. (1987). Response to an itch-producing substance in cat. II. Cutaneous receptor populations with unmyelinated axons. *Brain Res.* **413**, 513–30.

Vallbo, A., Olausson, H.., Wessberg, J., and Norrsell, U. (1993). A system of unmyelinated afferents for innocuous mechanoreception in the human skin. *Brain Res.* **628**, 301–4.

Valtorta, F., Fesce, R., Grohovaz, F., Haimann, C., Hurlbut, W.P., Iezzi, N., Torri-Tarelli, F., Villa, A., and Ceccarelli, B. (1990). Neurotransmitter release and synaptic vesicle recycling. *Neuroscience* **35**, 477–89.

Verge, V.M.K., Xu, Z.,, Xu, X-J., Wiesenfeld-Hallin, Z., and Hokfelt, T. (1992). Marked increase in nitric oxide synthase mRNA in rat dorsal root ganglia after peripheral axotomy: in situ hybridization and functional studies. *Proc. natl Acad. Sci., USA* **89**, 11617–21.

Vizzard, M.A., Erdman, S.L., and de Groat, W.C. (1933). Localization of NADPH-diaphorase in bladder afferent and postganglionic efferent neurons of the rat. *J. autonom. nerv. Syst.* **44**, 85–90.

Weddell, G., Palmer, E., and Pallie, W. (1955). Nerve endings in mammalian skin. *Biol. Rev.* **30**, 159–95.

Wei, J.Y. and Tuckett, R.P. (1991). Response of cat ventrolateral spinal axons to an itch-producing stimulus (cowhage). *Somatosens. Motor Res.* **8**, 227–39.

Whitear, M. (1974). The vesicle population in frog skin nerves. *J. Neurocytol.* **3**, 49–58.

Wong-Riley, M.T.T. and Kageyama, G.H. (1986). Localization of cytochrome oxidase in the mammalian spinal cord and dorsal root ganglia, with quantitative analysis of ventral horn cells in monkeys. *J. comp. Neurol.* **245**, 41–61.

Yeh, Y. and Byers, M.R. (1983). Fine structure and axonal transport labeling of intraepithelial sensory nerve endings in anterior hard palate of the rat. *Somatosens. Res.* **1**, 1–19.

Yeh, Y. and Kruger, L. (1984). Fine-structural characterization of the somatic innervation of the tympanic membrane in normal, sympathectomized, and neurotoxin-denervated rats. *Somatosens. Res.* **1**, 1–19.

Yokota, R. (1984). Occurrence of long non-myelinated axonal segments intercalated in myelinated, presumably sensory axons: electron microscopic observations in the dog atrial endocardium. *J. Neurocytol.* **13**, 127–43.

Zander, E. and Weddell, G. (1951). Observations on the innervation of the cornea. *J. Anat., London* **85**, 68–99.

Zimmermann, H. (1979). Vesicle recycling and transmitter release. *Neuroscience* **4**, 1773–804.

Zochodne, D.W. (1993). Epineurial peptides: a role in neuropathic pain? *Can. J. neurol. Sci.* **20**, 69–72.

3 Neurochemistry of cutaneous nociceptors

SALLY N. LAWSON

Introduction

Nociceptive information, that is, information about potentially damaging stimuli, from the skin of the limbs and the trunk, is carried to the spinal cord by several types of nociceptive dorsal root ganglion (DRG) neurones. The variety of cutaneous fibres that carry nociceptive information (about noxious mechanical, thermal, and chemical stimuli) have been well documented (Perl 1992). However, the study of the neurochemistry of these neurones is complicated by the presence of muscle and visceral as well as cutaneous neuronal somata, and the presence of nociceptive as well as non-nociceptive neuronal somata in DRGs. Unfortunately, there are no methods as yet of identifying all nociceptive neurones in the DRG.

As a result, there is little information to correlate the neurochemical phenotype of DRG neurones directly with their sensory properties, despite a considerable literature on the molecular phenotypes of DRG neuronal subpopulations (see review by Lawson 1992). It is the purpose of this chapter to consider the evidence for any of these molecules being expressed in nociceptive cutaneous afferent neurones. In view of the clinical desirability of selectively interfering with the functions of nociceptive afferent neurones, this chapter will examine neurochemical markers of neuronal subpopulations and exclude those common to all sensory neurones. I shall therefore review data on neurochemical expression in DRG neurones in order to identify molecules expressed in neurones with cell sizes that are appropriate for nociceptive neurones. This type of aproach examines circumstantial evidence only and can therefore provide only a guide as to which molecules may be more or less rewarding to study in future 'pain' research. I shall then examine the evidence that certain of these molecules are expressed in cutaneous afferent neurones. Finally, I shall examine the limited direct evidence on molecular expression in identified nociceptive cutaneous afferent neurones.

Neurochemistry of neurones in DRGs

Cell size and conduction velocity

The majority of cutaneous nociceptive afferent units have C or Aδ fibres, while a few also conduct in the Aβ range (Perl 1992). Also, most cutaneous afferent C fibres are nociceptive (see below). C-fibre neurones are known to have small cell bodies in rat, guinea-pig, and cat DRGs, and Aδ neurones are small- to medium-sized (Lee *et al.* 1986; Lawson and Waddell 1991; Lawson 1992; unpublished observations). Cutaneous nociceptive neurones should therefore mostly have small cell bodies in the DRG; their cell size distribution should have a peak of small cells and a diminishing tail of intermediate-sized neurones. This is also likely to be the case for nociceptive muscle and visceral afferent neurones.

Tables 3.2 and 3.3 list neurochemical markers. Abbreviations are listed in Table 3.1. The markers that label mainly small neurones (• in Tables 3.2 and 3.3) include, in Table 3.2, many peptides; glutamate and glutamine; peripherin (an intermediate filament); tyrosine kinase A (trkA; the high-affinity nerve growth factor (NGF) receptor); the enzymes tyrosine monophosphatase (TMP), fluoride-resistant acid phosphatase (FRAP), adenosine deaminase (ADA), β-glycerophosphatase monoamine oxidase, nitric acid synthase (NOS) and NADPH diaphorase; growth-associated protein 43 (GAP-43) and AB893 (an antibody against rat liver gap junctions). Table 3.3 shows that two groups of markers for oligosaccharides with galactose residues (antibodies against lactoseries carbohydrate groups and the groups of lectins that bind to galactose-extended oligosaccharides) label mainly small neurones in rat DRGs. From their cell size distributions, all the above markers probably label mainly slowly conducting neurones, and therefore may well be associated with nociceptors, but not necessarily exclusively since there are also non-nociceptive neurones with both C and Aδ fibres, see later.

Percentages of rat DRG neurones labelled

The approximate percentages of neurones labelled in rat DRGs (including skin, muscle, and visceral afferent neurones) are given in Tables 3.2 and 3.3 (for a review of further quantitative data for other species and for further discussion of most of these markers, see Lawson 1992). Presentation of these percentages is an oversimplification of the situation, snce they do not take into account rostrocaudal variations (most data is for lumbar DRGs), and since a few markers label all neurones, with a greater intensity in some. Nonetheless, they do provide a useful means of comparison between markers. Most reported percentages relate to all DRG neuronal profiles with nuclei or nucleoli. In rat lumbar DRGs about 54–60 per cent of all such profiles are neurofilament-poor (small dark neurones), the remainder being neurofilament-rich (large light neurones) (Perry *et al.* 1991). In rat DRGs, C-fibre somata are neurofilament-poor and A-fibre somata are neurofilament-rich (Lawson and Waddell 1991). A marker that labels about 55 per cent of all profiles and that labels predominantly small neurones must label a high proportion of small dark (C fibre) neurones, and could label all of them. (NB Using the dissector method to eliminate sampling bias in rat L5 DRGs, the percentage of small dark neurones was found to be closer to 70 per cent of all neurones Tandruff 1993).

Species differences

Some markers that label predominantly small neurones are expressed in DRG neurones of a variety of species. These include many peptides, intermediate filaments, certain enzymes (FRAP, NOS/NADPH diaphorase, acetyl choline esterase (AChE)), inter-mediate filaments, and galactose-extended oligosaccharides that bind to the lectins. There is, however, less evidence so far that the antibodies against lactoseries carbohy-drate groups label DRG neurones in species other than rat.

Neurochemical changes after peripheral axotomy

In some rat DRG neurones, changes in neuropeptide expression occur after peripheral axotomy (see Table 3.2). Peptides in DRGs have been classified (Hökfelt *et al.* 1994) as: type 1 peptides (including substance P, calcitonin gene-related peptide (CGRP),

Table 3.1 List of abbreviations

γMSH	Melanocyte-stimulating hormone
-LI	-like immunoreactivity
1B2	An anti-lactoseries carbohydrate antibody
2C5	An anti-lactoseries carbohydrate antibody
A5	An anti-lactoseries carbohydrate antibody
AB893	An antibody against rat liver gap junctions
AChE	Acetyl choline esterase
ADA	Adenosine deaminase
ANF	Atrial natriuretic factor
bFGF	Basic fibroblast growth factor
BSA-IB4 (GSA-IB4)	*Badeira Simplificolia (Grifonia simplicifolia)* agglutinin, a lectin (also called BSI-B4)
BOMB	Bombesin
CA	Carbonic anhydrase
CB	Cholera toxin B subunit
CCK	Cholecystokinin
CGRP	Calcitonin-gene related peptide
ChAT	Choline acetyl transferase
CRF	Corticotrophin-releasing factor
DRG	Dorsal root ganglion
DYN	Dynorphin
FRAP	Fluoride-resistant acid phosphatase
GAL	Galanin
GAP 43	Growth-associated protein, also known as neuromodulin or B50
GHRF	Growth hormone-releasing factor
GM1 (CB)	A ganglioside, a membrane receptor that binds to cholera toxin
HTM	High-threshold mechanoreceptor
LA4	Antibody against a lactoseries glycoconjugate
LCA	*Lens cularis* agglutinin, a lectin
LD2	Antibody aginst a lactoseries glycoconjugate
LENK	Leu-enkephalin
LTM	Low-threshold mechanoreceptor
mRNA	Messenger RNA
MSH	Melanocyte-stimulating hormone
NADPH d	NADPH diaphorase
NF	Neurofilament
NGF	Nerve growth factor
NKA	Neurokinin A
NOS	Nitric oxide synthase
NPY	Neuropeptide Y
Opioid rec	Opioid receptor
PKC	Phosphokinase C
PER	Peripherin
PNA	Peanut agglutinin
RCA I-β	*Ricinis communis* agglutinin, a lectin
rec	Receptor
RL 14.5 and 29	Endogenous lactose-binding lectins
SBA	Soybean (*Glycine max*) agglutinin

Table 3.1 *cont.*

SOM	Somatostatin
SSEA3/4	Stage-specific embryonic antigens 3 and 4 against globoseries glycoconjugates
TMP	Tyrosine monophosphatase
TOH	Tyrosine hydroxylase
trkA	Tyrosine kinase A (high-affinity NGF receptor)
trkB	Tyrosine kinase B (BDNF receptor)
trkC	Tyrosine kinase C (NT3 receptor)
VIP	Vasoactive intestinal polypeptide

somatostatin), normally expressed in substantial quantities, but are downregulated after peripheral axotomy, and are then detectable in fewer DRG neurones; type 2 peptides (for example, vasoactive intestinal peptide (VIP), galanin, cholecystokinin (CCK), neuropeptide Y (NPY)) as well as NOS, normally synthesized at a low level or not at all in adult rat DRGs, but are upregulated after peripheral axotomy and are then found in a much higher percentage of neurones. The increased synthesis of VIP, galanin, and NOS is mainly in small DRG neurones, whereas that for NPY and CCK and their receptor mRNAs occurs to a greater extent in larger neurones (Hökfelt *et al.* 1994; see Table 3.2). The immediate early gene c-*jun* and the growth-associated protein GAP-43 are also upregulated after axotomy.

From the percentages and cell sizes (Table 3.2), some slowly conducting DRG neurones (many of which may have nociceptive properties prior to axotomy) are probably involved in upregulating VIP, galanin, NOS, and/or GAP-43. However, neurones that upregulate NPY and CCK are more likely to be rapidly conducting. The exact sensory functions prior to axotomy of the neurones capable of upregulating their VIP and galanin production have yet to be determined. Some of the above changes may be important in nociceptive signalling since severing of the axon is likely to occur during major tissue damage.

Cutaneous afferent neurones

Spinal cord terminations of cutaneous afferent neurones

Cutaneous afferent neurones are known to have terminations in spinal cord laminae I, II, V, and X, while muscle and visceral afferents terminate in laminae, I, V, and X. Small-diameter primary afferent neurones terminate mainly in laminae I and II. Thus the localization of neurochemical markers of primary afferent terminals in lamina II is a further indication of the cutaneous projection of neurones with small-diameter fibres (Hunt *et al.* 1992). Lamina II labelling is seen by antibodies to substance P, CGRP, and somatostatin, as well as by FRAP, by antibodies against lactoseries carbohydrate groups, and by the lectins *Badeira simplificolia* agglutin (BSA-IB4), and soybean agglutinin (*Ricinus communis* agglutinin (RCA-1β) against galactose-extended oligosaccharides (Dodd and Jessell 1985; Lawson *et al.* 1985; Streit *et al.* 1985; Regan *et al.* 1986; Hunt *et al.* 1992). In the rat there is little overlap between labelling for these peptides (mainly laminal IIo) and FRAP, LA4, and BSA-IB4 (mainly lamina IIi) (Hunt *et al.* 1992).

Table 3.2 DRG cell size and neurochemical (non-carbohydrate) markers

Markers *	Cell sizes †	Species ‡	% rat normal §	After periph. axotomy % Change ¶	After periph. axotomy Sizes ‖	After periph. axotomy % **	Reference ††
Peptides							
Substance P • ‡‡	S m	r, m, g, c, h	20	↓			1, 2
NKA •	S	r, c, g					3,4
CGRP	S M l	r, g, c, h	40–60	↓			1
SOM •	S	r, (g), c, h	8	↓			1
DYN A & B •	S	(r), g, c, h	0 (7)				1
LENK •	S	(r), g, c	0 (7)				1
VIP/mRNA •	S m	r, g, c	0–few	↑	All	95	1, 5
GAL/mRNA •	S	r, c, p	Few	↑	S M	34	1, 6
BOMB/GRP •	S	r, (g), c	5	↑			1
CCK		r	0	↑	S	30	7
ANF	M L	g	(5)				1
NPY/mRNA	—	r	0–rare	↑	s M L	~25	6, 8
Amino acids							
Glutamate •	S m	m, r	30–70				9
Glutamine •	S	m, r	40				9
GABA	S M L	r	Many				10
Cytoskeletal proteins/intermediate filaments							
PER •	S m	r, h	74				1
NF	s M L	q, m, r, c, h	35				1, 3
Receptors							
NPY rec mRNA •	S m	r	20	↑	M L		11
GM1 (CB)	s M L	r	35				1
CCK$_B$ rec.				↑	S M L	7	
Opioid rec	?S	m	(8)				1
Histamine H1 rec	?S	m	(7)				1
Glucocorticoid rec	S M L	r					12
Growth factors and their receptors							
trkA •	S m	m, r	44 §§				13
trkB	S M L	m, r	27 §§				13
trkC	M L	m, r	17 §§				13
bFGF	S M L	r					14
Enzymes/hormones							
TMP •	S	m	35				1
FRAP •	S m	r, c, d, h	45	↓		6	1, 15, 16
ADA •	S	r	13				1
β-glycerophosphatase •	S	r					17
Monoamine oxidase •	S	r					17
NOS/mRNA or NADPH d •	S m	r, g, c	Few	↑	S M l		3, 7
CA	s M L	ch, r	30				1, 3
PKC	L	r	45				1
AChE	S M	r, c					1, 18
TOH	S	r, g	1				1, 3
GHRF	s	r	1				1
CRF		r					19
α-MSH	L	r	25				18
γ-MSH		h	Skin				20

Markers *	Cell sizes †	Species ‡	% rat normal §	% Change ¶	After periph. axotomy			
					Sizes ‖	% **	Reference ††

Markers *	Cell sizes †	Species ‡	% rat normal §	% Change ¶	Sizes ‖	% **	Reference ††
Other proteins							
AB893 •	S m l	r	14				21
GAP43/RNA •	s m l	r, c	16	↑	S M L	>95	1, 22, 23
Calbindin	S M L	ch, r	22				1
Parvalbumin	S M L	r	14				1
Calretinin	M L	ch					1

* Neurochemical markers for subpopulations of DRG neurones. In most cases the subpopulations of DRG neurones were identified by immunocytochemistry; thus the suffix -li (like immunoreactivity) is appropriate in these cases. mRNA data is from *in situ* hybridization techniques. For a list of abbreviations see Table 3.1. A bullet • following a marker indicates that it labels mainly small neurones.

† S, small; M, medium; L, large. Lower-case letters indicate relatively few positive neurones within that size range.

‡ f, frog; ch, chick; q, quail; m, mouse; r, rat; c, cat; d, dog; p, pig; g, guinea-pig; h, human. A letter in parentheses indicates that the marker was not found in that species.

§ Percentage of neurones labelled in normal adult rat DRGs (usually lumbar). Values in brackets are from other species.

¶ Changes in rat DRGs after peripheral axotomy. ↓, a decrease in the percentage of neurones labelled; ↑, an increase in the percentage of neurones labelled.

‖ S M L as in footnote †, but in this case they indicate the range of neurones newly expressing the peptide or mRNA.

** Percentage of DRG neurones labelled after axotomy.

†† References: 1, for references see Lawson 1992; 2, Henken *et al.* 1988; 3, personal observations; 4, Dalsgaard *et al.* 1985; 5, Shebab *et al.* 1986; 6, Noguchi *et al.* 1993; 7, Hökfelt *et al.* 1994; 8, Kashiba *et al.* 1994; 9, Battaglia and Rustioni 1988; 10, Szabat *et al.* 1992; 11, Zhang *et al.* 1994; 12, DeLeon *et al.* 1994; 13, McMahon *et al.* 1994; 14, Weise *et al.* 1992; 15, Tenser 1985; 16, Silverman and Kruger 1988*b*; 17, Kalina and Wolman 1970; 18, Dodd *et al.* 1983; 19, Skofitsch *et al.* 1985; 20, Johansson *et al.* 1991; 21, Carr *et al.* 1991; 22, Verge *et al.* 1990; 23, Wiese *et al.* 1992.

‡‡ Some of these studies may have used anti-substance P antibodies that also recognized NKA.

§§ For trkA, trkB, and trkC, the percentages are of neurones sending fibres into the sciatic nerve rather than in the whole DRG.

Nerve fibres in the skin

There is little known about the precise termination sites of nociceptive fibres in skin (Perl 1992), although many are thought to terminate as free nerve endings in the epidermis and dermis.

Epidermis

Nerve fibres penetrate the epidermis as far as the stratum spinosum in human skin (Kennedy and Wendelschafer-Crabb 1993). Nerve fibres with CGRP-like immunoreactivity (CGRP-LI) branch and exhibit terminals throughout the stratum spinosum in both glabrous and hairy skin of the rat (Kruger *et al.* 1989; also personal observations, see Fig. 3.1). Abundant fibres with melanocyte-stimulating hormone (γ-MSH-LI) penetrate the basal layers of human epidermis (Johansson *et al.* 1991). Sparse substance P-LI fibres (see Fig. 3.1) and somatostatin-LI fibres also penetrate the epidermis in human skin (Dalsgaard *et al.* 1983; Johansson and Vaalasti 1987).

Table 3.3   DRG cell size and neurochemical markers: oligosaccharides

Markers *	Cell sizes †	Species ‡	% rat normal §	Reference ¶
Lactoseries epitopes				
2C5 ●	S m	r, (g)	~40	1, 2, 3
LD2 ●	S	r	20–25	1, 3, 4
1B2 ●	S m		~35	1, 3
A5 ●	S m	r	40–45	3, 4
LA4 ●	S m	r, (g)	~45	1, 3
FC10.2 ●	S	r	5–10	4
anti-Lewis a ●	S	r	20	4
Globoseries epitopes				
SSEA3	S M L	r, g	9	1, 2, 4
SSEA4	S M L	r, g	11	1, 2, 4
RL 14.5	S m	r	46–63	3
RL 29	S m	r	56	3
SN1	S M L	ch, (m)	(40–90)	5
Lectins ‖				
Galactose extended ‖				
SBA ●	S m	r, g, c	33 **	1, 2, 6
PNA ●	S m	r, g	**	1, 2, 6
RCA I-β ●	S	r	**	1, 6
BSA-IB4 ●	S m	r, g	**	1, 2, 6
Non-galactose extended ‖				
GSAII	S M L Myelin	r		1, 6

* Markers that bind to olgosaccharides on subpopulations of DRG neurones. In most cases the subpopulations of DRG neurones were identified by immunocytochemistry. For a list of abbreviations see Table 3.1. For exact epitopes and binding sites see references. A bullet ● following a marker indicates that it labels mainly small neurones.

† S, small; M, medium; L, large. Lower-case letters indicate relatively few positive neurones within that size range.

‡ m, Mouse; r, rat; c, cat; g, guinea-pig; ch, chick. A letter in parentheses indicates that the marker was not found in that species.

§ Percentage of neurones labelled in normal adult rat DRGs (usually lumbar).

¶ References: 1, for references see Lawson 1992; 2, personal observations; 3, Regan *et al.* 1986; 4, Dodd and Jessell 1985; 5, Marusich *et al.* 1986; 6, Streit *et al.* 1985.

‖ Under lectins the headings galactose and non-galactose extended refer to the binding properties of the lectins.

** Streit *et al.* (1985) state that the galactose-specific lectins label about 75% of the smaller DRG cells, but no detailed quantitation is given.

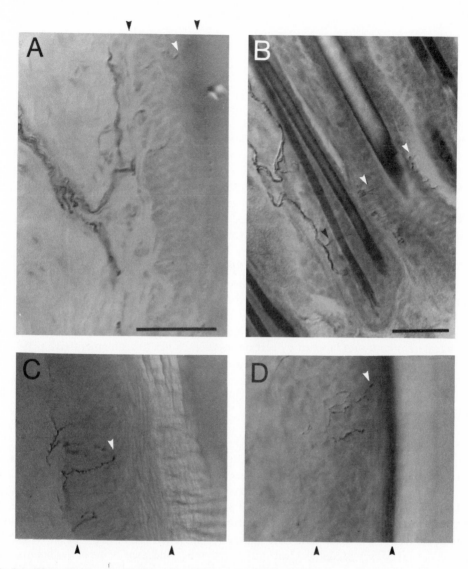

Fig. 3.1 Photomicrographs of frozen sections through Zamboni's fixed rat skin stained with the avidin–biotin complex method for: (A–C) CGRP-LI and (D) substance P-LI. Interference contrast optics are used.

(A), (C), and (D) show glabrous skin on the foot: scale bar in (A) = 50 μm; black arrowheads outside the photographs indicate the extent of the epidermal layer with dermis to the left of this and keratin layer to the right; white arrowheads indicate the greatest penetration of the fibre into the epidermis visible in each field. In (A) a group of nerve fibres branch near the dermal/epidermal border, and a few fibres are seen to penetrate the epidermis. In (C) and (D) greater detail of the penetration of epidermis by CGRP-LI or substance P-LI fibres is shown.

(B) Hairy skin: scale bar = 100 μm; several CGRP-LI positive fibres to the left; white arrowheads indicate CGRP-LI fibres appearing to wrap around the hair follicles.

Dermis

Many CGRP-LI and substance P-LI and fewer somatostatin-LI fibres run in the dermis and along the epidermal/dermal junction (see Fig. 3.1). In rat dermis, CGRP-LI fibres are frequent. Some end freely, others surround vascular loops in dermal papillae of glabrous skin; in hairy skin some terminate near Meissner's corpuscles or innervate each hair follicle (Kruger *et al.* 1989; also personal observations, see Fig. 3.1). γ-MSH fibres also innervate the base of hair follicles, Meissner's corpuscles, and run close to Merkel cells in human skin, but do not innervate most blood vessels (Johansson *et al.* 1991). As well as its probable association with nociceptive fibres, CGRP-LI is therefore also likely to be associated with some non-nociceptive A-fibres. The same may be true of the γ-MSH positive fibres, if they are all proved to be sensory. On the basis of studies in the tunica vasculosa of the rat testis, it was suggested that nerve fibres labelled by the lectin BSA-IB4 do not usually innervate blood vessels, in contrast to CGRP-LI fibres (Silverman and Kruger 1988*a*). This has yet to be demonstrated in skin.

Neurochemistry of DRG somata of cutaneous afferent neurones

The expression of certain markers has been studied directly in rat DRG neurones retrogradely labelled by the application of dye to cutaneous nerves or from dye injection into the skin. Table 3.4 summarizes the data from a number of studies, and also provides an indication of the percentages of neurofilament-rich and neurofilament-poor cutaneous afferent neurones labelled by certain markers. Since neurofilament-rich neurones in rat DRGs have myelinated fibres and neurofilament-poor neurones have unmyelinated fibres (Lawson and Waddell 1991), this provides an indication of the likely labelling of A-fibre and C-fibre neurones for these markers. A visual representation of this data is shown in Fig. 3.2.

Peptides

Somatostatin-LI is expressed almost exclusively in cutaneous afferent neurones (Table 3.4). It is released in response to noxious heat (see later), a type of stimulus encountered more frequently in skin than in muscle or visceral tissues. In contrast, both substance P-LI and CGRP-LI are found in about 20 per cent and 50–60 per cent, respectively, of cutaneous afferent neurones and are both present in higher proportions of muscle and splanchnic visceral afferent neurones (Lawson 1992). Substance P-LI, in particular, is present in far fewer cutaneous than muscle or visceral afferent neurones. This may be partly related to the important peripheral functions served by these peptides in influencing small blood vessels, functions that are important in tissues other than skin. Note that some of the anti-substance P antibodies used in these studies may also have labelled NKA (neurokinin A; see Lawson 1992).

Oligosaccharides and lectins

Both the lectin BSA-IB4 and, to a lesser extent, the antibody 2C5 labelled a much higher proportion of cutaneous than other afferent neurones (Table 3.4, Fig. 3.2). Both markers labelled around 40 per cent of cutaneous afferent neurones (Table 3.4). The majority (86 per cent) of 2C5-positive cutaneous afferent neurones were neurofilament (NF)-poor (that is, with probable C fibres) (see Table 3.4). The lectins PNA (peanut agglutinin) and SBA

Table 3.4 DRG cell markers and cutaneous afferent neurones

Marker *	Cutaneous afferents (%) †	Relative % C, M V ‡	NF (%) § Poor	NF (%) § Rich	References
Peptides					
Somatostatin	13	C ≫ M	20	0	O'Brien *et al.* 1989
Somatostatin	10	C ≫ M > V			Lawson 1992 ‖
Somatostatin	< 1				Molander *et al.* 1987 ¶
CGRP	49	M > C	50	49	O'Brien *et al.* 1987
CGRP	60	V > M > C			Lawson 1992 ‖
CGRP	~20	V ≫ M > C			Molander *et al.* 1987 ¶
Substance P	28	M > C	37	12	O'Brien *et al.* 1989
Substance P	20	V ≫ M ≫ C			Lawson 1992 ‖
Substance P	~10	V ≫ M > C			Molander *et al.* 1987 ¶
NPY	20	M ≫ C ≫ V		Most	Kashiba *et al.* 1994
Oligosaccharides					
2C5	44	C ≫ M > V	43	7	Lawson 1992 ‖
SSEA3	4	C = M > V			Lawson 1992 ‖
SSEA4	6	M > C > V			Perry & Lawson 1991 ‖
Lectins					
BSA-IB4	38	C ≫ M = V			Plenderleith & Snow 1993
PNA	55	C = V ≫ M	47	8	Perry & Lawson 1991 ‖
SBA	72	C = V = M	59	14	Perry & Lawson 1991 ‖
Enzymes					
FRAP	20	C = > M			Molander *et al.* 1987 ¶
TMP	52	C = M ≫ V	94	0	O'Brien *et al.* 1989
CA	6	M ≫ C > V			Peyronnard *et al.* 1988
CA	10				Perry & Lawson 1991 ‖
Calbindin	3	V ≫ C			Kashiba *et al.* 1992
Growth factor receptors					
trkA	48	V ≫ C ≫ M			McMahon *et al.* 1994
trkB	16	V ≫ M ≫ C			McMahon *et al.* 1994
trkC	10	M ≫ C > V			McMahon *et al.* 1994

* For a list of abbreviations see Table 3.1.
† This column gives the percentages of neurones in rat DRGs retrogradely labelled from skin nerves, which were also labelled by the marker indicated. Dye was applied to cut nerves either sural (Peyronnard *et al.* 1988) or saphenous (Molander *et al.* 1987; Perry and Lawson, in preparation) or to cutaneous branches of sinal nerves (Kashiba *et al.* 1992) or was injected into the skin (O'Brien *et al.* 1989), The dyes used were fluorogold (Kashiba *et al.* 1992), fast blue (Molander *et al.* 1987; O'Brien *et al.* 1989; Perry and Lawson, in preparation), or horseradish peroxidase (Peyronnard *et al.* 1988).
‡ This column relates to the relative percentages of cutaneous (C), muscle (M), and visceral (V) afferent neurones expressing the marker. ≫, Much greater than; ≪, much less than; =, similar to; = > very slightly greater than.
§ The percentages of neurofilament (NF)-poor (small dark cells with C-fibres) and NF-rich (large light cells with A-fibres) cutaneous afferent neurones expressing the marker.
¶ The earliest study (Molander *et al.* 1987) has lower percentages of cells labelled in the DRG overall and in cutaneous afferent neurones by all markers than found with recent improvement in techniques.
‖ Also Perry and Lawson, in preparation.
> Values for NPY were after peripheral nerve section, showing that NPY upregulation occurs in NF-rich neurones that is, with probable A fibres.

(soybean agglutinin) both labelled high proportions (55 per cent and 72 per cent) of cutaneous afferent neurones most of which were NF-poor and therefore probably had C-fibres. These lectins labelled similar percentages of visceral afferent neurones. In contrast to the above galactose-binding lectins and antibodies against lactoseries oligosaccharide groups, the antibodies SSEA3 and SSEA4, against globoseries carbohydrates, label small percentages of cutaneous afferent neurones, many of which are probably large neurones (Lawson 1992).

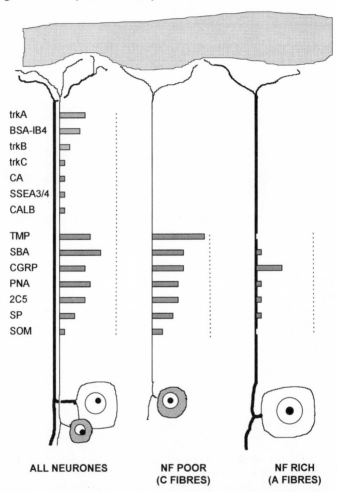

Fig. 3.2 A visual representation of the data given in Table 3.4. Column 1 gives the approximate percentages of all retrogradely labelled cutaneous afferent neurones also labelled by each marker. In the lower half of the diagram, the percentages of retrogradely labelled neurofilament-poor neurones (column 2) and neurofilament-rich neurones (column 3) labelled by each marker are indicated. The dotted lines in each case represent 100 per cent. SP, Substance P; all other abbreviations as in Table 3.

Enzymes

The enzymes FRAP and TMP are thought to be histochemical representations of the same enzyme (see Knyihar-Csillik *et al.* 1986). The reported percentage of FRAP-positive neurones was considerably lower than that of TMP in these experiments, which may have been due to variability inherent in the techniques for demonstrating the enzymes. All the TMP-positive cutaneous afferent somata were NF-poor, and thus probably all had C fibres. Since 94 per cent of the NF-poor neurones showed TMP activity, this group must include virtually all the cutaneous afferent C-fibre neurones, presumably including both nociceptive and non-nociceptive neurones.

In contrast, the enzyme carbonic anhydrase (CA) and calbindin were both expressed in few cutaneous afferent neurones and more afferent neurones projecting to other tissues. Both are expressed in large light as well as some small dark neurones and are thought to be expressed in some fast-conducting muscle afferent neurones (Lawson 1992). These neurones are therefore unlikely to be nociceptive.

Growth factor receptors

Each of the tyrosine kinase (trk) growth factor receptors (trkA, trkB, and trkC) labelled a subpopulation of cutaneous afferent neurones, but none labelled a higher percentage of cutaneous than of muscle or visceral afferent neurones (Table 3.4). By far the highest proportion was labelled by trkA. In view of the combination of the high percentage of cutaneous afferent neurones that expressed trkA and their cell size distributions, trkA is a strong candidate as a marker for at least a substantial proportion of cutaneous nociceptive afferent neurones (see below).

Figure 3.2 shows the overall patterns that emerge from these retrograde labelling studies. The pattern for the cutaneous afferent NF-poor neuronal somata (that is, with probable C fibres) will be considered first. Most of these expressed the enzyme TMP, more than half were labelled by the lectin SBA, and more than half showed CGRP-LI, about two-fifths were labelled by peanut agglutin (PNA), 2C5 or show substance P-LI; and one-fifth showed somatostatin-LI. All of these markers/molecules therefore have a strong likelihood of being expressed by cutaneous nociceptive neurones, but they may also be expressed by non-nociceptive neurones. From Fig. 3.2, it is clear that there must be co-localization of some of the markers shown in cutaneous afferent NF-poor neurones. It is known that in rat lumbar DRG neurones there is probably extensive co-localization between BSA-IB4, SBA, and PNA (see review in Lawson 1992), but little co-localization between substance P and any of the following: somatostatin, 2C5, or FRAP. Note that there is some evidence to indicate that FRAP and TMP may be the same enzyme (Knyihar-Csillik *et al.* 1986). Apparently in conflict with this, the data illustrated in Fig. 3.2 indicate some co-localization between both somatostatin-LI and substance P-LI with TMP in these cutaneous afferent neurones. A possible explanation is the variability in the histochemical methods for demonstrating TMP and FRAP.

The only neurochemical marker that was expressed in a substantial proportion of NF-poor (that is, probable A-fibre) cutaneous afferent neurones is the peptide CGRP. In rat lumbar DRG as a whole, both Aδ and Aα/β neurones express CGRP-LI, with a higher proportion of positive Aδ neurones (McCarthy and Lawson 1990). It is therefore likely that both types of A-fibre neurones express CGRP. There is some evidence (see below) to suggest that CGRP is expressed in both nociceptive and non-nociceptive A-fibre neurones.

If the total population of cutaneous afferent neurones is considered, regardless of neurofilament content or conduction velocity range, the percentages, ranked in order of magnitude, of all cutaneous afferent neurones labelled by these markers are:

75% > SBA > CGRP > PNA > TMP > 50% > trkA > 2C5 > BSA-IB4 > 25% = substance P > trkB.

Only three markers labelled much higher proportions of cutaneous than either muscle or visceral afferent neurones. These were, in order of the relative difference between cutaneous and other tissues, BSA-IB4 > somatostatin > 2C5. These markers may therefore be associated with an aspect or aspects of sensory neuronal function specific to skin and of less importance in the other tissues.

Dorsal horn release of peptides by cutaneous afferent fibres

Studies of the release of peptides into the dorsal horn of a variety of species have shown that some peptides are released in response to certain types of noxious stimuli applied to the skin. For instance, somatostatin was released in response to noxious heat but not noxious mechanical (Kuraishi *et al.* 1985) or noxious cold stimuli (Tiseo *et al.* 1990), while substance P was released by noxious mechanical stimuli (Kuraishi *et al.* 1985; Duggan *et al.* 1988) and noxious cold (Tiseo *et al.* 1990) but not by radiant heat stimuli to hairy skin (Kuraishi *et al.* 1985), although it was released by the more extreme stimulus of immersion of the entire hindlimb in hot water for 20 minutes at a time (Duggan *et al.* 1988), which would have affected both glabrous and hairy skin and possibly also subcutaneous units.

Electrophysiology of cutaneous afferent somata in DRGs

In rat and cat DRGs, cutaneous nociceptive A-fibre somata have distinctive active membrane properties, namely longer action potential and afterhyperpolarization durations (Ritter and Mendell 1992). Both substance P- and CGRP-LI-containing Aδ neurones in rat DRGs have significantly longer afterhyperpolarization durations than Aδ neurones without these peptides (Lawson, 1994), which may indicate that the majority of Aδ neurones with these peptides are nociceptive. However, not all the faster-conducting (Aα/β) CGRP-LI neurones have long afterhyperpolarization durations (Lawson *et al.* 1996). This is consistent with some of these being non-nociceptive as is also indicated by both the fibre termination sites in the skin (see above) and by direct studies on single units with identified receptor types (see below).

Sensory receptor types of cutaneous afferent fibres

The relative proportions of cutaneous afferent fibres with different sensory receptor types are hard to define since the size of the whole population depends on the initial search stimuli being adequate to stimulate all types of afferent fibres. Furthermore, there are clear differences between species, as well as between different parts of the body and between glabrous and hairy skin (Burgess and Perl 1973).

There are both nociceptive and non-nociceptive cutaneous C-fibre units (Table 3.5). For instance, in the rabbit ear preparation, the non-nociceptive units amounted to about 25 per cent of the total number of identified C-fibre units, although this figure is likely to vary both according to species and to the particular nerve examined. The largest subgroup of cutaneous C-fibre units in both rat and rabbit hairy skin were polymodal nociceptors, which respond to both noxious mechanical and noxious heat stimuli, and some of which respond to noxious chemical stimuli. Their proportion varies according to species and also is greater in nerves projecting to the distal parts of the limb (Burgess and Perl 1973). Certain aspects of polymodal nociceptors function are not uniform throughout the whole group. For instance, in rat hairy skin, 56 per cent responded to bradykinin (Lang *et al.* 1990), and had lower heat thresholds than the rest. Also in the rabbit ear preparation, sensitization by repeated noxious heat stimulation could be prevented by cyclo-oxygenase inhibitors in 50 per cent of polymodal units; it was therefore suggested that prostaglandins may be involved in sensitization in this subgroup (Cohen and Perl 1990). Thus, there are clear functional subdivisions within the polymodal nociceptor group. Smaller proportions of C fibres fall into the C high threshold mechanoreceptor (HTM) and C cold nociceptors or C cooling categories and C mechano units or C low-threshold mechanoreceptor (LTM) units.

Table 3.5 Percentage of C-fibre receptor types from fibre recordings

Preparation	C-fibre receptor types (%) * in			
	Rat	Rabbit ear	Cat	Monkey
C polymodals	73	66	30	> 90
C HTMs	5	7		
C mechano (LTM)	7	15		
Cold nociceptors	?4	3.2		
Cooling-sensitive		3		
Warming-sensitive		6		

* Percentages of C-fibre types reported from different preparations. References are as follows: rat, Lynn and Carpenter 1982; rabbit ear, Shea and Perl 1985; cat, Light and Perl 1993; monkey, Burgess and Perl 1973.

In monkey and cat, about 14–20 per cent of A-fibre units (mostly Aδ) were mechanical nociceptors, and a further group (a similar proportion of A-fibre units) have been classified as moderate pressure receptors and low-sensitivity mechanoreceptors, both groups with lower mechanical thresholds than the mechanical nociceptor class (Perl 1968). The rest of the A-fibre units are non-nociceptive mechanoreceptors. The Aδ group therefore includes mechanical nociceptors, moderate-pressure or low-sensitivity mechanoreceptors, D hair units (LTMs), and in some species (monkey and dog but not rat; see Hensel and Iggo 1971) cold receptors. The cold receptors comprised up to 8 per cent of A-fibre units in primate radial nerve (see Perl 1968).

The development of noxious heat sensitivity of cutaneous C-fibre units in young rats is thought to be NGF-dependent (Lewin and Mendell 1994; Mendell, Chapter 19, this volume). It has also been proposed (Lewin *et al.* 1992) that NGF is necessary for the normal development into D hair units instead. If NGF is essential to the development of A-fibre nociceptor units, and that, in the absence of NGF, these develop of C polymodal and A-fibre nociceptor units, it might be expected that these units express the NGF receptor (trkA) at least during development.

About 70 per cent of cutaneous afferent C-fibre units in rat hairy skin are polymodal nociceptors. This can be compared with the numerical neurochemical data on cutaneous afferent neurones in rat (Table 3.4). Since about 95 per cent of retrogradely labelled NF-poor rat DRG neurones are labelled by TMP, 60 per cent by SBA, 50 per cent by PNA, and 50 per cent by CGRP, these are all possible candidates for labelling a large part of the polymodal nociceptor population. Substance P and 2C5 label only about 37 per cent and 43 per cent respectively, of the NF-poor cutaneous afferent population in the rat. Thus neither is a candidate for labelling the whole polymodal population, and from these numbers, either may label mainly non-polymodal subpopulations. Somatostatin labels an even smaller population. Clearly, from Tables 3.2 and 3.3, there are a number of further candidates that could label a high percentage of the polymodal nociceptor population. This type of numerically based comparison does not differentiate between the different classes of receptor type. To identify the chemical phenotypes of each different type of nociceptor (polymodal nociceptors, C HTM units, cold nociceptors, A-fibre nociceptors) and to establish how these differ from those of non-nociceptive neurones, studies on individual neurones are needed (see below).

Neurochemistry of cutaneous afferent neurones with identified sensory receptor types

Only four studies have combined intracellular recording in DRG neurones, identification of the cutaneous sensory receptor type, dye injection, and subsequent immunochemisty on the neuronal soma. All have studied peptide-LI. Because the data bears so directly on the subject of this chapter, I shall briefly review each such study.

The first (Leah *et al.* 1985) was on cat DRG neurones, pretreated with 20 per cent colchicine. C-fibre units were divided into three classes (with 1–8 cells in each class) responding to: noxious mechanical plus noxious heat; noxious mechanical stimulus alone; and innocuous mechanical stimulus plus skin cooling. Neither substance P-LI or somatostatin-LI were found in more nociceptive than non-nociceptive units. The only C-fibre neurone with VIP-LI was non-nociceptive. No Aδ-neurones (two nociceptive units and three D hair units) showed substance P-LI or somatostatin-LI but two of three D hair units showed VIP-LI. Some of these data may have been affected by: (1) the colchicine treatment that blocks axonal transport, and may therefore mimic the effects of axotomy (upregulation of VIP, downregulation of other peptides, see Table 3.2); (2) the high currents (4–40 nA. min of hyperpolarizing charge) used to eject the dye, which may have abolished peptide-LI in some cells. It was subsequently shown (Scharfman *et al.* 1989) that currents of 15–60 nA. min to eject lucifer yellow abolished the peptide-LI in hippocampal CA1 neurones. These factors, together with the broad categories of receptor type used and the small numbers of neurones, may have contributed to the lack of correlation found between peptide content and sensory modality.

The second study was an abstract (Zhang and Hoffert 1986) on cat lumbar DRG A-fibre neurones: two of three myelinated mechanical nociceptors. However, none of the following cells showed SP-LI. Three type II LTMs, one type I LTMs, and one D hair unit had substance P-LI in DRG somata. Again, very small numbers of units were studied.

A third study (Hoheisel *et al.* 1994) found no correlation between CGRP-LI content and cutaneous sensory modality in identified rat DRG neurones. Units were classified as HTM, LTM and hair follicle units, but since no noxious heat tests were used, no distinction between C polymodal and C HTM units was possible. Of the cutaneous units tested, the only C-fibre cell (either HTM or polymodal) was positive. No cutaneous A-fibre HTM units were tested, but one of 11 hair follicle none of 11 LTM units were positive, indicating the presence of CGRP in a few non-nociceptive A-fibre units. The percentage of CGRP-LI positive neurones in the ganglia was low (20 per cent) compared with the usual level of 40–60 per cent in the rat. This, with the very high levels (mean value calculated to be about 75 nA˙min) of hyperpolarizing intracellular currents used to eject dye (5–20 nA˙pulses at 1.7 Hz over 2–15 min, which I calculate to cover a range of 6 to 175 nA˙min) could have resulted in false negatives.

In the fourth study, we have examined substance P-LI in relation to sensory modality in guinea-pig (L6-S1) DRG neurones (Lawson *et al.* 1993, 1994). Intracellular dye injections were made with currents of 0.3 nA, with a total current of 0.5–1.5 nA˙min (much lower than currents used in the above studies). A greater number of sensory type categories have been used. Although the identified units with substance P-LI were nociceptive, substance P-LI was not detectable in all C-fibre or A-fibre nociceptive units. Approximately half the C-fibre somata with identified receptive fields had substance P-LI (an appropriate percentage for guinea-pig skin). The positive C-fibre units included many C HTM units (both cutaneous and subcutaneous units) and subcutaneous C mechanoheat units, but only about half the polymodal nociceptor units with receptive fields in hairy and glabrous skin and glabrous skin mechanoheat units). As regards substance P-LI in non-nociceptive C-fibre neurones, it was absent from most cooling sensitive units, and warm sensitive units were not tested. In A-fibre somata, substance P-LI was found in subcutaneous (but not superficial) cutaneous mechanical nociceptor units and in mechanoheat sensitive units. No A-fibre LTM units (D hair, or more rapidly conducting units) showed substance P-LI.

Preliminary data on CGRP-LI in the guinea-pig, show similar patterns to these of substance P-LI, although some hair follicle afferent neurones also showed CGRP-LI (Lawson *et al.*, in press), consistent with previous findings (Hoheisel *et al.* 1994) and with the distribution of CGRP-LI fibres seen in skin (see Fig. 3.2).

There is little data of this type on markers for oligosaccharide groups on DRG neurones. However, some preliminary data indicate that the anti-globoseries antibodies SSEA3 and SSEA4 label a subgroup of A-fibre mechanical nociceptor somata in guinea-pig DRGs (Perl 1991).

Conclusions

The evidence reviewed in this chapter indicates that neurochemical markers are related to certain aspects of neuronal structure and function. These include: cell size/probable conduction velocity (see Tables 3.2 and 3.3); the type of tissue to which the neurone projects (see Table 3.4); the electrophysiological properties of the neurones (for example, substance P and CGRP); sensory receptor type (substance P); and spinal cord termination sites.

There is considerable circumstantial evidence indicating probable correlations of particular molecular structures and cutaneous nociceptor neurones, but, as yet, limited direct evidence for such correlation with precisely defined receptor types. Neurochemical markers expressed predominantly in small DRG neurones include many peptides, glutamate and glutamine, peripherin, trkA, NOS, and FRAP/TMP, and galactose-extended oligosaccharides. Of these, substance P, CGRP, somatostatin, TMP, trkA, and galactose-extended oligosaccharides are known to label subpopulations of cutaneous afferent neurones in rat DRGs with small, neurofilament-poor somata and most of which therefore probably have C fibres. Single-neurone studies have defined which types of cutaneous afferent neurones express substance P; these may be limited almost entirely to nociceptive afferent neurones, but do not include all nociceptive neurones. CGRP is probably present in most substance P-containing as well as some non-substance P-containing cutaneous afferent neurones, including some non-nociceptive A-fibre neurones. Further single-neurone studies are needed to establish the precise relationship of other aspects of the neurochemical phenotype with sensory receptor properties in these neurones.

Acknowledgements

Thanks for technical help go to Barbara Carruthers. Work from this laboratory was supported by the MRC (UK) and by the Wellcome Trust.

References

Battaglia, G. and Rustioni, A. (1988). Coexistence of glutamate and substance P in dorsal root ganglion neurons of the rat and monkey. *J. comp. Neurol.* **277**, 302–12.

Burgess, P.R. and Perl, E.R. (1973). Cutaneous mechanoreceptors and nociceptors. In *Handbook of sensory physiology*, Vol. 2. *Somatosensory systems* (ed. A. Iggo), pp. 29–78. Springer-Verlag, Berlin.

Carr, P.A., Yamamoto, T., Karmy, G., and Nagy, J.I. (1991). Cytochemical relationships and central terminations of a unique population of primary afferent neurons in rat. *Brain Res. Bull.* **26**, 825–43.

Cohen, R.H. and Perl, E.R. (1990). Contributions of arachidonic acid derivatives and substance P to the sensitisation of cutaneous nociceptors. *J. Neurophysiol.* **64**, 457–64.

Dalsgaard, C.-J., Jonsson, C.-E., Hökfelt, T., and Cuello, A.C. (1983). Localisation of substance P-immunoreactive nerve fibres in the human digital skin. *Experientia* **39**, 1018–20.

Dalsgaard, C.-J., Haegerstrand, A., Theodorrson-Norheim, E., Brodin, E., and Hökfelt, T. 1985). Neurokinin A-like immunoreactivity in rat primary sensory neurones: coexistence with substance P. *Histochemistry* **83**, 37–9.

De Leon, M., Covenas, R., Chadi, G., Narvaez, J.A., Fuxe, K., and Cintra, A. (1994). Subpopulations of primary sensory neurons show coexistence of neuropeptides and glucocorticoid receptors in the rat spinal and trigeminal ganglia. *Brain Res.* **636**, 338–42.

Dodd, J. and Jessell, T.M. (1985). Lactoseries carbohydrates specify subsets of dorsal root ganglion neurones projecting to the superficial dorsal horn of rat spinal cord. *J. Neurosci.* **5**, 3278–94.

Dodd, J., Jahr, C.E., Hamilton, P.N., Heath, M.J.S., Mathew, W.D., and Jessell, T.M. (1983). Cytochemical and physiological properties of sensory and dorsal horn neurones that transmit cutaneous sensation. *Cold Spring Harbour Symp. quantitat. Biol.* **XLVVII**, 685–95.

Duggan, A.W., Hendry, I.A., Morton, C.R., Hutchison, W.D., and Zhao, Z.O. (1988). Cutaneous stimuli releasing immunoreactive substance P in the dorsal horn of the cat. *Brain Res.* **451**, 261–73.

Henken, D.B., Tessler, A., Chesselet, M.F., Hudson, A., Baldino, F. Jr, and Murray, M. (1988). In situ hybridization of mRNA for beta-preprotachykinin and preprosomatostatin in adult rat dorsal root ganglia: Comparison with immunocytochemical localization. *J. Neurocytol.* **17R, 671–81.**

Hensel, H. and Iggo, A. (1971). Analysis of cutaneous warm and cold fibres in primates. *Pflügers Arch.* **329,** 1–8.

Hoheisel, U., Mense, S., and Scherotzke, R. (1994). Calcitonin gene-related peptide immunoreactivity in functionally identified primary afferent neurones in the rat. *Anat. Embryol.* **189,** 41–9.

Höfelt, T., Zhang, X., and Wiesenfeld-Hallin, Z. (1994). Messenger plasticity in primary sensory neurones following axotomy and its functional implications. *Trends Neurosc.* **17,** 22–30.

Hunt, S.P., Mantyh, P.W., and Priestley, J.V. (1922). The organisation of biochemically characterised sensory neurons. In *Sensory neurons, diversity, development and plasticity* (ed. S.A. Scott), pp. 60–76. Oxford University Press, New York.

Johansson, O. and Vaalasti, A. 1987). Immunohistochemical evidence for the presence of somatostatin-containing sensory nerve fibres in the human skin. *Neurosci. Lett.* **73,** 225–30.

Johansson, O., Ljungberg, A., Han, S.W., and Vaalasti, A. (1991). Evidence for gamma-melanocyte stimulating hormone containing nerves and neutrophilic granulocytes in the human skin by indirect immunofluorescence. *J. Invest. Dermatol.* **96,** 852–6.

Kalina, M. and Wolman, M. 1970). Correlative histochemical and morphological study on the maturation of sensory ganglion cells in the rat. *Histochemie* **22,** 100–108.

Kashiba, H., Senba, E., Ueda, Y., and Tohyama, M. (1992). Co-localized but target-unrelated expression of vasoactive intestinal polypeptide and galanin in rat dorsal root ganglion neurons after periperal nerve crush injury. *Brain Res.* **582,** 47–57.

Kashiba, H., Noguchi, K., Ueda, Y., and Senba, E. (1994). Neuropeptide Y and galanin are coexpressed in rat large type A sensory neurons after peripheral transection. *Peptides* **15,** 411–16.

Kennedy, W.R. and Wendelschafer-Crabb, G. 1993). The innervation of human epidermis. *J. neurol. Sci.* **115,** 184–90.

Knyihar-Csillik, E., Bezzegh, A., Boti, S., and Csillik, B. 1986). Thiamine monophosphatase: A genuine marker for transganglionic regulation of primary sensory neurones. *J. Histochem. Cytochem.* **34,** 363–71.

Kruger, L., Silverman, J.D., Mantyh, W., Sternini, C., and Brecha, N.C. (1989). Peripheral patterns of calcitonin-gene-related peptide general somatic sensory innervation: cutaneous and deep terminations. *J. comp. Neurol.* **280,** 291–302.

Kuraishi, Y., Hiroto, N., Sato, Y., Hino, Y., Satoh, M., and Takagi, H. (1985). Evidence that substance P and somatostatin transmit separate information related to pain in the spinal dorsal horn. *Brain Res.* **325,** 294–8.

Lang, E., Novak, A., Reeh, P.W., and Handwerker, H.O. (1990). Chemosensitivity of fine afferents from rat skin in vitro. *J. Neurophysiol.* **63,** 887–901.

Lawson, S.N. (1994). Morphological and biochemical cell types of sensory neurones. In *Sensory neurones: diversity, development and plasticity* (ed. S.A. Scott), pp. 27–59. Oxford University Press, New York.

Lawson, S.N. (1996). Neuropeptides in morphologically and functionally identified primary afferent neurones root ganglia: substance P, CGRP and somatostatin. *Prog. Brain Res.* **104,** 161–73.

Lawson, S.N. and Waddell, P.J. (1991). Soma neurofilament immunoreactivity is related to cell size and fibre conduction velocity in rat primary sensory neurons. *J. Physiol.* **435,** 41–63.

Lawson, S.N., Harper, E.I., Harper, A.A., Garson, J.A., Coakham, H.B., and Randle, B.J. (1985). Monoclonal antibody 2C5: a marker for a subpopulation of small neurones in rat dorsal root ganglia. *Neuroscience* **16,** 365–74.

Lawson, S.N., Crepps, B., Bao, J., Brighton, B.W., and Perl, E.R. (1993). Differential correlation of substance P-like immunoreactivity (SP-LI) with the type of C-fiber sensory receptor. *Soc. Neurosci. Abstr.* **19,** 136.6.

Lawson, S.N., McCarthy, P.W., and Prabhakar, E. (1995). Electrophysiological properties of neurones with CGRP-like immunoreactivity in rat dorsal root ganglia. *J. comp. Neurol.* **365,** 355–66.

Lawson, S.N., Crepps, B., Bao, J., Brighton, B.W., and Perl, E.R. (1994). Substance P-like immunoreactivity (SP-LI) in guinea pig dorsal root ganglia (DRGs) is related to sensory receptor type in A and C fibre neurons. *J. Physiol.* **476P**, 39P (abstract).

Lawson, S.N., Crepps, B., Buck, H., and Perl, E.R. (in press). Correlation of CGRP-like immunoreactivity (CGRP-LI) with sensory receptor properties in dorsal root ganglion (DRG) neurones in guinea pigs, *J. Physiol.* (abstract) (in press).

Leah, J.D., Cameron, A.A., and Snow, P.J. (1985). Neuropeptides in physiologically identified mammalian sensory neurones. *Neurosci. Lett.* **56**, 257–63.

Lee, K.H., Chung, K., Chung, J.M., and Coggeshall, R.E. (1986). Correlation of cell body size, axon size, and signal conduction velocity for individually labelled dorsal root ganglion cells in the cat. *J. comp. Neurol.* **243**, 335–46.

Lewin, G.R. and Mendell, L.M. (1994). Regulation of cutaneous C-fiber heat nociceptors by nerve growth factor in the developing rat. *J. Neurophysiol.* **71**, 941–9.

Lewin, G.R., Ritter, A.M., and Mendell, L.M. (1992). On the role of nerve growth factor in the development of myelinated nociceptors. *J. Neurosci.* **12**, 1896–905.

Light, A.R. and Perl, E.R. (1993). Peripheral sensory systems. In *Peripheral neuropathy* (ed. P.J. Dyck, P.K. Thomas, J.W. Griffin, P.A. Low, and J.F. Poduslo), pp. 149–65. W.B. Saunders Co, Philadelphia.

Lynn, B. and Carpenter, W.E. (1982). Primary afferent units from the hairy skin of the rat hind limb. *Brain Res.* **238**, 29–43.

McCarthy, P.W. and Lawson, S.N. (1990). Cell type and conduction velocity of rat primary sensory neurons with calcitonin gene-related peptide-like immunoreactivity. *Neuroscience* **34**, 623–32.

McMahon, S.B., Armanini, M.P., Ling, L.H., and Phillips, H.S. (1994). Expression and coexpression of Trk receptors in subpopulations of adult primary sensory neurons projecting to identified peripheral targets. *Neuron* **12**, 1161–71.

Marusich, M.F., Pourmehr, K., and Weston, F.A. (1986). The development of an identified subpopulation of avian sensory neurones is regulated by interaction with the periphery. *Develop. Biol.* **118**, 505–10.

Molander, C., Ygge, Y., and Dalsgaard, C.-J. (1987). Substance P-, Somatostatin- and calcitonin gene-related peptide-like immunoreactivity and fluoride resistant phosphatase activity in relation to retrogradely labelled cutaneous, muscular and visceral primary sensory neurones in the rat. *Neurosci. Lett.* **74**, 37–42.

Noguchi, K., De Leon, M., Nahin, R.L., Senba, E., and Ruda, M.A. (1993). Quantification of axotomy-induced alteration of neuropeptide mRNAs in dorsal root ganglion neurons with special reference to neuropeptide Y mRNA and the effects of neonatal capsaicin treatment. *J. Neurosci. Res.* **35**, 54–66.

O'Brien, C., Woolf, C.J., Fitzgerald, M., Lindsay, R.M., and Molander, C. (1989). Differences in the chemical expression of rat primary afferent neurons which innervate skin, muscle or joint. *Neuroscience* **32**, 493–502.

Perl, E.R. (1968). Myelinated afferent fibres innervating in the primate skin and their response to noxious stimuli. *J. Physiol.* **197**, 593–615.

Perl, E.R. (1991). Specificity in characteristic of fine primary afferent fibres. In *Information processing in the somatosensory processing* (ed. O. Franzen and J. Westman), pp. 383–98. Macmillan Academic and Professional Ltd, Basingstoke.

Perl, E.R. (1992). Function of dorsal root ganglion neurons: An overview. In *Sensory neurons: diversity, development and plasticity* (ed. S.A. Scott), pp. 3–23. Oxford University Press, New York.

Perry, M.J. and Lawson, S.N. (1991). Immunocytochemical properties of rat dorsal root ganglion (DRG) neurones innervating muscle, skin or viscera. *Soc. Neurosci. Abstr.* **17**, 105 (Abstract).

Perry, M.J., Lawson, S.N., and Robertson, J. (1991). Neurofilament immunoreactivity in populations of rat primary afferent neurones: a quantitative study of phosphorylated and non-phosphorylated subunits. *J. Neurocytol.* **20**, 746–58.

Peyronnard, J.M., Charron, L., Lavoie, J., Messier, J.P., and Dubreuil, M. (1988). Carbonic anhydrase and horseradish peroxidase: double labelling of rat dorsal root ganglion neurones innervating motor and sensory peripheral nerves. *Anat. Embryol.* **177**, 353–9.

Plenderleith, M.B. and Snow, P.J. (1993). The plant lectin Bandeira Simplicifolia I-B4 identifies a subpopulation of small diameter primary sensory neurones which innervate the skin in the rat. *Neurosci. Lett.* **159**, 17–20.

Regan, L.J., Dodd, J., Barondes, S.H., and Jessell, T.M. (1986). Selective expression of endogenous lactose-binding lectins and lactoseries glycoconjugates in subsets of rat sensory neurones. *Proc. natl Acad. Sci. USA* **83**, 2248–52.

Ritter, A.M. and Mendell, L.M. (1992). Somal membrane properties of physiologically identified sensory neurons in the rat: Effects of nerve growth factor. *J. Neurophysiol.* **68**, 2033–41.

Scharfman, H.E., Kunkel, D.D., and Schwartzkroin, P.A. (1989). Intracellular dyes mask immunoreactivity of hippocampal interneurons. *Neurosci. Lett.* **96**, 23–8.

Shea, V.K. and Perl, E.R. (1985). Sensory receptors with unmyelinated (C) fibres innervating the skin of the rabbit's ear. *J. Neurophysiol.* **54**, 491–501.

Shebab, S.A.S., Atkinson, M.E., and Payne, J.N. (1986). The origins of the sciatic nerve and changes in neuropeptides after axotomy: a double labelling study using retrograde transport of true blue and vasoactive intestinal polypeptide immunohistochemistry. *Brain Res.* **376**, 180–5.

Silverman, J.D. and Kruger, L. (1988). Lectin and neuropeptide labeling of separate populations of dorsal root ganglion neurons and associated 'nociceptor' thin axons in rat testis and cornea whole-mount preparations. *Somatosens. Res.* **5**, 259–67.

Silverman, J.D. and Kruger, L. (1988). Acid phosphatase as a selective marker for a class of small sensory ganglion cells in several mammalian species: spinal cord distribution, histochemical properties, and relation to fluoride-resistant acid phosphatase (FRAP) of rodents. *Somatosens. Res.* **5**, 219–46.

Skofitsch, G., Zamir, N., Helke, C.J., Savitt, J.M., and Jacobowitz, D.M. (1985). Corticotrophin releasing factor-like immunoreactivity in sensory ganglia and capsaicin sensitive neurons of the rat central nervous system: colocalisation with other neuropeptides. *Peptides* **6**, 307–18.

Streit, W.J., Schulte, B.A., Balentine, J.D., and Spicer, S.S. (1985). Histochemical localisation of galactose-containing glycoconjugates in sensory neurons and their processes in the central and peripheral nervous system of the rat. *J. Histochem. Cytochem.* **33**, 1042–52.

Szabat, E., Soinila, S., Häppölä, O., Linnala, A., and Virtanen, I. (1992). A new monoclonal antibody against the GABA-protein conjugate shows immunoreactivity in sensory neurons of the rat. *Neuroscience* **47**, 409–20.

Tandruff, T. (1993). A method for unbiased and efficient estimation of number and mean volume of specified neuron subtypes in rat dorsal root ganglion. *J. comp. Neurol.* **329**, 269–76.

Tenser, R.B. (1985). Sequential changes of sensory neuron (fluoride resistant) acid phosphatase in dorsal root ganglion neurons following neurectomy and rhizotomy. *Brain Res.* **332**, 386–9.

Tiseo, P.J., Adler, M.W., and Liu-Chen, L-Y. (1990). Differential release of substance P and somatostatin in the rat spinal cord in response to noxious cold and heat; effect of dynorphin A(1–17). *J. Pharmacol. exp. Ther.* **252**, 539–45.

Verge, V.M.K., Tetzlaff, W.,, Richardson, P.M., and Bisby, M.A. (1990). Correlation between GAP43 and nerve growth factor receptors in rat sensory neurons. *J. Neurosci.* **10**, 926–34.

Weise, B., Unsicker, K., and Grothe, C. (1992). Localization of basic fibroblast growth factor in a subpopulation of rat sensory neurons. *Cell Tissue Res.* **267**, 125–30.

Wiese, U.H., Ruth, J.L., and Emson, P.C. (1992). Differential expression of growth-associated protein (GAP-43) mRNA in rat primary sensory neurons after peripheral nerve lesion: A non-radioactive in situ hybridisation study. *Brain Res.* **592**, 141–56.

Zhang, S. and Hoffert, M. (1986). Substance P is contained in myelinated mechanical nociceptors. *Soc. Neurosci. Abstr.* **12**, 538P.

Zhang, X., Wiesenfeld-Hallin, Z., and Hökfelt, T. (1994). Effect of peripheral axotomy on expression of neuropeptide Y receptor mRNA in rat lumbar dorsal root ganglia. *Eur. J. Neurosci.* **6**, 43–57.

4 Comparative and evolutionary aspects of nociceptor function

EDGAR T. WALTERS

By definition, all nociceptors must perform two basic functions: they must detect actual or imminent injury, and they must generate neural signals that can inform the central nervous system (CNS) about the injury or impending injury. In addition, nociceptors may be modified after nearby injury so that they become more sensitive, thus aiding in the defence of the injured site (see Walters 1994). Because of their importance for human pain, nociceptors have received intensive study. However, most studies have focused on only a few mammalian species (primarily domestic cat and dog, laboratory rats, and macaque monkeys), selected for their physiological similarity to humans and for their experimental convenience. This narrow focus has made it difficult to assess the general biological significance of properties found in mammalian nociceptors. As a first step in examining general solutions to biological problems associated with nociception, this chapter will compare selected nociceptors innervating the surface (skin and cornea) of mammals to surface nociceptors in a few invertebrates: notably the medicinal leech, *Hirudo medicinalis*, and the marine snail, *Aplysia californica*. Most of the invertebrate work to be reviewed has been performed on the N ('noxious') and P ('pressure') sensory neurones found in each segmental ganglion of the leech (Nicholls and Baylor 1968) and on mechanosensory neurones of *Aplysia* found in the ('LE') cluster of the abdominal ganglion (Byrne *et al.* 1974) and ventrocaudal ('VC') cluster in each pleural ganglion (Walters *et al.* 1983*a*). These invertebrate sensory neurones, like somatic sensory neurones of mammals, have their somata located in discrete central ganglia, connected to their peripheral receptive fields by long axons.

Evolutionary considerations

Physiology largely (although not exclusively) reflects the operation of biological adaptations (Diamond 1993). Biological adaptations are inherited traits that have been selected during the course of evolution by enhancing the bearers' reproductive success (Darwin 1872; Skelton 1990). Particularly potent selection pressures are those that prevent an animal from surviving long enough to reproduce. Bodily injury has a key position among selection pressures affecting survival because it is the final mediator of many of these selection pressures (Walters 1994). Survival-related pressures include both non-biological hazards (for example, radiation, extreme temperatures, and aquatic turbulence) and biological hazards (competition, predation, parasitism, and disease—see Vermeij 1987). The impact of biological hazards on the evolution of contemporary adaptations is likely to have been especially strong (Darwin 1872; Fisher 1958; Vermeij 1987). Injury produced by biological and non-biological hazards will not only hinder survival, but may compromise an animal's ability to reproduce, even if it survives the injury (for example, Maiorana 1977).

These considerations indicate that, during most of the course of animal evolution, very strong selection pressures have been operating on processes that minimize the likelihood and severity of bodily injury (Habgood 1950; Walters 1994). During the 700 million years or so of animal evolution many opportunities would have been available for the independent development (analogous evolution) of novel defensive mechanisms in divergent animal groups. Indeed, adaptations that aid in the avoidance and minimization of injury are displayed by virtually all animals, and these defensive adaptations are remarkably diverse (Edmunds 1975; Endler 1986; Evans and Schmidt 1990; Walters 1994). However, certain functional aspects of injury are quite similar, and probably have long been similar, throughout the animal kingdom. Recognition of functional similarities in injury responses may divulge basic physical and biological constraints that have shaped outwardly similar adaptations to injury in diverse organisms.

Outwardly similar nociceptive adaptations in divergent lineages could reflect either (1) convergent evolution of similar solutions to common physical and biological problems associated with injury or (2) conservation of fundamental mechanisms associated with injury that appeared very early in the course of evolution and resisted change. Although our understanding of the enormous differences in apparent rates of evolution of different biological traits is limited (see, for example, Campbell 1990), a trait may be assumed to resist evolutionary change if there is little change in the selection pressures that originally shaped it, or if the trait is basic to so many processes in the organism that there is almost no chance the organism can live or reproduce after any significant change in the trait. Clearly, there are many enzyes and metabolic pathways (for example, cytochrome *c* and the electron transport chain) that have resisted change for over a billion years, as indicated by their occurrence in nearly identical form in virtually all living organisms. An interesting task for investigators of nociception and nociceptive plasticity is to determine which aspects of nociceptor design and function have been malleable during evolution, and which have been highly constrained.

Injury detection

Very little is known about peripheral mechanisms of injury detection in vertebrates or invertebrates, primarily because the terminal regions of nociceptors are quite small and impractical for intracellular recording. In principle, a nociceptor could detect actual or imminent tissue injury by responding to: (1) forces or energy levels, such as extreme pressures or temperatures, that do not immediately injure the receptor, but would damage the tissue if sustained; (2) intrinsic signs of the nociceptor's own injury, such as massive depolarization, Ca^{2+} influx, or cytoskeletal disruption; (3) extrinsic chemical signals, such as K^+, H^+, amino acids, prostaglandins, and neuropeptides, released from nearby cells that have been injured or activated by injury; and (4) extrinsic chemical signals, such as cytokines, released from inflammatory or host defence cells that migrate to a site of injury.

Because many mechanonociceptors in both vertebrates and invertebrates can be activated immediately by pressures that are unlikely to produce tissue damage (see below), these nociceptors probably respond directly to increases in pressure, perhaps via the same mechanical transduction processes used in vertebrate and invertebrate stretch receptors (for example, Hunt 1990; Wilson and Paul 1990; Erxleben 1993). Interestingly, mechanically sensitive channels are found in virtually all cells (Sachs 1991), including bacteria (for example, Sukharev *et al.* 1994) and protozoans (for example, Wood 1989). Many of these non-specific cation channels (Sachs 1991) and thus could, in principle, be used in a nociceptor to produce a depolarizing generator potential during mechanical strain. Because damage to individual cells in organ culture or dissociated cell culture can directly activate sensory neurones, it is likely that at least one factor contributing to activation of nociceptors during tissue injury is rapid depolarization of nociceptor branches as a result of direct injury to those branches. Heat-activated nociceptors in mammals, like mechanonociceptors, often respond before tissue is actually damaged. This suggests that initially they respond directly to elevated temperature rather than to products of tissue injury (although indirect activation might still occur via substances released from other cells that are heat-sensitive). Recently, the first heat-sensitive nociceptor in an invertebrate was found: high-threshold N cells in the leech are activated by temperatures $\geqslant 39°C$ (Belmonte *et al.* 1994; Pastor, Soria, and Belmonte, in press). The absence of other reports of heat-activated sensory neurones in invertebrates (for example, Nicholls and Baylor 1968; Byrne *et al.* 1974) may reflect a minor role for heat injury in the biology of aquatic (especially marine) animals, which are heavily represented in the few invertebrate species in which nociceptive physiology has been studied.

The ability to isolate and examine individually identified nociceptors, such as the leech N cell or *Aplysia* VC cells, *in vitro* offers hope that mechanisms by which noxious stimuli are transduced into neuronal signals can be explored directly in cells of known function. Analyses of transduction events in easily accessible nociceptor somata or large neurites in dissociated cell culture can lead to specific hypotheses about peripheral transduction events, which may then be tested in more natural (although less tractable) semi-intact preparations. An encouraging sign for this type of analysis in both vertebrates and invertebrates is striking parallels between sensory neurone somata and peripheral receptors in their discharge properties (especially the degree of accommodation) and the effects of various neuromodulators on excitability (for example, Baccaglini and Hogan 1983; Billy and Walters 1989*b*; Hammer *et al.* 1989; Bevan and Yeats 1991; Harper 1991).

Many nociceptors are activated by chemical signals released by tissue injury. Early evidence for such activation was the long latency to discharge of some afferents following noxious stimulation (for example, Hogg 1935) and the ability of extracts from minced frog skin to activate cutaneous afferents when applied to the underside of intact frog skin (Habgood 1950). Bessou and Perl (1969) first characterized what has proven to be the most common nociceptor in vertebrates—the unmyelinated C polymodal nociceptor, named for its responsiveness not only to mechanical stimuli but also to heat and certain chemicals. Bessou and Perl found that, in contrast to myelinated high-threshold mechanonociceptors (Burgess and Perl 1967), the C polymodal nociceptors were activated by 'irritant chemicals', specifically, several kinds of dilute acid. While C polymodal nociceptors can be activated by injection or vascular perfusion of various chemicals into the largely intact organism (reviewed by Besson and Chaouch 1987), the clearest results have come from simplified preparations in which effects secondary to alterations in blood flow can be eliminated. Studies of polymodal nociceptors in *in vitro* preparations of rat skin and dog testis and in the avascular cornea of the intact cat have shown activation by low concentrations of bradykinin and by higher concentrations of serotonin, histamine, prostaglandin E_2, and capsaicin (the algesic agent in red peppers) (Mizumura *et al.* 1987; Lang *et al.* 1990; Belmonte *et al.* 1994). Polymodal nociceptors are also activated by hypertonic NaCl, and by moderate elevations of K^+ or H^+ ions (for example, Kumazawa and Mizumura 1980; Kumazawa *et al.* 1987; Steen *et al.* 1992; Gallar *et al.* 1993).

In contrast to our knowledge of chemical activators of vertebrate nociceptors, until recently it was not even known whether chemical activation occurs in invertebrate nociceptors. Studies of the leech N cells initially failed to find responses to cutaneous application of solutions with altered pH or osmolarity (Nicholls and Baylor 1968). However, leech N cells can be activated by applying acetic acid (pH3.3 or lower) or NaCl crystals to the surface of the skin—if the overlying mucus is first removed (Pastor *et al.*, in press; Belmonte *et al.* 1994). The same authors found that, unlike the T and P sensory neurones, one of the two types of N cells could be activated by high concentrations of capsaicin ($\sim 10^4$M). It would be interesting to know if capsaicin is more potent when injected intradermally than topically in the leech, as it is in mammals (for example, Baumann *et al.* 1991). Pastor and colleagues found that the soma of the same N cells is excited by similarly high concentrations of capsaicin, but the density of the involved channels or receptors might be much lower in the soma than in peripheral branches. The effects of potential chemical activators on *Aplysia* nociceptors have not yet been reported. However, preliminary observations indicate that acid and hypertonic saline can sometimes activate peripheral branches of LE siphon sensory neurones (P. Illich and E. Walters, unpublished observations). Although the effects of capsaicin have not been examined on *Aplysia* sensory neurones, it is intriguing that relatively high concentrations of capsaicin ($\geq 10^{-4}$M activate unidentified neurones in isolated ganglia of this animal (Erdelyi *et al.* 1986).

The only other invertebrate nociceptor known by this author to be activated by chemical stimuli is the S ('sensory') cell in the nudibranch mollusc, *Tritonia*. It is not yet known if these cells are primary or secondary sensory neurones but, like the other sensory neurones considered here, they have a centrally located soma, a peripheral axon, and a well-defined receptive field on the body surface that responds preferentially to intense mechanical stimulation (Getting 1976). The unusual feature of these neurones is that they display a particularly intense, slowly adapting discharge in response to chemicals sensed during contact with the major predator of adult *Tritonia*—the voracious sea star, *Pycnopodia*. Equivalent contact with other sea stars fails to activate the S cells or to initiate escape behaviour. The S cells strongly excite neural networks that produce local withdrawal and vigorous escape swimming (Getting 1977). These sensory neurones, unlike the potentially homologous VC nociceptors in *Aplysia* (Walters *et al.* 1983a), also show brisk activation by NaCl crystals or concentrated NaCl solution outside the skin (Getting 1976). While the significance of the activation by external salt is unclear, the dramatic responses to a single species of sea star suggest that this nociceptive system has been tuned during evolution to chemicals identifying what may have been a predominant source of injury to adult *Tritonia*.

Nociceptive coding

A major issue in nociceptive physiology concerns the codes by which nociceptors inform the CNS about peripheral injury. In mammals there is strong evidence for both the specificity and intensity (or pattern) theories of nociceptive coding (for example Cervero and Jänig 1992). High-threshold mechanonociceptors are specifically activated by mechanical forces strong enough to threaten tissue injury (Fig. 4.1 (A)), thus providing labelled lines from the skin to the CNS. Any activity in these lines can therefore signify only one thing—that the receptive field is damaged or about to be damaged. On the

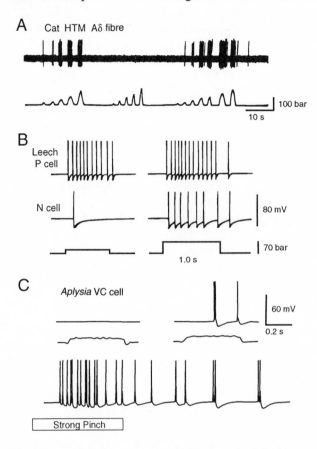

Fig. 4.1 Examples of nociceptor responses to strong mechanical stimulation in a mammal and two invertebrates. (A) Myelinated high-threshold mechanoreceptor (HTM) innervating hairy skin of cat. Series of progressively higher forces (lower trace) were delivered via a 1-mm^2 probe to three spots. Graded spiking responses to stimulation of two responsive spots are seen during the first (left) and third (right) series of stimuli. Reproduced with permission from Kruger *et al.* (1981). (B) Identified nociceptive (N) and pressure-sensitive (P) mechanoreceptors innervating leech skin. Responses were recorded simultaneously from the two cells during indentation of the skin by a 0.2-mm stylus attached to a 7- or 21-g spring. The bars indicate the relative spring force rating, not the recorded force. Reproduced with permission from Nicholls and Baylor (1968). (C) Wide-dynamic-range nociceptor from the pleural ventrocaudal (VC) cluster innervating *Aplysia* tail. Three responses are shown. The top two are responses to von Frey hair indentation (reproduced with permission from Billy and Walters 1989*a*). The lower part of the first two traces shows immediate (prior to reflexive contraction) changes in tension of the tail during bending of 6 mN (left) and 10 mN (right) von Frey hairs (exerting pressures of about 3 and 3.5 bars, respectively). The 6-mN hair failed to elicit spikes, whereas the 10-mN hair elicited a burst of three spikes. The third trace shows the intense response (24 spikes) of another VC cell to strong pinch (reproduced with permission from Clatworthy and Walters 1993). Note the afterdischarge.

other hand, many nociceptors (including many unmyelinated C fibres and some myelinated Aδ fibres) can also respond to weak, innocuous forces (Table 4.1). Burgess and Perl (1967) first described high-threshold Aδ mechanonociceptors in cat hairy skin, which had mechanical thresholds > 30 mN, as measured by thin von Frey filaments. Bessou and Perl (1969) then showed that the median threshold of C polymodal nociceptors in the same preparation was only ~6 mN, and some had von Frey thresholds as low as 2 mN. Subsequent investigations in various preparations revealed that Aδ- and C-fibre nociceptors show a large range of thresholds (Table 4.1), with many activated below the threshold level for human pain. Depending upon the duration, total area, and site of stimulation, humans first report cutaneous pain at pressure thresholds of 3–8 bars, or von Frey hair forces of 20–100 mN (for example, Hardy *et al.* 1952; Burgess and Perl 1967). Some nociceptors innervating very delicate structures, such as the cornea, have much lower thresholds (Table 4.1; Belmonte and Giraldez 1981; Gallar *et al.* 1993), equivalent to those of low-threshold receptors tuned to innocuous stimuli in tougher tissues. Nevertheless, corneal mechanoafferents, like the other sensory neurones discussed here, are properly considered nociceptors because they show a graded increase in discharge to increasing pressures, with maximal activation occurring in response to pressures that cause tissue damage (see also Kumazawa 1990). In wide-dynamic-range nociceptors intense (but not weak) activity can signify that the cell's receptive field is being damaged.

Table 4.1 Comparison of selected surface nociceptors

Property	Rat skin *		Cat cornea †		Leech ‡	*Aplysia* §
	Aδ fibres	C fibres	Aδ fibres	C fibres	N cells	VC, LE cells
Receptive field area (mm²)	0.3–100	0.3–10	20–200	1–50	50–150	5–500
Mechanical force threshold (mN)	10–400	5–500	0.1–1	0.1–3	10–30	0.3–50
Heat activation	Uncommon	Yes	Yes	Yes	Yes	No
Chemical activation	Uncommon	Yes	Yes	Yes	Yes	?
Afterdischarge	Yes	Yes	Yes	Yes	Yes	Yes
Spontaneous activity	No	Uncommon	No	Uncommon	Yes Low rate	No
Sensitization to mechanical stimuli	Yes	'Waking'	No	No	?	Yes
Sensitization to heat	Yes	Yes	Yes	Yes	Yes	?

* Handwerker *et al.* 1987, 1991; Reeh *et al.* 1987; Kessler *et al.* 1992; Light 1992; Steen *et al.* 1992; Leem *et al.* 1993.
† Tower 1950; Belmonte and Giraldez 1981; Gallar *et al.* 1993; Belmonte *et al.* 1994.
‡ Nicholls and Baylor 1968; Blackshaw *et al.* 1982; Belmonte *et al.* 1994; J. Pastor, B. Soria, and C. Belmonte, unpublished observations.
§ Byrne *et al.* 1974; Walters *et al.* 1983*a*; Clatworthy and Walters 1993; E. Walters, A. Billy, and P. Illich, unpublished observations.

Wide-dynamic-range, polymodal nociceptors are more numerous than high-threshold mechanonociceptors, especially in deeper tissues. Indeed, it has been argued that viscera may not be innervated by any high-threshold mechanonociceptors, with nociceptive information carried solely by polymodal nociceptors (McMahon and Koltzenburg 1990; but see also Cervero 1994; Cervero, Chapter 9, this volume). Because many high-threshold mechanonociceptors have rapidly conducting, myelinated axons whereas most polymodal nociceptors have slowly conducting, unmyelinated axons, and the latter are much more responsive to chemical signs of inflammation and injury, it has been suggested that the former serve an early warning and rapid defence function, while activity in the latter provides continuing information about the state of an injury that can aid in recuperative behaviour (for example, Lynn 1984).

The first nociceptor identified in invertebrates was the leech N cell, which is activated preferentially by injurious stimuli such as pinching or cutting the skin (Fig. 4.1 (B); Nicholls and Baylor 1968). Pastor *et al.* (in press) examined the N-cell threshold systematically using thin von Frey filaments, and found it to be about 19 and 17 mN for the lateral and medial N cells, respectively (Table 4.1). The latter group did not give the diameters of the filaments they used but, assuming a filament diameter of 0.15 mm, their threshold pressure would have been about 10 bar. This indicates that the N cells have a wide dynamic range and, along with their chemical and heat sensitivity (see above), suggests that the N cells may be similar to mammalian polymodal nociceptors. Like many C polymodal nociceptors, the N cells show relatively little adaptation to prolonged mechanical stimulation, display afterdischarge following stimulus offset, and sometimes fire spontaneously at low rates (~ 0.2 Hz). Another leech mechanoreceptor, the P cell (Fig. 4.1 (B), has been assumed to lack a nociceptive function because it responds well to innocuous pressures (the threshold is about 30 per cent of that of the N cells; Nicholls and Baylor 1968; Pastor *et al.*, in press). Although the response properties of the P cell have not been explored systematically, P-cell responses are graded with the intensity of stimulation and may peak at noxious levels. It is interesting that 'writhing' behaviour, evoked selectively by strong noxious stimulation, requires activity in P cells for full expression (Kristan *et al.* 1982). Similarly, intracellular stimulation of either a single N or P cell can evoke escape swimming (Debski and Friesen 1987). This suggests that strong activation of P cells can contribute nociceptive information.

Mechanosensory neurones identified in *Aplysia*, like the leech P cells, were initially assumed to have no nociceptive function because their thresholds were relatively low. Byrne *et al.* (1974) found a mean threshold of 0.13 bar in LE sensory neurones using a 0.5-mm probe applied to a tightly pinned out, sensitized (see below) siphon preparation. Jets of seawater exerting pressures of 0.25 bar caused weak activation of some LE cells and no activation of others (Byrne *et al.* 1978). Responses increased with increasing pressures, but only a small range of pressures (up to 0.4 bar) were examined system-atically, which caused relatively little discharge (up to 7 spikes for a 0.8 s stimulus). Despite these observations of weak or moderate discharge elicited by innocuous stimuli, recent studies have found that the LE cells display much higher frequency and more prolonged discharge in response to noxious stimuli such as pinching or cutting the siphon (Illich and Walters, 1995). It is noteworthy that the LE cells, like the equally sensitive corneal nociceptors (Table 4.1), innervate very delicate tissue. Clearly, the threshold of an effective nociceptor needs to be matched to the range of forces that can potentially damage the tissue, and different tissues vary enormously in their suscept-ibility to mechanical damage.

Somewhat higher thresholds were found in similar mechanosensory neurones in *Aplysia*, the VC cells (Fig. 4.1 (C); Walters *et al.* 1983*a*), which have receptive fields in the thicker body wall (relative to the thin siphon tissue) covering most of the ipsilateral half of the body. Systematic examination of VC-cell mechanosensory thresholds using von Frey filaments revealed a mean threshold of about 4.5 bar for all the VC cells except those innervating the anterior tentacles, which had a mean threshold of about 3.5 bar (Billy and Walters 1989*a*; Dulin, Billy, and Walters, in preparation). Moderate-intensity stimuli (2–8 bar) produce short-lasting VC-cell discharge that is graded according to the intensity of the stimulus. Strong, noxious stimuli, such as intense pinch, produce higher-frequency immediate activation and sometimes also produce afterdischarge that can last several seconds and comprise > 30 spikes (Fig. 4.1 (C); Clatworthy and Walters 1993).

Additional evidence for the nociceptive functions of LE and VC mechanosensory neurones comes from their morphology. Using an antibody to a sensory neurone-specific peptide, I. Steffensen and C. Morris (personal communication) have shown that the peripheral terminals of VC and LE cells are spindle-like structures that coil around muscle fibres underneath the skin. Although the receptors are associated with superficial muscle, they are never activated by strong contractions produced by intracellular stimulation of motor neurones or reflexly by stimulation of other sites on the body (Byrne *et al.* 1974; Walters *et al.* 1983*a*; Walters, unpublished observations). Therefore, they are not proprioceptors. Their location in subcutaneous layers is consistent with a defensive function in which they sense sharp indentations sufficient to radically deform the underlying muscle. Such forces would be exerted by the claws or mouthparts of various potential predators (lobsters, crabs, carnivorous molluscs) that have been observed to attack *Aplysia* (Walters *et al.* 1993). Another reason that the LE siphon sensory neurones were initially found to display very low thresholds is that they were probably sensitized by the dissection and testing procedures. Unlike studies of the pleural VC cells (for example, Walters *et al.* 1983*a*; Billy and Walters 1989*a*), the early studies of the LE cells were conducted in preparations that had been dissected from animals in the absence of anaesthesia. Furthermore, the test stimuli were usually applied to a tightly pinned out siphon (greatly reducing its compliance) in which most receptive fields were impaled by one or more pins. Recent results show that von Frey thresholds are significantly lower in pinned out siphons prepared without anaesthesia than in freely moving siphons prepared under anaesthesia (Illich and Walters, 1995).

In conclusion, initial studies of identified mechanosensory neurones in invertebrates have revealed nociceptive properties resembling those of many nociceptors in mammals. One cell type that was initially compared to high-threshold Aδ mechanonociceptors in mammals, the leech N cell, is probably more similar to C polymodal nociceptors because of its wide dynamic range, heat and chemical sensitivity, spontaneous activity, and sensitization to heat stimuli (Table 4.1, and see below). In *Aplysia* both the pleural VC and abdominal LE cells show a wide dynamic range, like many C polymodal nociceptors. However, these cells may be more similar to Aδ nociceptors (Table 4.1). They are insensitive to noxious heat (something that is not encountered by most marine organisms), they lack spontaneous activity in the absence of injury, and they display pronounced sensitization to mechanical stimuli (see below). Although the range of forces that a nociceptor responds to will reflect the special properties of the tissue that the receptor is situated in, and the behavioural ecology of the species, the wide dynamic range and relatively low thresholds of these invertebrate nociceptors indicate that intensity codes have been important during the course of animal evolution for conveying information to the CNS about actual and imminent bodily injury. These preliminary observations do not, however, exclude an important role for specificity codes as well.

Short-term nociceptive sensitization

Most mammalian nociceptors show enhanced responses (sensitization) at some stage during or shortly after noxious stimulation (for example, Treede *et al*. 1992; Meyer *et al*., Chapter 15, this volume). Analysis has focused on nociceptors' responses to noxious heat stimulation, which typically causes threshold to decrease and discharge to increase during subsequent stimulation of both myelinated and unmyelinated nociceptors. Sensitization of responses to mechanical stimulation (which is of greater interest for broad phylogenetic comparisons of nociceptive systems, especially those involving aquatic animals) has been more difficult to observe, even though mechanical hypersensitivity is prominent during cutaneous hyerglasia in man (Lewis 1942; Hardy *et al*. 1952). Bessou and Perl (1969) showed that heat injury lowers mechanical thresholds of C polymodal nociceptors. Reeh and colleagues (1987) found strong mechanical sensitization of high-threshold mechanoreceptors in the rat following mild mechanical trauma of the tail, expressed as a drop in von Frey thresholds of Aδ nociceptors (Fig. 4.2 (B)) but not of C-fibre nociceptors. Several groups have shown that a major contribution to mechanical sensitization probably results from injury and inflammation enabling (or 'waking') the mechanical responsiveness of C polymodal nociceptors that are mechanically insensitive or 'sleeping' under normal conditions (Schaible and Schmidt 1988; Habler *et al*. 190; Handwerker *et al*. 1991; Meyer *et al*. 1991). Previous attempts to study mechanical sensitization would have overlooked these silent nociceptors because nociceptive afferents were typically selected for study on the basis of their responses to mechanical search stimuli. Many extracellular chemical signals have been identified that can sensitize responses to heat or responses to chemical activators such as bradykinin. Direct sensitizers of nociceptors include serotonin, adenosine, prostaglandins E$_2$ and I$_2$, lipoxygenase products of arachidonic acid, and protons, while indirect sensitizers include bradykinin, leukotriene B4, nerve growth factor, nerve-growth factor-derived octapeptide, interleukin 1β, interleukin 8, and peptide fragments from bacterial cell wall proteins and the complement cascade (reviewed by Tweede *et al*. 1992; Levine *et al*. 1993; see also Cunha *et al*. 1991; Lewin and Mendell 1993). Lowered pH appears to be particularly important, as it is to date the only chemical factor that has been shown to produce mechanical sensitization (Steen *et al*. 1992). The intracellular pathways mediating these sensitizing effects have been difficult to explore because of the inaccessibility of peripheral terminals. However, pharmacological studies have implicated cyclic adenosine monophosphate (cAMP) and protein kinase A (PKA) in the pathway for the direct sensitizing actions of serotonin, adenosine, prostaglandin E2, and the lipoxygenase product 8R,15S, diHETE (Taiwo and Levine 1991; Taiwo *et al*. 1992). Protein kinase C (PKC) has been implicated as a mediator of bradykinin's effects (Dray *et al*. 1988.

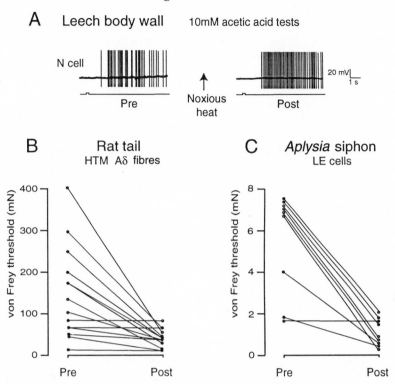

Fig. 4.2 Sensitization of nociceptor responses in diverse animal groups. (A) Heat enhances discharge in leech N cell elicited by chemical test stimulus (a drop of 10 mM acetic acid, pH 3.3). The skin was heated in three 15-s cycles to 46°C, and returned to 26°C before the post-test reading. Reproduced with permission from Belmonte *et al.* (1994). (B) Strong mechanical stimulation decreases von Frey hair threshold of high-threshold (Aδ) mechanoreceptors on rat tail. Noxious stimulation was a series of four 120-s constant-pressure stimuli (1.6, 2.4, 3.2, and 1.2 bar) delivered to the receptive fields of the tested fibres with a 25-mm² probe. Reproduced with permission from Reeh *et al.* (1987). (C) Strong mechanical stimulation decreases the von Frey hair threshold of LE mechanoreceptors on the delicate *Aplysia* siphon. The LE cells were tested in a reduced but freely moving siphon preparation. The noxious stimulus was focal, noxious pinch (> 50 bar) to the receptive fields of the tested cells. Unpublished observations from P. Illich and E. Walters.

Relatively little is known about nociceptor sensitization in the leech. Indeed, mechanical sensitization of leech nociceptors following noxious stimulation has not yet been described. However, Pastor *et al.* (in press) found that repeated heating of the skin above 39°C at 10-min intervals (but not shorter intervals) sensitized N-cell responses to subsequent heating and to application of acetic acid (Fig. 4.2 (A)) or capsaicin. Interestingly, peripheral serotonin application increases the number of spikes evoked by mechanical stimulation in P ('pressure') and low-threshold T ('touch') sensory neurones (Gascoigne and McVean 1991), but the effects on N cells were not described. A potential problem in the leech is that the surgically reduced, restrained preparations used to study sensory physiology might, as in *Aplysia* (see above), themselves produce background sensitization that could obscure the effects of planned sensitizing manipulations.

The wide-dynamic-range nociceptors in the pleural VC and abdominal LE clusters of

Aplysia show strong sensitization, involving both the central and peripheral parts of the neurone. Noxious shock to the tail transiently enhances the discharge of VC cells to tap stimuli near the site of noxious stimulation, and moderate intensity tail shocks repeated at 5-s intervals cause a progressive 'wind-up' of discharge to each shock (Clatworthy and Walters 1993). A small increase in the number of spikes evoked in LE cells by siphon tap was initially observed after either stimulation of an interganglionic connective or application of serotonin to the siphon (Klein *et al.* 1986). Recently, P. Illich and E. Walters (1995) showed that siphon pinch causes a profound decrease in the von Frey threshold of LE cells (Fig. 4.2 (C)). These effects might involve release of serotonin or a molluscan cardioactive peptide, since injection of either into the tail reduced the threshold of VC cells innervating the injection site (Billy and Walters 1989*b*).

Not only does nociceptive sensitization involve increased sensitivity of nociceptors to their inputs, but, in mammals and *Aplysia*, noxious stimulation is also likely to increase the synaptic output of nociceptors. This possibility has been difficult to study in mammals, but is supported by evidence that synapses from primary afferent neurones express long-term potentiation (LTP). This spinal LTP appears to be mediated by *N*-methyl-D-asparate (NMDA)-receptor-dependent mechanisms which, in the hippocampus (where they have been intensively analysed) may involve an enhancement of neurotransmitter release (that is, presynaptic facilitation; see Bliss and Collingridge 1993). A review of the evidence for NMDA-receptor-dependent hyperalgesia and facilitation of dorsal horn interneurone responses is beyond the scope of this chapter. However, the behavioural and interneuronal facilitation may be mediated in part by the NMDA-receptor-dependent LTP of mono- and polysynaptic excitatory post synaptic potentials (e.p.s.p.s) from primary afferents to dorsal horn interneurones (Randic *et al.* 1993), and this might involve presynaptic facilitation of nociceptors.

Injury-related facilitation of the synaptic output of nociceptors in *Aplysia* has received far more attention than the potentially corresponding facilitation in mammals. Heterosynaptic facilitation of abdominal LE cell synapses was first shown by stimulating an interganglionic connective (Castellucci *et al.* 1970), an effect that on the basis of quantal analysis, appeared to be due to a presynaptic change (Castellucci and Kandel 1976). Relatively few studies have examined the effects on *Aplysia* sensory neurone synapses of noxious cutaneous stimulation. Stimulating the tail with a stiff von Frey hair facilitated synapses between pleural VC cells and pedal motor neurones (Walters *et al.* 1983*b*). Noxious tail shock causes rapid heterosynaptic facilitation of VC and LE cells that are not activated by the shock. However, tail shock produces 2–4 times as much facilitation if the tested sensory neurones are activated during the tail shock (Hawkins *et al.* 1983; Walters and Byrne 1983; Walters 1987*b*). Thus, the greatest facilitation occurs in nociceptors strongly activated by a noxious stimulus (Walters 1987*b*), and this activity-dependent facilitation provides a mechanism for site-specific sensitization. This sensitization is functionally equivalent to primary *hyperalgesia* in humans, while the decrease in peripheral threshold should contribute to the equivalent of *allodynia* (Walters 1987*a*, 1992). Noxious stimulation also enhances the excitability of the sensory neurone soma, an effect that increases the likelihood that afterdischarge will be generated in the soma during subsequent responses (Clatworthy and Walters 1993; see also Walters and Byrne 1985; Klein *et al.* 1986; Walters 1987*b*). This allows the soma to act as an amplifier of peripherally generated discharge, increasing the output of the sensory neurone. Interestingly, in mammalian nociceptors generation of additional spikes within the soma may also occur under some conditions (Wall and Devor 1983; Kajander *et al.* 1992).

Mechanisms underlying synaptic facilitation and hyperexcitability of the soma in *Aplysia* nociceptors have been examined primarily with the aid of serotonin, which mimics most of the modulatory effects of noxious stimulation on these cells, including presynaptic facilitation and soma hyperexcitability (reviewed by Walters 1994; Walters and Ambron 1995). Serotonin also apears to be required for some sensitizing effects in the intact animal (Glanzman *et al.* 1989). Briefly, serotonin broadens the sensory neurone spike, which increases transmitter release when it occurs in or near the presynaptic terminals (Klein and Kandel 1978; Hochner *et al.* 1986*a*). Spike broadening is produced by a reduction of at least two K^+ currents (Klein *et al.* 1982; Baxter and Byrne 1989; Goldsmith and Abrams 1992). Synaptic facilitation also involves processes independent of spike broadening, perhaps a direct effect on transmitter mobilization (Gingrich and Byrne 1985; Hochner *et al.* 1986*b*). The effects on both synaptic facilitation and excitability may involve several different protein kinases, with PKA and PKC being particularly prominent (for example, Goldsmith and Abrams 1992; Sugita *et al.* 1992; Braha *et al.* 1993). Activity-dependent enhancement of presynaptic facilitation involves a Ca^{2+}-dependent amplification of adenylate cyclase activity, which increases cAMP levels and PKA activity (Ocorr *et al.* 1985; Abrams and Kandel 1988; Abrams *et al.* 1991). However, it seems likely that other mechanisms are also involved in activity-dependent facilitation.

An unexpected activity-dependent mechanism for enhancing synaptic transmission from *Aplysia* nociceptors was recently discovered in dissociated cell culture. Lin and Glanzman (1994*a*) found that several brief trains of high-frequency discharge evoked by intracellular stimulation of a single pleural VC cell caused LTP of the stimulated synapse lasting at least 80 min. Similar observations had been made previously in isolated ganglia by Walters and Byrne (1985), but these authors could not rule out the possibility that the LTP was due to activity-dependent enhancement of the effects of extrinsic neuromodulators such as serotonin released by interneurones activated by the stimulated sensory neurones. Because Lin and Glanzman only had two cells in culture (a tail nociceptor and a siphon motor neurone), release of extrinsic neuromodulators could not occur. Of particular interest was the observation that the LTP could be blocked by hyperpolarizing the postsynaptic motor neurone, as has been shown in mammalian hippocampus. Moreover, the LTP in *Aplysia*, like some forms of hippocampal and spinal LTP in mammals, could be produced by pairing presynaptic activity with postsynaptic depolarization, and could be blocked by bath application of an NMDA receptor antagonist or by injection of a Ca^{2+} chelator into the postsynaptic cell (Lin and Glanzman 1994*b*). Similar properties have recently been revealed at synapses between VC tail nociceptors and tail motor neurones in intact ganglia (Cui and Walters 1994). These findings, along with evidence that glutamate is the primary neurotransmitter of the sensory neurones (Dale and Kandel 1993), suggest that NMDA-receptor-dependent LTP mechanisms are much more primitive than previously assumed and that in *Aplysia* they might contribute to the enhanced sensitivity around a wound (that is, to the equivalent of primary hyperalgesia). Because LTP mechanisms might have evolved very early in response to injury-related selection pressures, it will be very interesting to see if similar mechanisms exist in nociceptive systems of other species.

Long-term nociceptive sensitization and axon injury

LTP in mammals and *Aplysia* is typically examined for only a few hours. However, enhanced sensitivity around an injury may last for as long as the wound takes to heal (perhaps weeks) or even longer under certain pathological conditions. Persistent alterations of nociceptors have rarely been examined after deliberate tissue injury, but have been studied after experimental manipulations that mimic two of the most important effects of naturally occurring bodily injury: nerve damage and inflammation.

Several persisting alterations have been observed in mammalian afferents following peripheral injury or inflammation. One is the appearance of spontaneous activity, which has been described after axotomy (Wall and Devor 1983), loose ligation of the sciatic nerve (Kajander *et al.* 1992), and subcutaneous injection of the inflammatory agent, carageenan (Kocher *et al.* 1987). Another alteration that has been observed after axotomy is an increase in the excitability of the sensory neurone soma (Gallego *et al.* 1987; Gurtu and Smith 1988). Dramatic morphological alterations—collateral sprouting—can occur in the periphery, which compensate for loss of function after injury and could contribute to the sensitization of a wounded region. Collateral sprouting into territory denervated after nerve transection has been described in rats, rabbits, and humans (Weddell *et al.* 1941; Devor *et al.* 1979; Nixon *et al.* 1984; Doucette and Diamond 1987; Inbal *et al.* 1987; Kingery and Vallin 1989). Finally, long-term morphological changes have also been implicated in the central terminals of mammalian afferents. Although the commonly used nerve transection procedures typically cause death and degeneration of some afferents (perhaps because the number of axons transected is far greater than would normally be damaged during survivable injury—see Walters 1994), Cameron and colleagues (1992) found evidence that C fibres extend into laminae not normally occupied following peripheral axotomy. Similar sprouting into 'novel' laminae occurred in large myelinated afferents after axotomy (Woolf *et al.* 1992). These results suggest that in mammals, as in *Aplysia* (see below), peripheral injury may trigger the growth of central as well as peripheral branches of affected sensory neurones. Growth of central synaptic terminals might increase the number of release sites per postsynaptic target, contributing to persistent presynaptic facilitation. The signals that initiate these long-term changes in mammalian sensory neurones have not yet been identified.

In the leech, axotomy of N, P, and T cells is usually followed by regeneration of peripheral receptive fields (Van Essen and Jansen 1977). Regeneration is accompanied by exuberant sprouting of N cells at the crush site and within the central ganglion (Bannatyne *et al.* 1989). The latter study did not find electrophysiological alterations in the somata of N or T cells. It seems premature, however, to conclude that axotomy has no effect on the excitability of nociceptors in the leech because this study did not examine some of the properties that show the largest alterations in *Aplysia* (specifically, peripheral excitability and repetitive firing and spike threshold in the central soma— see below), and it did not examine the P cells. No studies of possible effects of bodily injury on central or peripheral properties have been reported. However, a potential for injury-related receptive field expansion in the adult leech was suggested by the finding that destruction of three of four N cells within a ganglion (by injection of pronase) caused the receptive field of the surviving N cell to expand into the denervated territory (Blackshaw *et al.* 1982).

In *Aplysia*, LE and VC nociceptors show very long-lasting peripheral and central changes associated with intense or prolonged noxious stimulation. Billy and Walters (1989*a*) found that 1 to 3 weeks after a cut injury to the tail the *peripheral* mechanosensory thresholds of VC cells had decreased and their receptive fields had expanded in the region of the cut. Dulin *et al.* (1995) showed that regenerating receptive fields of VC cells (following nerve crush—see below) had significantly depressed von Frey thresholds. Most attention, however, has been paid to the long-term *central* alterations of *Aplysia* sensory neurones. The first long-term change reported was an increase in active zones, vesicles, synaptic varicosities, and branches in the central arbour of LE cells after prolonged noxious stimulation that did not activate the tested cells (Bailey and Chen 1983, 1988). Frost and colleagues (1985) found that, 1 day after delivering the last of 64 intense shocks spread over 4 days, e.p.s.p.s from abdominal LE sensory neurones (which were not activated by the shocks) were doubled in amplitude. Using a protocol designed to mimic primary hyperalgesia, Walters (1987*b*) showed as much or more synaptic facilitation in pleural VC sensory neurones after only a 2-min sequence of cutaneous shock (e.p.s.p.s in the activated cells were double those in unactivated cells; synaptic connections in unsensitized animals were not examined). This shows that, as with short-term sensitization, nociceptors activated by noxious stimulation are modified for the long term much more readily than nociceptors that are not activated.

Again, as with the analysis of short-term sensitization mechanisms in *Aplysia*, the analysis of long-term sensitization has relied heavily on the application of serotonin to mimic noxious stimulation, and many of the studies have been performed on dissociated pairs of sensory and motor neurones regrown in culture. Thus far, studies of long-term alterations in culture have not addressed the activity dependence of the alterations seen in the intact animal and semi-intact preparations; that is, they have not examined the effects of sensory neurone activation during serotonin application. One day after repeated serotonin application in culture, sensorimotor synapses show presynaptic facilitation (Montarolo *et al.* 1986; Dale *et al.* 1988) and the sensory neurone somata are hyperexcitable (Dale *et al.* 1987). In dissociated cell culture (Schacher *et al.* 1988) or cultured ganglia (Scholz and Byrne 1988), 1-day facilitation can be produced by application of cAMP analogues or injection of cAMP into the soma. Appropriate serotonin treatment or cAMP treatment also induces growth of central branches and varicosities of LE and VC sensory neurones (Nazif *et al.* 1991; Bailey *et al.* 1992). The 1-day serotonin-induced effects and cAMP-induced effects on e.p.s.p. amplitude, excitability, and the growth of varicosities require gene transcription and new protein synthesis (Montarolo *et al.* 1986; Dale *et al.* 1987; Schacher *et al.* 1988; Bailey *et al.* 1992). Considerable effort has gone into identifying molecular pathways underlying the long-term effects (reviewed by Walters 1994; Walters and Ambron—see Fig. 4.3). Long-term, serotonin-induced synaptic facilitation in culture depends upon phosphorylation by PKA of a cAMP-responsive element-binding (CREB) protein in the nucleus (Dash *et al.* 1990), which then activates one or more immediate-early genes to regulate transcription of various effector genes (for example, Barzilai *et al.* 1989; Eskin *et al.* 1989; Kaang *et al.* 1993). A critical immediate-early gene in this pathway is CCAAT enhancer-binding protein, C/EBP (Alberini *et al.* 1994). This pathway may, among other things, increase proteolysis of the regulatory subunit of PKA (perhaps by upregulating synthesis of a protease), which would have a facilitating effect by increasing free levels of the catalytic subunit of PKA (Bergold *et al.* 1992).

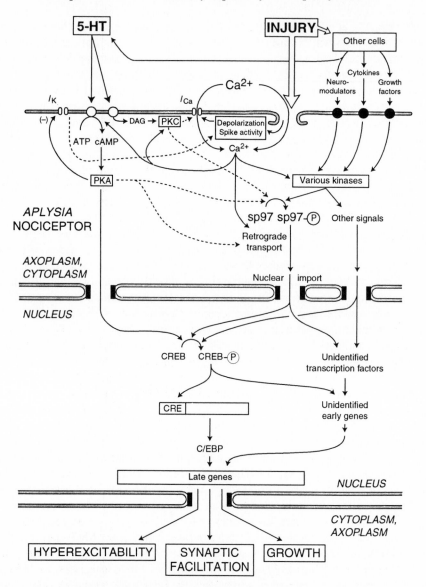

Fig. 4.3 Intracellular pathways that have been implicated in triggering long-term sensitization of *Aplysia* nociceptors. Many of the signals in the axonal injury pathway (right side) remain hypothetical. Arrows do not necessarily indicate direct effects. Dashed lines indicate potential effects of 5-hydroxytryptamine (5-HT) on events associated with axonal injury. Roles in the induction of long-term alterations by many other potential effects of 5-HT and injury (for example, effects on phosphatases, proteases, and other enzymes) have not yet been examined in these cells. I, current; C/EBP,CCAAT enhancer-binding protein; CRE, cAMP response element; CREB, CRE-binding protein; DAG, diacylglycerol; PKA, protein kinase A; PKC, protein kinase C; sp97, 97-kDa protein recognized by antibody to a signal peptide containing a nuclear localization signal (see text). Modified with permission from Walters and Ambron (1995).

A few years ago it was found that very long-lasting increases in synaptic transmission and soma excitability of *Aplysia* nociceptors could be produced under conditions in which serotonin and spike activity were unlikely to contribute (Walters *et al.* 1991). Pedal nerves containing nerves of VC cells were crushed in the intact animal while it was cooled to 0°C and infused with $MgCl_2$ solution. There were no signs of behavioural or neural sensitization for about 2 days, but within 3 days and persisting for 1–2 months the sensory neurones showed hyperexcitability and synaptic facilitation. The changes were not expressed in nociceptors whose axons were not crushed, even if the nociceptor soma was quite close to the crush site (Clatworthy and Walters 1994). The nociceptors also responded to axonal injury with dramatic regenerative growth and sprouting of new axons that entered aberrant, uninjured nerves (Dulin *et al.* 1995; Steffensen *et al.* 1995). Similar changes in excitability were seen after inducing an inflammatory reaction around undamaged pedal nerves (loosely ligating string around the nerve, causing a foreign body reaction) (Clatworthy *et al.* 1994*a*), or by applying the cytokine, interleukin-1, which appears to be present in *Aplysia* amoebocytes (Clatworthy *et al.* 1994*b*). Thus, one of many possible initiating signals for long-term sensory plasticity available during injury may be cytokines from inflammatory cells attracted to damaged tissue and injured nerves. Using *in vitro* preparations, Gunstream and colleagues(1994, 1995) showed that persistent nociceptor hyperexcitability produced by axonal injury was blocked by blocking protein synthesis or gene transcription, and that the initiating signals did not depend on spike activiy, neurotransmitter release, or an interruption of retrograde transport of trophic factors. Instead, long-term hyperexcitability required the retrograde transport of positive axonal injury signals. Under their conditions, inflammatory signals were unlikely to contribute, suggesting that some initiating signals may be generated directly in damaged axons. Ambron and colleagues (1995) showed that nerve injury activates axonal signal proteins by unmasking nuclear localization sequences in the proteins, which cause them to be transported back to the soma and imported into the nucleus (Schmied *et al.* 1993). When axoplasm enriched in activated signal proteins was injected into VC sensory neurones, it produced the same long-lasting hyperexcitability and spike broadening that has been observed after nerve crush, noxious shock, or serotonin application (Ambron *et al.* 1995). It will be very interesting to see where the signal transduction pathways used to produce these outwardly similar forms of plasticity converge (Fig 4.3). Because adaptive reactions to cell injury may be quite primitive, these pathways may have been highly conserved and could be important in mammalian nociceptors as well.

Conclusions

Parallels between the physiology of nociceptors in mammals, the leech, and *Aplysia* suggest that functional similarities in nociceptive systems may reflect the conservation of very primitive injury-related processes. If so, the comparative study of nociceptors in diverse species will help identify fundamental nociceptive mechanisms that may be involved in human pain and perhaps basic substrates of some types of memory. The preliminary comparisons made in this chapter point to the general importance of several features in nociceptors. These include a wide dynamic range, responsiveness to injury-related chemical signals as well as to mechanical forces, a capacity for rapid peripheral sensitization (perhaps involving primitive roles for serotonin, protons, and cAMP), a capacity for potentiating central synaptic connections of the nociceptor (perhaps involving NMDA-receptor-mediated LTP), collateral as well as regenerative growth of peripheral branches in a region of injury, and growth of central synaptic terminals (with both forms of growth contributing to long-term sensitization). It will be particularly interesting to see if certain stimulus transduction pathways and transcriptional regulatory systems are preferentially involved in triggering adaptive reactions to injury in nociceptors. The identification of such pathways is now becoming possible in favourable vertebrate and invertebrate nociceptor preparations.

Acknowledgements

The preparation of this chapter was supported by grants MH38726 from the NIMH and IBN-9210268 from the National Science Foundation. The author is grateful to P. Illich for helpful comments, and to C. Belmonte, C. Morris, J. Pastor, B. Soria, and I. Steffensen for sharing unpublished observations.

References

Abrams, T.W. and Kandel, E.R. (1988). Is contiguity detection in classical conditioning a system or a cellular property? Learning in *Aplysia* suggests a possible molecular site. *Trends Neurosci.* **11**, 128–35.

Abrams, T.W., Karl, K.A., and Kandel, E.R. (1991). Biochemical studies of stimulus convergence during classical conditioning in *Aplysia*: Dual regulation of adenylate cyclase by Ca^{2+}-calmodulin and transmitter. *J. Neurosci.* **11**, 2655–65.

Alberini, C.M., Ghirardi, M., Metz, R., and Kandel, E.R. (1994). C/EBP is an immediate-early gene required for the consolidation of long-term facilitation in *Aplysia*. *Cell* **76**, 1099–114.

Ambron, R.T., Dulin, M.F., Zhang, X-P., Schmied, R., and Walters, E.T. (1955). Axoplasm enriched in a protein mobilized by nerve injury elicits memory-like alterations in *Aplysia* neurons. *J. Neurosci.* **15**, 3440–6.

Baccaglini, P.L. and Hogan, P.G. (1983). Some rat sensory neurones in culture express characteristics of sensory cells. *Proc. natl Acad. Sci., USA* **80**, 594–8.

Bailey, C.H. and Chen, M (1983). Morphological basis of long-term habituation and sensitization in *Aplysia*. *Science* **220**, 91–3.

Bailey, C.H. and Chen, M. (1988). Long-term memory in *Aplysia* modulates the total number of varicosities of single identified sensory neurons. *Proc. natl Acad. Sci. USA* **85**, 2373–7.

Bailey, C.H., Montarolo, P., Chen, M., Kandel, E.R., and Schacher, S. 1992). Inhibitors of protein and RNA synthesis block structural changes that accompany long-term heterosynaptic plasticity in *Aplysia*. *Neuron* **9**, 749–58.

Bannatyne, B.A., Blackshaw, S.E., and McGregor, M. (1989). New growth elicited in adult leech mechanosensory neurones by peripheral axon damage. *J. exp. Biol.* **143**, 419–34.

Barzilai, A., Kennedy, T.E., Sweatt, J.D., and Kandel, E.R. (1989). 5-HT modulates protein synthesis and the expression of specific proteins during long-term facilitation in *Aplysia* sensory neurons. *Neuron* **2**, 1577–86.

Baumann, T.K., Simone, D.A., Shain, C.N., and LaMotte, R.H. (1991). Neurogenic hyperalgesia: the search for the primary cutaneous afferent fibers that contribute to capsaicin-induced pain and hyperalgesa. *J. Neurophysiol.* **66**, 212–27.

Baxter, D.A. and Byrne, J.H. (1989). Serotonergic modulation of two potassium currents in the pleural sensory neurons of *Aplysia. J. Neurophysiol.* **62**, 665–79.

Belmonte, C. and Giraldez, F. (1981). Responses of cat corneal sensory receptors to mechanical and thermal stimulation. *J. Physiol.* **321**, 355–68.

Belmonte, C., Gallar, J., Lopez-Briones, L.G., and Pozo, M.A. (1994). Polymodality in nociceptive neurons: experimental models of chemotransduction. In *Cellular mechanisms of sensory processing* (ed. L. Urban), pp. 87–117. Springer-Verlag, Berlin.

Bergold, P.J., Beushausen, S.A., Sacktor, T.C., Cheley, S., Bayley, H., and Schwartz, J.H. (1992). A regulatory subunit of the cAMP-dependent protein kinase down-regulated in aplysia sensory neurons during long-term sensitization. *Neuron* **8**, 387–97.

Besson, J.M. and Chaouch, A. 1987). Peripheral and spinal mechanisms of nociception. *Physiol. Rev.* **67**, 67–186.

Bessou, P. and Perl, E.R. (1969). Response of cutaneous sensory units with unmyelinated fibers to noxious stimuli. *J. Neurophysiol.* **32**, 1025–43.

Bevan, S. and Yeats, J. (1991). Protons activate a cation conductance in a subpopulation of rat dorsal root ganglion neurones. *J. Physiol.* **433**, 145–61.

Billy, A.J. and Walters, E.T. (1989a). Long-term expansion and sensitization of mechanosensory receptive fields in *Aplysia* support an activity-dependent model of whole-cell sensory plasticity. *J. Neurosci.* **9**, 1254–62.

Billy, A.J. and Walters, E.T. (1989b). Modulation of mechanosensory threshold in *Aplysia* by serotonin, small cardioactive peptide$_B$ (SCP$_B$), FMRFamide, acetylcholine, and dopamine. *Neurosci. Lett.* **105**, 200–4.

Blackshaw, S.E., Nicholls, J.G., and Parnas, I. (1982). Expanded receptive fields of cutaneous mechanoreceptor cells after single neuron deletion in leech central nervous system. *J. Physiol.* **326**, 261–8.

Bliss, T.V.P. and Collingridge, G.L. (1993). A synaptic model of memory: long-term potentiation in the hippocampus. *Nature* **361**, 31–9.

Braha, O., Edmonds, B., Sacktor, T., Kandel, E.R., and Klein, M. (1993). The contributions of protein kinase A and protein kinase C to the actions of 5-HT on the L-type Ca^{2+} current of the sensory neurons of *Aplysia. J. Neurosci.* **13**, 1839–51.

Burgess, P.R. and Perl, E.R. (1967). Myelinated afferent fibers responding specifically to noxious stimulation of the skin. *J. Physiol., London* **190**, 541–62.

Byrne, J., Castellucci, V., and Kandel, E.R. (1974). Receptive fields and response properties of mechanoreceptor neurons innervating siphon skin and mantle shelf in *Aplysia. J. Neurophysiol.* **37**, 1041–64.

Byrne, J.H., Castellucci, V.F., Carew, T.J., and Kandel, E.R. (1978). Stimulus–response relations and stability of mechanoreceptor and motor neurons mediating defensive gill-withdrawal reflex in *Aplysia. J. Neurophysiol.* **41**, 402–17.

Cameron, A.A., Pover, C.M., Willis, W.D., and Coggeshall, R.E. (1992). Evidence that fine primary afferent axons innervate a wider territory in the superficial dorsal horn following peripheral axotomy. *Brain Res.* **575**, 151–4.

Campbell, N.A. (1990). *Biology.* Benjamin/Cummings Publishing Co, Redwood, California.

Castellucci, V. and Kandel, E.R. (1976). Presynaptic facilitation as a mechanism for behavioral sensitization in *Aplysia. Science* **194**, 1176–81.

Castellucci, V., Pinsker, H., Kupfermann, I., and Kandel, E.R. (1970). Neuronal mechanisms of habituation and dishabituation of the gill-withdrawal reflex in *Aplysia. Science* **167**, 1745–8.

Cervero, F. (1994). Sensory innervation of the viscera: peripheral basis of visceral pain. *Physiol. Rev.* **74**, 95–138.

Cervero, F. and Jänig, W. (1992). Visceral nociceptors: a new world order? *Trends Neurosci.* **15**, 374–8.

Clatworthy, A.L. and Walters, E.T. (1993). Rapid amplification and facilitation of mechanosensory discharge in *Aplysia* by noxious stimulation. *J. Neurophysiol.* **70**, 1181–94.

Clatworthy, A.L. and Walters, E.T. (1994). Comparative analysis of hyperexcitability and synaptic facilitation induced by nerve injury in two populations of mechanosensory neurones of *Aplysia californica*. *J. exp. Biol.* **190**, 217–38.

Clatworthy, A.L., Castro, G.A., Budelmann, B.U., and Walters, E.T. (1994a). Induction of a cellular defense reaction is accompanied by an increase in sensory neuron excitability in *Aplysia*. *J. Neurosci.* **14**, 3263–70.

Clatworthy, A.L., Hughes, T.K., Budelmann, B.U., Castro, G.A., and Walters, E.T. (1994b). Cytokines may act as signals for the induction of injury-induced hyperexcitability in nociceptive sensory neurons of *Aplysia*. *Soc. Neurosci. Abstr.* **20**, 557.

Cui, M. and Walters, E.T. (1994). Homosynaptic LTP and PTP of sensorimotor synapses mediating the tail withdrawal reflex in *Aplysia* are reduced by postsynaptic hyperpolarization. *Soc. Neurosci. Abstr.* **20**, 1071.

Cunha, F.O., Lorenzetti, B.B., Poole, S., and Ferreira, S.H. (1991). Interleukin-8 as a mediator of sympathetic pain. *Br. J. Pharmacol.* **104**, 756–7.

Dale, N. and Kandel, E.R. (1993). L-glutamate may be the fast excitatory transmitter of *Aplysia* sensory neurons. *Proc. natl Acad. Sci., USA* **90**, 7163–7.

Dale, N., Kandel, E.R., and Schacher, S. (1987). Serotonin produces long-term changes in the excitability of *Aplysia* sensory neurons in culture that depend on new protein synthesis. *J. Neurosci.* **7**, 2232–8.

Dale, N., Schacher, S., and Kandel, E.R. (1988). Long-term facilitation in *Aplysia* involves increase in transmitter release. *Science* **239**, 282–5.

Darwin, C. (1872). *The origin of species by natural selection or the preservation of favored races in the struggle for life.* Colliers, New York.

Dash, P.K., Hochner, B., and Kandel, E.R. (1990). Injection of the cAMP-responsive element into the nucleus of *Aplysia* sensory neurons blocks long-term facilitation. *Nature* **347**, 718–21.

Debski, E.A. and Friesen, W.O. 1987). Intracellular stimulation of sensory cells elicits swimming activity in the medicinal leech. *J. comp. Physiol.* **A160**, 447–57.

Devor, M., Schonfeld, D., Seltzer, Z., and Wall, P.D. (1979). Two modes of cutaneous reinnervation following peripheral nerve injury. *J. comp. Neurol.* **185** 211–20.

Diamond, J. (1993). Evolutionary physiology. In *The Logic of Life: The Challenge of Integrative Physiology* (ed. C.A.R. Boyd and D. Noble), pp. 89–111. Oxford University Press, Oxford.

Doucette, R. and Diamond, J. (1987). Normal and precocious sprouting of heat nociceptors in the skin of adult rats. *J. comp. Neurol.* **261**, 592–603.

Dray, A., Bettaney, J., Forster, P., and Perkins, M.N. (1988). Bradykinin-induced stimulation of afferent fibers is mediated through protein kinase C. *Neurosci. Lett.* **91**, 301–8.

Dulin, M.F., Steffensen, I., Morris, C.E., and Walters, E.T. (1995). Recovery of function, peripheral sensitization, and sensory neurone activation by novel pathways following axonal injury in *Aplysia*. *J. exp. Biol.* **198**, 2055–66.

Edmunds, M. (1975). *Defence in animals: a survey of anti-predator defences.* Longman, London.

Endler, J.A. (1986). Defense against predators. In *Predator-prey relationships* (ed. M.E. Feder and G.V. Lauder), pp. 1–198. University of Chicago Press, Chicago.

Erdelyi, L., Such, G., and Nedeljkovic, G. (1986). Effects of capsaicin on molluscan neurons: an intracellular study. *Comp. Biochem. Physiol.* **85**, 313–17.

Erxleben, C.F. (1993). Calcium influx through stretch-activated cation channels mediates adaptation by potassium current activation. *Neuroreport* **4**, 616–18.

Eskin, A., Garcia, K.S., and Byrne, J.H. (1989). Information storage in the nervous system of *Aplysia*: specific proteins affected by serotonin and cAMP. *Proc. natl Acad. Sci., USA* **86**, 2458–62.

Evans, D.L. and Schmidt, J.O. (ed.) (1990). *Insect defenses: adaptive mechanisms and strategies of prey and predators,* SUNY Series in Animal Behavior. State University of New York Press, Albany.

Fisher, R.A. (1958). *The genetical theory of natural selection.* Dover, New York.

Frost, W.N., Castellucci, V.F., Hawkins, R.D., and Kandel, E.R. (1985). Monosynaptic connections made by the sensory neurons of the gill- and siphon-withdrawal reflex in *Aplysia* participate in the storage of long-term memory for sensitization. *Proc. natl. Acad. Sci., USA* **82**, 8266–9.

Gallar, J., Pozo, M.A., Tuckett, R.P., and Belmonte, C. (1993). Response of sensory units with unmyelinated fibres to mechanical, thermal, and chemical stimulation of the cat's cornea. *J. Physiol.* **468**, 609–22.

Gallego, R., Ivorra, I., and Morales, A. (1987). Effects of central or peripheral axotomy on membrane properties of sensory neurones in the petrosal ganglion of the cat. *J. Physiol., London* **391**, 39–56.

Gascoigne, L. and McVean, A. (1991). Neuromodulatory effects of acetylcholine and serotonin on the sensitivity of leech mechanoreceptors. *Comp. Biochem. Physiol.* **C99**, 369–74.

Getting, P.A. (1976). Afferent neurons mediating escape swimming of the marine mollusc, Tritonia. *J. comp. Physiol.* **110**, 271—86.

Getting, P.A. (1977). Neuronal organization of escape swimming in Tritonia. *J. comp. Physiol.* **121**, 325–42.

Gingrich, K.J. and Byrne, J.H. (1985). Simulation of synaptic depression, posttetanic potentiation, and presynaptic facilitation of synaptic potentials from sensory neurons mediating gill–withdrawal reflex in *Aplysia*. *J. Neurophysiol.* **53**, 652–69.

Glanzman, D.L., Mackey, S.L., Hawkins, R.D., Dyke, A.M., Lloyd, P.E., and Kandel, E.R. (1989). Depletion of serotonin in the nervous system of *Aplysia* reduces the behavioral enhancement of gill withdrawal as well as the heterosynaptic facilitation produced by tail shock. *J. Neurosci.* **9**, 4200–13.

Goldsmith, B.A. and Abrams, T.W. (1992). cAMP modulates multiple K^+ currents, increasing spike duration and excitability in *Aplysia* sensory neurons. *Proc. natl Acad. Sci., USA* **89**, 11481–5.

Gunstream, J.D., Castro, G.A., and Walters, E.T. (1994). Injury-induced hyperexcitability of *Aplysia* sensory neurons depends on retrograde axonal transport, gene transcription, and protein synthesis. *Soc. Neurosci. Abstr.* **20**, 230.

Gunstream, J.D., Castro, G.A., and Walters, E.T. (1995). Retrograde transport of plasticity signals in *Aplysia* sensory neurons following axonal injury. *J. Neurosci.* **15**, 439–48.

Gurtu, S. and Smith, P.A. (1988). Electrophysiological characteristics of hamster dorsal root ganglion cells and their response to axotomy. *J. Neurophysiol.* **59**, 408–23.

Habgood, J.S. (1950). Sensitization of sensory receptors in the frog's skin. *J. Physiol., London* **111**, 195–213.

Habler, H.J., Jänig, W., and Koltzenburg, M. (1990). Activation of unmyelinated afferent fibres by mechanical stimuli and inflammation of the urinary bladder in the cat. *J. Physiol.* **425**, 545–62.

Hammer, M., Cleary, L.J., and Byrne, J.H. (1989). Serotonin acts in the synaptic region of sensory neurons in *Aplysia* to enhance transmitter release. *Neurosci. Lett.* **104**, 235–40.

Handwerker, H.O., Anton, F., and Reeh, P.W. (1987). Discharge patterns of afferent cutaneous nerve fibers from the rat's tail during prolonged noxious mechanical stimulation. *Exp. Brain Res.* **65**, 493–504.

Handwerker, H.O., Kilo, S., and Reeh, P.W. (1991). Unresponsive afferent nerve fibres in the sural nerve of the rat. *J. Physiol.* **435**, 229–42.

Hardy, J.D., Wolff, H.G., and Goodell, H. (1952). Pain sensations and reactions. Williams & Wilkins, Baltimore.

Harper, A.A. (1991). Similarities between some properties of the soma and sensory receptors of primary afferent neurones. *Exp. Physiol.* **76**, 369–77.

Hawkins, R.D., Abrams, T.W., Carew, T.J., anl Kandel, E.R. (1983). A cellular mechanism of classical conditioning in *Aplysia*: activity-dependent amplification of presynaptic facilitation. *Science* **219**, 400–04.

Hochner, B., Klein, M., Schacher, S., and Kandel, E.R. (1986a). Action-potential duration and the modulation of transmitter release from the sensory neurons of *Aplysia* in presynaptic facilitation and behavioral sensitization. *Proc. natl Acad. Sci., USA* **83**, 8410–14.

Hochner, B., Klein, M., Schacher, S., and Kadel, E.R. (1986*b*). Additional component in the cellular mechanism of presynaptic facilitation contributes to behavioral dishabituation in *Aplysia*. *Proc. natl Acad. Sci., USA* **83**, 8794–8.

Hogg, B.M. (1935). Slow impulses from the cutaneous nerves of the frog. *J. Physiol., London* **84**, 250–8.

Hunt, C.C. (1990). Mammalian muscle spindle: peripheral mechanisms. *Physiol. Rev.* **70**, 643–63.

Illich, P.A. and Walters, E.T. (1995). Nociceptive responses and sensitization of LE siphon sensory neurons in *Aplysia*. *Soc. Neurosci. Abstr.* **21**, 1679.

Inbal, R., Rousso, M., Ashur, H., Wall, P.D., and Devor, M. (1987). Collateral sprouting in skin and sensory recovery after nerve injury in man. *Pain* **28**, 141–54.

Kaang, B.K., Kandel, E.R., and Grant, S.G. (1993). Activation of cAMP-responsive genes by stimuli that produce long-term facilitation in *Aplysia* sensory neurons. *Neuron* **10**, 427–35.

Kajander, K.C., Wakisaka, S., and Bennett, G.J. (1992). Spontaneous discharge originates in the dorsal root ganglion at the onset of a painful peripheral neuropathy in the rat. *Neurosci. Lett.* **138**, 225–8.

Kessler, W., Kirchhoff, C., Reeh, P.W., and Handwerker, H.O. (1992). Excitation of cutaneous afferent nerve endings in vitro by a combination of inflammatory mediators and conditioning effect of substance P. *Exp. Brain Res.* **91**, 467–76.

Kingery, W.S. and Vallin, J.A. (1989). The development of chronic mechanical hyperalgesia, autotomy and collateral sprouting following sciatic nerve section in rat. *Pain* **38**, 321–32.

Klein, M. and Kandel, E.R. (1978). Presynaptic modulation of voltage-dependent Ca^{2+} current: mechanism for behavioral sensitization in *Aplysia californica*. *Proc. natl Acad. Sci., USA* **75**, 3512–16.

Klein, M., Camardo, J., and Kandel, E.R. (1982). Serotonin modulates a specific potassium current in the sensory neurons that show presynaptic facilitation in *Aplysia*. *Proc. natl. Acad. Sci., USA* **79**, 5713–17.

Klein, M., Hochner, B., and Kandel, E.R. (1986). Facilitatory transmitters and cAMP can modulate accommodation as well as transmitter release in *Aplysia* sensory neurons: Evidence for parallel processing in a single cell. *Proc. natl. Acad. Sci., USA* **83**, 7994–8.

Kocher, L., Anton, F., Reeh, P.W., and Handwerker, H.O. (1987). The effect of carrageenan-induced inflammation on the sensitivity of unmyelinated skin nociceptors in the rat. *Pain* **29**, 363–73.

Kristan, W.B., McGirr, S.J., and Simpson, G.V. (1982). Behavioural and mechanosensory neurone responses to skin stimulation in leeches. *J. exp. Biol.* **96**, 143–60.

Kruger, L., Perl, E.R., and Sedivec, M.J. (1981). Fine structure of myelinated mechanical nociceptor endings in cat hairy skin. *J. comp. Neurol.* **198**, 137–54.

Kumazawa, T. (1990). Functions of the nociceptive primary neurons. *Jap. J. Physiol.* **40**, 1–14.

Kumazawa, T. and Mizumura, K. (1980). Chemical responses of polymodal receptors of the scrotal contents in dogs. *J. Physiol., London* **299**, 219–31.

Kumazawa, T., Mizumura, K., and Sato, J. (1987). Response properties of polymodal receptors studied using *in vitro* testis superior spermatic nerve preparations of dogs. *J. Neurophysiol.* **57**, 702–11.

Lang, E., Novak, P., Reeh, P.W., and Handwerker, H.O. (1990). Chemosensitivity of fine afferents from rat skin in vitro. *J. Neurophysiol.* **63**, 887–901.

Leem, J.W., Willis, W.D., and Chung, J.M. (1993). Cutaneous sensory receptors in the rat foot. *J. Neurophysiol.* **69**, 1684–99.

Levine, J.D., Fields, H.I., and Basbaum, A.I. (1993). Peptides and the primary afferent nociceptor. *J. Neurosci.* **13**, 2273–86.

Lewin, G.R. and Mendell, L.M. (1993). Nerve growth factor and nociception. *Trends Neurosci.* **16**, 353–9.

Lewis, T. (1942). *Pain*. Macmillan Co, New York.

Light, A.R. (1992). *The initial processing of pain and its descending control: spinal and trigeminal systems*. Karger, Basel.

Lin, X.Y. and Glanzman, D.L. (1994*a*). Long-term potentiation of *Aplysia* sensorimotor synapses in cell culture: regulation by postsynaptic voltage. *Proc. R. Soc. London* **B255**, 113–18.

Lin, X.Y. and Glanzman, D.L. (1994*b*). Hebbian induction of long-term potentiation of *Aplysia* synapses: partial requirement for activation of an NMDA-related receptor. *Proc. R. Soc. London* **B255**, 215–21.

Lynn, B. (1984). Cutaneous nociceptors. In *The neurobiology of pain* (ed. A.V. Holden and W. Winlow), pp. 97–107 Manchester University Press, Manchester.

McMahon, S. and Koltzenburg, M. (1990). The changing role of primary afferent neurones in pain. *Pain* **43**, 269–72.

Maiorana, V.C. (1977). Tail autotomy, functional conflicts and their resolution by a salamander. *Nature* **265**, 533–5.

Meyer, R.A., Davis, K.D., Cohen, R.H., Treede, R.D., and Campbell, J.N. (1991). Mechanically insensitive afferents (MIAs) in cutaneous nerves of monkey. *Brain Res.* **561**, 252–61.

Mizumura, K., Sato, J., and Kumazawa, T. (1987). Effects of prostaglandins and other putative intermediaries on the activity of canine testicular polymodal receptors studied in vitro. *Pflügers Arch.* **408**, 565–72.

Montarolo, P.G., Goelet, P., Castellucci, V.F., Morgan, J., Kandel, E.R., and Schacher, S. (1986). A critical period for macromolecular synthesis in long-term heterosynaptic facilitation in *Aplysia*. *Science* **234**, 1249–54.

Nazif, F.A., Byrne, and Cleary, L.I. (1991). cAMP induces long-term morphological changes in sensory neurons of *Aplysia*. *Brain Res.* **539**, 324–7.

Nicholls, J.G. and Baylor, D.A. (1968). Specific modalities and receptive fields of sensory neurons in cns of the leech. *J. Neurophysiol.* **31**, 740–56.

Nixon, B.I., Doucette, R., Jackson, P.C., and Diamond, J. (1984). Impulse activity evokes precocious sprouting of nociceptive nerves into denervated skin. *Somatosens. Res.* **2**, 97–126.

Ocorr, K.A., Walters, E.T., and Byrne, J.H. (1985). Associative conditioning analog selectively increases cAMP levels of tail sensory neurons in *Aplysia*. *Proc. natl Acad. Sci., USA* **82**, 2548–52.

Pastor, J., Soria, B., and Belmonte, C. (1996). Properties of the nociceptive neurons of the leech segmental ganglion. *J. Neurophysiol.* (in press).

Randic, M., Jiang, M.C., and Cerne, R. (1993). Long-term potentiation and long-term depression of primary afferent neurotransmission in the rat spinal cord. *J. Neurosci.* **13**, 5228–41.

Reeh, P.W., Bayer, J., Kocher, L., and Handwerker, H.O. (1987). Sensitization of nociceptive cutaneous nerve fibers from the rat tail by noxious mechanical stimulation. *Exp. Brain Res.* **65**, 505–12.

Sachs, F. (1991). Mechanical transduction by membrane ion channels: a mini review. *Mol. Cell. Biochem.* **104**, 57–60.

Schacher, S., Castellucci, V.F., and Kandel, E.R. (1988). cAMP evokes long-term facilitation in *Aplysia* sensory neurons that requires new protein synthesis. *Science* **240**, 1667–9.

Schaible, H.G. and Schmidt, R.F. (1988). Time course of mechanosensitivity changes in articular afferents during a developing experimental arthritis. *J. Neurophysiol.* **60**, 2180–96.

Schmied, R., Huang, C-C., Zhang, X-P., Ambron, D.A., and Ambron, R.T. (19993). Endogenous axoplasmic proteins and proteins containing nuclear localization signal sequences use the retrograde axonal transport/nuclear import pathway in *Aplysia* neurons. *J. Neurosci.* **313**, 4064–771.

Scholz, K.P. and Byrne, J.H. (1988). Intracellular injection of cAMP induces a long-term reduction of neuronal K^+ currents. *Science* **240**, 1664–6.

Skelton, P.W. (1990). Adaptation. In *Paleobiology: a synthesis* (ed. D.E.G. Briggs and P.R. Crowther), pp. 139–46. Blackwell Scientific, Oxford.

Steen, K.H., Reeh, P.W., Anton, F., and Handwerker, H.O. (1992). Protons selectively induce lasting excitation and sensitization to mechanical stimulation of nociceptors in rat skin, in vitro. *J. Neurosci.* **12**, 86–95.

Steffensen, I., Dulin, M.F., Walters, E.T., and Morris, C.E. (1995). Peripheral regeneration and central sprouting of sensory neurone axons in *Aplysia* following nerve injury. *J. exp. Biol.* **198**, 2067–78.

Sugita, S., Goldsmith, J.R., Baxter, D.A., and Byrne, J.H. (1992). Involvement of protein kinase C in serotonin-induced spike broadening and synaptic facilitation in sensorimotor connections of *Aplysia*. *J. Neurophysiol.* **68**, 643–51.

Sukharev, S.I., Blount, P., Martinac, B., Blattner, F.R., and Kung, C. (1994). A large-conductance mechanosensitive channel in *E. coli* encoded by mscL alone. *Nature* **368**, 265–8.

Taiwo, Y.O. and Levine, J.D. (1991). Further confirmation of the role of adenyl cyclase and of cAMP-dependent protein kinase in primary afferent hyperalgesia. *Neuroscience* **44**, 131–5.

Taiwo, Y.O., Heller, P.H., and Levine, J.D. (1992). Mediation of serotonin hyperalgesia by the cAMP second messenger system, *Neuroscience* **48**, 479–83.

Tower, S.S. (1940). Unit for sensory reception in cornea. *J. Neurophysiol.* **3**, 486–500.

Treede, R.D., Meyer, R.A., Raja, S.N., and Campbell, J.N. (1992). Peripheral and central mechanisms of hyperalgesia. *Prog. Neurobiol.* **38**, 397–421.

Van Essen, D.C. and Jansen, J. (1977). The specificity of reinnervation by identified sensory and motor neurons in the leech. *J. comp. Neurol.* **171**, 433–54.

Vermeij, G.J. (1987). *Evolution and escalation: an ecological history of life*. Princeton University Press, Princeton, New Jersey.

Wall, P.D. and Devor, M. (1983). Sensory afferent impulses originate from dorsal root ganglia as well as from the periphery in normal and nerve injured rats. *Pain* **17**, 321–39.

Walters, E.T. (1987*a*). Site-specific sensitization of defensive reflexes in *Aplysia*: a simple model of long-term hyperalgesia. *J. Neurosci.* **7**, 400–7.

Walters, E.T. (1987*b*). Multiple sensory neuronal correlates of site-specific sensitization in *Aplysia*. *J. Neurosci.* **7**, 408–17.

Walters, E.T. (1992). Possible clues about the evolution of hyperalgesia from mechanisms of nociceptive sensitization in *Aplysia*. In *Hyperalgesia and allodynia* (ed. W.D. Willis), pp. 45–58. Raven Press, New York.

Walters, E.T. (1994). Injury-related behavior and neuronal plasticity: an evolutionary perspective on sensitization, hyperalgesia and analgesia. *Int. Rev. Neurobiol.* **36**, 325–427.

Walters, E.T. and Ambron, R.T. (1995). Long-term alterations induced by injury and by 5-HT in *Aplysia* sensory neurons: convergent pathways and common signals? *Trends Neurosci.* **18**, 137–42.

Walters, E.T. and Byrne, J.H. (1983). Associative conditioning of single sensory neurons suggests a cellular mechanism for learning. *Science* **219**, 405–8.

Walters, E.T. and Byrne, J.H. (1985). Long-term enhancement produced by activity-dependent modulation of *Aplysia* sensory neurons. *J. Neurosci.* **5**, 662–72.

Walters, E.T., Byrne, J.H., Carew, T.J., and Kandel, E.R. 1983*a*). Mechanoafferent neurons innervating tail of *Aplysia*. I. Response properties and synaptic connections. *J. Neurophysiol.* **50**, 1522–42.

Walters, E.T., Byrne, J.H., Carew, T.J., and Kandel, E.R. 1983*b*). Mechanoafferent neurons innervating tail of *Aplysia*. II. Modulation by sensitizing stimulation. *J. Neurophysiol.* **50**, 1543–59.

Walters, E.T., Alizadeh, H., and Castro, G.A. (1991). Similar neuronal alterations induced by axonal injury and learning in *Aplysia*. *Science* **253**, 797–9.

Walters, E.T., Illich, P.A., and Hickie, C. (1993). Inking and siphon response plasticity in *Aplysia*: anti-predator and alarm signal functions. *Soc. Neurosci. Abstr.* **19**, 578.

Weddell, G., Guttmann, L., and Guttmann, E. (1941). The local extension of nerve fibers into denervated areas of skin. *J. Neurol. Neurosurg.* **4**, 206–25.

Wilson, L.J. and Paul, D.H. (1990). Functional morphology of the telson-uropod stretch receptor in the sand crab *Emerita analoga*. *J. comp. Neurol.* **296**, 343–58.

Wood, D.C. (1989). Localization of mechanoreceptors in the protozoan, *Stentor coeruleus*. *J. comp. Physiol.* **A165**, 229–35.

Woolf, C.J., Shortland, P., and Coggeshall, R.E. (1992). Peripheral nerve injury triggers central sprouting of myelinated afferents. *Nature* **355**, 75–8.

PART 2
Nociceptors and the signalling of injury

5 Cutaneous nociceptors

JAMES N. CAMPBELL AND RICHARD A. MEYER

Introduction

The cutaneous nociceptor, the subject of this chapter, has been the centrepiece of research on peripheral nociceptive mechanisms. This is for three reasons: (1) it is relatively easy to apply temperature, chemical, and mechanical stimuli to the skin; (2) the skin is accessible both in animals and man for psychophysical studies; (3) the nerve fibres that lead to the skin may be recorded with facility.

Several other chapters in this book deal with the cutaneous nociceptor. The focus here will be on knowledge gleaned from single-fibre recordings in normal skin. To reduce redundancy we concentrate in particular on research conducted in our own laboratories, an admittedly parochial view. Unless otherwise specified, the properties discussed pertain to nociceptor studies in the primate, specifically monkey. The properties of nociceptors in the monkey parallel what is known about nociceptors studied in humans with the technique of microneurography. Injury may sensitize nociceptors, and this plays a fundamental role in the development of hyperalgesia. This topic will only be briefly covered as sensitization and hyperalgesia are covered in detail in other chapters.

In the broadest terms cutaneous sensory receptors may be subdivided into four categories. First, there are the predominantly myelinated afferents that respond to gentle deformations of the skin. These afferents are referred to as low-threshold mechanor-eceptors (LTMs) and provide information to the brain regarding texture and shape (for example, Johnson 1983). A second class of afferents are those that are sensitive selectively to gentle cooling stimuli. These 'cold fibres' signal sensations of cold (for example, Johnson et al. 1973). The third category, 'warm fibres', are C fibres that respond to mild heat stimuli and account for the sensation of warmth (for example, Darian-Smith et al. 1979; Johnson et al. 1979). The fourth group, the subject of this chapter, is a heterogeneous population of high-threshold receptors. These afferents are thought to be responsible for the sensations of pain, itch, and prickle. Because these receptors respond preferentially to noxious stimuli, they are termed nociceptors (Sherrington 1906).

Several different criteria may be used to classify nociceptors: (1) unmyelinated (C fibre) versus myelinated (A fibre) parent nerve fibre; (2) adequate stimulus; (3) type of response (for example, quickly adapting versus slowly adapting). Identification of the adequate stimuli (that is, the stimuli that most readily activate the afferent) and determination of the conduction velocity serve most commonly as the basis for identifying the afferent type.

Electrophysiological techniques

To understand currently used nomenclature, it is useful to note how physiological recordings are done. The technique used to record from afferent peripheral nerve fibres in animal studies is termed the 'teased-fibre' preparation (Burgess and Perl 1967). A cut-down procedure is done on the nerve of interest, and a well is created into which a non-conducting agent such as mineral oil is placed. Using a dissecting microscope, the epineurium is opened. The perineurium is then opened on one of the fascicles. Proximally, a small group of fibres is severed and rotated on to a small dissection platform. Jeweller's forceps are used to tease away small bundles of nerve fibres. These are placed on to a unipolar recording electrode. Action potentials are amplified and differentially recorded using standard electrophysiological techniques.

There are several constraints and possible sources of bias with this recording configuration. Under normal circumstances there are three types of afferents that have ongoing activity: cold fibres; warm fibres; and muscle spindles. Nociceptive fibres 'speak only when spoken to'. The technique described here involves a random sampling of the nerve for nerve fibres of interest for recording. There is no way to identify a nociceptive fibre except by activating it in some way and then noting the action potential discharge.

A fibres have larger electrical signals than C fibres, and, consequently, it is easier to record from A fibres. With some practice and proper equipment, however, it is possible to record readily from C fibres. In order to have an ideal recording, it is best to have a situation where there are no spontaneously active fibres. The receptive field should be in an area such that presentation of the stimulus of interest only activates one receptor.

An alternative technique for studying nociceptors involves the use of microneurography (for example, Hagbarth *et al.* 1970; Torebjörk 1974). This involves the placement of a microelectrode into a nerve. The principal advantage of this technique is that it can be used in humans. The recording constraints are similar to those described above for the teased fibre preparation. There are, however, additional constraints. The technique is in many ways more difficult than the teased-fibre recording. The recordings of C-fibres can be very unstable. Accordingly, in the teased-fibre technique it is common to be able to record from fibres over several hours. Long recording sessions with the microneurography technique are very difficult for the subject and the investigator. The recording quality in terms of signal to noise ratio is generally inferior to that achieved with the teased-fibre technique. In human studies the subjects are awake and thus nociceptive stimuli used in the experiments induce pain, a problem circumvented for the animals since they are anaesthetized. The range of noxious stimuli used in the microneurography technique tends to be constrained for this reason. Another more puzzling problem is that, for unclear reasons, A-fibre nociceptors are difficult to identify and record using the microneurography technique. Psychophysical studies on cold sensation and first pain sensation (see later) suggest that the reason for this does not relate to the paucity of A-δ fibres. Finally, in microneurography studies there is a risk, albeit small, of nerve injury.

In conducting physiological studies in animals we invoke the cross-species assumption. We assume that the properties of nociceptors in anaesthesized animals are similar to those in awake humans. Microneurography has played an important role in confirming that human nociceptors, so far as we can tell, behave the same as non-human primate (monkey) nociceptors. What can be done uniquely in microneurography studies is to microstimulate (for example, Lundberg *et al.* 1992). Small groups of axons can be stimulated, and the human subject can be asked what he feels. Such experiments have provided corroborative evidence that nociceptors signal pain, and they also have been important in demonstrating that in hyperalgesic conditions other afferent types, such as the low-threshold mechanoreceptor, acquire the capacity to evoke pain.

Effects of anaesthetics

In order to correlate neurophysiological data obtained in anaesthetized monkeys with the results of psychophysical data obtained from awake humans, it is necessary to know what effects anaesthetics have on the properties of nociceptors. We studied the effects of pentobarbital, halothane, and nitrous oxide on nociceptors in monkey (Campbell *et al.* 1984). Halothane was shown to sensitize reversibly both C-fibre and Aδ-fibre nociceptors to heat stimuli. An example in a single fibre is shown in Fig. 5.1. These effects were shown to be independent of vascular and sympathetic effects and probably represent direct action on the nociceptor. Pentobarbital and narcotics (Raja *et al.* 1986), in contrast, had no effect on nociceptor response properties. Therefore, in studies performed in our laboratory, pentobarbital or a pentobarbital/morphine mixture is used as the preferred anaesthetic.

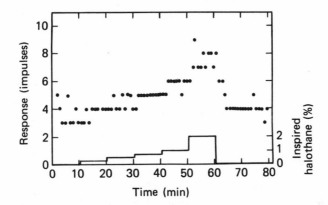

Fig. 5.1 Effects of halothane on the heat responses of a C-fibre mechano-heat-sensitive nociceptor (CMH). A 47°C, 3-s stimulus was delivered to the receptive field every 60 s. Halothane was administered as shown. The responses of the CMH increased as halothane was increased. When halothane was stopped, the response of the CMH decreased to near baseline response. Anaesthesia was maintained by a constant infusion of pentobarbitol sodium. From Campbell *et al.* (1984) with permission.

Classification of nociceptors

CMHs and AMHs

Once a small strand of axons is placed on the recording electrode, the task is to identify the receptive field of the nociceptors. The easiest way to do this is with mechanical search stimuli (firm pinching of the skin may be used, for example). Once the mechanically responsive receptve field is located, other stimulus modalities may be applied. Unlike other types of C afferents, nociceptors, more often than not, respond to multiple stimulus modalities including mechanical, heat, chemical, and—to some extent—cold stimuli. In situations where responses to three stimulus modalities are demonstrated, it is appropriate to label the afferents polymodal nociceptors. However, in many of the early studies of nociceptors, heat and mechanical stimuli were used as the only stimuli. C fibres responsive to mechanical and heat stimuli were referred to as *CMHs*. A fibres responsive to mechanical and heat stimuli were referred to as *AMHs*. When the terms CMH and

AMH were first used, it was not clear how many of these fibres responded to chemical stimuli. However, CMHs and AMHs in general do respond to chemical stimuli (Davis *et al.* 1993). Thus, CMHs and AMHs are indeed polymodal nociceptors. However, nociceptors differ widely with regard to the chemicals to which they respond. One could argue that each chemical in a sense constitutes another modality. In light of this and because of the relative simplicity of the terms, we prefer to use the acronyms CMH and AMH.

Type I and type II AMHs

CMHs as a group respond similarly to heat and mechanical stimuli. The AMHs, however, respond in two distinctly different ways to heat. *Type I AMHs*, found in both hairy and glabrous skin, have relatively high thresholds to heat stimuli and sensitize to a burn injury. *Type II AMHs*, which account for first pain sensation, occur only in hairy skin and have lower heat thresholds (mean, 46°C; Treede *et al.* 1995). Type I AMHs are also termed high-threshold mechanoreceptors in the literature (HTMs; Perl 1968). The contrasting properties of type I and type II AMHs are summarized in Table 5.1 and will be discussed in more detail subsequently.

Table 5.1 Comparison of type I and type II AMHs

Property	Type I AMHs	Type II AMHs
Location of receptive field	Glabrous and hairy skin	Hairy skin only
Median threshold to 1-s heat stimulus	$> 53°C$	46°C
Latency of first action potential to a 53°C, 30-s heat stimulus	Majority > 400 ms	All < 400 ms
Latency of peak response to a 53°C, 30-s heat stimulus	All > 2 s	Nearly all < 1 s
Profile of heat response	Wind-up	Slowly adapting
Sensitization to heat stimuli	Prominent	Desensitization
Mean conduction velocity	25 m/s	15 m/s
Role in sensation	Hyperalgesia in response to burn stimulus on hand	First pain sensation in response to heat

MIAs

Another group of nociceptors has a relatively high threshold to mechanical stimuli and thus eluded analysis in early studies of nociceptors. It is not yet clear that this group of fibres has a distinctive physiological role. These receptors, which may be termed mechanically insensitive afferents (MIAs), will be discussed in more detail below. Mechanically sensitive afferents (CMHs and AMHs) will sometimes be referred to as 'conventional' nociceptors in this chapter.

Some A fibres and C fibres do not respond to even intense heat stimuli. These C and A high-threshold mechanoreceptors account for less than 10 per cent of the total population of nociceptors (Georgopoulos 1976; Treede *et al.* 1995). A distinctive physiological role for these receptors has not been elucidated. There are also occasional low-threshold C-fibre mechanoreceptors that do not respond to heat (Nordin 1990). They are not seen on the glabrous skin of the hand, but have been reported in other areas of the body. No one knows what their physiological role is, and these fibres will not be discussed further.

Organization of receptive field and general properties

The responses to heat stimuli of type I AMHs when compared to those of type II AMHs are strikingly different, as already discussed. The mechanical threshold of glabrous skin CMHs is higher than that of the other groups, but the heat threshold of glabrous and hairy skin CMHs is about the same (Treede *et al.* 1995). The heat threshold of type II AMHs is higher than that of CMHs. The conduction velocity of glabrous skin AMHs (all type I) is higher than that of hairy skin type I AMHs, which is in turn higher than that of type II AMHs (all hairy skin).

The mechanically responsive receptive field of CMHs that innervate human (Torebjörk 1974; Van Hees and Gybels 1981) and monkey (Beitel and Dubner 1976; Kumazawa and Perl 1977; Canpbell and Meyer 1983) hairy skin is typically organized into discrete areas of mechanosensitivity that are variably termed 'hot spots', 'sensitive spots', or 'receptive points'. The number of sensitive spots was determined to range from 1 (observed in one-third of the CMHs studied) to 11, with a median of 3 (Treede *et al.* 1990). The receptive field to mechanical stimuli in glabrous skin CMHs does not have the same punctate areas of sensitivity.

The size of the receptive field ranges from single punctate spots (less than 1 mm in diameter) to multiple spots covering an expanse as large as several centimetres. The mean ($\pm$SD) receptive field size of A-fibre and C-fibre nociceptors on hairy skin is 40 ± 53 and 18 ± 9 mm^2 (Treede *et al.* 1995). The area of the receptive field that responds to mechanical stimuli has been found to correspond to the area that responds to heat stimuli (Treede *et al.* 1990). Thus, the mechanical and heat transducers are probably located on the same or nearby receptor endings. However, the transducer elements that account for mechanosensitivity are probably different from those responsible for heat sensitivity, since topical capsaicin treatment of the cornea results in an alteration in the heat response but not in the mechanical response of C-fibre polymodal nociceptors (Belmonte *et al.* 1991).

The mean radius of the heat-receptive fields in CMHs extends more than 2 mm beyond the centres of highest mechanical sensitivity (that is, outside the mechanical receptive field defined by near-threshold stimuli) but correlates well with the region responsive to a suprathreshold (10-bar von Frey hair) mechanical stimulus (Treede *et al.* 1990). This finding implies that the punctate nature of sensitivity to mechanical stimuli does not mean that transduction is confined to those spots, but rather that transduction to mechanical stimuli also occurs in the zones between these 'hot spots'.

Responses of CMHs to heat stimuli

The heat threshold of CMHs in primates is typically greater than 38°C, but less than 50°C. The response of a typical CMH to a random sequence of heat stimuli ranging from

41 to 49°C is shown in Fig. 5.2. It can be seen that the response increases monotonically with stimulus intensity over this temperature range, which encompasses the pain threshold in humans.

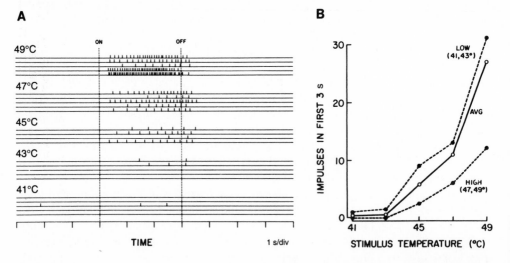

Fig. 5.2 Responses of a CMH to a random presentation of heat stimuli ranging from 41 to 49°C. Each stimulus was presented five times and was preceded by every other stimulus an equal number of times. Within these constraints, stimulus temperature was randomized. Base temperature was 38°C, and the interstimulus interval was 25 s. (A) Action potential replicas of responses on each trial (horizontal line) with trials grouped by the temperature of the stimulus delivered. Within each temperature group, trials are arranged in order of random presentation within the run. (B) Intensity functions constructed from the data shown in left panel. The solid line represents the mean cumulative action potential count during each stimulus averaged for all presentations of the same intensity. The dotted lines represent the stimulus–response functions obtained when the preceding stimulus was of low (41 and 43°C) or high (47 and 49°C) intensity. From LaMotte and Campbell (1978) with permission.

Fatigue

A prominent property in CMHs is fatigue, which can be characterized as a decrement in neural response with repeated stimuli. The response of a typical CMH to a repeated 53°C stimulus is shown in Fig. 5.3. The first response is characterized by a short burst of action potentials followed by adaptation. With subsequent trials the burst is no longer evident. Moreover, the response latency is shorter and the cumulative response is greater in the first trial. Stimulus interaction effects persist for several minutes. As shown in Fig. 5.4, the recovery cycle exceeds 5 minutes.

The family of stimulus–response functions shown in Fig. 5.2 illustrates how fatigue varies with stimulus history. The stimulus–response functions were calculated by determining the response to each temperature as a function of the intensity of the preceding stimulus. A greater response was observed when the preceding stimulus was of low intensity.

Dependence of the CMH heat threshold on temperature at the depth of the receptor

Ramped heat stimuli are often used to determine heat threshold of nociceptors. However, the surface temperature at threshold for CMHs is strongly dependent on

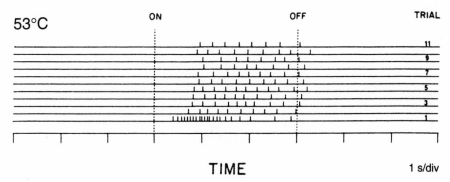

Fig. 5.3 Fatigue of a CMH in response to repeated presentations of a heat stimulus. A 53°C, 3-s stimulus was applied with an interstimulus interval of 25 s (base temperature was 38°C). Each horizontal line represents one trial. Each small vertical mark is a single nerve impulse. The dotted vertical lines mark the time between onset of the stimulus and the onset of passive cooling 3 s later. From LaMotte and Campbell (1978) with permission.

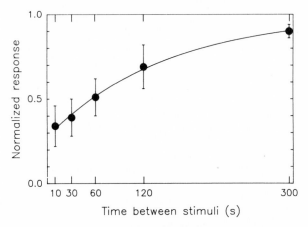

Fig. 5.4 Suppression of the response of C-fibre nociceptors to repeated heat stimuli depends on time interval between stimuli. Two identical heat stimuli were presented to the receptive field of 13 CMHs. The response to the second stimulus is expressed as a fraction of the response to the first stimulus (mean ± SD). Suppression was greatest at the short interstimulus intervals. Full recovery takes more than 5 min. Adapted from Tillman (1992) with permission.

the rate of temperature change (Bessou and Perl 1969; Lynn 1979; Tillman *et al.* 1995*a*). This dependence is illustrated in Fig. 5.5 for a typical CMH. In this example the surface temperature at threshold was 41.9°C when the ramp rate was 5.8°C/s, but was 39.6°C when the ramp rate was 0.095°C/s. Thus, surface temperature at threshold varies inversely with rate of temperature change.

To account for this phenomenon, it is necessary to consider how subsurface temperature at the depth of the receptor varies as a function of surface temperature. Figure 5.6 illustrates this phenomenon with calculations derived from a three-layer, heat-transfer model of skin. Temperature at a specified depth is clearly dependent on surface temperature, as well as on the rate of temperature change at the surface. The faster the rate of temperature change at the surface, the greater the disparity will be between the surface and the subsurface.

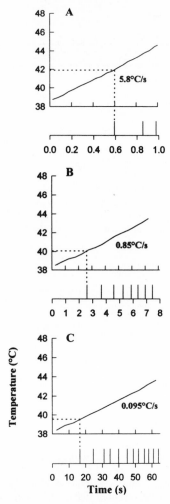

Fig. 5.5 The heat thresholds of CMHs are dependent on the rate of change of temperature at the skin surface. This typical CMH was exposed to heat stimuli at three different ramp rates. Under each stimulus waveform is the response of this CMH to that stimulus. (A) For a stimulus ramp rate of 5.8°C/s, the surface temperature at threshold was 41.9°C. (B) For a stimulus ramp rate of 0.85°C/s, the surface temperature at threshold was 40.1°C. (C) For a stimulus ramp rate of 0.095°C/s, the surface temperature at threshold was 39.6°C. (Note: the time-scale is different for each figure.) From Tillman *et al.* (1995*a*) with permission.

Let us assume for the moment that temperature alone at the depth of the receptor (without consideration of rate of temperature change) is the sole determinant of CMH threshold. The surface temperature needed to reach this threshold temperature would depend on the rate of change of surface temperature. As illustrated in Fig. 5.6 (B), if the receptor were located at 100 μm below the surface and had a heat threshold of 43°C, the surface temperature at threshold would be 43.5°C for a ramp rate of 0.85°C/s, but 46.4°C for a ramp rate of 5.8°C/s. Thus the apparent dependence of heat threshold on ramp rate (for example, Fig. 5.5) can be explained by the thermal inertia of the skin and the depth of the receptor.

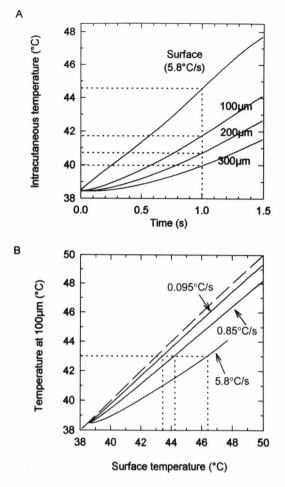

Fig. 5.6 Intracutaneous temperature profiles predicted by a three-layer heat-transfer model of skin. (A) Intracutaneous temperature profiles at three different depths. The surface temperature waveform was a 5.8°C/s ramp. At any instant (for example, at 1 s as indicated by the dotted lines), the temperature decreased with depth. (B) Predicted intracutaneous temperature profiles at three different stimulus ramp rates. Temperature at a depth of 100 μm is plotted versus surface temperature. Note that the surface temperature required to attain an intracutaneous temperature of 43°C (dotted lines) increases as the stimulus ramp rate increases. From Tillman *et al.* (1995*a*) with permission.

A similar analysis can be used to predict the depth of the receptor and the threshold at the receptor from data on the surface temperature at threshold as a function of ramp rate. To investigate this, three ramp rates of heating were applied to the skin surface, and the time of the first action potential was recorded. Long interstimulus intervals were used (10 min) to avoid stimulus interaction effects, and latencies for the first action potential were corrected for conduction distance. Using a three-layer, heat-transfer model of the skin, it is possible, for each ramp rate, to calculate temperature as a function of depth at the time of the first action potential. If the temperature at the receptor is the sole determinant of the time of this action potential, the three temperature versus depth curves derived in this way should intersect at a single point. This point should correspond to the depth and heat threshold of the receptor.

This prediction was confirmed in a study of 23 CMHs. The results for four representative CMHs are shown in Fig. 5.7. The temperature shown for the '0' depth corresponds to the surface threshold. This is the value that would ordinarily be considered as the 'threshold'. Notably, the surface temperature threshold was highest for the highest ramp rate. The steepest profile shown in this figure corresponds to the highest ramp.

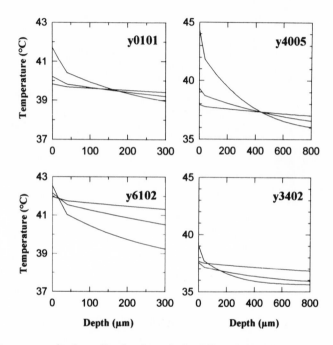

Fig. 5.7 Temperature versus depth profiles for data obtained from four typical CMHs. Intracutaneous temperature predicted from a three-layer heat-transfer model is plotted versus depth for the instant at which the first action potential occurred. Each curve corresponds to the profile for a different ramp rate. Ramp rates of 5.8°C/s, 0.85°C/s, and 0.095°C/s were used. The locus of intersections of the three curves corresponds to the predicted depth of the receptor and threshold temperature for activating the receptor. Adapted from Tillman *et al.* (1995*a*) with permission.

Estimated receptor depths derived from these data ranged from 20 to 570 μm with a mean of 201 ± 173 (± SD) μm. The mean receptor threshold was 40.4 ± 2.2°C. These threshold levels are nearly equal to the surface heat threshold values determined at the slowest ramp rate (0.095°C/s.

When stepped (as opposed to ramp) stimuli are applied to the skin surface, the surface temperature at threshold is found to vary inversely with base temperature, and to vary directly with stimulus duration (Tillman *et al.* 1995*a*). When the stepped temperature increase was applied with a base temperature of 35°C, the threshold was higher than if the base temperature was 38° (42.4°C versus 41.4°C, $n = 9$). When the duration of the stepped temperature stimulus was 30 s, the threshold was lower than if the stimulus was 1 s in duration (40.1°C versus 41.4°C, $n = 16$). These findings support the conclusion that threshold is specified by the temperature at the receptor located at some discrete location underneath the skin surface. At the higher base temperature, a smaller stepped increase in surface temperature is needed to reach the threshold temperature at a given depth. Similarly, a smaller stepped increase in surface temperature will be needed to achieve the intracutaneous threshold temperature if the duration of the stimulus is prolonged.

Thus, surface threshold is only a good indicator of receptor threshold when the stimulus ramp rate is very slow or the stimulus duration is very long. In this same study, we determined that receptor depth does not correlate with mechanical and thermal threshold, receptive field size, or conduction velocity (Tillman *et al.* 1995*a*). Thus, differences in thermal and mechanical threshold of CMHs are not simply a result of some endings being deeper than others.

Suprathreshold responses to ramped heat stimuli

The prior discussion suggests that temperature rather than rate of temperature change governs threshold for the first action potential in CMHs. Of note, however, is the finding that rate of temperature change *does* influence peak discharge rate (Tillman *et al.* 1995*b*). This is illustrated in Fig. 5.8 for a typical CMH. The discharge rate is highest for the fastest stimulus ramp rate. This is remarkable because thermal modelling reveals that intracutaneous temperature lags surface temperature more for faster stimulus ramp rates (Fig. 5.6).

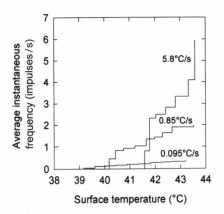

Fig. 5.8 The peak discharge of CMHs increases with ramp rate. The response of a typical CMH to heat stimuli at three different ramps is shown. Average instantaneous frequency is plotted versus surface temperature so that the responses to the three different stimulus ramp rates can be compared. Although the surface temperature for the initial response was lower for the slower ramp rate, the peak response frequency was much higher for the faster ramp rate. Bin widths were 0.05, 0.5, and 5.0 s for the 5.8, 0.85, and 0.095°C/s ramp rates, respectively. From Tillman *et al.* (1995*b*) with permission.

As shown in Fig. 5.9, the surface temperature threshold goes up with ramp rate, but at the same time peak frequency correlates positively with ramp rate. To account for these findings it is necessary to invoke separate mechanisms for nociceptor threshold and peak frequency response. Peak frequency, but not threshold, is rate-sensitive. The molecular basis for these differing transduction mechanisms is not known at present.

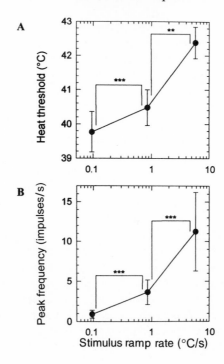

Fig. 5.9 Responses of CMHs to ramped heat stimuli. (A) The surface temperature at threshold for initiating an action potential increased with ramp rate ($n = 13$, mean $\pm$ SEM). (B) The peak frequency during the ramp increased with ramp rate. From Tillman *et al.* (1955*b*) with permission.

Responses of AMHs to heat

Two different types of AMHs have been identified on the basis of their responses to stepped heat stimuli (Fig. 5.10; Meyer *et al.* 1985*a*; Treede *et al.* 1995). For type II AMHs, the peak response is reached early in the stimulus, and adaptation occurs over the next several seconds. In type I AMHs the response winds up and reaches a peak late in the stimulus. Figure 5.11 is a scatter plot of the time of peak discharge as a function of response latency for the first action potential for 46 AMHs in hairy skin of the monkey. The same stimulus, 53°C for 30 s, was applied to each unit. Type II AMHs form a cluster at short response latencies and short peak latencies. Type I AMHs have longer latencies for peak response and for first response.

Type II AMHs do not exist on the glabrous skin of the hand. However, both type I and type II AMHs occur on the hairy skin. Another difference between the fibre types pertains to the property of sensitization to heat stimuli. Type II AMHs are desensitized by a burn injury to their receptive field, whereas type I AMHs are sensitized (Fitzgerald and Lynn 1977; Campbell *et al.* 1979; Treede *et al.* 1995).

It might be argued that the extremely long onset latency of action potentials in type I AMHs is due to a location of the nerve endings deep in the skin. This is unlikely, however, because, even at a depth of about 0.5 mm, skin temperature is near equilibrium after about 6 s (Hensel 1950), and the response latency of most type I AMHs is longer than 6 s.

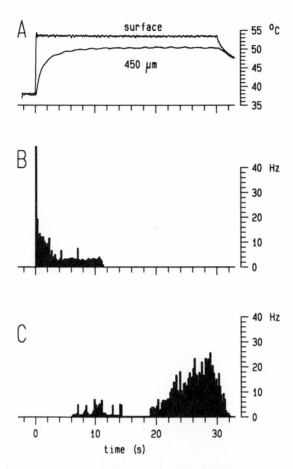

Fig. 5.10 Typical examples of the responses of type I and type II AMHs to a stepped heat stimulus. (A) Temperature recordings from the skin surface (radiometer) and at a depth of about 450 μm (thermocouple) for the 53°C, 30-s heat stimulus. (B) Peristimulus frequency histogram of the response of an AMH in hairy skin (bin width, 0.2 s; conduction velocity, 14 m/s; mechanical threshold, 3.3 bar; heat threshold, 44°C, 1 s). Due to its short response latency of 52 ms and peak latency of 0.1 s, this fibre was classified as a type II AMH. (C) Peristimulus frequency histogram from a different AMH fibre in hairy skin (conduction velocity, 46 m/s; mechanical threshold, 1.3 bar; heat threshold with 1-s stimulus duration, > 53°C). For this type I AMH, the response latency was about 6100 ms, and the peak latency was about 29 s. From Treede *et al.* (1995) with permission.

It is likely that the majority of what were termed high-threshold mechanoreceptors (HTMs) in previous studies in cat, rabbit, and monkey (for example, Perl 1968; Fitzgerald and Lynn 1977; Roberts and Elardo 1985) were in fact what we term here type I AMHs. The slowly increasing discharge of type I AMHs during the sustained heat stimulus might represent heat sensitization. Arguments can be made either way as to whether to call these fibres type I AMHs or HTMs. The important point to note is that these fibres do have the capacity to transduce heat.

CMHs resemble type II AMHs with regard to heat response, though the mean heat threshold in type II AMHs is higher (Treede *et al.* 1995). The neural response latency was recorded to be as short as 15 ms for CMHs. Because this latency includes the time for heat transmission to the receptor, the actual transduction process may be in the sub-millisecond range for both fibre types. This makes it unlikely that release of a chemical mediator is involved in the activation of these nociceptors by heat stimuli.

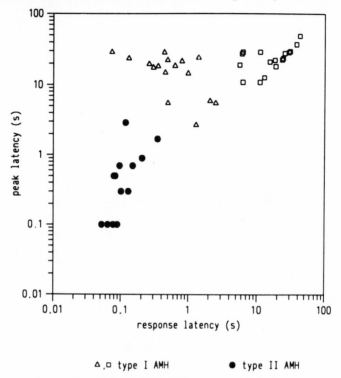

△,□ type I AMH   ● type II AMH

Fig. 5.11 Heat response properties of A-fibre nociceptors in the hairy skin of the monkey. Scatter plot of time of peak discharge as a function of time of first action potential is plotted for 46 AMHs in response to a 53°C, 30-s heat stimulus. Type II AMHs (filled symbols) had short response latencies and short peak latencies. Type I AMHs (open symbols) had long response latencies and long peak latencies. From Treede *et al.* (1995) with permission.

Evidence that heat pain is signalled by activity in nociceptors

CMHs signal pain from heat stimuli to glabrous skin

We now examine the evidence that CMHs signal pain. In normal glabrous skin of the hand, two types of fibres, the CMH nociceptors (not AMHs) and the warm fibres, respond to heat stimuli at temperatures near the pain threshold in humans (that is, around 45°C). It is of interest, therefore, to compare how warm fibres and CMHs encode information about noxious heat stimuli. Warm fibres respond vigorously to gentle warming of the skin (Konietzny and Hensel 1975; Darian-Smith *et al.* 1979). An example of the response of a warm fibre to stimuli in the noxious heat range is shown in Fig. 5.12. The response of warm fibres is not monotonic over this temperature range. In the example shown in Fig. 5.12, the total evoked response at 49°C was less than that at 45°C. Psychophysical studies done in man demonstrate that pain increases monotonically with stimulus intensities between 40 and 50°C (LaMotte and Campbell 1978; Meyer and Campbell 1981*b*). Because the responses of CMHs increase monotonically over this temperature range (Fig. 5.2) and the responses of warm fibres do not (Fig. 5.12), it follows that CMHs signal the sensation of heat pain to the glabrous skin of the hand (LaMotte and Campbell 1978).

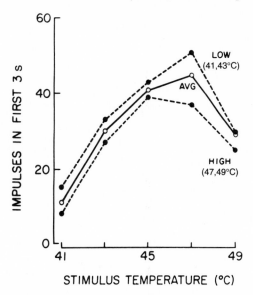

Fig. 5.12 Non-monotonic response of a warm fibre to heat stimuli in the noxious range. Stimulus presentation paradigm same as for Fig. 5.2. The total response during the 3-s stimulus interval is plotted as a function of stimulus temperature. From LaMotte and Campbell (1978) with permission.

Other evidence in support of a role of CMHs in pain sensation includes: (1) human judgements of pain in response to stimuli over the range 41–49°C correlate well with the activity of CMH nociceptors over this range (Meyer and Campbell 1981*b*); (2) selective A-fibre ischaemic blocks or C-fibre (local anaesthetic) blocks indicate that C-fibre function is necessary for thermal pain perception near the pain threshold (Sinclair and Hinshaw 1950; Torebjörk and Hallin 1973); (3) stimulus interaction effects observed in psychophysical experiments (LaMotte and Campbell 1978) are also observed in recordings from CMHs; (4) the latency to pain sensation on glabrous skin following step temperature changes is long and consistent with input from CMHs (Campbell and LaMotte 1983); (5) in patients with congenital insensitivity to pain, microscopic examination of the peripheral nerves indicates the absence of C fibres (Bischoff 1979).

In addition, the following evidence from microneurographic studies in humans points to the capacity of activity in CMHs to evoke pain: (1) intraneural electrical stimulation of presumed single identified CMHs in humans elicits pain (Torebjörk and Ochoa 1980); (2) the heat threshold for activation of CMHs recorded in awake humans is just below the pain threshold (Gybels *et al.* 1979; Van Hees and Gybels 1981); (3) a linear relationship exists between responses of CMHs recorded in awake humans and ratings of pain over the temperature range 39–51°C (Torebjörk *et al.* 1984).

AMHs and pain

As shown in Fig. 5.13, a long-duration heat stimulus applied to the glabrous skin of the hand in human subjects evokes substantial pain for the duration of the stimulus. CMHs have a prominent discharge during the early phase of the stimulus, but this response adapts within seconds to a low level. In contrast, type I AMHs are initially unresponsive, but then discharge vigorously. Therefore, type I AMHs probably contribute to the pain during a sustained high-intensity heat stimulus (Meyer and Campbell 1981*a*).

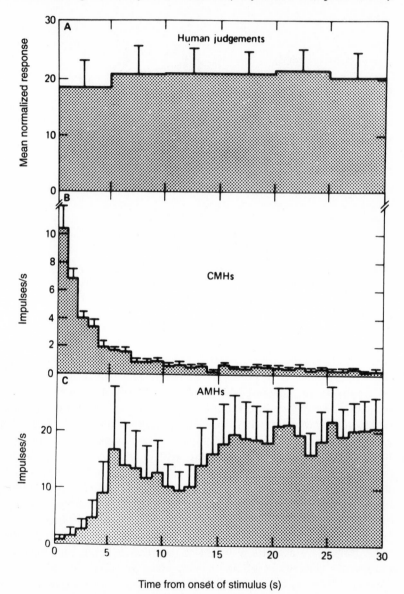

Fig. 5.13 Ratings of pain by human subjects during a long-duration, intense-heat stimulus (53°C, 30 s) applied to the glabrous hand are compared with responses of CMHs and type I AMHs. (A) Pain was intense throughout the stimulus ($n=8$). (B) The brisk response of the CMHs at the beginning of the stimulus changed to a low rate of discharge after 5 s ($n=15$). (C) The response of the type I AMHs increased during the first 5 s and remained high throughout the stimulus ($n=14$). From Meyer and Campbell (1981*a*) with permission.

In the hairy skin, stepped heat stimuli evoke a double pain sensation (Lewis and Pochin 1937; Campbell and LaMotte 1983). The first perception is of a sharp pricking sensation, and the second sensation felt is a burning feeling that occurs after a momentary lull during which little if anything is felt. Myelinated afferent fibres must signal the first pain, since the latency of response to first pain is too quick to be carried by slowly conducting C fibres (Campbell and LaMotte 1983). Type II AMHs (Fig. 5.10) are ideally suited to signal this first pain sensation for the following reasons: (1) the thermal threshold is near the threshold temperature for first pain (Dubner *et al.* 1977); (2) the receptor utilization time (time between stimulus onset and receptor activation) is short (Meyer *et al.* 1985a; Treede *et al.* 1995); and (3) the burst of activity at the onset of the heat stimulus is consistent with the perception of a momentary pricking sensation. The absence of a first pain sensation in response to heat stimuli applied to the glabrous skin of the human hand (Campbell and LaMotte 1983) correlates with the failure to find type II AMHs on the glabrous skin of the hand in monkey.

A dual pain sensation is also perceived in response to sharp mechanical stimuli presented to both hairy and glabrous skin. The first pain is probably signalled by activity in a subset of A-fibre nociceptors.

The preceding discussion indicates that nociceptors may signal pain. However, two caveats are in order. First, this does not mean that activity in CMHs always signals pain. It is clear that low-level discharge rates in nociceptors do not always lead to sensation (for example, Van Hees and Gybels 1981; Adriaensen *et al.* 1984). Central mechanisms for attention quite obviously play a crucial role in whether and how much nociceptor activity leads to the perception of pain. Second, it is probable that receptors other than nociceptors signal pain in certain circumstances. For example, the pain in response to light touch that occurs after certain nerve injuries or with tissue injury appears to be signalled by activity in low-threshold mechanoreceptors (Campbell *et al.* 1988).

Mechanical response properties of nociceptors

Conventional nociceptors, as defined in the section, 'Classification of nociceptors', respond to both heat and mechanical stimuli. The mechanical threshold is usually determined by using a set of hand-held nylon monofilaments (that is, von Frey probes) that produce a peak force when the monofilament bends (for example, Anesthesiometer Set, Stoelting Autogenics Co). The distribution of mechanical thresholds for conventional AMH and CMH nociceptors on the hairy skin of the monkey is shown in Fig. 5.14. The mean ($\pm$SD) mechanical threshold for CMHs that innervate hairy skin (2.2 ± 1.3 bar) is not significantly different from that for AMHs that innervate hairy skin (2.7 ± 2.1 bar; from Meyer *et al.* 1991). In contrast, the mean mechanical threshold for nociceptors on glabrous skin is significantly higher (CMHs, 5.6 ± 2.3 bar; AMHs, 3.8 ± 2.4 bar; from Treede *et al.* 1995). (Note that 1 bar $= 100$ kPa $= 10$ g/mm^2.)

CMH and AMH nociceptors exhibit a slowly adapting response to stepped increases in force. As shown in Fig. 5.15, the frequency of discharge at the beginning of the constant force stimulus is higher than at the end of the stimulus. For most AMHs, the response increases as the applied force increases. In contrast, for many C-fibre nociceptors the response appears to reach a plateau level at relatively low forces (for example, Garell and Greenspan 1994; Slugg *et al.* 1994; Reeh, personal communication). In addition, A-fibre nociceptors tend to exhibit a greater response to a given stimulus than do the C-fibre nociceptors.

Cutaneous nociceptors

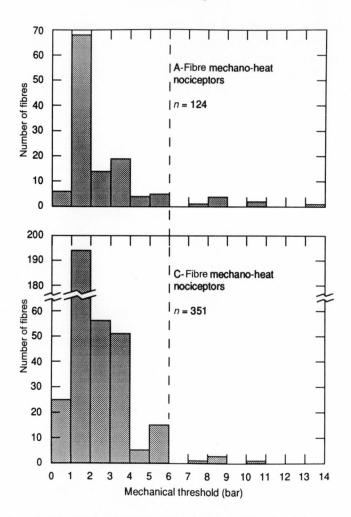

Fig. 5.14 Histogram of mechanical thresholds for A-fibre (top) and C-fibre (bottom) mechanoheat-sensitive nociceptors. The threshold was determined using calibrated von Frey probes. These nociceptors come from studies in which a pinching stimulus was used to locate the receptive field. Only fibres that innervated hairy skin were included. Eight (of 124) A fibres and five (of 351) C fibres had a mechanical threshold greater than 6 bars. From Meyer *et al.* (1991) with permission.

As with heat stimuli, a marked suppression is observed in response to mechanical stimuli that are presented to the same location in the receptive field at short interstimulus intervals. For example, the response of a C fibre to a second 10-g stimulus applied 15 s after the first 10-g stimulus was almost half the response to the first stimulus. Full recovery requires a stimulus-free interval of greater than 5 min for C-fibre nociceptors, but of only 2 min for A-fibre nociceptors (Slugg *et al.* 1994).

A paradox with regard to mechanically induced pain is that a mechanical stimulus that evokes the same level of activity in a C-fibre nociceptor as that evoked by a heat stimulus evokes less pain than the heat stimulus (for example, Van Hees and Gybels

1981). In addition, the mechanical threshold for activating nociceptors is well below the pain threshold. This apparent discrepancy could be due to the spatial summation (that is, recruitment of more nociceptors) associated with the larger area heat stimulus. Alternatively, the co-activation of low-threshold mechanoreceptors with the mechanical stimulus, but not the heat stimulus, could result in suppression of pain.

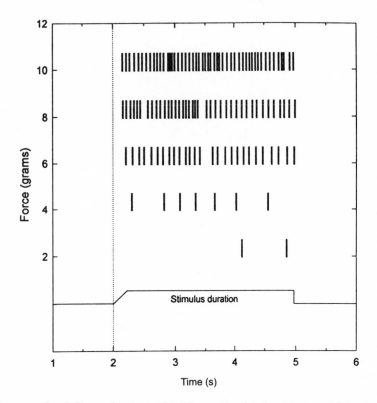

Fig. 5.15 Response of an A-fibre nociceptor on the glabrous skin of the hand to stepped force stimuli. A- and C-fibre nociceptors exhibit a slowly adapting response to stepped force stimuli. The response of this A-fibre nociceptor increased as the stimulus force increased. Each vertical line corresponds to the time of occurrence of an action potential. Each horizontal line corresponds to the response obtained at the given force level. The stimulus profile consisted of a 0.2-s ramp to a controlled force, and a 2.8-s hold at that force. An ascending series of controlled force stimuli (2, 4, 6, 8, 10 g) with an interstimulus interval of 60 s were applied with a 0.4-mm diameter cylindrical probe to one of the most sensitive spots in the receptive field. From Schneider *et al.* (1995) with permission.

In psychophysical experiments using cylindrical probes of various diameters, Greenspan and McGillis (1991) found that, as force increased, perception changed from dull presssure to sharp pressure to sharp pain. As the probe area increased, the sharpness and pain thresholds increased inversely with probe circumference (not probe area). This suggests that nociceptors respond best at the edge of the cylindrical probe where the strain concentration of the stimulus is largest. The one-dimensional map of the receptive field of an A-fibre nociceptor shown in Fig. 5.16 is consistent with this hypothesis. For this map, a 400-μm diameter cylindrical probe was moved in 100-μm increments across one of the punctate spots within the receptive field. Two distinct maxima were seen in the response which correspond to the situation when one edge or the other edge of the cylindrical probe was aligned with the punctate spot.

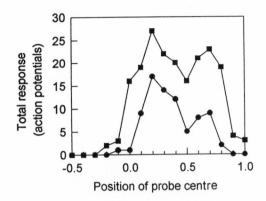

Fig. 5.16 A one-dimensional map of the receptive field for an A-fibre nociceptor on the glabrous skin of the distal phalanx. The total response to a stepped force stimulus is plotted as a function of probe position. The 400-μm diameter cylindrical probe was moved in 100-μm increments along the *x*-axis which was aligned with a ridge on the finger-tip. Each stimulus was of 3-s duration. The first run was with a 10-g stimulus and a 60-s interstimulus interval (filled circles). The second run was with a 20-g stimulus and a 120-s interstimulus interval (filled squares). From Schneider *et al.* (1995) with permission.

When a capsaicin analogue was injected into the volar forearm of human subjects, heat pain was completely abolished whereas the threshold for sharpness and mechanically induced pain was not significantly altered (Davis *et al.* 1995). This dissociated loss of heat but not mechanical pain sensibility may be due to: (1) a selective action of capsaicin on heat transduction in nociceptors responsive to both heat and mechanical stimuli (Belmonte *et al.* 1991); or (2) an insensitivity to capsaicin of the subset of nociceptors responsible for signalling mechanically evoked pain and sharpness (for example, A-fibre nociceptors).

Mechanically insensitive afferents in the skin

The CMHs and AMHs discussed up to this point might be considered 'conventional' nociceptors. Conventional nociceptors are initially found by firmly squeezing the skin. These nociceptors are easy to find and a large literature has accumulated across many species that establishes in some detail their properties. The distribution of the mechanical thresholds of conventional nociceptors was shown in Fig. 5.14. Very few nociceptors had thresholds above 6 bar. The data shown in this figure correspond to values reported in other studies. Kumazawa and Perl (1977), for example, reported a mean threshold of 1.1 ± 0.7 bar in CMHs.

However, nociceptors that are not sensitive to mechanical stimuli may be important in cutaneous sensation. For example, intradermal injection of capsaicin produces an intense pain in human subjects, but results in a weak response in conventional nociceptors. Mechanically insensitive afferents have been reported in knee joint

(Schaible and Schmidt 1985), viscera (Häbler *et al.* 1988), and the cornea (Tanelian 1991).

To find mechanically insensitive afferents (MIAs) in the skin ideally would require the use of a technique that did not involve the use of an adequate stimulus. We previously showed that electrical stimuli did not have enduring effects on the response properties of nociceptors. We therefore investigated how electrical stimuli might be used to identify putative receptive fields.

When an electrical stimulus is applied to the skin, neural activity will be provoked in fibres of passage provided the stimulus intensity is sufficient. As the electrical stimulus is applied more distally, the electrical stimulus will in due course be applied to the area where the nociceptor terminates in the skin. Nociceptors taper as they terminate in the skin. Two electrical poperties are expected to change as a result of this:

1. The electrical threshold is expected to decrease as the fibre reaches a more superficial position.
2. The latency to response at the threshold electrical stimulus should increase in the region of the receptive field. This is because the diameter of nociceptive terminals becomes small, and therefore the conduction velocity becomes slow.

These predictions were indeed upheld. Figure 5.17 is a schematic drawing that shows how the electrical receptive field (eRF) was obtained. Typically, as the search electrode was moved distally along the course of the nerve, the action potential latency increased gradually. A region was usually found in which the suprathreshold latency no longer increased as the probe was moved distally. In this region, the latency at threshold usually increased abruptly and the electrical threshold decreased. An example of this is shown in Fig. 5.18 (A) for an A-fibre nociceptor. The eRF was defined as the region of maximum latency at threshold and minimum electrical threshold. Subsequent testing with mechanical stimuli (17 bar) in the region of the eRF revealed that this area was responsive to intense mechanical stimuli in the region indicated by the horizontal bar. The threshold for activation at the most sensitive spot within this zone was 7.3 bar. This afferent did not respond to a 51°C, 1-s heat stimulus but did respond (five action potentials) to a 53°C, 1-s stimulus.

As shown in Fig. 5.18 (B), the latency decreased in discrete steps as the electrical stimulation intensity at position 0 in Fig. 5.18 (A) increased. These stepwise latency shifts are also observed with electrical stimulation of the RF of conventional C- and A-fibre nociceptors. The collision experiments of Matthews (1977) suggest that these discrete steps in latency are due to the activation of successively larger and more proximal terminal branches of the receptor structure as the stimulus strength increases. Discrete drops in latency do not occur when the axon trunk is stimulated. The finding of these stepwise drops thus supports the contention that the eRF corresponds to the terminal endings of the nerve fibre in the skin.

Given a technique to identify fibres independent of the use of adequate stimuli, we are now able to characterize fibre types without necessarily biasing the sample toward afferents that respond to firm squeezing stimuli. MIAs are arbitrarily defined as fibres whose mechanical threshold is at least two standard deviations beyond the mean mechanical threshold of conventional nociceptors (Fig. 5.14; Meyer *et al.* 1991). Thus, fibres with thresholds greater than 6 bar are considered MIAs.

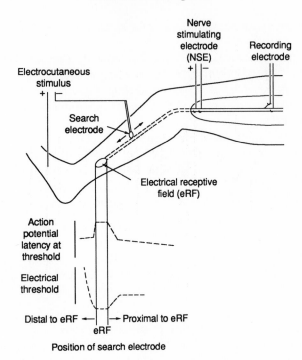

Fig. 5.17 Schematic drawing of electrical search technique. (Top) A bipolar electrode (cathode proximal) was placed on the nerve approximately 40 mm distal to the teased fibre recording electrode and was used to determine the number of fibres on the recording electrode. The electrocutaneous search was performed with a saline-soaked cotton swab search electrode (cathode) and remote needle return electrode (anode). (Bottom) As the search electrode was moved distally along the course of the nerve, the action potential latency at threshold gradually increased. In the vicinity of the electrical receptive field (eRF), the latency usually increased abruptly accompanied by a decrease in the electrical threshold. From Meyer *et al.* (1991) with permission.

Figure 5.19 shows how the properties of MIAs compare to those of mechanically sensitive afferents (MSAs). Ten of 23 C fibres (43 per cent) were classified as MIAs. Of the 10 MIA C fibres (excluding thermoreceptors), only two had no response whatsoever to mechanical stimuli. One of these responded to heat stimuli and the other responded to chemical stimuli. Thus, there were no C fibres that had no response to natural stimuli. Of 28 A-fibre nociceptors, 16 (57 per cent) were classified as MIAs. Of the 16 MIAs, five had no response to mechanical stimuli, but only one of these had no response to natural stimuli. This fibre developed mechanical sensitivity after exposure to a chemical stimulus. Two A-fibre MIAs were responsive only to chemical stimuli on initial testing. Cutaneous MIAs have also been reported in the rat (Handwerker *et al.* 1991) and pig (Lynn *et al.* 1995) skin. Recently, Schmidt *et al.* (1995) demonstrated that cutaneous C-fibre MIAs also exist in humans (see also Torebjörk *et al.*, Chapter 14, this volume).

The role of MIAs in sensation is unclear. The major interest in these fibres has been to investigate whether they may play a role in hyperalgesia. These fibres do indeed sensitize. The frequency of sensitization to heat and mechanical stimuli after chemical injury appears to be less in MIAs, however (Davis *et al.* 1993).

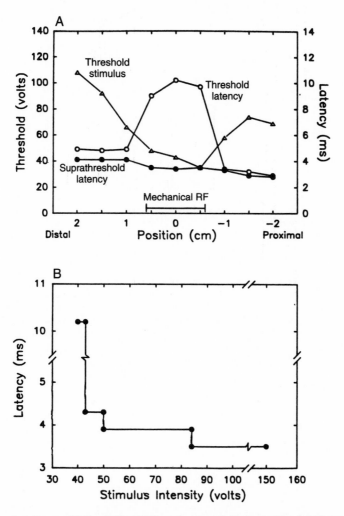

Fig. 5.18 Latency data from an Aδ-fibre MIA. (A) The action potential latency at threshold (open circles) and the suprathreshold latency (closed circles) are plotted as a function of distance from the centre of the electrical receptive field. In addition, the threshold voltage (open triangles) at each location is shown (stimulus duration was 0.1 ms). The horizontal bar indicates the location of a mechanical receptive field mapped with a 17-bar von Frey probe. As predicted in Fig. 5.17, the latency at threshold was higher and the threshold was lower in the region of the cutaneous RF. The 0 position was 85 mm from the recording electrode. (B) The action potential latency is plotted as a function of stimulus strength for the search electrode placed at the 0 position. As the stimulus strength increased, the latency decreased in a stepwise manner. From Meyer *et al.* (1991) with permission.

Responses to chemical stimuli

One thought about MIAs was that these fibres may be particularly important in mediating responses to chemical stimuli. To investigate this, we developed a mixture of inflammatory mediators thought to be important in pain that stems from tissue injury (bradykinin, serotonin, histamine, and prostaglandin E_1). We tested the responses of MIAs and MSAs to this inflamatory 'soup' (Davis *et al.* 1993).

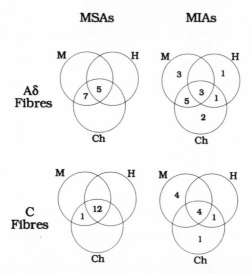

Fig. 5.19 Subclassification of fibres based on the stimulus modality to which the fibre responds. Chemo-sensitivity was based on response to a 10-μl injection of a mixture of inflammatory mediators (bradykinin, serotonin, histamine, and prostaglandin). Sensitivity to heat and mechanical stimuli was based on responses obtained before the chemical injection. The number of fibres in each submodality are indicated. M, mechanical stimuli; H, heat stimuli; Ch, chemical mixture. From Davis *et al.* (1993) with permission.

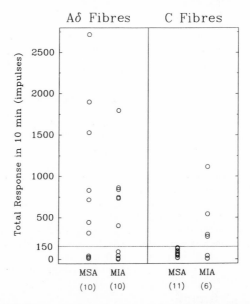

Fig. 5.20 Summary of chemically evoked activity. As a measure of the chemically evoked response, the total response during the 10 min after injection of the chemical mixture was computed. Each symbol represents the response of a single Aδ-fibre (left) or C-fibre (right) mechanically sensitive afferent (MSA) or mechanically insensitive afferent (MIA). Only those fibres that responded to the injection (that is, chemoresponsive) are shown. All of the C-fibre MSAs had a weak response to the chemical mixture (< 150 action potentials). In contrast, many of the C-fibre MIAs and most of the Aδ-fibre MIAs and MSAs had a strong response. From Davis *et al.* (1993) with permission.

Figure 5.20 shows the spectrum of the total neural response of individual MIAs and MSAs during the 10 min after injection of the soup. The largest responses were seen in Aδ MSAs, and the weakest responses were seen in conventional CMHs. MIAs had intermediate responses.

Coupling

Somatosensory fibres have generally been assumed to have no chemical or electrical synapses with one another outside the central nervous system. However, crosstalk between nerve fibres, presumably due to electrical coupling, has been observed in various forms of nerve injury. This prompted us to examine whether similar interactions between fibres might occur in normal peripheral nerves.

We used the teased-fibre preparation and added both distal (DSE) and proximal (PSE) stimulating electrodes (Fig. 5.21). In 3 per cent of cases we found evidence of coupling (Meyer *et al.* 1985*b*). Collision techniques (Fig. 5.21) establish that the coupling of action potential activity between two peripheral nerve fibres accounts for this phenomenon. In most cases the coupling is demonstrated between two C fibres. A single receptive field was identified and the responses at the receptive field indicated that a conventional CMH is involved in most cases. The action potential occurred with a fixed latency, suggesting ephaptic conduction rather than a chemical synapse. Procaine applied at the receptive field of the identified CMH temporarily abolished the coupling. Thus coupling was likely to occur at the receptive field. Two types of evidence corroborated the conclusion that the cutaneous receptor was associated with the coupled action potential produced by stimulation at the PSE. Mechanical stimulation of the receptive field, but not the surrounding skin, resulted in an increase in the latency of the coupled action potential from proximal electrode stimulation. Electrical simulation at the proximal site resulted in a subsequent decrease in response of the receptor to that stimulus. Sympathetic stimulation and sympathetic ablation experiments demonstrated that the sympathetic nervous system is not involved in this coupling.

The function of coupling is not clear. One noteworthy possibility is that coupling provides a basis for the flare response. The flare is part of the axon reflex and has been thought to result from antidromic invasion of axon branches after nociceptor activation.

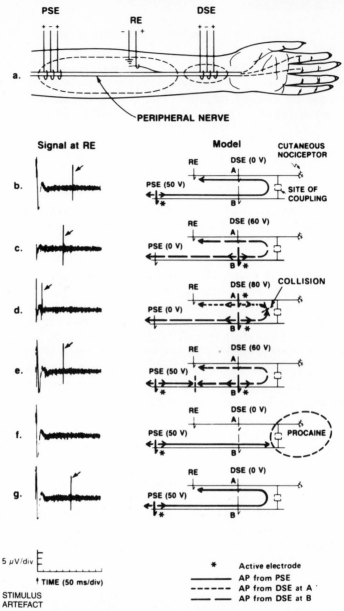

Fig. 5.21 Demonstration of action potential coupling between unmyelinated fibres in the normal peripheral nerve of the monkey. (a) Location of recording electrode (RE), proximal stimulating electrode (PSE), and distal stimulating electrode (DSE). All stimulus durations were 0.1 ms. (b) Electrical stimulation at the PSE resulted in an action potential (AP) at a latency of 280 ms (arrow points to the AP). On the right is the model we propose to explain the observation. The AP reached the RE via coupling between the fibres labelled A and B. (c) stimulation at the DSE at 60 V led to stimulation of fibre B only. The same AP occurred at a latency of 220 ms as a result of coupling between the fibres. (d) When the voltage at the DSE was increased to 80 v, the same AP occurred at a latency of 46 ms, which corresponded to the directly conducted AP. As depicted in the model, the coupled AP was not observed as a result of collision. Near the threshold for this directly conducted AP, the observed latency alternated between 46 and 200 ms. Two APs were never observed. (e) When the DSE (at 60 V) and PSE were activated simultaneously, a single AP occurred at the 220-ms latency. Near the DSE threshold for activation of fibre B, the observed latency alternated between 280 and 220 ms. Again, two APs were never observed. (f) A cutaneous receptor was associated with this AP, which had characteristics of a nociceptor. Intracutaneous injection of procaine (2 per cent, 0.05 ml) at the receptive field eliminated the coupled activity after PSE stimulation. (g) Forty minutes after this procaine injection, the coupled response returned. From Meyer *et al.* (1985) with permission.

Acknowledgements

We appreciate the assistance of J.L. Turnquist and T.V. Hartke. This research was supported by NIH grants NS-14447 and NS-32386 and a research grant from the Bristol-Myers Squibb Corporation.

References

Adriaensen, H., Gybels, J., Handewerker, H.O., and Van Hees, J. (1984). Suppression of C-fiber discharges upon repeated heat stimulation may explain characteristics of concomitant pain sensations. *Brain Res.* **302**, 203–11.

Beitel, R.E. and Dubner, R. (1976). Response of unmyelinated (C) polymodal nociceptors to thermal stimuli applied to monkey's face. *J. Physiol.* **39**, 1160–75.

Belmonte, C., Gallar, J., Pozo, M.A., and Rebollo, I. (1991). Excitation by irritant chemical substances of sensory afferent units in the cat's cornea. *J. Physiol., London* **437**, 709–25.

Bessou, P. and Perl, E.R. (1969). Response of cutaneous sensory units with unmyelinated fibers to noxious stimuli. *J. Neurophysiol.* **32**, 1025–43.

Bischoff, A. (1979). Congenital insensitivity to pain with anhidrosis. A morphometric study of sural nerve and cutaneous receptors in the human prepuce. In *Advances in pain research and therapy* (ed. J.J. Bonica, J.C. Liebeskind, and D.G. Albe-Fessard), pp. 53–65. Raven Press, New York.

Burgess, P.R. and Perl, E.R. (1967). Myelinated afferent fibres responding specifically to noxious stimulation of the skin. *J. Physiol. London* **190**, 541–62.

Campbell, J.N. and LaMotte, R.H. (1983). Latency to detection of first pain. *Brain Res.* **266**, 203–8.

Campbell, J.N. and Meyer, R.A. (1983). Sensitization of unmyelinated nociceptive afferents in the monkey varies with skin type. *J. Neurophysiol.* **49**, 98–110.

Campbell, J.N., Meyer, R.A., and LaMotte, R.H. (1979). Sensitization of myelinated nociceptive afferents that innervate monkey hand. *J. Neurophysiol.* **42**, 1669–79.

Campbell, J.N., Raja, S.N., and Meyer, R.A. (1984). Halothane sensitizes cutaneous nociceptors in monkeys. *J. Neurophysiol.* **52**, 762–70.

Campbell, J.N., Raja, S.N., Meyer, R.A., and Mackinnon, W.E. (1988). Myelinated afferents signal the hyperalgesia associated with nerve injury. *Pain* **32**, 89–94.

Darian-Smith, I., Johnson, K.O., LaMotte, C., Shigenaga, Y., Kenins, P., and Champness, P. (1979). Warm fibers innervating palmar and digital skin of the monkey: responses to thermal stimuli. *J. Neurophysiol.* **42**, 1297–315.

Davis, K.D., Meyer, R.A., and Campbell, J.N. (1993). Chemosensitivity and sensitization of nociceptive afferents that innervate the hairy skin of monkeys. *J. Neurophysiol.* **69**, 1071–81.

Davis, K.D., Meyer, R., Turnquist, L.L., Filloon, T.G., Pappagallo, M., and Campbell, J.N. (1995). Cutaneous injection of the capsaicin analogue, NE-21610, produces analgesia to heat but not to mechanical stimuli in man. *Pain* **61**, 17–26.

Dubner, R., Price, D.D., Beitel, R.E., and Hu, J.W. (1977). Peripheral nural correlates of behavior in monkey and human related to sensory-discriminative aspects of pain. In *Pain in the trigeminal region* (ed. D.J. Anderson and B. Matthews), pp. 57–66. Elsevier, Amsterdam.

Fitzgerald, M. and Lynn, B. 1977). The sensitization of high threshold mechanoreceptors with myelinated axons by repeated heating. *J. Physiol.* **265**, 549–63.

Garell, P.C. and Greensan, J.D. (1994). A comparison of the mechanical response properties of myelinated vs. unmyelinated nociceptors and their relationship to perception. *Proc. Neurosci. Abstr.* **19**, 324.

Georgopoulos, A.P. (1976). Functional properties of primary afferent units probably related to pain mechanisms in primate glabrous skin. *J. Neurophysiol.* **39**, 71–83.

Greenspan, J.D. and McGillis, S.L.B. (1991). Stimulus features relevant to the perception of sharpness and mehanically evoked cutaneous pain. *Somatosens. Motor Res.* **8**, 137–47.

Gybels, J., Handwerker, H.O., and Van Hees, J. (1979). A comparison between the discharge of human nociceptive nerve fibers and the subjects ratings of his sensations. *J. Physiol., London* **292**, 193–206.

Häbler, H.-J., Jänig, W., and Koltzenburg, M. 1988). A novel type of unmyelinated chemosensitive nociceptor in the acutely inflamed urinary bladder. *Agents Actions* **25**, 219–21.

Hagbarth, K.E., Hongell, A., Hallin, R.G., and Torebjörk, H.E. (1970). Afferent impulses in median nerve fascicles evoked by tactile stimuli of the human hand. *Brain Res.* **24**, 423–42.

Handwerker, H.O., Kilo, S., and Reeh, P.W. (1991). Unresponsive afferent nerve fibres in the sural nerve of the rat. *J. Physiol.* **435**, 229–42.

Hensel, H. (1950). Die intracutane Temperaturbewegung bei Einwirkung äusserer Temperaturreize. *Pflüger's Archiv,* **252**, 146–64.

Johnson, K.O. (1983). Neural mechanisms of tactual form and texture discrimination. *Fed. Proc.* **42**, 2542–7.

Johnson, K.O., Darian-Smith, I., and LaMotte, C. (1973). Periperal neural determinants of temperature discrimination in man: a correlative study of responses to cooling skin. J. Neurophysiol. **36**, 347–70.

Johnson, K.O., Darian-Smith, I., and LaMotte, C., Johnson, B., and Oldfield, S. (1979). Coding of incremental changes in skin temperature by a population of warm fibers in the monkey: correlation with intensity discrimination in man. *J. Neurophysiol.* **42**, 1332–53.

Konietzny, F. and Hensel, H. 1975). Warm fiber activity in human skin nerves. *Eur. J. Physiol.* **359**, 265–7.

Kumazawa, T. and Perl, E.R. (1977). Primate cutaneous sensory units with unmyelinated (C) fibers. *J. Neurophysiol.* **40**, 1325–38.

LaMotte, R.H. and Campbell, J.N. (1978). Comparison of responses of warm and nociceptive C-fiber afferents in monkey with human judgements of thermal pain. *J. Neurophysiol.* **41**, 509–28.

Lewis, T. and Pochin, E.E. (1937). The double pan response of the human skin to a single stimulus. *Clin. Sci.* **3**, 67–76.

Lundberg, L.E.R., Jorum, E., Holm, E., and Torebjörk, H.E. (1992). Intra-neural electrical stimulation of cutaneous nociceptive fibres in humans: effects of different pulse patterns on magnitude of pain. *Acta physiol. scand.* **146**, 41–8.

Lynn, B. 1979). The heat sensitization of polymodal nociceptors in the rabbit and its independence of the local blood flow. *J. Physiol.* **287**, 493–507.

Lynn, B., Faulstroh, K., and Pierau, F.-K. (1995). The classification and properties of nociceptive afferent units from the skin of the anaesthetized pig. *Eur. J. Neurosci.* **7**, 431–7.

Matthews, B. (1977). Responses of intradental nerves to electrical and thermal stimulation of teeth in dogs. *J. Physiol., London* **264** 641–64.

Meyer, R.A. and Campbell, J.N. (1981*a*). Myelinated nociceptive afferents account for the hyperalgesia that follows a burn to the hand. *Science* **231**, 1527–9.

Meyer, R.A. and Campbell, J.N. (1981*b*). Peripheral neural coding of pain sensation. *Johns Hopkins appl. Phys. Lab. tech. Digest* **2**, 164–71.

Meyer, R.A., Campbell, J.N., and Raja, S.N. (1985*a*). Peripheral neural mechanisms of cutaneous hyperalgesia. In *Advances in pain research and therapy*, Vol. 9 (ed. H.L. Fields, R. Dubner, and F. Cervero), pp. 53–71. Raven Press, New York.

Meyer, R.A., Raja, S.N., and Campbell, J.N. (1985*b*). Coupling of action potential activity between unmyelinated fibers in the peripheral nerve of monkey. *Science* **227**, 184–7.

Meyer, R.A., Davis, K.D., Cohen, R.H., Treede, R.-D., and Campbell, J.N. (1991). Mechanically insensitive afferents (MIAs) in cutaneous nerves of monkey. *Brain Res.* **562**, 252–61.

Nordin, M. (1990). Low-threshold mechanoreceptive and nociceptive units with unmyelinated (C) fibres in the human supraorbital nerve. *J. Physiol., London* **426**, 229–40.

Perl, E.R. (1968). Myelinated afferent fibres innervating the primate skin and their response to noxious stimuli. *J. Physiol., London* **197**, 593–615.

Raja, S.N., Meyer, R.A., Campbell, J.N., and Khan, A.A. (1986). Narcotics do not alter the heat response of unmyelinated primary afferents in monkeys. *Anesthesiology* **65**, 468–73.

Roberts, W.J. and Elardo, S.M. (1985). Sympathetic activation of A-delta nociceptors. *Somatosens. Res.* **3**, 33–44.

Schaible, H.G. and Schmidt, R.F. (1985). Effects of an experimental arthritis on the sensory properties of fine articular afferent units. *J. Neurophysiol.* **54**, 1109–22.

Schmidt, R., Schmelz, M., Forster, C., Ringkamp, M., Torebjörk, H.E., and Handwerker, H.O. (1995). Novel classes of responsive and unresponsive C nociceptors in human skin. *J. Neurosci.* **15**, 333–41.

Schneider, W., Slugg, R.M., Turnquist, B.P., Meyer, R.A., and Campbell, J.N. (1955). An electromechanical stimulator system for neurophysiological and psycophysical studies of pain. *J. Neurosci. Meth.* **60**, 135–40.

Sherrington, C.S. (1906). *The integrative action of the nervous system.* Scribner, New York.

Sinclair, D.C. and Hinshaw, J.R. (1950). A comparison of the sensory dissociation produced by procaine and by limb compression. *Brain* **73**, 480–98.

Slugg, R.M., Meyer, R.A., and Campbell, J.N. (1994). Suppression of response of cutaneous C- and A-fiber nociceptors in the monkey to repeated mechanical stimuli differs. *Soc. Neurosci. Abstr.* **20**, 1570.

Tanelian, D.L. (1991). Cholinergic activation of a population of corneal afferent nerves. *Exp. Brain Res.* **86**, 414–20.

Tillman, D.B. (1992). Heat response properties of unmyelinated nociceptors. Unpublished D.Phil. dissertation, Johns Hopkins University, Baltimore, Maryland.

Tillman, D.B., Treede, R.-D., Meyer, R.A., and Campbell, J.N. (1955a). Response of C-fiber nociceptors in the anesthetized monkey to heat stimuli: estimates of receptor depth and threshold. *J. Physiol.* **485**(3), 753–65..

Tillman, D.B., Treede, R.-D., Meyer, R.A., and Campbell, J.N. (1955b). Response of C-fiber nociceptors in the anesthetized monkey to heat stimuli: correlation with pain threshold in humans. *J. Physiol.* **485**(3), 766–74.

Torebjörk, H.E. (1974). Afferent C units responding to mechanical thermal and chemical stimuli in human non-glabrous skin. *Acta Physiol. Scand.* **92**, 374–90.

Torebjörk, H.E. and Hallin, R.G. (1973). Perceptual changes accompanying controlled pre-ferential blocking of A and C fibre responses in intact human skin nerves. *Exp. Brain Res.* **16**, 321–32.

Torebjörk, E. and Ochoa, J. (1980). Specific sensations evoked by activity in single identified sensory units in man. *Acta Physiol. Scand.* **110**, 445–7.

Torebjörk, H.E., LaMotte, R.H., and Robinson, C.J. (1984). Peripheral neural correlates of magnitude of cutaneous pain and hyperalgesia: simultaneous recordings in humans of sensory judgements of pain and evoked responses in nociceptors with C-fibers. *J. Neurophysiol.* **51**, 325–39.

Treede, R.-D., Meyer, R.A., and Campbell, J.N. (1990). Comparison of heat and mechanical receptive fields of cutaneous C-fiber nociceptors in monkey. *J. Nerophysiol.* **64**, 1502–13.

Treede, R.-D., Meyer, R.A., Raja, S.N., and Campbell, J.N. (1995). Evidence for two different heat transduction mechanisms in nociceptive primary afferents innervating monkey skin. *J. Physiol.* **483**, 747–58.

Van Hees, J. and Gybels, J.C. (1981). Nociceptor activity in human nerve during painful and non-painful skin stimulation. *J. Neurol. Neurosurg. Psychiat.* **44**, 600–7.

6 Corneal nociceptors

CARLOS BELMONTE AND JUANA GALLAR

Introduction

Early studies on corneal innervation and sensitivity played an important role in our present understanding of the neurobiology of peripheral pain. In 1894, von Frey stated that different modalities of cutaneous sensation were subserved by morphologically distinct populations of sensory fibres and that unspecialized free nerve terminals were the origin of pain. This early version of the 'specificity theory' of sensory discrimination was partly based on the observation that pain was the sole sensation that could be evoked from the cornea which was innervated exclusively by free nerve endings. von Frey's theory was challenged by Weddell and colleagues (Weddell and Zander 1950; Zander and Weddell 1951; Lele and Weddell 1956, 1959), again using the cornea as a model. These authors concluded that different qualities of sensations were evoked by the stimulation of the human cornea with various forms of energy, in spite of the unspecialized morphological and functional characteristics of corneal afferents (Lele and Weddell 1956, 1959). The capacity of apparently identical nerve fibres to evoke different sensations was taken as a key argument to support the alternative 'pattern theory' of sensory discrimination. According to this view, non-noxious and noxious stimuli were distinguished in the central nervous system by the different temporal course of nerve discharges evoked at non-specialized peripheral terminals. On the basis of their electrophysiological data obtained in corneal free nerve endings, it was proposed that 'an effective stimulus will cause spatially as well as temporally dispersed pattern of activity to be transmitted to the central nervous system. Sensory discrimination may, therefore, be dependent upon the central analysis of the space-time pattern of this activity' (Lele and Weddell 1956, 1959). About a decade later, the alternative possibility that the detection of injurious stimuli depends on a functionally specific population of sensory fibres, the nociceptors (Iggo 1963; Bessou and Perl 1969), gained progressive support (Light 1992; see Perl, Chapter 1, this volume). Nevertheless, the cornea remained an apparent and unexplored 'exception' to this rule. It took another decade to prove experimentally that corneal sensory afferents are functionally similar to nociceptive fibres innervating the skin and other territories of the body (Giraldez *et al.* 1979; Belmonte and Giraldez 1981).

The cornea is an avascular tissue of ectodermal origin, with a very simple structure (Maurice 1962). The external surface is formed by a polystratified epithelium, while a single-layered endothelium covers the internal surface. The stroma or substantia propria, represents about 90 per cent of the tissue and consists of collagen and of large, flattened fibroblasts (keratocytes or stromal cells).

The cornea is the first optical medium for the transmission of the light to the retina. It also represents the outermost barrier for the defence of the eye against injury and infection. Therefore, it is not surprising that the cornea possesses the most dense sensory innervation of the body: it has been estimated that the cornea contains 300–600 times more sensory endings than the skin and 20–40 times more than the tooth pulp (Rózsa and Beuerman 1982). As is discussed below, most of this innervation appears to be nociceptive in nature. This abundance in nociceptive terminals, together with the absence of blood vessels and the structural simplicity of the supporting tissues, makes the cornea a good model for analyzing the morphological and functional properties of peripheral nociceptors (Belmonte *et al.* 1994).

Corneal trigeminal neurones

The cornea is almost exclusively innervated by sensory fibres in trigeminal ganglion neurones (Arvidson 1977; Marfurt 1981; Lehtosalo 1984; Morgan *et al.* 1987). Using fluorescence techniques that label adrenergic structures, a few sympathetic fibres have been also reported in the cornea (Laties and Jacobowitz 1964; Ehinger 1966). The existence of a weak parasympathetic innervation of the cornea, suggested by old histological studies but denied later (Palkama *et al.* 1986), has been recently confirmed in the rat (Marfurt and Jones 1995).

In mammalian species (mouse, rat, guinea-pig, cat, and monkey), about 95 per cent of trigeminal neurones innervating the cornea are located in the anteromedial side (ophthalmic division) of the ganglion (Arvidson 1977; Morgan *et al.* 1978, 1987; Kuwayama *et al.* 1987; Marfurt and DelToro 1987; Marfurt and Echtenkamp 1988; Tusscher *et al.* 1988; Ichikawa *et al.* 1993; Passagia *et al.* 1993); the remaining 4 per cent are found in the maxillary region (Morgan *et al.* 1978, 1987; Marfurt and Echtenkamp 1988). Retrograde labelling studies have shown that the number of corneal trigeminal cells varies between 100 and 900 depending on the staining technique and the animal employed. The total number of neurones in the trigeminal ganglion has been estimated to be around 50 000 in the rat and cat (Dixon 1963; Gregg and Dixon 1973); thus, corneal neurones represent less than 2 per cent of this total. Most corneal sensory neurones are small (diameter of less than 20 μm; mean surface, 200–400 μm^2) and with dark cytoplasm (type B, Duce and Keen 1977), while a small proportion (about 11 per cent) are medium-sized neurones, with clear cytoplasm (diameter, 20–33 μm; mean surface, 500-800 μm^2) (Martin and Dolivo 1983; Sugimoto *et al.* 1988). Both small- and medium-sized cells belong to the group of primary sensory neurones with unmyelinated or thin myelinated peripheral axons.

About 40 per cent of trigeminal neurones innervating the cornea and conjunctiva are tachykinin-positive (Lehtosalo 1984; Lehtosalo *et al.* 1984; Ichikawa *et al.* 1993; LaVail *et al.* 1993). Among rat trigeminal cells, identified as ocular by retrograde labelling with cholera toxin introduced in the anterior chamber, 18.5 per cent were reactive to substance P (SP), 40.4 per cent to calcitonin gene-related peptide (CGRP), and 2.7 per cent to cholecystokinin (CCK) (Kuwayama *et al.* 1987). This relative incidence of peptides in ocular trigeminal cells is similar for sensory neurones in the rat ganglion as a whole (Lee *et al.* 1985); in this species, virtually all ocular SP-containing cells are also reactive to CGRP (Terenghi *et al.* 1985).

Nerve pathways to the cornea

The peripheral axons of sensory neurones innervating the cornea leave the trigeminal ganglion as a part of the ophthalmic nerve and travel to the eye with the nasociliary nerve. According to morphological studies, a small proportion of corneal nerve fibres in monkeys and presumably also in humans reach the cornea through the maxillary nerve (Marfurt and Echtenkamp 1988). The ophthalmic nerve gives off the long ciliary nerves through the nasociliary branch and a sensory root to the ciliary ganglion, which in turn reach the eye through the short ciliary nerves (Attias 1912). Long and short ciliary nerves mix while travelling to the eye and pierce the sclera as 10–20 fine nerve trunks at the posterior pole of the eyeball, around the optic nerve; nevertheless there is a considerable anatomical variability among species in the number and point of entrance into the eye of the ciliary nerves (Grimes and von Sallmann 1960). In these nerve trunks, sensory fibres of small diameter (2–4 µm) and some of larger size (about 6 µm) are mixed with sympathetic axons supplied by neurones of the superior cervical ganglion, and with parasympathetic fibres originating in the ciliary and the pterygopalatine ganglia. These autonomic fibres innervate blood vessels, secretory epithelia, and muscle fibres within the eye and correspond to the vast majority of unmyelinated axons found in the ciliary nerves.

Nerve trunks entering the eye run anteriorly in the suprachoroidal space or the scleral substance to innervate scleral tissue, ciliary body, iris, and cornea. Most corneal fibres enter this tissue at the level of the sclera, forming large nerve bundles; a few fibres penetrate the cornea more superficially, some of them from nerve trunks running in the subconjunctiva and others from nerves in the episcleral tissue. These superficial fibres join with branches from the corneal scleral bundles and form at the transition zone between the conjunctiva and the cornea (the limbus) an episcleral pericorneal plexus (Zandell and Weddell 1951).

Pattern of neural organization in the cornea

Between 10 and 80 large nerve trunks, depending on the species, penetrate radially the collagenous stromal substantia propria at various sites around the corneal circumference. They represent the main neural supply to the cornea in non-primate species. Thinner nerve bundles arising from the pericorneal plexus also enter the most superficial layers of the stroma (Zandell and Weddell 1951; Lim and Ruskell 1978; (Fig. 6.1 (A), (B)).

Corneal nerve strands contain thin myelinated and unmyelinated axons. Myelinated fibres lose their myelin sheath early (Zander and Weddell 1951). When approaching the central region, axons branch off repeatedly to form the subepithelial plexus (Fig. 6.1). Axon terminals ascend from this plexus toward the stroma–epithelium interface, losing the perineural sheath. No nerve terminals have been found innervating the corneal endothelium. Ascending nerve filaments give off collaterals that run for long distances, predominantly in one direction within the basal epithelial layer, offering the characteristic appearance of a 'leash'. The leashes, formed by a few up to several dozen strands, run for long distances (0.2–2.5 mm) and produce extensions that ascend vertically, branching both vertically and horizontally, to reach the outer epithelial layers (Fig. 6.1 (B), (C)). They end as terminal enlargements or boutons between the wing cells, at a few microns of the corneal surface. Axons in the subepithelial plexus also produce terminals that ascend vertically, with or without branching, and reach the most superficial layers of the cornea. Some fibres ending as naked terminals in the anterior and medium portions of the stroma have also been described (Zander and Weddell 1951; Whitear 1960).

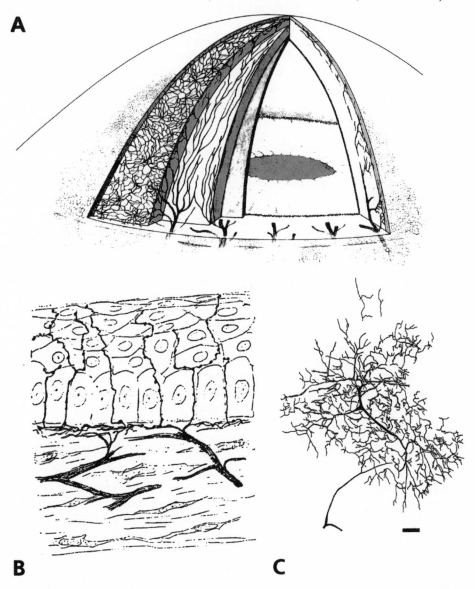

Fig. 6.1 (A) Representation of corneal innervation, showing the distribution of nerves in the different planes of the cornea. From R. Beuerman, in Maurice (1984). (B) Diagram illustrating the innervations of the corneal epithelium by ascending nerve filaments that show varicosities and end as terminal boutons at the level of wing cells. From Ramón y Cajal (1899). (C) Camera lucida drawing of the branching pattern of a parent axon in the epithelium of the mouse cornea. Scale bar, 0.1 mm. Courtesy of F. de Castro.

In the limbus of cat, monkey, and man (Whitear 1960; Lim and Ruskell 1978), fibres that are finer and more numerous than the deep stromal trunks form the episcleral plexus. Branches of this plexus are more superficial than the deep, radial stromal nerves and penetrate the cornea at the basal epithelial cell layer and immediately below the epithelial basement membrane (Chan-Ling 1989). In monkey, it has been suggested that most of the innervation of the corneal epithelium is provided by the limbal subepithelial plexus (Lim and Ruskell 1978). In the limbal area adrenergic fibres are frequently found, most of them innervating the blood vessels and other penetrating for short distances within the corneal tissue (see below). Also, endings with morphological specializations (Krause corpuscles) have been described in the limbus (Lawrenson and Ruskell 1991).

Fine structure of corneal nerve terminals

Electron microscopy studies (Whitear 1960; Matsuda 1968; Hoyes and Barber 1976; T. Tervo and Palkama 1978*a*, *b*; Beckers *et al.* 1992, 1993; Müller *et al.* 1996) have confirmed that nerve bundles running in the stroma contain several fibres (10–20) wrapped in a Schwann cell. The fibre diameters vary between 0.15 and 2 μm. Axon terminals traversing the epithelium-stroma interface are devoid of Schwann cells and present varicosities along their trajectory as well as at branching points (Fig. 6.2). In the basal layer of the epithelium, nerve fibres are invaginated into the epithelial cells in deep grooves containing one to more than one dozen axons. In the more superficial cells, thin nerve terminals (0.25 μm or less) run between epithelial cells and sometimes in a groove. There, the epithelial cells are in as close a relationship to the nerve fibres as are the Schwann cells in nerve bundles (Whitear 1960). Nerve varicosities contain neurotubuli, neurofilaments, and dark mitochondria in abundance. Numerous clear and incidental vesicles with small granules were also seen (Matsuda 1968; Hoyes and Barber 1976; Beckers *et al.* 1992; Müller *et al.* 1996). Terminals containing granular vesicles are more often observed near the limbus and are rare in the central cornea. They disappear after sympathectomy, which suggests that they belong to the scarce adrenergic fibres found in the avascular cornea (T. Tervo and A. Palkama 1978*a*).

Density of corneal innervation

Data on the number of nerve fibres present in the cornea are scarce, because of the difficulty involved in their quantification. The number of parent axons entering the cornea has been estimated to be 1200 in the human, each of which will produce 50 fibres subserving the epithelium (Lele and Weddell 1956). In the stroma of the rat, an average number of 60 nerve bundles and its branches were measured per mm^2 of cornea. The density was lower in the centre than in the periphery, possibly reflecting the penetration of the epithelium by stromal branches before they reach the central cornea (Ishida *et al.* 1984).

Rózsa and Beuerman (1982) reported a total of 6570 ± 1709 nerve endings in all layers of the epithelium in rabbits. The highest number of terminals was found in the wing cells layer, which almost double those present in the basal layer and the wing-superficial layer. Also, the innervation density was greater in the central cornea than in the periphery in agreement with the stromal nerve density data.

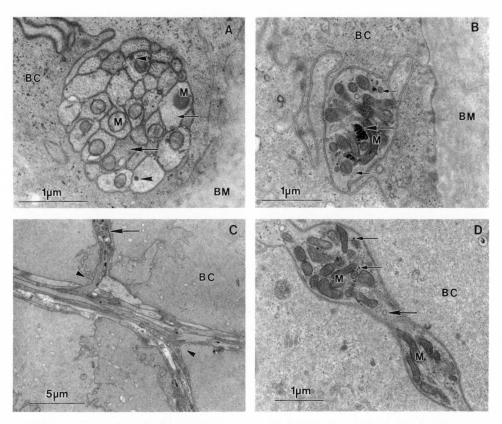

Fig. 6.2 Electron microscopy images of nerve fibres in the epithelium of the human cornea. (A) Cross-section through a nerve bundle, showing mitochondria (M), vesicles (arrowheads), microtubules (large arrow), and neurofilaments (small arrow). Magnification, $19\,712 \times$. (B) Cross-section of a single nerve fibre at the level of a bead, showing numerous mitochondria (M), glycogen particles (large arrow), and vesicles (small arrow). Magnification, $16\,576 \times$. (C) Frontal section of a nerve filament that bifurcates at the points indicated by the arrowheads. The single fibre running in the upper part of the picture has a bead filled with mitochondria (large arrow). Magnification, $3000 \times$. (D) Frontal section of a single fibre, showing two beads filled with numerous dark mitochondria (M), glycogen particles (small arrows), and vesicles (large arrow). Magnification, $12\,544 \times$. BC, Basal cell; BM, Bowman's membrane. Courtesy of Linda J. Müller; photographs (B)–(D) taken from Müller *et al.* (1996).

Histochemical heterogeneity of corneal nerves

The presence of SP-immunoreactive nerves in the cornea of various animal species including man is now well documented (Miller *et al.* 1981; K. Tervo *et al.* 1981; Stone *et al.* 1982; T. Tervo *et al.* 1982; Bynke *et al.* 1984; Lehtosalo 1984; Beckers *et al.* 1993}. The differences in density of SP innervation among reports is prominent, possibly due to technical difficulties and to poor penetration of antibodies (K. Tervo 1981). Corneal SP fibres originate in peptidergic neurones present in the trigeminal ganglion, because they disappear by maxillary and ophthalmic neurotomy (K. Tervo *et al.* 1982; T. Tervo *et al.* 1983). CGRP-immunoreactive nerves have been observed in the stroma and epithelium of the mammalian cornea and are eliminated by sensory denervation (Colin and Kruger

1986; Stone *et al.* 1986, 1987; Stone and McGlinn 1988; Beckers *et al.* 1992; see also Kruger and Halata, Chapter 2, this volume). Also, galanin-containing fibres, that disappear after combined superior cervical ganglion removal and intracranial transection of the ophthalmomaxillary nerve have been reported (Marfurt and Jones 1995). Finally, neurokinin A/neurokinin B immunoreactivity has been detected in corneal tissue (Beding-Barnekow *et al.* 1988).

Capsaicin, a toxin that depletes neuropeptides from sensory nerve terminals (see Buck and Burks 1986), eliminates SP and CGRP from the cornea as well as from corneal fibres immunoreactive to these peptides when administered neonatally (Gamse *et al.* 1981; Terenghi *et al.* 1986). However, the reduction in the number of corneal nerves varies greatly from one species to another and is often followed in later stages by hyper-reinnervation (K. Tervo 1981; Bynke *et al.* 1984; Fujita *et al.* 1984; Olgilvy and Borges 1990; Marfurt *et al.* 1993). This effect appears to be due in part to sprouting of capsaicin-resistant sensory nerves that include CGRP-containing sensory fibres (Marfurt *et al.* 1993).

As was mentioned above, the existence of a small number of corneal nerve fibres of sympathetic origin was repeatedly suggested by optical and electron microscopy studies (Laties and Jacobowitz 1964; Ehinger 1966; T. Tervo 1977; Terenghi *et al.* 1986; Marfurt and Ellis 1993). These fibres appear to be more abundant in prenatal stages (Ehinger and Sjöberg 1971; K. Tervo *et al.* 1978), but are present in adult corneas in a variety of animal species, including the human (Toivanen *et al.* 1987; Marfurt and Ellis 1993). Ocular adrenergic fibres apparently contain neuropeptide Y, because nerves immunoreactive to this peptide disappeared from the rat cornea after extirpation of the superior cervical ganglion (Stone 1986; Marfurt and Jones 1995).

In the rat, limbal and corneal vasoactive intestinal peptide (VIP)- and Met-enkephalin-immunoreactive nerve fibres have also been detected. These fibres were not affected by sympathetic and sensory denervation. Moreover, retrograde transport of wheat germ agglutinin–horseradish peroxidase (WGA–HRP) from the central cornea labels neurones in the ciliary ganglion and in the optic nerve sheath miniganglia, thus suggesing a parasympathetic origin for these corneal fibres (Marfurt and Jones 1995).

Development of corneal innervation

In mammals, invasion of corneal tissue by sensory nerves takes place at the early stages of embryonic development, although corneal innervation is not fully developed at birth (Lukas and Dolezel 1975; Ozanics *et al.* 1977; K. Tervo and T. Tervo 1981). Penetration of the epithelium by nerve processes occurs late in the fetal period and during the first postnatal days, as demonstrated by the increased number of neurites extending upward from the stroma toward the epithelium seen postnatally in the rat. Moreover, the electron microscopic appearance of corneal nerve terminals during the fetal period suggests that complete maturation of nerve endings is not achieved before birth (Ozanics *et al.* 1977; K. Tervo and T. Tervo 1981).

The time course of corneal innervation has been followed in detail in the developing avian cornea (Bee 1982; Bee *et al.* 1986, 1988). Initially (embronic day 5), nerves extend around the cornea to enclose it within a perilimbal ring. In a second phase (embryonic day 11), nerves penetrate radially into the midcorneal stroma, branch extensively, and innervate the epithelium at embryonic day 12. Nerves display extensive homology of position within the developing nerve ring, indicating that they follow specific pathways around the cornea. When bifurcation points of radial nerves are joined to its nearest neighbour on a line parallel of the cornea, a series of regular, non-overlapping, concentric circles is revealed (Bee *et al.* 1986). This suggests that the position of intracorneal nerve branching is also designated by the intracorneal milieu (Bee *et al.* 1986). Furthermore, the rate of radial growth of the eye and cornea determines the extension of nerves into the stroma (Bee and Locke 1992).

Corneal sensory nerves appear to be dependent on nerve growth factor (NGF) for their maturation as occurs with primary sensory neurones innervating other ectodermal tissues. NGF is produced by peripheral tissues and taken up by tyrosin kinase A (trkA), a high-affinity receptor present in sensory nerve terminals (Meakin and Shooter 1992). In transgenic mice deficient in trkA receptor (Smeyne *et al.* 1994), a very low number of corneal fibres was found. Furthermore, the blinking response of these animals to noxious mechanical stimuli, to saline at 0°C or 60°C, and to 10 mM acetic acid or 33 mM capsaicin was severely reduced (de Castro *et al.* 1995). Conversely, transgenic mice displaying an overproduction of NGF exhibited a hyperinnervation with a high density of abnormally thick corneal nerves (Crouch *et al.* 1995). This suggests that most corneal nociceptive neurones are NGF-dependent, although there is a small proportion of them that apparently do not depend on NGF for their development and behave functionally as polymodal nociceptive neurones (see below).

Functional types of corneal sensory neurones

General properties

Tower (1940) was the first to record the electrical activity of ocular sensory units evoked by mechanical stimulation of the cat corneal surface. Since then electrophysiological studies on corneal sensory afferents have been relatively scarce. Recordings have been performed mainly in anaesthetized cats (Lele and Weddell 1959; Giraldez *et al.* 1979; Belmonte and Giraldez 1981; Belmonte *et al.* 1991; Pozo *et al.* 1992; Gallar *et al.* 1993; Chen *et al.* 1995*a*) or rabbits (Tanelian and Beuerman 1984). Other experimental models include '*in vitro*' preparations of the isolated and perfused cornea of rat (Mark and Maurice 1977) or rabbit (Tanelian and MacIver 1990; MacIver and Tanelian 1993*a, b*) as well as preparations of the excised eye globe of the cat (Lele and Weddell 1959) or rat (Trimarchi 1967), or of the excised mouse eye conected to its trigeminal ganglion (López de Armentia *et al.* 1995).

Mechanical stimulation has been employed routinely to localize the corneal receptive area of nerve filaments displaying multiple- or single-unit activity. Each of the ciliary nerves containing corneal sensory fibres covers a quadrant or more of the cornea and a variable area of the adjacent conjunctiva, with a considerable overlap (Tower 1940; Lele and Weddell 1959; Mark and Maurice 1977; Giraldez *et al.* 1979). Single units dissected from these nerve trunks also have large receptive fields with a size of 50–200 mm^2 in the cat (Tower 1940) and 5–20 per cent of the corneal surface in the rabbit (Tanelian and Beuerman 1984). Receptive fields extend in most cases to the adjacent episclera, and partially overlap with those of neighbouring units. Figure 6.3 (A) shows the relative incidence of sensory fibres of the cat's cornea with small receptive fields restricted to the cornea (about 30 per cent) or with large receptive fields that extend into the limbus and adjacent episclera (70 per cent). Pure corneal fibres had slightly slower conduction velocities and gave a smaller response to acidic stimulation but were otherwise functionally similar to corneoscleral fibres (Belmonte *et al.* 1991).

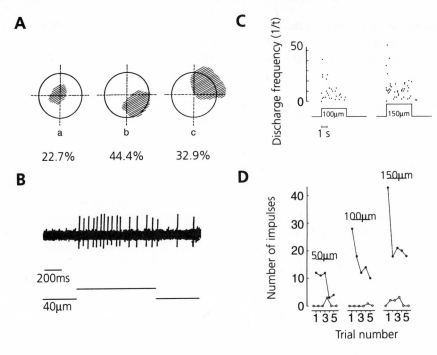

Fig. 6.3 Mechanical response of corneal nociceptors. (A) Location and relative incidence of the receptive area of single corneal mechanosensory units. (B) Sample record of the impulse response evoked by a square-wave indentation of the cornea. Note the postdischarge at the end of the stimulus. (C) Instantaneous frequency response of a single unit to two square-wave indentations of increasing amplitude. (D) Fatigue of the mechanical response of the unit represented in (C). The number of impulses evoked per stimulus (black circles) is plotted versus the stimulus order for three different series of 5-s square-wave indentations at the amplitudes indicated by each bar. The interval was 5 s between successive pulses of the same amplitude and 3 min between two series at different amplitudes. White circles represent the number of impulses fired during the interstimulus periods. From Giraldez (1979) and Belmonte and Giraldez (1981).

Spontaneous ongoing activity is always present in multiunit recordings of the ciliary nerves (Tower 1940; Lele and Weddell 1959; Belmonte *et al.* 1971; Mark and Maurice 1977). As will be discussed later, the contribution to this ongoing activity of the various functional classes of corneal sensory fibres is different. Furthermore, spontaneous activity also appears associated with the occurrence of corneal injury (see below).

Mechanosensory units

The existence of corneal units that respond exclusively to mechanical forces has been reported in the corneas of the cat and rabbit (Lele and Weddell 1959; Tanelian and Beuerman 1984; Belmonte *et al.* 1991; MacIver and Tanelian 1993*b*). These units belong to the highest conduction velocity group of corneal fibres and give large-amplitude, fast action potentials. Pure mechanosensory units represent about 30 per cent of the population of the thin myelinated fibres innervating the cat's cornea (Lele and Wedell 1959; Belmonte *et al.* 1991). In this species, the mechanical threshold of corneal mechanosensory fibres ranges between 0.11 and 1.96 mN with a mean value of 0.64 mN, which corresponds to a corneal indentation of about 40 μm. The mechanical threshold of these fibres in the rabbit is 3–4 times higher (mean, 2.2 mN with a range between 1.7 and 2.5 mN; Tanelian and Beuerman 1984; MacIver and Tanelian 1993*b*). Mechanosensory fibres are more easily excited by a moving stimulus than by a sustained indentation (Mosso and Kruger 1973; Belmonte and Giraldez 1981). When indentations of increasing force are applied, the impulse response is composed of an accelerating discharge of spikes, whose duration, latency, and instantaneous frequency are roughly proportional to the amplitude and velocity of the stimulus (Fig. 6.3). In most units, long-lasting mechanical pulses cause a complete adaptation of the response.

Within the receptive field of a mechanosensitive unit, there are differences in threshold between the centre and the periphery. In corneo-episcleral units of the cat, the threshold is usually lowest in the limbus and is 2–3 times higher as the stimulus is moved into the sclera (Belmonte *et al.* 1991). Using selective electrical stimulation, MacIver and Tanelian (1993*a*) showed that the receptive fields of mechanosensory units have an elongated shape that corresponds to the trajectory of the fibre. Stimuli moving parallel to the long axis of the receptive area produced maximal activation, while perpendicular stimuli were less effective. This organization may provide a certain degree of directional sensitivity to this type of fibre.

Polymodal units

The existence of a separate population of Aδ and C corneal units responding to mechanical forces, temperature changes, and chemical agents was established through the application of controlled mechanical, thermal, and chemical stimuli to the cat's cornea while recording single-unit activity of Aδ and C ciliary nerve afferents (Giraldez *et al.* 1979; Belmonte and Giraldez 1981; Belmonte *et al.* 1991; Gallar *et al.* 1993; Chen *et al.* 1995*a*). This class of fibres is the most abundant type of corneal sensory unit found in this species. Corneal polymodal units have large receptive fields (about 25 mm^2), that often cover the adjacent episclera. They are usually silent at rest but may fire occasional spikes at very low frequency (0.06/s in Aδ fibres; 0.1/s in C-fibres) in the absence of intended stimulation or of corneal damage.

Response to mechanical forces

Polymodal units respond to mechanical stimulation of the cornea with an irregular discharge of impulses as do pure mechanosensory fibres. However, polymodal afferents often show spontaneous activity and a slightly lower mechanical threshold than that of mechanosensory units. Also, in response to a sustained mechanical indentation, they give a tonic, irregular discharge that persists throughout the stimulus with a variable degree of adaptation and whose frequency is roughly proportional to the intensity of the applied force. They also show a postdischarge after high-intensity stimuli and fatigue when these are repeated at short intervals (Fig. 6.3). All these response characteristics—tonic discharge, fatigue, and long-lasting postdischarge—are more prominent in unmyelinated (C) than in thin myelinated (Aδ) polymodal units (Gallar *et al.* 1993).

Response to temperature changes

Heating of the cornea excites both Aδ and C polymodal units when temperatures over 38–39°C are attained. The response to a sudden, suprathreshold temperature elevation consists of an accelerating train of impulses, whose frequency reaches a peak and then decays gradually to a lower, maintained level (Fig. 6.4 (A)). During sustained heating of the cornea, this impulse discharge is irregular. Temperature increases between threshold and noxious levels are encoded by proportional elevations of the mean firing frequency of the impulse discharge (Fig. 6.4 (D)). Returning to basal temperature stops firing transiently. Nevertheless, when noxious thermal levels have been exceeded, activity resumes a few seconds later as an irregular, low-frequency background impulse discharge (Fig. 6.4 (B, C); Giraldez *et al.* 1979; Belmonte and Giraldez 1981; Belmonte *et al.* 1991; Gallar *et al.* 1993).

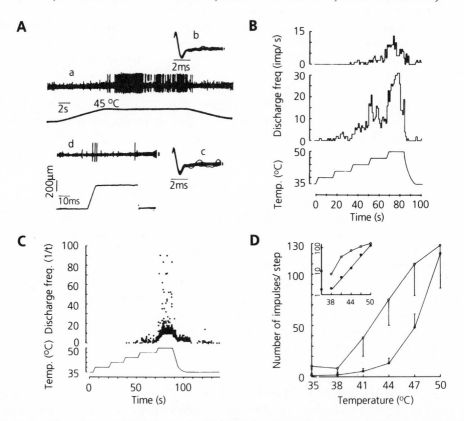

Fig. 6.4 Response of corneal nociceptors to heating. (A) Sample recording of the impulse discharge of a corneal unit evoked by a temperature elevation of the corneal surface to 45°C. The same unit (as judged by the shape of the action potential shown at higher speed) was also recruited by a mechanical indentation applied to the receptive area. (C) Instantaneous frequency of the impulse discharge evoked in a corneal unit by a stepwise heating. Note the postdischarge at the end of the stimulus, after a brief silent period. (B) Peristimulus time histograms obtained in the same corneal unit showing the first (upper) and the second (lower) response to two identical stepwise heat stimuli separated by 3 min. (D) Mean stimulus–response relation of a population of eight corneal units in response to the first (black circles) and the second (open circles) stepwise heating. Bars are SEM. In the inset, the same data are plotted in a log-linear scale. From Belmonte and Giraldez (1981).

Cold is usually ineffective in activating corneal polymodal units. Only a small proportion of Aδ fibres were weakly excited in the cat by temperature decreases within the noxious range (Belmonte and Giraldez 1981). In fact, temperature decreases below 20°C tend to diminish or silence background activity of polymodal afferents.

Response to chemicals

In the cat's cornea, afferent units exhibiting sensitivity to mechanical stimuli (and to heat, when this stimulus was tested) were classified as polymodal when they responded also to acid and/or hyperosmotic NaCl (Fig. 6.5 (A), (C)). The usefulness of NaCl in predicting the sensitivity of nociceptive terminals to other chemical agents, such as those acting as putative excitants during injury or inflammation (Handwerker 1991), is questionable. Possibly, the high concentration of extracellular Na^+ depolarizes small nerve terminals directly, by altering the distribution of charges across the membrane. In fact, only a fraction of corneal fibres that respond to NaCl are also excited by acid (Belmonte *et al.* 1991; Gallar *et al.* 1993).

Protons appear to be a more selective stimulus for nociceptive endings. In the skin, low-threshold mechanosensory fibres are not consistently excited by application of acid, but acid causes a sustained excitation of thin sensory fibres and strong pain (Lindahl 1961; Keele 1962; Steen *et al.* 1992). Local decreases in pH have been obtained in the cornea by topical application on the corneal surface of solutions of increasing concentrations of acetic acid (down to pH 4.5), or of a gas jet of CO_2 whose combination with water produces carbonic acid locally (Chen *et al.* 1995a). About 60 per cent of corneal fibres exhibiting mechanosensitivity also respond to acidic stimulation after a short latency, with an immediate discharge of impulses (Fig. 6.5 A,B) whose frequency is nearly proportional to proton concentration (Belmonte *et al.* 1991). Furthermore, when CO_2 stimulation is employed, in addition to fibres that respond immediately, a small number of units produces an impulse discharge that appeared after a latency of several seconds (Chen *et al.* 1995a).

The site of action of protons in corneal nerve endings has not been established. Buffered solutions of the same pH made with acetic acid (which penetrates the cell membrane easily) or with less permeable citric acid have comparable excitatory effects on corneal nerve endings, suggesting an extracellular binding site for protons, presumably a nonselective cationic channel (Belmonte *et al.* 1991). It has been hypothesized that capsaicin and protons may act at the same membrane site of the nociceptive ending (Rang 1991; Bevan and Geppetti 1994). In the cornea, capsaicin has an excitatory effect on both Aδ and C corneal polymodal units (Fig. 6.5 (D); Green and Tregear 1964; Belmonte *et al.* 1991; Gallar *et al.* 1993; Chen *et al.* 1996). At low concentrations (10^{-7} M) this excitatory action is not followed by inactivation. When higher doses (up to 33×10^{-3} M) are used, a complete inactivation to subsequent applications of the toxin and to mechanical stimulation, heat, or acid was observed in C-fibres (Belmonte *et al.* 1988, 1991; Gallar *et al.* 1993), while Aδ units retained their mechanosensitivity but lost the responsiveness to thermal and chemical stimulation (Fig. 6.8 (A)–(C); Belmonte *et al.* 1988, 1991). These data suggest that, in corneal polymodal nociceptors, sensitivity to protons and to mechanical stimuli are subserved by separate transduction mechanisms. On the other hand, the response of corneal polymodal units to low concentrations of capsaicin but not to protons, was blocked by capsazepine, a chemical analogue of capsaicin that acts as a competitive antagonist (Chen *et al.*, 1996). This observation speaks in favour of a distinct mechanism for the excitatory effects of protons and capsaicin on corneal polymodal fibres (see Garcia-Hirschfeld *et al.* 1995).

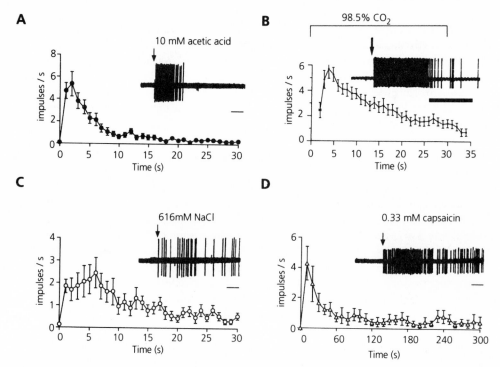

Fig. 6.5 Chemical response of corneal nociceptors. Frequency curves obtained with the pooled data of individual polymodal units responding to topical application to the cornea of: (A) acetic acid, 10 mM ($n = 31$); (B) a 98.5 per cent CO_2 pulse for 30 s ($n = 48$); (C) 616 mM NaCl ($n = 22$); (D) 0.33 mM capsaicin ($n = 14$). Time-scales: 0.5 s for (A) and (C); 4 s for B; 5 s for (D). From Gallar *et al.* 1993, Chen *et al.* 1995.

In addition to protons, other chemical agents that may be released during corneal injury and/or inflammation exert a direct excitatory effect on polymodal terminals. Bradykinin (BK) is a kinin produced during inflammation with an apparently prominent role in the genesis of pain. It excites consistently polymodal nociceptive endings of the skin, muscle, joints, and testis. Similarly, in the cornea of the cat, topical BK (10^{-5} M) evokes an impulse discharge in about 80 per cent of Aδ and C-polymodal fibres. This response outlasts the stimulation period and has a long latency and a slow onset, compared with other chemical stimuli, such as acid. Although a certain degree of tachyphylaxis is present, it does not seem to be as prominent in corneal nociceptors as in other preparations (Belmonte *et al.* 1994).

In the skin, the excitatory effects on nociceptors of inflammatory exudates have been reproduced with a mixture of BK, 5-hydroxytryptamine (5-HT), histamine, prostaglandin E_2 (PGE_2), SP (all at 10^{-5} M), and K^+ (7×10^{-3}M), at a pH of 7.0 (called inflammatory soup (IS); Kessler *et al.* 1992). As expected, application of IS to the cornea also excites polymodal nociceptors, in a more consistent and vigorous manner than when BK alone was applied.

SP and CGRP are contained in sensory nerve terminals of the cornea and are presumably released antidromically during nerve excitation (Unger 1990; also see below). Although SP seems to contribute to the local inflammatory reaction, no impulse activity was evoked in Aδ and C corneal polymodal nociceptive fibres by topical application of SP at concentrations up to 10^{-3} M. Moreover, responses to mechanical and chemical stimuli or sensitization to heat were not changed by pretreatment with this neuropeptide. The SP antagonists spantide and SP-150 did not vary neural activity or responsiveness of corneal nociceptors to acidic stimulation (Rebollo and Belmonte 1988). CGRP was equally ineffective in modifying spontaneous or evoked discharges of corneal polymodal units (Belmonte *et al.* 1994).

Mechanoheat units

The term mechanoheat nociceptor has been employed to characterize cutaneous nociceptors that are presumably polymodal, but in which chemosensitivity was not systematically explored (Meyer *et al.* 1994). In the cornea of the cat a small proportion of Aδ units presenting mechanical and thermal sensitivity but failing to respond initially to chemicals have been described. These fibres exhibited a high mechanical threshold and developed sensitivity to acid after repeated noxious heating (Fig. 6.6; Belmonte *et al.* 1991). Similarly, Aδ 'bimodal afferents', responding to high-intensity mechanical forces

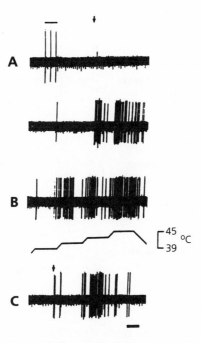

Fig. 6.6 Response of a mechanoheat unit to mechanical, chemical, and thermal stimulation and development of chemosensitivity by repeated heating. (A) Response to stimulation with a von Frey hair (horizontal bar) and absence of firing after the application of a drop of 10 mM acetic acid on the receptive area (arrow). (B) First (upper) and a second (lower) impulse response to two identical stepwise heat stimuli separated by 3 min. The lower trace shows the stimulus waveform. (C) Response to 10 mM acetic acid applied after heating. Time-scales for (A) and (B), 10 s; for C, 5 s. From Belmonte *et al.* (1991).

and to heat, but not to acetylcholine (ACh) have been reported in the rabbit cornea (MacIver and Tanelian 1993*b*). The comparatively high mechanical threshold of mechanoheat fibres of the cornea may indicate that they are in reality polymodal nociceptors whose endings are more deeply located into the epithelium or in the stroma (Lele and Weddell 1956). If this is true, mechanoheat units would represent the fraction of polymodal nociceptors with the highest chemical threshold, rather than a specific subpopulation of nociceptive fibres (Adriaensen *et al.* 1983; Belmonte *et al.* 1991).

Cold units

Changes in multiunit activity of corneal nerves induced by temperature reductions were described in early reports (Lele and Weddell 1959; Trimarchi 1967; Mark and Maurice 1977). Tanelian and Beuerman (1984), using a saline jet at controlled temperature, detected the existence in the rabbit cornea of sensory units conducting in the C range that responded to decreases in temperature. Similar units have been identified in the cat's cornea, where their functional properties have been studied in detail (Gallar *et al.* 1993). Cold-sensitive units are unmyelinated and fire spontaneously at the resting temperature of the cornea (around 33°C), giving an irregular discharge of impulses (0.75/s in the cat). They respond to cooling steps with a vigorous impulse discharge during the temperature drop, whose frequency is roughly proportional to the magnitude of the corneal

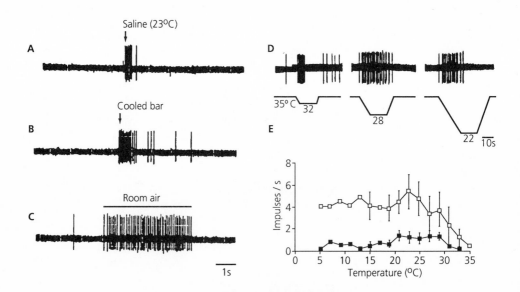

Fig. 6.7 Response of 'cold' nociceptive units. (A)–(C) Firing response of a single unit in response to: (A) a drop of isotonic saline a 23°C; (B) touching with an ice-cooled bar (arrow indicates the moment of stimulus application, which is maintained throughout the remaining recording time); and (C) blowing with an air jet at room temperature. (D) impulse discharge in a 'cold' nociceptive unit in response to constant-velocity cooling pulses of increasing amplitude applied with a contact thermode. (E) Average response of eleven units stimulated as in (D). Open squares: Response during the ramp. Filled squares: response during the steady-state part of the temperature pulse. From Gallar *et al.* (1993).

temperature reduction (Fig. 6.7 (D), (E)). However, sustained low temperatures gave similar impulse discharges irrespective of their value, indicating that these fibres do not encode steady-state corneal temperatures. In accordance with these response characteristics, cold units fire repeatedly when cold air is blown to the cornea, or when a drop of cold saline is applied (Fig. 6.7 (A)–(C)).

The receptive fields of corneal cold units (about 10 mm^2) are smaller than those of polymodal units and are preferentially found in the periphery of the cornea. Cold fibres do not respond consistently to mechanical stimulation, but have a weak response to acid and to hypertonic NaCl and are inactivated by 0.33 mM capsaicin.

Other types of corneal sensory units

The existence in the rabbit cornea of a specific population of chemosensory fibres, insensitive to mechanical or thermal stimuli has been suggested by Tanelian (1991) and MacIver and Tanelian (1993*b*). The chemosensitivity of such corneal fibres was based upon their excitation by ACh and also by a large battery of drugs that, in principle, cannot be considered natural chemical stimuli for corneal nociceptors (glutamate, *N*-methyl-D-aspartate (NMDA)), associated with an absence of response to subsequent mechanical stimulation or heat. Unfortunately, the authors do not provide information on the conduction velocity of the explored fibres, or on the magnitude and duration of the evoked impulse response; neither do they report whether several drugs were assayed in the same unit and what doses were employed. Therefore, it is difficult to exclude the possibility that depolarizations were still obtained through the excitation by a drug of the regenerative area of the axon, in spite of a blockade of the transducing region of the fibre to other stimuli. It has long been known that unmyelinated fibres (such as those of the cornea) are more susceptible to chemicals than the myelinated ones, because their regenerative region is more exposed (Paintal 1964). When responsiveness to CO_2 was systematically explored in the cat's cornea in a population of 62 Aδ and C fibres, only three sensory units initially sensitive to a jet of CO_2 could not be recruited by mechanical stimulation of the receptive field (Chen and Belmonte, unpublished results). With the available information, it seems premature to conclude that either these or the ACh-sensitive units found in the rabbit cornea represent pure chemosensory afferents, similar to mechanically insensitive (MIAs) or 'silent' nociceptors described in other territories (Schaible and Schmidt 1985; Meyer *et al.* 1994).

Limbal units

As was noted above, the margin of scleral conjunctiva immediately adjacent to the cornea (that is, the limbus) is innervated by collaterals of corneal axons (sclerocorneal units). Therefore, stimulation of the limbal portion of their receptive field excites both mechanosensory and polymodal sclerocorneal units. In addition, a small number of low-threshold mechanosensory units (mechanical threshold about 0.1 mN) have been found in the cat's eye. These units have a very small receptive field, almost restricted to the limbus, and a comparatively high conduction velocity (about 20 m/s). They adapt rapidly, giving only 2–4 impulses in response to a sustained stimulation and are insensitive to heat or cold (Gallar 1991). It can be speculated that nerve fibres with specialized terminals described in the limbus (Lawrenson and Ruskell 1991) are the morphological correlate of limbal, low-threshold mechanosensory units.

Also, cold fibres with functional properties somewhat different from those found in the cornea have been described in the limbal border and adjacent sclera of the cat's eye (Gallar *et al.* 1993). Such cold units have small receptive fields (of about 4 mm^2) and fire rhythmically at rest (33°C). They exhibit a dynamic and a tonic component in the impulse response caused by a sustained temperature reduction, thus resembling cold afferents of other territories (Hensel *et al.* 1960). Limbal cold receptors belong either to the low range of the Aδ or to the C-fibre type and, in contrast with corneal cold units, they are insensitive to chemical stimulation.

Relationship between the morphological and functional characteristics of corneal afferents

No morphological specialization has been found in corneal nerve terminals associated with the various functional classes of corneal afferents. Neither has it been feasible to correlate the functional types of corneal afferents with their neuropeptide content, while there is only a broad relationship between sensory modality and the size and myelinization of afferent fibres of the cornea: the mechanosensory units of cat and rabbit are always myelinated, while corneal 'cold' sensitive units are unmyelinated in both species (Tanelian and Beuerman 1984; Belmonte *et al.* 1991; Gallar *et al.* 1993). Nevertheless, polymodal fibres of the cat can be either thin myelinated or unmyelinated; this is only reflected in minor differences in responsiveness, which appear to be mainly associated with the size of the branching tree and with the diameter of the axon terminals but not with the transducing properties of the ending's membrane (Gallar *et al.* 1993).

On the other hand, the branching pattern and diameter of corneal afferents determine some of the functional characteristics of their receptive field. This has been demonstrated through the combination of epifluorescence microscopy of living nerve endings with electrophysiological recordings of single fibres (MacIver and Tanelian 1993*a*). Living nerve terminals originating in identified Aδ fibres, ran horizotally after traversing the basal lamina and formed elongated horizontal endings. Excitability maps in these fibres were composed of two to three continuous ridges that ran over the entire length of the elongated nerve endings observed by microscopy. On the other hand, C fibres produced nerve endings that form short branching clusters within the epithelium and end between the most superficial epithelial cells. In accordance with this morphological arrangement, the excitability map of C fibres was composed of spots that corresponded to clusters of nerve terminals separated by insensitive areas, with a variable density and number of excitability peaks per fibre.

Transduction mechanisms in corneal nociceptors

Corneal nociceptors possibly share common transduction mechanisms with nociceptors of other territories, as suggested by their morphological and functional similarities. Molecular and cellular processes involved in the transduction by nociceptive terminals of different territories to the various modalites of stimuli are still unknown to a great extent (Belmonte *et al.* 1994). The same is true for corneal nociceptors, where the evidence, albeit indirect, suggests that separate mechanisms exists for the transduction of chemical and mechanical stimuli (see above). As was proposed for other nociceptors, it is conceivable that non-selective cationic channels are responsible for the depolarization of corneal terminals by noxious chemical and mechanical stimuli (Shepherd 1991).

Modification by injury and inflammation of corneal nociceptor responses

Once the cornea is damaged, a cascade of events results in an enhanced responsiveness of nociceptors (sensitization). The main difference between the cornea and other territories is that the absence of blood vessels prevents the rapid access of blood-borne substances to the injured area. However, polymorphonuclear leucocytes (PMNs) and mononuclear cells appear in the edges of corneal wound as early as 2–3 h after injury (Bazan 1990). Also, as a consequence of the insult, several biochemical changes take place in corneal tissue including the formation of several mediators of inflammation. The metabolites of arachidonic acid (AA) are generated through two major pathways, cyclooxygenase and lipooxygenase. However, epoxidation of AA by a microsomal cytochrome P450-dependent mixed-function oxidase system has been also described in the cornea (Schwartzman *et al.* 1985, 1987). The basal synthesis of eicosanoids in the cornea is greatly increased after injury. Cyclooxygenase metabolites augment in the stroma and epithelium 2 h after a cryogenic injury of the cornea. The main metabolites in the epithelium are $PGF_{2\alpha}$ and PGE_2, while activated keratocytes of the stroma produce mainly PGI_2 and thromboxane A_2 (TXA_2). A rapid increase of the lipoxygenase metabolites, 5-HETE and 12-HETE, particularly in the epithelium has been detected after injury (Bazan 1990). Epoxyeicosatrienoid acids are generated in the cornea through the cytochrome P450 system. Finally, synthesis of platelet-activating factor (PAF) occurs soon after corneal lesioning.

Sensitization of corneal nociceptors

The lipid inflammatory mediators generated by corneal cells, together with those released by activated PMNs and macrophages, are expected to contribute to nociceptor sensitization, as occurs in other territories (Handwerker and Reeh 1991). However, experimental information about the effect of these substances on corneal nociceptors is very scarce.

Sensitization of corneal nociceptors *in vivo* is seen in the cat when repeated 'staircase' heating pulses are applied to the receptive field of corneal polymodal units (Belmonte and Giraldez 1981; Gallar *et al.* 1993). In about 70 per cent of the Aδ and C corneal polymodal units, repetition of heat pulses over 40–45°C led to a 2–3 fold increase of the number of impulses evoked by a given temperature and a decrease of threshold of about 3°C. Also, poststimulus background activity appears (Fig. 6.4 (C)). No changes in mechanical threshold are apparent in heat-sensitized units. A proportion of the polymodal units do not develop sensitization or become totally or partially inactivated after repeated heating; this phenomenon is more prominent in C polymodal units.

Calcium ions seem to be necessary for sensitization to heat. When corneal nociceptors were superfused with a calcium-free medium, firing activity evoked by acid was preserved, but responses to heat and sensitization disappeared (Chen *et al.* 1994; Belmonte *et al.* 1994). Whether this is an effect on the nerve ending itself, on the epithelial cell, or on both cannot be inferred from these experiments.

Corneal mechanoheat fibres are also sensitized by repeated heating. Under these circumstances, they become responsive to topical application of acetic acid (Fig. 6.6). This observation lends support to the hypothesis that mechanoheat units are polymodal nociceptors with a weak chemical sensitivity (Belmonte *et al.* 1991).

Only a few of the known mediators of corneal inflammation have been tested for their sensitizing effect on nociceptive nerve fibres of the cornea. PGE_2 (10^{-7} to 10^{-4} M) increased spontaneous activity of Aδ and C polymodal nociceptors of the cat in a dose-dependent manner (Gallar and Belmonte 1990). Furthermore, responses to topical application of 10 mM acetic acid were significantly enhanced after PG administration, thus suggesting that endogenous PGE_2 released during corneal injury may be one of the substances contributing to sensitization of corneal polymodal nociceptors. The role of leukotrienes, PAF, and other putative inflammatory mediators generated during corneal inflammation in the sensitization process is still unexplored.

Electrical activity in corneal afferents following injury

Acute mechanical injury of the cornea elicits a high-frequency discharge in corneal polymodal nociceptors that is followed by a long-lasting afterdischarge. Immediately after damage, threshold and near-threshold responses were depressed, but renewal of the ongoing activity was often produced by mild periliminal stimulation. Similar effects were observed when a strong acid (0.1 N HCl) was applied to the corneal surface (Belmonte and Giraldez 1981). At longer periods of time after mechanical wounding of the rabbit cornea (up to 7 days), spontaneous corneal nerve activity was not found to be markedly increased, although mild mechanical or chemical stimuli of the wound margin would elicit spontaneous firing that persisted for several hours. Also, an abnormal responsiveness to mechanical, thermal, and chemical stimuli was noticed: the borders of the wound showed an enhanced response to mechanical stimuli, whereas sensitivity was decreased in the centre of the wound. Application of hypertonic NaCl or 40°C saline evoked a vigorous impulse response that outlasted the stimulus, whereas cold saline silenced this activity (Beuerman *et al.* 1985). It is conceivable that this abnormal activity originated from neuromas of the injured axons, from sprouting nerve endings, or from sensitized intact terminals. Depending on the depth of a corneal wound, the magnitude of corneal nerve damage will be different (Beuerman and Kupke 1982) and, when the stroma is also affected, nerve trunks of the subepithelial plexus are presumably injured. Sprouting terminals arising from undamaged nerves as well as neuromas formed by severed axons are present in the margin of the lesioned area (see below). It would be interesting to determine the relative contribution of these fibres to nerve activity in damaged corneas. Also, more detailed studies are required to establish the responsiveness of the different subtypes of corneal nociceptors affected by injury.

Corneal sensory afferents may also be excited by tissue disturbances not accompanied by direct nerve damage. For instance, acute ocular hypertension evokes an activation of corneal sensory units (Zuazo *et al.* 1986). Also hypoxia and hypoglycaemia increase the spontaneous discharge of corneal unmyelinated fibres (MacIver and Tanelian 1992).

Plasticity and regeneration of corneal nerve fibres after injury

The continuous shedding of corneal epithelium cells influences the arrangement and dynamics of corneal nerve terminals. Examination of corneal nerve afferents innervating a selected territory of the intact corneal surface of mice after staining the nerves with the fluorescent dye 4-Di-2-ASP showed an extensive rearrangement of nerve terminals with time. Over a period of 24 h, changes in the position and appearance of epithelial endings were clear, although an overall similarity to initial configuration was retained. After 1 week, the architecture of terminal arborizations bears no resemblance with the initial branching pattern. In contrast, stromal nerves maintained a constant position (Harris and Purves 1989).

Sensory nerves of the cornea contain 43 kDa growth-assoctiated protein (GAP-43), a protein that is expressed in developing and regenerating neurones. This is co-localized with nerve-cell adhesion molecule (N-CAM). Moreover, an increase in the GAP-43 content of the corneal epithelium was noted after 24–48 h in corneas subjected to mild alkali injury. These data are interpreted as indicative of a synthesis of these proteins in the soma of sensory neurones to be carried by axonal transport to the cornea, where they will be involved in the continuous remodelling of corneal nerves (Martin and Bazan 1992).

Rearrangement of corneal sensory innervation also occurs when nerves are damaged by corneal injury or after experimental manipulations. Several studies have been devoted to analysing the remodelling of stromal and epithelial corneal nerves following corneal injury caused by epithelial wounding or by various surgical procedures developed for treatment of a heterogeneous group of ocular diseases (cataract removal, refraction defects, corneal opacities) that involve perilimbal or intracorneal incisions (radial or circular, with or without removal of a corneal bouton).

Small epithelial wounds of the cornea are covered in about 48 h by basal cells that migrate from the wound margin over the denuded area. In this type of wound (for instance, those produced by mechanical abrasion or by application of *n*-heptanol, which destroys only epithelium and intraepithelial nerves), a few terminals arriving from the subepithelial plexus outside the wound penetrate the wound in 2 days. Newly formed terminals originating at long distances occur irregularly around the wound margin in a radial fashion. Their density at the wound margin increases with time (from 39 fibres/mm on day two to 55 fibres/mm by day seven; Beuerman and Kupke 1982; de Leeuw and Chan 1989). These fibres result from sprouting of fibres of the subepithelial and deeper stromal nerves located outside the wound area. With time, regenerating axons progress at the basoepithelial level towards the wound centre, either as single axons or adopting a leash-like pattern oriented towards the centre of the wound. Partial regeneration of the epithelial nerves is completed after 3–4 weeks with no further improvements up to 10 weeks afer wounding (Beuerman and Kupke 1982; Beuerman and Rózsa 1984; de Leeuw and Chan 1989).

When stromal corneal wounds are performed, 24 hours later the wound margins are completely surrounded by long, large-calibre sprouts, originating in neighbouring intact axons, that course perpendicularly to the wound border. They reach a maximum density in about 72 h (54 terminals/mm). A second wave of regeneration takes place at around 7 days, now originating in transected axons of the subepithelial plexus. This process is accompanied by secondary degeneration of the collateral sprouts of intact axons (Rózsa *et al.* 1983; Beuerman and Rózsa 1984). A reduced nerve density in relation to the intact cornea was still observed months afterwards. Essentially similar results have been described in nerve lesions caused by photokeratectomy, in which an accurate excision of the corneal superficial stroma is performed with an excimer laser to modify the refractive power of the cornea (Pallicaris *et al.* 1990). In this case though, there is an increase in density of reinnervation in comparison with manually debrided or control corneas, with wider and longer leashes and a thicker subepithelial plexus, so that nerve density was significantly higher than normal 35 days after excimer laser surgery (Ishikawa *et al.* 1994; Trabucchi *et al.* 1994). This was accompanied by a significant enhancement of corneal sensitivity to mechanical stimulation (Ishikawa *et al.* 1994).

When penetrating perilimbal incisions covering half of the cornea are performed, such as those used in cataract or glaucoma surgery, the reinnervation process is much slower and incomplete. Nerve fibres distal to the lesion degenerate. New fibres enter the denervated area through the scar tissue, with minor contribution of axons originating in the innervated cornea (Rózsa *et al.* 1983). An abnormal and incomplete pattern of reinnervation persists more than 2 years later. Thus, it appears that the more proximal the nerve lesion, the more delayed and incomplete is the regeneration process. Also, in pure corneal incisions, the depth of the cut appears to be important in determining the degree of regeneration; this is incompletely achieved when it exceeds 50 per cent of the total corneal thickness (Chan-Ling *et al.* 1987, 1990). Similarly, corneal transplants in humans often remain devoid of nerve fibres for years and are invaded very slowly and incompletely by a reduced number of axons when reinnervation takes place (T. Tervo *et al.* 1985). This is not solely due to misalignment of Schwann cell channels by introduction of grafted tissue, because limited reinnervation also happens in cats in which a penetrating circular keratotomy was made. The formation of scar tissue appears to be a major obstacle for normal reinnervation (Chan-Ling *et al.* 1990).

Trophic interactions between the cornea and its innervation

The cornea, like other peripheral target tissues, appears to contribute to the survival and development of its sensory and autonomic innervation. Convincing experimental evidence of this trophic dependence of sensory neurones on corneal tissue was first obtained by Chan and Haschke (1981, 1982, 1985). These authors showed that neurone survival and neurite outgrowth were promoted by corneal and conjunctival epithelial cells co-cultured with trigeminal neurones (see also Garcia-Hirschfeld *et al.* 1994). This effect was attributed to the secretion by the epithelial cell of an 'epithelial neurono-trophic factor' (ENF), which also stimulated protein synthesis in cultured trigeminal neurones. A 2–4 times increase in the secretion of this ENF was reported after corneal wounding; such elevation was not parallel to the epithelial regeneration taking place during the first week of the wound closure process, but to the regeneration of intraepithelial nerves, which took place about 3 weeks after wounding (Chan *et al.* 1987).

There is additional experimental evidence supporting the promoting effect of corneal tissue on neurite outgrowth of corneal trigeminal neurones. *In vivo*, epithelial implants placed into the corneal stroma attract nerve spouts from deep stromal nerves and from the subepithelial plexus. These growing neurites penetrate the implant and form nerve terminals around epithelial cells, similar to those observed in normal epithelium (Emoto and Beuerman 1987). Also, when an epithelial lesion is made in the centre of the cornea, the subepithelial nerve leashes that in the intact rabbit cornea are predominantly oriented towards the nasal-most limbus, change their direction towards the wound margin, thus suggesting that a wound-derived factor is attracting the regenerating neurites (de Leeuw and Chan 1989). Finally, substance P appears in avian corneal nerves concomitantly with their penetration into the epithelium (Bee *et al.* 1988), thus suggesting that the signal for the production of this neuropeptide by corneal sensory neurones is given by corneal epithelium.

Molecules influencing the development of neurones belong to various classes of agents, including: the neurotrophin family NGF; brain-derived neurotrophic factor (BDNF); and neurotrophins -3, -4, and -5 (NT-3, NT-4, NT-5)); ciliary neurotrophic factor (CNTF); other growth factors (for example, fibroblast growth factor (FGF), epidermal growth factor (EGF), platelet-derived growth factor (PDGF)); cell adhesion molecules (for example, N-CAM, cadherins); and components of the extracellular matrix (for example, fibronectin, laminin, collagens, thrombospondin, tenascin) (Hagg *et al.* 1993; Korsching 1993). Therefore, with the available evidence, it is difficult to determine the correspondence of the ENF described by Chan and Haschke with any of the identified trophic molecules, although these authors suggested that it was not identical to NGF or to extracellular matrix proteins that promote neurite extension. As mentioned above, NGF seems to play an important role in the development of corneal innervation in prenatal stages (de Castro *et al.* 1995). Whether this is also true for the survival and regeneration of adult corneal sensory neurones remains to be determined.

An inverse trophic dependence, namely, of the corneal epithelium cells on their sensory innervation, was suspected for a long time after the clinical observation that damage of the corneal innervation in human patients, either for therapeutic purposes (Gasserian ganglionectomy) or by accident, led to the appearance of severe lesions in the corneal epithelium called keratitis neuroparalytica (Pannabecker 1944). Also, destruction of corneal sensory neurones in more controlled experimental conditions has shown that several disturbances appear in the corneal epithelium: impaired cell attachment and altered epithelium structure (Alper 1976; Beuerman and Schimmelpfennig 1980; Araki *et al.* 1994); decreased mitotic rate (Sigelman and Friedenwald 1954; Mishima 1957); increased permeability (Beuerman and Schimmelpfennig 1980); reduction of glycogen content (Gilbard and Rossi 1990); and delayed wound healing rate (Araki *et al.* 1994). These alterations are conducive to recurrent corneal erosion of denervated corneas (Alper 1976).

The existence of trophic influences of sensory neurones on corneal epithelial cells has been shown experimentally in co-cultures of trigeminal neurones with corneal epithelial cells. When co-cultured with trigeminal sensory neurones, corneal epithelial cells increase their mitotic rate and number (Garcia-Hirschfeld *et al.* 1994) and express type VII collagen, a component of anchoring fibrils that adhere epithelial cells of the cornea to their basement membrane (Baker *et al.* 1993).

Indirect evidence suggests that such neurotrophic influences may be mediated at least in part, by neuropeptides contained in corneal sensory terminals. During embryonic development, the opaque cornea becomes transparent, a process that depends on the pumping of water by the epithelium cells; this phenomenon takes place in parallel with the appearance of SP in the nerves of the avian cornea (Bee *et al.* 1988). Capsaicin administered neonatally destroys a large amount of small peptidergic neurones in the trigeminal ganglion including those innervating the cornea; in these animals, the loss of an important part of SP- and CGRP-containing nerves is accompanied by corneal signs of neuroparalytic keratitis; the severity of corneal lesions goes in parallel with the reduction of peptide-containing nerves (Buck *et al.* 1983; Fujita *et al.* 1984; Ogilvy and Borges 1990; Marfurt *et al.* 1993). Moreover, the healing rate of corneal epithelium wounds is delayed after retrobulbar injection of capsaicin (Gallar *et al.* 1990), a manoeuvre that blocks axoplasmic transport of neuropeptides in corneal nerves (Bynke 1983), while the healing rate is promoted by exogenous application of SP (Reid *et al.* 1990). Finally, SP enhanced the mitotic rate of corneal epithelium cells in culture (as did their co-culture with trigeminal neurones), while CGRP reduced it (Garcia-Hirschfeld *et al.* 1994). Therefore, there is experimental support for the possibility that SP and CGRP contained in sensory afferents modulate the functional activity of epithelial cells in the cornea, perhaps through antagonistic effects, thus contributing to the integrity of the normal cornea.

As was mentioned above, a sparse sympathetic innervation of the cornea has also been demonstrated by histochemical methods. Adrenergic fibres are abundant at the periphery of the cornea, where they innervate limbal blood vessels. However, their functional role in the avascular cornea is unknown. While sympathectomy modifies corneal mitotic rate and corneal ion transport (Butterfield and Neufeld 1977; Klyce *et al.* 1985), electrical stimulation of the cervical sympathetic nerve for prolonged periods of time delays the healing time of experimental corneal wounds (Pérez *et al.* 1987). *In vitro*, corneal epithelial cells increase their mitotic rate when they are co-cultured for long periods of time with sympathetic neurones (Garcia-Hirschfeld *et al.* 1994). These results suggest that sympathetic neurones may also participate in the trophic maintenance of corneal epithelium cells. In sympathectomized animals, a marked increase in CGRP immunoreactivity was observed, while in tissue subjected to sensory denervation the reverse was found (Unger *et al.* 1988). Moreover, in capsaicin-treated animals, a hyperreinnervation of the cornea by sympathetic sprouts has been described (Marfurt *et al.* 1993). This would reflect a trophic competition between sensory and adrenergic fibres in the cornea, as occurs in other territories (Kessler *et al.* 1983).

'Efferent' actions of corneal nociceptors

Corneal irritation and wounding is often accompanied by corneal oedema and also by miosis, aqueous humour flare, photophobia, conjunctival vasodilatation, lid oedema, and lacrimation. A part of these symptoms are attributable to neurogenic inflammation, caused by antidromic release by corneal nerves of neuropeptides (SP and CGRP) that enhance local inflammatory processes (Jancsó *et al.* 1966; Unger 1990). Topical application to the cornea of capsaicin or nitrogen mustard evokes this irritation response, which can be attenuated by denervation or blockade of corneal nerves with local anaesthetics or tetrodotoxin (Jampol *et al.* 1975; Szolcsányi *et al.* 1975; Camras and Bito 1980*a*, *b*; Gonzalez *et al.* 1993, 1995). Diltiazem, which blocks the responsiveness of corneal fibres to chemical irritants, also reduces corneal neurogenic inflammation (Pozo *et al.* 1992; Gonzalez *et al.* 1993, 1995; Gallar *et al.* 1995). Corneal nerve fibres branching into the perilimbal conjunctiva and the root of the iris (Zuazo *et al.* 1986) may become excited antidromically during corneal irritation and contribute to the intense conjunctival and iridal reaction developed during corneal injury. Also, photophobia (pain caused by light) following corneal injuries is possibly mediated by these fibres, which will cause neurogenic inflammation and sensitization of nociceptive endings of the iris (Mintenig *et al.* 1995).

Effect of drugs on corneal nociceptors

Topical anaesthetic agents are used routinely to obtain corneal anaesthesia. These include among others tetracaine, procaine, benoxinate, and proxymetacaine (proparacaine) (Ritchie and Greene 1985). These agents eliminate propagated action potentials through their well-known blocking effects on axonal Na^+ channels (Hille 1994). Interestingly, it has been reported that, in the cornea, lidocaine at low doses reduced multiunit, tonic discharges elicited by a corneal injury, while nerve impulses evoked by supramaximal electrical shocks persisted (Tanelian and MacIver 1991). However, this evidence is still insufficient to conclude that lidocaine at low concentrations has, in addition to the conventional blockade of propagated impulses, an additional selective effect on the ionic channels involved in the transduction process.

In spite of their usefulness for acute superficial anaesthesia, local anaesthetics have serious toxic effects on corneal epithelium and cannot be employed for prolonged elimination of neural activity evoked by a corneal wound. Pain is the main clinical problem in acute corneal lesions. Moreover, the recent development of refractive surgery techniques, which include extensive damage to corneal nerves, has prompted the demand for topical drugs to reduce the intense pain caused by this surgery. Non-steroidal anti-inflammatory drugs (NSAIDs) and morphine have been claimed to attenuate corneal pain when applied topically (Payman *et al.* 1994; Epstein and Laurence 1994). There is conflicting evidence about a decrease of mechanical sensitivity of the cornea caused by topical administration of these agents to humans (Gwon *et al.* 1994; Peyman *et al.* 1994; Szerenyi *et al.* 1994). Flurbiprofen, diclofenac, and indomethacin applied to the cornea of the cat reduced spontaneous activity of polymodal nociceptors and their response to chemical stimulation with CO_2 (Chen *et al.* 1995*b*). The effect appeared several minutes after application of the drugs and augmented with time (about 1 h); thus, the possibility exists that the decrease in the excitability of nociceptors was caused by a reduction in the production of arachidonic acid metabolites. A minor increase of mechanical threshold was also noticed in these experiments, which suggests an additional non-specific anaesthetic effect of these drugs. Morphine (0.5–5 mg/ml), applied topically, has been reported to diminish corneal sensibility in humans (Peyman *et al.* 1994). In the cat, topical morphine at 0.05–5 mg/ml concentrations reduced the mechanical and chemical responsiveness of both polymodal and mechanonociceptive corneal fibres, thus indicating that this drug has an anaesthetic effect on corneal sensory fibres (Chen *et al.* 1995*c*). Diltiazem, a calcium antagonist, at high concentrations (1 mM) blocks chemical responsiveness to acid of corneal polymodal units, without apparently reducing their mechanosensitivity (Pozo *et al.* 1992; Fig. 6.8 (D) (E)). This drug also decreases behavioural signs of pain evoked by irritant chemicals applied to the rabbit's eye (Gonzalez *et al.* 1993). However, its efficacy on human ocular pain remains to be established.

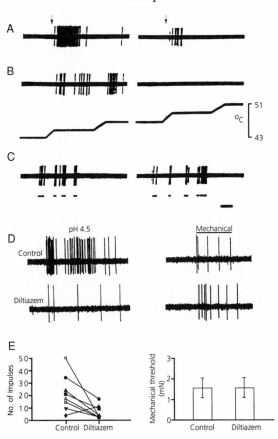

Fig. 6.8 The effects of capsaicin and diltiazem on the response of Aδ polymodal nociceptors to mechanical, chemical, and thermal stimulation. (A–C) Left, impulse discharges evoked in an intact fibre by: (A) 10 mM acetic acid; (B) stepwise heating; and (C) mechanical stimulation during the period indicated by the horizontal bar. Right, response of the unit to the same stimuli, applied after a 5-min pretreatment with 0.33 mM capsaicin. (D) Impulse discharge evoked by application of a pH 4.5 solution (left) or a mechanical stimulation (right) before and after pretreatment with 1 mM diltiazem. (E) Left, change in total number of impulses elicited by acid during a 30-s period, before and after 1 mM diltiazem in nine polymodal units; right, average mechanical threshold in the same units, before and after diltiazem.
Error bars are SEM. Time-scale in nerve recordings, 5 s. From Belmonte *et al.* (1991) and Pozo *et al.* (1992).

Relationship between corneal nerves and sensation

It is a common experience that touching the cornea causes a brisk sensation of pain. However, the question whether other qualities of sensation could be evoked from the cornea by lower-intensity mechanical stimuli or by temperature changes, which was at the centre of the controversy over specificity of pain sensations, has not been answered completely. Psychophysical studies on corneal sensation are complicated by the extreme apprehension produced in experimental subjects by the approximation of any device to the front of the eye. Furthermore, any noxious stimuli of the cornea causes immediate and unavoidable blinking, even before the unpleasantness of the stimulus is consciously felt. Sensations experienced as a result of corneal stimulation are very difficult to describe and to compare with those elicited by analogous stimuli applied to the skin or mucosae.

The loss of corneal sensibility has serious consequences for the integrity of corneal tissues; for this reason, clinicians have been mainly preoccupied by gross disturbances of corneal sensitivity. This interest prompted the development of several instruments aimed at quantifying corneal sensibility to mechanical stimuli. The most commonly used corneal aesthesiometers (Boberg-Ans 1956; Cochet and Bonnet 1960) are based on von Frey's principle that the force required to buckle a long hair when it is pushed axially against the corneal surface is constant and proportional to the diameter of the hair and its length (von Frey 1922). Other, more sophisticated instruments have been developed to define with greater accuracy the magnitude of the mechanical force required to evoke a corneal sensation (Schirmer 1963a; Larson 1970; Draeger 1984; Weinstein *et al*. 1992). These used various types of probes directly placed on the cornea or an air jet, to apply a controlled force on the corneal surface. In all instances, the objective was to determine threshold to punctate mechanical stimulation of the different regions of the cornea or of the bulbar conjunctiva and its variations in a number of normal or pathological conditions.

The results of the numerous studies dedicated to this problem are essentially similar (Draeger 1984): Application of a mechanical probe to the cornea evokes an unpleasant sensation of touching that, with high intensities, becomes a sharp, jabbing pain outlasting the stimulus. The centre of the cornea has a lower mechanical threshold than the periphery and even more than the conjunctiva, with minor regional differences between the superior and inferior regions of the cornea (Boberg-Ans 1956; Cochet and Bonnet 1960; Millodot 1973; Norn 1973). These variations in corneal sensitivity appear to correlate well with the density of corneal innervation (Millodot *et al*. 1978; Rózsa and Beuerman 1982; Chan-Ling 1989). Also, mechanical sensitivity of the cornea decreases with age and, surprisingly, is higher in blue-eyed subjects (Millodot 1975). It is reduced at night and during pregnancy and menstruation in women, possibly associated to the presence of corneal oedema (Millodot and Lamont 1974; Millodot 1977). It is also lower in contact lens wearers (Schirmer 1963b), presumably due to a certain degree of corneal oedema due to chronic hypoxia and perhaps also to peripheral or central adaptation to continuous subthreshold stimulation of mechanosensory nerve fibres (Polse 1978; Millodot and O'Leary 1980; Tanelian and Beuerman 1980).

Corneal sensitivity is altered in a variety of clinical circumstances in which corneal innervation is disturbed. These include diabetes (Schwartz 1974), herpes simplex, herpes zoster, corneal and scleral inflammation (Lyne 1977; Metcalf 1982), corneal wounds (Zander and Weddell 1951) and ocular surgery accompanied by damage to corneal nerves, such as cataract extraction, radial keratotomy, excimer laser keratectomy (Biermann *et al*. 1992; Campos *et al*. 1992), or corneal transplantation (Zorab 1971; Rao *et al*. 1985). In these cases, reduction of corneal sensitivity is correlated with the degree of nerve damage and with the success of the regeneration of corneal nerves in the injured tissue (de Leeuw and Chan 1989; Mathers *et al*. 1988). Nevertheless, as noted above, transient (1–3 months) corneal hypersensitivity has been detected in the centre of excimer laser wounds, in spite of the fact that no intraepithelial neurites had reached the central wound at this time (Ishikawa *et al*. 1994). This may reflect abnormal sensitivity to mechanical stimuli of regenerating nerve fibres entering the wounded area as well as sensitization of surrounding intact nerve fibres.

The abundant research on clinical alterations of corneal mechanosensitivity was not accompanied by a parallel interest in corneal sensations evoked by other modalities of stimuli. Only a few papers have been devoted to this topic in the literature of the last 40 years.

Lele and Weddell (1956) used warmed and cooled copper cylinders in direct contact with the cornea, air jets at different temperatures, and infrared radiation to stimulate the cornea of human volunteers and claimed that subjects were able to distinguish the temperature (warm or cold) of the applied stimulus. Kenshalo (1960) re-examined the corneal sensibility to temperature by applying to the human cornea, conjunctiva, and forehead skin the bulb of a warmed or cooled laboratory thermometer. Sensations evoked from the cornea by temperatures ranging between 20°C and 55°C were always described in terms of irritation and not of temperature, although subjects reported changes in the quality of the sensation at certain points of the temperature continuum, namely, when descending below 31°C and when reaching temperatures over 42°C. In oral reports, high temperature was experienced as a very sharp and irritating sensation, not unlike the one experienced by heating the skin but without a thermal component. Sensation experienced with cold appears to be very different; it was described as rather sharp but possessing a quality different from high temperatures. Yet, subjects refused to identify this different quality as the cool they experienced by stimulation of the skin or the conjunctiva. These observations were confirmed by Beuerman and co-workers (Beuerman *et al.* 1977; Beuerman and Tanelian 1979). They applied a jet of warmed or cooled saline to the eye, which was submerged in a bath, and showed that only sensations of irritation were evoked when the stimulus was restricted to the cornea.

Controlled chemical stimulation of the cornea has rarely been attempted. Diluted capsaicin has been dropped into the eye to determine the threshold concentration necessary to elicit a sensation of irritation; that was established at 6.0×10^{-8}M (Dupuy *et al.* 1988). Also, hypertonic saline has been applied to detect ophthalmic nerve impairment (Mandahl 1993). A more accurate method has been developed by applying to the cornea a jet of CO_2 at different concentrations (between 10 and 90 per cent) (Chen *et al.* 1995a). With this technique, a sensation of stinging pain was evoked when a threshold concentration around 40 per cent CO_2 was attained. Higher concentrations produced a more intense sensation, which was also proportional to the duration of the stimulus.

A tentative correlation can be made between the functional type of corneal units recruited by the different modalities of stimuli in animal experiments and the corresponding evoked sensation in psychophysical experiments in humans. Irritation elicited by mechanical stimulation is presumably due to the excitation of mechanosensory and polymodal nociceptive fibres. Both types of units have quite similar mechanical thresholds. Thus, undefined sensations of contact elicited by borderline mechanical stimulation appear to be due to a low firing frequency in the fraction of these two classes of fibres having the lowest mechanical threshold. Only mechanosensory limbal fibres appear to be suited to discriminate very-low-intensity, non-noxious mechanical stimuli but, because of their small receptive field and fast adaptation properties, they seem to be limited to detecting rapid stimuli, such as those produced by the sliding of the upper lid over the front of the eye.

Heat recruits mechanoheat and polymodal units, while protons are expected to stimulate only polymodal fibres. In both cases, the sensation evoked is one of irritation. A good correspondence exists between the firing frequency in polymodal units of the cat cornea and the intensity of the sensations experienced in humans, both for increasing CO_2 concentrations and for corneal temperature elevations (Fig. 6.9). On the other hand, thermal stimulation with temperatures below 30°C recruits exclusively 'cold' corneal units and evokes a different kind of unpleasant sensation, suggesting that activation of the specific population of cold nociceptors is responsible for the peculiar irritation sensation evoked by low corneal temperatures. In contrast, sensations of cooling evoked by low temperatures acting more extensively on the front of the eye are presumably mediated by the abundant specific cold receptors, present in the limbal and perilimbal conjunctiva.

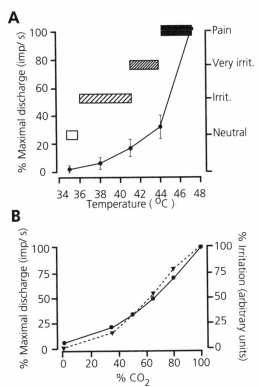

Fig. 6.9 The relationship between the amplitude of the noxious stimulus, the impulse frequency of polymodal fibres, and corneal sensation. (A) The stimulus–response curve obtained by stepwise heating of the cornea in nine corneal polymodal units of the cat (Belmonte and Giraldez 1981) has been plotted together with the verbal response profiles for the same temperature values obtained in humans by Beuerman *et al.* (1977; Beuerman and Tanelian 1979). (B) The mean firing response evoked by CO_2 pulses of increasing concentration in 13 corneal polymodal fibres (circles) has been plotted together with the mean sensation of irritation measured with a visual analogue scale (triangles), evoked by the same CO_2 pulses in seven human volunteers. From Belmonte *et al.* 1994; Chen *et al.* 1995a.

Concluding remarks

The cornea of the eye is innervated by unspecialized terminals of trigeminal sensory neurones, which show close functional similarities with the various subclasses of nociceptors described in other ectodermal tissues. Mechanonociceptors, polymodal nociceptors, and 'cold' nociceptors have been identified electrophysiologically in the cornea. Distinct types of irritation sensations are evoked by noxious mechanical, chemical, and thermal stimulation of the human cornea. These differences in the quality of pain sensation might be associated with a variable activation of the various subpopulations of corneal nociceptive afferents.

Furthermore, significant trophic interactions appear to exist between corneal sensory neurones and corneal tissue. The corneal epithelium appears to be a source of neurotrophic factors for its trigeminal sensory neurones. On the other hand, there is evidence that afferent nerve fibres contribute to maintain the integrity of the intact cornea and also participate in the repair processes activated by injury, both enhancing the inflammatory reaction (neurogenic inflammation) and stimulating the recovery of damaged tissues (migration and mitosis of epithelium cells). Substance P and CGRP, two neuropeptides that are present in corneal sensory fibres and are released upon injury, may possibly contribute to these effects.

Corneal irritation and pain are common problems associated with many clinical situations (accidental injury, surgery, contact lens wearing). Their incidence justifies a deeper knowledge of peripheral neural mechanisms involved in their genesis. The cornea is, in addition, an excellent model for morphological, biochemical, and electrophysiological studies of the peripheral terminals of nociceptive neurones. Its structural simplicity and the absence of blood vessels facilitates the experimental manipulation of the nociceptive endings in a comparatively uncomplicated environment and makes the cornea an attractive preparation for this type of study.

Acknowledgements

The authors wish to express their deep appreciation to Drs Jennifer Laird and Fernando Cervero for helpful criticism and correction of the manuscript. Supported by the Plan Nacional de Investigación Científica y Desarrollo Tecnológico (SAF93-0267), Spain.

References

Adriaensen, H., Gybels, J., Handwerker, H.O., and van Hees, J. (1983). Response properties of thin myelinated (A-delta) fibers in human skin nerves. *J. Neurophysiol.* **49**, 111–22.

Alper, M.G. (1976). The anesthesic eye: an investigation of change in the anterior ocular segment of the monkey caused by interrupting the trigeminal nerve at various levels along its course. *Trans. Am. Ophthalmol. Soc.* **72**, 323–65.

Araki, K., Ohashi, Y., Kinoshita, S., Hayashi, K., Kuwayama, Y., and Tano, Y. (1994). Epithelial wound healing in the denervated cornea. *Curr. Eye Res.* **13**, 203–11.

Arvidson, B. (1977). Retrograde axonal transport of horseradish peroxidase from cornea to trigeminal ganglion. *Acta neuropathol., Berlin* **38**, 49–52.

Attias, G. (1912). Die Nerven der Hornhaut des Menschen. *v. Graefe's Arch. Ophthalmol.* **83**, 14–316.

Baker, K.S., Anderson, S.C., Romanowski, E.G., Thoft, R.A., and SundarRaj, N. (1993). Trigeminal ganglion neurons affect corneal epithelial phenotype. Influence on type VII collagen expression in vitro. *Invest. Ophthalmol. Vis. Sci.* **34**, 137–144.

Bazan, H.E.P. (1990). Response of inflammatory lipid mediators following corneal injury. In *Lipid mediators in eye inflammation* (ed. N.G. Bazan), pp. 1–11. Karger, Basel.

Beckers, H.J.M., Klooster, J., Vrensen, G.F.J.M., and Lamers, W.P.M.A. (1992). Ultrastructural organization of trigeminal nerve endings in the rat cornea and iris. *Invest, Ophthalmol. Vis. Sci.* **33**, 1979–86.

Beckers, H.J.M., Klooster, J., Vrensen, G.F.J.M., and Lamers, W.P.M.A. (1993). Substance P in rat corneal and iridal nerves: An ultrastructural immunohistochemical study. *Ophthalmic Res.* **25**, 192–200.

Beding-Barnekow, Brodin, E., and Håkanson, R. (1988). Substance P, neurokinin A and neurokinin B in the ocular responses to injury in rabbits. *Br. J. Pharmacol.* **95**, 259–67.

Bee, J.A. (1982). The development and pattern of innervation of the avian cornea. *Develop. Biol.* **92**, 5–11.

Bee, J.A. and Roche, S.M. (1992). Reducing intraocular pressure by intubation elicits precocious development and innervation of the embryonic chick cornea. *Invest. Ophthalmol. Vis. Sci.* **33**, 3469–78.

Bee, J.A. Hay, R.A., Lamb, E.M., Devore, J.J., and Conrad, G.W. (1986). Positional specificity of corneal nerves during development. *Invest. Ophthalmol. Vis. Sci.* **27**, 38–43.

Bee, J.A., Kuhl, U., Edgar, D., and von der Mark, K. (1988). Avian corneal nerves: co-distribution with collagen type IV and acquisition of substance P immunoreactivity. *Invest. Ophthalmol. Vis. Sci.* **29**, 101–7.

Belmonte, C. and Giraldez, F. (1981). Responses of cat corneal sensory receptors to mechanical and thermal stimulation. *J. Physiol.* **321**, 355–68.

Belmonte, C., Simon, J., and Gallego, A. (1971). Effects of intraocular pressure changes on the afferent activity of the ciliary nerves. *Exp. Eye Res.* **12**, 342–55.

Belmonte, C., Gallar, J., Pozo, M.A., and Rebollo, I. (1988). Effects of capsaicin on the neural discharge of corneal sensory fibres in the anaesthetized cat. *J. Physiol.* **401**, 57P.

Belmonte, C., Gallar, J., Pozo, M.A., and Rebollo, I. (1991). Excitation by irritant substances of sensory afferent units in the cat's cornea. *J. Physiol.* **437**, 709–25.

Belmonte, C., Gallar, J., Lopez-Briones, L.G., and Pozo, M.A. (1994). Polymodality in nociceptive neurons: Experimental models of chemotransduction. In *Cellular mechanisms of sensory processing*, NATO series, Vol. H 79 (ed. L. Urban), pp. 87–117. Springer-Verlag, Berlin.

Bessou, P. and Perl, E.R. (1969). Response of cutaneous sensory units with unmyelinated fibers to noxious stimuli. *J. Neurophysiol.* **32**, 1025–43.

Beuerman, R.W. and Kupke, K. (1982). Neural regeneration following experimental wounds of the cornea in the rabbit. In *The structure of the eye* (ed. J.G. Hollyfield), pp. 319–30. Elsevier North Holland, Amsterdam.

Beuerman, R.W. and Rózsa, A.J. (1984). Collateral sprouts are replaced by regenerating neurites in the wounded corneal epithelium. *Neurosci. Lett.* **44**, 99–104.

Beuerman, R.W. and Schimmelpfennig, B. (1980). Sensory denervation of the rabbit cornea affects epithelial properties. *Exp. Neurol.* **69**, 196–201.

Beuerman, R.W. and Tanelian, D.L. (1979). Corneal pain evoked by thermal stimulation. *Pain* **7**, 1–14.

Beuerman, R.W., Maurice, D.M., and Tanelian, D.L. (1977). Thermal stimulation of the cornea. In *Pain in the trigeminal region* (ed. D. Anderson and B. Matthews), pp. 422–3. Elsevier, Amsterdam.

Beuerman, R.W., Rózsa, A.J., and Tanelian, D.L. (1985). Neurophysiological correlates of post traumatic acute pain. In *Advances in pain research and therapy*, Vol. 9 (ed. H.L. Fields, R. Dubner, and F. Cervero), pp. 73–81. Raven Press, New York.

Bevan, S. and Geppetti, P. (1994). Protons: small stimulants of capsaicin-sensitive sensory nerves. *Trends Neurosci.* **17**, 509–12.

Biermann, H., Grabner, G., Baumgartner, I., and Reim, M. (1992). Zur Hornhautsensibilität nach Epikeratophakie. *Klin. Mbl. Augenheilk.* **201**, 18–21.

Boberg-Ans, J. (1956). On the corneal sensitivity. *Acta Ophthalmol.* **34**, 149–62.

Buck, S.H. and Burks, T.F. (1986). The neuropharmacology of capsaicin: review of some recent observations. *Pharmacol. Rev.* **38**, 179–226.

Buck, S.H., Walsh, J.H., Davis, T.P., Brown, M.R., Yamamura, H.I., and Burks, T.F. (1983). Characterization of the peptide and sensory neurotoxic effects of capsaicin in the guinea pig. *J. Neurosci.* **3**, 2064–74.

Butterfield, L.C. and Neufeld, A.H. (1977). Cyclic nucleotides and mitosis in the rabbit cornea following superior cervical ganglionectomy. *Exp. Eye Res.* **25**, 427–33.

Bynke, G. (1983). Capsaicin pretreatment prevents disruption of the blood-aqueous barrier in the rabbit eye. *Invest. Ophthalmol. Vis. Sci.* **24**, 744–8.

Bynke, G., Håkanson, R., and Sundler, F. (1984). Is substance P necessary for corneal nociception? *Invest. Ophthalmol. Vis. Sci.* **24**, 744–8.

Campos, M., Hertzog, L., Garbus, J.J., and McDonnell, P.J. (1992). Corneal sensitivity after photorefractive keratectomy. *Am. J. Ophthalmol.* **114**, 51–4.

Camras, C.B. and Bito, L.Z. (1980*a*). The pathophysiological effects of nitrogen mustard on the rabbit eye. I. The biphasic intraocular pressure response and the role of prostaglandins. *Exp. Eye Res.* **30**, 41–52.

Camras, C.B. and Bito, L.Z. (1980*b*). The pathophysiological effects of nitrogen mustard on the rabbit eye. II. The inhibition of the initial hypertensive phase by capsaicin and the apparent role of substance P. *Invest. Ophthalmol. Vis. Sci.* **19**, 423–8.

Chan, K.Y. and Haschke, R.H. (1981). Action of a trophic factor(s) from rabbit corneal epithelial culture on dissociated trigeminal neurons. *J. Neurosci.* **1**, 1155–62.

Chan, K.Y. and Haschke, R.H. (1982). Isolation and culture of corneal cells and their interactions with dissociated trigeminal neurons. *Exp. Eye Res.* **35**, 137–56.

Chan, K.Y. and Haschke, R.H. (1985). Specificity of a neuronotrophic factor from rabbit corneal epithelial cell cultures. *Exp. Eye Res.* **41**, 687–99.

Chan, K.Y., Jones, R.R., Brak, D.H., Swift, J., Parker, J.A., and Haschke, R.H. (1987). Release of neuronotrophic factor from rabbit corneal epithelium during wound healing and nerve regeneration. *Exp. Eye Res.* **45**, 633–46.

Chan-Ling, T. (1989). Sensitivity and neural organization of the cat cornea. *Invest Ophthalmol. Vis. Sci.* **30**, 1075–82.

Chan-Ling, T., Tervo, K., Tervo, T., Vannas, A., Holden, B., and Eränkö, L. (1987). Long-term neural regeneration in the rabbit following 180° limbal incision. *Invest. Ophthalmol. Vis. Sci.* **28**, 2083–8.

Chan-Ling, T., Vannas, A., Holden, B.A., and O'Leary, D.J. (1990). Incision depth affects the recovery of corneal sensitivity and neural regeneration in the cat. *Invest. Ophthalmol. Vis. Sci.* **31**, 1533–41.

Chen, X., Gallar, J., and Belmonte, C. (1994). Influence of calcium ions on excitation and sensitisation of corneal nociceptors. *Eur. J. Neurosci.* **Suppl. 7**, 133.

Chen, X., Gallar, J., Pozo, M.A., Baeza, M., and Belmonte, C. (1995*a*). CO_2 stimulation of the cornea: a comparison between human sensation and nerve activity in polymodal nociceptive afferents of the cat. *Eur. J. Neurosci.* **7**, 1154–63.

Chen, X., Gallar, J., and Belmonte, C. (1995*b*). Effects of nonsteroidal antiinflammatory drugs on chemical sensitivity of corneal nociceptors. *Eur. J. Neurosci.* **Suppl. 8**, 31.

Chen, X., Gallar, J., and Belmonte, C. (1995*c*). Effects of morphine on the response of pain corneal fibers to chemical and mechanical stimulation. JERMOV Meeting, Montpellier, France.

Chen, X., Belmonte, C., and Rang, H.P. (1996). Capsaicin and carbon dioxide act by distinct mechanisms on sensory nerve terminals in the cat cornea. *Pain* (submitted).

Cochet, P. and Bonnet, R. (1960). L'esthésie cornéene. *La Clin. Ophthalmol.* **4**, 3–27.

Colin, S. and Kruger, L. (1986). Peptidergic nociceptive axon visualisation in whole-mount preparations of cornea and tympanic membrane in rat. *Brain Res.* **398**, 199–203.

Crouch, D.S., Davis, B.M., Albers, K.M., and Rickman, D.W. (1995). Nerve growth factor regulation of corneal sensory innervation. *Invest. Ophthalmol. Vis. Sci.* **36** (suppl.), 574.

de Castro, F., Silos-Santiago, I., Lopez de Armentia, M., Barbacid, M., and Belmonte, C. (1995). Corneal innervation in mice lacking nerve growth factor (NGF) receptor (*trkA* knockouts). *Invest. Ophthalmol. Vis. Sci.* **36** (suppl.), 574.

de Leeuw, M. and Chan, K.Y. (1989). Corneal nerve regeneration. Correlation between morphology and restoration of sensitivity. *Invest. Ophthalmol. Vis. Sci.* **30**, 1980–90.

Dixon, A.D. (1963). Fine structure of nerve-cell bodies and satellite cells in the trigeminal ganglion. *J. dent. Res'.* **42**, 990–9.

Draeger, J. (1984). *Corneal sensitivity: measurement and clinical importance.* Springer Verlag, Vienna.

Duce, I.R. and Keen, P. (1977). An ultrastructural classification of the neuronal cell bodies of the rat dorsal root ganglion using zinc iodide–osmium impregnation. *Cell Tissue Res.* **185**, 263–77.

Dupuy, B., Thompson, H., and Beuerman, R.W. (1988). Capsaicin: a psychophysical tool to explore corneal sensitivity. *Invest. Ophthalmol. Vis. Sci.* **29** (suppl.), 454.

Ehinger, B. (1966). Ocular and orbital vegetative nerves. *Acta physiol. scand.* **67** (suppl.), 1–35.

Ehinger, B. and Sjöberg, N.-O. (1971). Development of the ocular adrenergic nerve supply in man and guinea pig. *Z. Zelllforsch.* **118**, 579–92.

Emoto, I. and Beuerman, R.W. (1987). Stimulation of neurite growth by epithelial implants into corneal stroma. *Neurosci. Lett.* **82**, 140–4.

Epstein, R.L. and Laurence, E.O. (1994). Effect of topical diclofenac solution on discomfort after radial keratotomy. *J. Cataract Refract. Surg.* **20**, 378–80.

Fujita, S., Shimizu, T., Izumi, K., Fukuda, T., Sameshima, M., and Ohba, N. (1984). Capsaicin-induced neuroparalytic-like corneal changes in the mouse. *Exp. Eye Res.* **38**, 165–75.

Gallar, J. (1991). Caracterización electrofisiólogica de los receptores sensoriales del ojo del gato. Unpublished PhD thesis, University of Alicante, Spain.

Gallar, J. and Belmonte, C (1990). Modulation by prostaglandins of nervous activity in corneal nociceptors. *Invest. Ophthalmol. Vis. Sci.* **31** (suppl.), 514.

Gallar, J., Pozo, M.A., Rebollo, I., and Belmonte, C (1990). Effects of capsaicin on corneal wound healing. *Invest. Ophthalmol. Vis. Sci.* **31**, 1968–74.

Gallar, J., Pozo, M.A., Tuckett, R.P., and Belmonte, C (1993). Response of sensory units with unmyelinated fibres to mechanical, thermal and chemical stimulation of the cat's cornea. *J. Physiol.* **468**, 609–22.

Gallar, J., Garcia de la Rubia, P., Gonzalez, G.G., and Belmonte, C (1995). Irritation of the anterior segment by ultraviolet radiation: influence of nerve blockade and calcium antagonists. *Curr. Eye Res.* **14**, 827–35.

Gamse, R., Leeman, S., Holzer, P., and Lembeck, F. (1981). Differential effects of capsaicin on the content of somatostatin, substance P and neurotensin in the nervous system of the rat. *Naunyn-Schmiedberg's Arch. Pharmacol.* **317**, 140–8.

Garcia-Hirschfeld, J., Lopez-Briones, L.G., and Belmonte, C. (1994). Neurotrophic influences on corneal epithelial cells. *Exp. Eye Res.* **59**, 597–605.

Garcia-Hirschfeld, J., Lopez-Briones, L.G., Belmonte, C., and Valdeolmillos, M. (1995). Intracellular free calcium responses to protons and capsaicin in cultured trigeminal neurons. *Neuroscience* **67**, 235–43.

Gilbard, J.P. and Rossi, S.R. (1990). Tear film and ocular surface changes in a rabbit model of neurotrophic keratitis. *Ophthalmology* **97**, 308–12.

Giraldez, F. (1979). Estudio electrofisiológico de los receptores sensoriales de la córnea del gato. Unpublished PhD thesis. University of Valladolid, Spain.

Giraldez, F., Geijo, E., and Belmonte, C. (1979). Response characteristics of corneal sensory fibers to mechanical and thermal stimulation. *Brain Res.* **177**, 571–6.

Gonzalez, G.G., Garcia de la Rubia, P., Gallar, J., and Belmonte, C. (1993). Reduction of capsaicin-induced ocular pain and neurogenic inflammation by calcium antagonists. *Invest. Ophthalmol. Vis. Sci.* **34**, 3329–35.

Gonzalez, G.G., Gallar, J., and Belmonte, C. (1995). Influence of diltiazem on the ocular irritative response to nitrogen mustard. *Exp. Eye Res.* **61**, 205–12.

Gotz, R. (1972). Zwei neue Instrumente für die Untersuchung der Hornhautsensibilität. *Klin. Mbl. Augenheilk* **161**, 469–74.

Green, D.M. and Tregear, R.T. (1964). The action of sensory irritants on the cat's cornea. *J. Physiol.* **175**, 37P.

Gregg, J.M. and Dixon, A.D. (1973). Somatotopic organization of the trigeminal ganglion in the rat. *Arch. oral Biol.* **18**, 487–98.

Grimes, P. and von Sallmann, L. (1960). Comparative anatomy of the ciliary nerves. *Arch. Ophthalmol.* **64**, 81–91.

Gwon, A., Vaughan, E.R., Cheetham, J.K., and DeGryse, R. (1994). Ocufen (Flurbiprofen) in the treatment of ocular pain after radial keratotomy. *CLAO J.* **20**, 131–8.

Hagg, T., Louis. J-C., and Varon, S. (1993). Neurotrophic factors and CNS regeneration. In *Neuroregeneration* (ed. A. Gorio), pp. 265–87. Raven Press, New York.

Handwerker, H.O. (1991). What peripheral mechanisms contribute to nociceptive transmission and hyperalgesia? In *Towards a new pharmacology of pain* (ed. A.I. Basbaum and J.M. Besson), pp. 5–19. John Wiley & Sons, New York.

Handwerker, H.O. and Reeh, P.W. (1991). Pain and inflammation. In *Pain research and clinical management* Proceedings of the 6th World Congress on Pain, Vol. 4, pp. 59–70. (ed. M.R. Bond, J.E. Charlton, and C.J. Wolf). Elsevier, Amsterdam.

Harris, L.W. and Purves, D. (1989). Rapid remodelling of sensory endings in the corneas of living mice. *J. Neurosci.* **9**, 2210–14.

Hensel, H., Iggo, A., and Witt, I. (1960). A quantitative study of sensitive cutaneous thermo-receptors with C afferent fibres. *J. Physiol.* **153**, 113–26.

Hille, B. (1994). *Ionic channels of excitable membranes.* Sinauer, Sunderland, Massachusetts.

Hoyes, A.D. and Barber, P. (1976). Ultrastructure of corneal nerves in the rat. *Cell Tissue Res.* **172**, 133–44.

Ichikawa, H., Mitani, S., Hijiya, H., Nakago, T., Jacobowittz, D.M., and Sugimoto, T. (1933). Calretinin-immunoreactivity in trigeminal neurons innervating the nasal mucosa of the rat. *Brain Res.* **629**, 231–8.

Iggo, A. (1963). An electrophysiological analysis of afferent fibres in primate skin. *Acta Neuroveg.* **24**, 225–40.

Ishida, N., del Cerro, M., Rao, G.N., Mathe, M., and Aquavella, J.V. (1984). Corneal stromal innervation. A quantitative analysis of distribution. *Ophthalmic Res.* **16**, 139–44.

Ishikawa, T., del Cerro, M., Liang, F-Q., Loya, N., and Aquavella, J.V. (1994). Corneal sensitivity and nerve regeneration after laser ablation. *Cornea* **13** 225–31.

Jampol, L.M., Neufeld, A.H., and Sears, M.L. (1975). Pathways of the response of the eye to injury. *Invest. Ophthalmol. Vis. Sci.* **14**, 184–9.

Jancsó, N., Jancsó-Gabor,, A., and Szolcsányi, J. (1966). The role of sensory nerve endings in neurogenic inflammation induced in human skin and in the eye and paw of the rat. *Br. J. Pharmacol. Chemother.* **33**, 32–41.

Keele, C.A. (1962). The common chemical sense and its receptors. *Arch. int. Pharmacodyn.* **139**, 547–57.

Kenshalo, D.R.(1960). Comparison of thermal sensitivity of the forehead, lip, conjunctiva and cornea. *J. appl. Physiol.* **15**, 987–91.

Kessler, J.A., Bell, W.O., and Black, I.O. (1983). Interactions between the sympathetic and sensory innervation of the iris. *J. Neurosci.* **3**, 1301–07.

Kessler, W., Kirchhoff, C., Reeh, P.W., and Handwerker, H.O. (1992). Excitation of cutaneous afferent nerve endings in vitro by a combination of inflammatory mediators and conditioning effect of substance P. *Exp. Brain Res.* **91**, 467–76.

Klyce, S.D., Beuerman, R.W., and Crosson, C.E. (1985). Alteration of corneal epithelial ion transport by sympathectomy. *Invest. Ophthalmol. Vis. Sci.* **26**, 434–42.

Korsching, S. (1993). The neurotrophic factor concept: a re-examination. *J. Neurosci.* **13**, 2739–48.

Kuwayama, Y., Terenghi, G., Polak, J.M., Trojanowski, J.Q., and Stone, R.A. (1987). A quantitative correlation of substance P-, calcitonin gene-related peptide- and cholecystokinin-like immunoreactivity with retrogradely labelled trigeminal ganglion cells innervating the eye. *Brain Res.* **405**, 220–6.

Larson, W.L. (1970). Electro-mechanical corneal esthesiometer. *Br. J. Ophthalmol.* **54**, 342–7.

Laties, A. and Jacobowitz, D. (1964). A histochemical study of the adrenergic and cholinergic innervation of the anterior segment of the rabbit eye. *Invest. Ophthalmol. Vis. Sci.* **3**, 592–600.

LaVail, J., Johnson, W.E., and Spencer, L.C. (1993). Immunohistochemical identification of trigeminal ganglion neurons that innervate the mouse cornea: relevance to intercellular spread of herpes simplex virus. *J. comp. Neurol.* **327**, 133–40.

Lawrenson, J.G. and Ruskell, G.L. (1991). The structure of corpuscular nerve endings in the limbal conjunctiva of the human eye. *J. Anat.* **177**, 75–84.

Lee, Y., Kawai, Y., Shiosaka, S., Takami, K., Kiyama, H., Hillyard, C.J., Girgis, S., MacIntyre, I., Emson, P.C., and Tohyama, M. (1985). Coexistence of calcitonin gene-related peptide and substance P-like in single cells of the trigeminal ganglion of the rat: immunohistochemical analysis. *Brain Res.* **330R, 194–6.**

Lehtosalo, J.I. (1984). Substance P-like immunoreactive trigeminal ganglion cells supplying the cornea. *Histochemistry* **80**, 273–6.

Lehtosalo, J.I., Uusitalo, H., Stjernschantz, J., and Palkama, A. (1984). Substance P-like immunoreactivity in the trigeminal ganglion. A fluorescence, light and electron microscope study. *Histochemistry* **80**, 421–7.

Lele, P.P. and Weddell, G. (1956). The relationship between neurohistology and corneal sensibility. *Brain* **19**, 119–54.

Lele, P.P. and Weddell, G. (1959). Sensory nerves of the cornea and cutaneous sensibility. *Exp. Neurol.* **1**, 334–59.

Light, A.R. (1992). *The initial processing of pain and its descending control: spinal and trigeminal systems.* Pain and headache, Vol. 12 (ed. Ph.L. Gidenberg). Karger, Basel.

Lim, C.H. and Ruskell, G.L. (1978). Corneal nerve access in monkey. *Albrecht v. Graefes Arch. klin. exp. Ophthal.* **208**, 15—23.

Lindahl, O. (1961). Experimental skin pain induced by injection of water-soluble substances in humans. *Acta Physiol. Scand.* **suppl. 179**, 1–89.

López de Armentia, M., Gallar, J., and Belmonte, C. (1995). An *in vitro* preparation of the eye–trigeminal ganglion of the mouse for intracellular recording of corneal neurons. *Invest. Ophthalmol. Vis. Sci.* **36** (suppl.), 575.

Lukás, Z. and Dolezel, S. (1975). A histochemical study on the development of the innervation of the rabbit cornea. *Folia Morpholog.* **23**, 272–6.

Lyne, A.J. (1977). Corneal sensation in scleritis and episcleritis. *Br. J. Ophthalmol.* **61**, 650–4.

MacIver, M.B. and Tanelian, D.L. (1992). Activation of C fibers by metabolic perturbations associated with tourniquet ischemia. *Anesthesiology* **76**, 617–23.

MacIver, M.B. and Tanelian, D.L. (1993a). Free nerve ending terminal morphology is fiber type specific for A-delta and C fibers innervating rabbit corneal epithelium. *J. Neurophysiol.* **69**, 1779–83.

MacIver, M.B. and Tanelian, D.L. (1993b). Structural and functional specialization of A-delta and C fiber free nerve endings innervating rabbit corneal epithelium. *J. Neurosci.* **13** 4511–24.

Mandahl, A. (1993). Hypertonic saline test for ophthalmic nerve impairment. *Acta Ophthalmol.* **71**, 556–9.

Marfurt, C.F. (1981). Somatotopic organization of the cat trigeminal ganglion as determined by the horseradish peroxidase technique. *Anat. Rec.* **201**, 105–18.

Marfurt, C.F. and DelToro, D.R. (1987). Corneal sensory pathway in the rat: a horseradish peroxidase tracing study. *J. comp. Neurol.* **261**, 450–9.

Marfurt, C.F. and Echtenkamp, S.F. (1988). Central projections and trigeminal ganglion location of corneal afferent neurons in the monkey, *Macaca fascicularis*. *J. comp. Neurol.* **272**, 370–82.

Marfurt, C.F. and Ellis, L.C. (1993). Immunohistochemical localization of tyrosine hydroxylase in the corneal innervation of five mammalian species, including human. *J. comp. Neurol.* **336**, 517–31.

Marfurt, C.F. and Jones, M.A. (1995). Parasympathetic innervation of the rat cornea. *Invest. Ophthalmol. Vis. Sci.* **36** (Suppl.), S576.

Marfurt, C.F., Ellis, L.C., and Jones, M.A. (1993). Sensory and sympathetic nerve sprouting in the rat cornea following neonatal administration of capsaicin. *Somatosens. Mot. Res.* **10**, 377–98.

Mark, D. and Maurice. D. (1977). Sensory recording from isolated cornea. *Invest. Ophthalmol. Vis. Sci.* **16**, 541–5.

Martin, R.E. and Bazan, N.G. (1992). Growth-associated protein GAP-43 and nerve cell adhesion molecule in sensory nerves of the cornea. *Exp. Eye Res.* **55**, 307–14.

Martin, X. and Dolivo, M. (1983). Neuronal and transneuronal tracing in the trigeminal system of the rat using the herpes virus suis. *Brain Res.* **273**, 253–76.

Mathers, W.D., Jester, J.V., and Lemp, M.A. (1988). Return of human corneal sensitivity after penetrating keratoplasty. *Arch. Ophthalmol.* **106**, 210–15.

Matsuda, H. (1968). Electron microscopic study of the corneal nerve with special reference to the nerve endings. *Acta soc. ophthalmol. Jap.,* **72**, 860.

Maurice, D.M. (1962). The cornea and sclera. In *The eye. Vegetative physiology and biochemistry,* Vol. (ed. H. Davson), pp. 289–368. Academic Press, New York.

Meakin, S.O. and Shooter, E.M. (1992). The nerve growth factor family of receptors. *Trends Neurosci.* **15**, 323–31.

Metcalf, J.F. (1982). Corneal sensitivity and neuro-histochemical studies of experimental herpetic keratitis in the rabbit. *Exp. Eye Res.* **35**, 231–7.

Meyer, R.A., Campbell, J.N., and Raja, S.N. (1994). Peripheral neural mechanisms of nociception. In *Textbook of pain* (ed. P.D. Wall and R. Melzack), pp. 13–44. Churchill Livingstone, Edinburgh.

Miller, A., Costa, M., Furness, J.B., and Chubb, I.W. (1981). Substance P immunoreactive sensory nerves supply to the rat iris and cornea. *Neurosci. Lett.* **23**, 243–9.

Millodot, M. (1973). Objective measurement of corneal sensitivity. *Acta ophthalmol.* **51**, 325–34.

Millodot, M (1975). Do blue-eyed people have more sensitive corneas than brown-eyed people? *Nature* **255**, 151–2.

Millodot, M. (1977). The influence of pregnancy on the sensitivity of the cornea. *Br. J. Ophthalmol.* **61**, 646–9.

Millodot, M. and Lamont, M. (1974). Influence of menstruation on corneal sensitivity. *Br. J. Ophthalmol.* **58**, 752–6.

Millodot, M. and O'Leary, D.J. (1980). Effect of oxygen deprivation on corneal sensitivity. *Acta opththalmol.* **58**, 434–9.

Millodot, M., Lim, C.H., and Ruskell, G.L. (1978). A comparison of corneal sensitivity and nerve density in albino and pigmented rabbits. *Ophthalmic Res.* **10**, 307.

Mintenig, G., Sanchez-Vives, M.V., Martin, C., Gual, A., and Belmonte, C. (1995). Sensory receptors in the anterior uvea of the cat's eye. An *in vitro* study. *Invest. Ophthalmol. Vis. Sci.* **36**, 1615–24.

Mishima, S. (1957). The effects of denervation and stimulation of the sympathetic and the trigeminal nerve on the mitotic rate of the corneal epithelium in the rabbit. *Jap. J. Ophthalmol.* **1**, 65–73.

Morgan, C.W., Nadelhaft, I., and deGroat, W.C. (1978). Anatomical localization of corneal afferent cells in the trigeminal ganglion. *Neurosurgery* **2**, 252–7.

Morgan, C., Jannetta, P.J., and deGroat, W.C. (1987). Organization of corneal afferent axons in the trigeminal nerve root entry zone in the cat. *Exp. Brain Res.* **68**, 411–16.

Mosso, J.A. and Kruger, L. (1973). Receptor categories represented in trigeminal nucleus caudalis. *J. Neurophysiol.* **36**, 472–88.

Müller, L.J., Pels, L., and Vrensen, G.F.J.M. (1996). Ultrastructure of human corneal nerves. *Invest. Ophthalmol. Vis. Sci.* (in press).

Norn, M.S. (1973). Conjunctival sensitivity in normal eyes. *Acta ophthalmol.* **51**, 58–66.

Ogilvy, C.S. and Borges, L.F. (1990). Changes in corneal innervation during postnatal development in normal rats and in rats treated with capsaicin. *Invest. Ophthalmol. Vis. Sci.* **31**, 1810–15.

Ozanics, V., Rayborn, M., and Sagun, D. (1977). Observations on the morphology of the developing primate cornea: epithelium, its innervation and anterior stroma. *J. Morph. et al.* **153**, 263–98.

Paintal, A.S. (1964). Effects of drugs on vertebrate mechanoreceptors. *Pharmacol. Rev.* **16**, 341–80.

Palkama, A., Uusitalo, H., and Lehtosalo, J. (1986). Innervation of the anterior segment of the eye: with special reference to functional aspects. In *Neurohistochemistry: modern methods and applications.* (ed. P. Panula, H. Paivarinia, and S. Soinila), pp.587–615. Alan R. Liss, New York.

Pallikaris, I.G., Papatzanaki, M.E., Georgiadis, A., and Frenschok, O. (1990). A comparative study of neural regeneration following corneal wounds induced by argon fluoride excimer laser and mechanical methods. *Lasers Light Ophthalmol.* **3**, 89–95.

Pannabecker, C.L. (1944). Keratitis neuroparalytica: corneal lesion following operations for trigeminal neuralgia. *Arch. Ophthalmol.* **32**, 456–63.

Passagia, J.G., Benabid, A.L., and Chirossel, J.P. (1993). Approche de la topie cornéenne dans le ganglion trigéminal du rat. *Bull. Assoc. Anatomistes* **77**, 73–8.

Pérez, E., López-Briones, L.G., Gallar, J., and Belmonte, C. (1987). Effects of chronic sympathetic stimulation on corneal wound healing. *Invest. Ophthalmol. Vis. Sci.* **28**, 221–4.

Peyman, G.A., Rahimy, M.H., and Fernandes, M.L. (1994). Effects of morphine on corneal sensitivity and epithelial wound healing: implications for topical analgesia. *Br. J. Ophthalmol.* **78**, 138–41.

Polse, A. (1978). Etiology of corneal sensitivity changes accompanying contact lens wear. *Invest. Ophthalmol. Vis. Sci.* **78**, 1202–6.

Pozo, M.A., Gallego, R., Gallar, J., and Belmonte, C. (1992). Blockade by calcium antagonists of chemical excitation and sensitization of polymodal nociceptors in the cat's cornea. *J. Physiol.* **450**, 179–89.

Ramón y Cajal, S. (1899). *Textura del sistema nervioso del hombre y de los vertebrados.* Vidal Leuca, Alicante.

Rang, H.P. (1991). The nociceptive afferent neurone as a target for new types of analgesic drug. *Pain Research and Clinical Management (Proceedings of the 6th World Congress on Pain)* **4**, 119–27.

Rao, G., John, T., Ishida, N., and Aquavella, J.V. (1985). Recovery of corneal sensitivity in grafts following penetrating keratoplasty. *Ophthalmology* **92**, 1408–11.

Rebollo, I. and Belmonte, C. (1988). Effects of substance P and SP-antagonists on the neural activity of corneal sensory fibers. *Proceedings of the 8th International Congress of Eye Research,* (ed. M.R. Bond, J.E. Charlton and C.J. Woolf), p. 110.

Reid, T.W., Murphy, C.J., Twahashi, C., Malfroy, B., and Mannis, M.J. (1990). The stimulation of DNA synthesis in epithelial cells by substance P and CGRP. *Invest. Ophthalmol. Vis. Sci.* **31** (suppl.), 2.

Ritchie, J.M. and Greene, M.N. (1985). Local anesthetics. In *Goodman and Gilman's pharmaco-logical basis of therapeutics* (ed. A.G. Gilman, L.S. Goodman, T.W. Rall, and F. Murad), pp. 302–21. McMillan, New York.

Rózsa, A.J. and Beuerman, R.W. (1982). Density and organization of free nerve endings in the corneal epithelium of the rabbit. *Pain* **14**, 105–20.

Rózsa, A.J., Guss, R.B., and Beuerman, R.W. (1983). Neural remodelling following experimental surgery of the rabbit cornea. *Invest. Ophthalmol. Vis. Sci.* **24**, 1033–51.

Schaible, H-G. and Schmidt, R. (1985). Effect of an experimental arthritis on the sensory properties of the fine articular afferent units. *J. Neurophysiol.* **54**, 1109–22.

Schirmer, K.E. (1963a). Assessment of corneal sensitivity. *Br. J. Ophthalmol.* **47**, 488–92.

Schirmer, K.E. (1963b). Corneal sensitivity and contact lenses. *Br. J. Ophthalmol.* **47**, 493–5.

Schwartz, D.E. (1974). Corneal sensitivity in diabetics. *Arch. Ophthalmol.* **91**, 174–8.

Schwartzman, M.L., Abraham, N.G., Masferrer, J., Dunn, M.W., and McGiff, J.C. (1985). Cytochrome P-450 dependent metabolism of arachidonic acid in bovine corneal epithelium. *Biochem. Biophys. Res. Commun.* **132**, 343–51.

Schwartzman, M.L., Balazy, M., Masferrer, J., Abraham, N.G., McGiff, J.C., and Murphy, R.C. (1987). 12(R)-hydroxyicosatetranoic acid: a cytochrome P450-dependent arachidonate metabolite that inhibits Na⁺K⁺-ATPase in the cornea. *Proc. natl Acad. Sci., USA* **84**, 8125–9.

Shepherd, G.M. (1991). Sensory transduction: entering the mainstream of membrane signalling. *Cell* **67**, 845–51.

Sigelman, S. and Friedenwald, J.S. (1954). Mitotic and wound-healing activities of the corneal epithelium. *Arch. Ophthalmol.* **52**, 46–57.

Smeyne, R.J., Klein, R., Schnapp, A., Long, L.K., Bryant, S., Lewin, A., Lira, S.A., and Barbacid, M. (1994). Severe sensory and sympathetic neuropathies in mice carrying a disrupted Trk/NGF receptor gene. *Nature* **368**, 246–9.

Steen, K.H., Reeh, P.W., Anton, F., and Handwerker, H.O. (1992). Protons selectively induce lasting excitation and sensitization to mechanical stimulation of nociceptors in the rat skin. *J. Neurosci.* **12**, 86–95.

Stone, R.A. (1986). Neuropeptide Y and the innervation of the human eye. *Exp. Eye Res.* **42**, 349–55.

Stone, R.A. and McGlinn, A.M. (1988). Calcitonin gene-related peptide immunoreactive nerves in human and rhesus monkey eyes. *Invest. Ophthalmol. Vis. Sci.* **29**, 305–10.

Stone, R.A., Laties, M.A., and Brecha, N.C. (1982). Substance P-like immunoreactive nerves in the anterior segment of the rabbit, cat and monkey eye. *Neuroscience* **7**, 2459–68.

Stone, R.A., Kuwayama, Y., Terenghi, G., and Polak, J.M. (1986). Calcitonin gene-related peptide: occurrence in corneal sensory nerves. *Exp. Eye Res.* **43**, 279–83.

Stone, R.A., Kuwayama, Y., and Laties, A.M. (1987). Regulatory peptides in the eye. *Experientia* **43**, 791–800.

Sugimoto, T., Takemura, M., and Wakisaka, S. (1988). Cell size analysis of primary neurons innervating the cornea and tooth pulp of the rat. *Pain* **32**, 375–81.

Szerenyi, K., Sorken, K., Garbus, J.J., Lee, M., and McDonnell, P.J. (1994). Decrease in human corneal sensitivity with topical diclofenac sodium. *Am. J. Ophthalmol.* **118**, 312–15.

Szolcsányi, J., Jancsó-Gábor, A., and Joó, F. (1975). Functional and fine structural characteristics of the sensory neuron blocking effect of capsaicin. *Naunyn-Schmiedebergs Arch. Pharmacol.* **287**, 157–69.

Tanelian, D.L. (1991). Cholinergic activation of a population of corneal afferent nerves. *Exp. Brain Res.* **86**, 414–20.

Tanelian, D.L. and Beuerman, R.W. (1980). Recovery of corneal sensation following hard contact lens wear and the implication for adaptation. *Invest. Ophthalmol. Vis. Sci.* **19**, 1391–4.

Tanelian, D.L. and Beuerman, R.W. (1984). Responses of rabbit corneal nociceptors to mechanical and thermal stimulation. *Exp. Neurol.* **84**, 165–78.

Tanelian, D.L. and MacIver, M.B. (1990). Simultaneous visualization and electrophysiology of corneal A-delta and C fiber afferents. *J. Neurosci. Meth.* **32**, 213–22.

Tanelian, D.L. and MacIver, M.B. (1991). Analgesic concentrations of lidocaine suppress tonic A-delta and C fiber discharges produced by acute injury. *Anesthesiology* **74**, 934–6.

Terenghi, G., Polak, J.M., Ghatei, M.A., Mulderry, P.K., Butler, J.M., Unger, W.G., and Bloom, S.R. (1985). Distribution and origin of calcitonin gene-related peptide (CGRP) immunoreactivity in the sensory innervation of the mammalian eye. *J. comp. Neurol.* **233**, 506–16.

Terenghi, G., Zhang, S.-Q., Unger, W.G., and Polak, J.M. (1986). Morphological changes of sensory CGRP-immunoreactive and sympathetic nerves in periperal tissues following chronic denervation. *Histochemistry* **86**, 89–95.

Tervo, K. (1981). Effect of prolonged and neonatal capsaicin treatments on the substance P immunoreactive nerves in the rabbit eye and spinal cord. *Acta ophthalmol.* **59**, 737–46.

Tervo, K. and Tervo, T. (1981). The ultrastructure of rat corneal nerves during development. *Exp.. Eye Res.* **33**, 393–402.

Tervo, K., Tervo, T., and Palkama, A. (1978). Pre- and postnatal development of catecholamine-containing and cholinesterase-positive nerves of the rat cornea and iris. *Anat. Embryol.* **154**, 253–65.

Tervo, K., Tervo, T., Eränko, L., and Eränko, O. (1981). Substance P immunoreactive nerves in the rodent cornea. *Neurosci. Lett.* **25**, 95–7.

Tervo, K., Tervo, T., Eränko, L., Eränko, O., Valtonen, S., and Cuello, C. (1982). Effect of sensory and sympathetic denervation on substance P immunoreactivity in nerve fibres of the rabbit eye. *Exp. Eye Res.* **34**, 577–85.

Tervo, T. (1977). Consecutive demonstration of nerves containing catecholamine and acetylcholinesterase in the rat cornea. *Histochemistry* **50**, 291–9.

Tervo, T. and Palkama, A. (1978a). Innervation of the rabbit cornea. A histochemical and electronmicroscopic study. *Acta Anat.* **102**, 164–75.

Tervo, T. and Palkama, A. (1978b). Ultrastructure of the corneal nerves after fixation with potassium permanganate. *Anat. Rec.* **190**, 851–60.

Tervo, T., Tervo, K., Eränkö, L., Vannas, A., Cuello, C., and Eränkö, O. (1982). Substance P-immunoreactive nerves in the human cornea and iris. *Invest. Ophthalmol. Vis. Sci.* **23**, 671–4.

Tervo, T., Tervo, K., Eränkö, L., Vannas, A., Eränkö, O., and Cuello, C. (1983). Substance P immunoreaction and acetylcholinesterase activity in the cornea and gasserian ganglion. *Ophthalmic Res.* **15**, 280–8.

Tervo, T., Vannas, A., Tervo, K., and Holden, B.A. (1985). Histochemical evidence of limited reinnervation of human corneal grafts. *Acta ophthalmol.* **63**, 207–10.

Toivanen, N., Tervo, T., Partanen, M., Vannas, A., and Hervanen, A. (1987). Histochemical demonstration of adrenergic nerves in the stroma of human cornea. *Invest. Ophthalmol. Vis. Sci.* **28**, 398–400.

Tower, S. (1940). Unit for sensory reception in cornea. With notes on nerve impulses from sclera, iris and lens. *J. Neurophysiol.* **3**, 486–500.

Trabucchi, G., Brancato, R., Verdi, M., Carones, F., and Sala, C. (1994). Corneal nerve damage and regeneration after excimer laser photokeratectomy in rabbit eyes. *Invest. Ophthalmol. Vis. Sci.* **35**, 229–35.

Trimarchi, F. (1967). La sensibilità corneale alle variazioni termiche. *Ann. Oftal.* **93**, 592–8.

Tusscher, M.P.M. ten, Klooster, J., and Vrensen, G.F.J.M. (1988). The innervation of the rabbit's anterior eye segment: a retrograde tracing study. *Exp. Eye Res.* **46**, 717–30.

Unger, W.G. (1990). Review: mediation of the ocular response to injury. *J. ocular Pharmacol.* **6**, 337–52.

Unger, W.G., Terenghi, G., Zhang, S.-Q., and Polak, J.M. (1988). Alteration in the histochemical presence of tyrosine hydroxylase and CGRP-immunoreactivities in the eye following chronic sympathetic or sensory denervation. *Curr. Eye Res.* **7**, 761–9.

von Frey, M. (1894). Beiträge zur Physiologie des Schmerzsinnes. In *Berichte über die Verhandlungen der königlich-sächsischen Gesellschaft der Wissenschaften zu Leipzig mathematische Klasse*, pp. 185–96. Hirzel, Leipzig.

von Frey, M. (1922). Die Sensibilität der Hornhaut und Bindehaut des menschlichen Auges. *Dtsch. med. Wschr.* **48**, 212–25.

Weddell, G. and Zander, E. (1950). A critical evaluation of methods used to demonstrate tissue neural elements, illustrated by reference to the cornea. *J. Anat.* **84**, 168–99.

Weinstein, S., Drozdenko, R., and Weinstein, C. (1922). A new device for corneal esthesiometry: clinical significance and application. *Clin. Eye Vision Care* **4**, 123–8.

Whitear, M. (1960). An electron microscope study of the cornea in mice, with special reference to the innervation. *J. Anat.* **94**, 387–409.

Zander, E. and Weddell, G. (1951). Observations on the innervation of the cornea. *J. Anat., London* **85**, 68–99.

Zorab, E.C. (1971). Corneal sensitivity after grafting. *Proc. R. Soc. Med.* **64**, 117–18.

Zuazo, A., Ibañez, J., and Belmonte, C. (1986). Sensory nerve responses elicited by experimental ocular hypertension. *Exp Eye Res.* **43**, 759–69.

7 Nociceptors in skeletal muscle and their reaction to pathological tissue changes

SIEGFRIED MENSE

Neurophysiology of slowly conducting afferent units from skeletal muscle

Functional properties of muscle nociceptors under physiological conditions

Discharge behaviour

A nociceptor has been defined as a receptive ending that is activated by noxious (tissue-threatening, subjectively painful) stimuli, is capable by its response behaviour of distinguishing between innocuous and noxious events, and encodes the intensity of noxious stimuli (Perl 1984; Besson and Chaouch 1987). Recordings of the electrical activity of single muscle afferent units in anaesthetized cats and rats have shown that in these species muscle nociceptors as defined above are present. When tested with graded natural stimuli (mechanical, chemical, thermal), these receptors do not respond to stimuli such as occur during the normal activity of the muscle (for example, weak local pressure, contractions, and stretches within the physiological range) but require noxious intensities of stimulation for activation (Fig. 7.1; Bessou and Laporte 1960; Paintal 1960; Mense and Meyer 1985). A liminal activation of a muscle nociceptor may occur if the intensity of stimulation approaches noxious levels without being tissue damaging, for example, during unphysiological stretch or during strong contractions elicited by electrical stimulation of the muscle nerve. Teleologically, this property is important, since a nociceptor is supposed not only to signal tissue damage but also to prevent its occurrence.

Conduction velocity

In the gastrocnemius–soleus (GS) muscle of the cat, the conduction velocity of nociceptive afferent units spans the entire spectrum of group III and IV units (from 0.3 to 30 m/s; Paintal 1960; Iggo 1961; Mense and Meyer 1985; Mense 1986). Nociceptors have been found to be more frequent among group IV than among group III units (43 versus 33 per cent; Mense and Meyer 1985).

Resting activity

In contrast to the skin where nociceptors usually have no resting or background activity (defined as discharges in the absence of intentional stimulation), a small proportion of cat muscle nociceptors (approximately 25 per cent) have been found to exhibit such an activity (Berberich *et al.* 1988). The discharges typically consist of single impulses at irregular intervals; the mean frequency is very low and does not exceed a few impulses per minute in a surgically exposed but otherwise intact muscle. Because of its low frequency the resting discharge will probably not elicit subjective sensations. Single impulses in (cutaneous) nociceptive fibres have been reported not to reach consciousness level (Torebjörk 1985).

Nociceptive Unit (Group III)

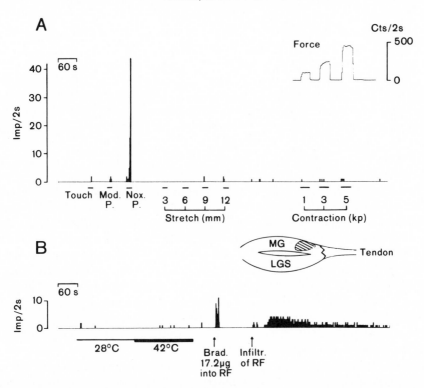

Fig. 7.1 Response behaviour of a muscle nociceptor supplied by a thin myelinated (group III) fibre, conduction velocity 12.0 m/s. The location of the receptive ending is marked by the hatched area on the medial gastrocnemius (MG) muscle. LGS, lateral gastrocnemius–soleus muscle. In the histogram of the fibre's activity the impulses per counting interval (2 s) are plotted on the ordinate against time on the abscissa. The duration of the stimuli used is indicated by the length of the bars underneath the histogram. Touch, touching the muscle with an artist's brush; Mod. p., Moderate, innocuous pressure; Nox. p., noxious pressure; temperature values in (B) indicate the temperature of water circulating through a thermode in contact with the muscle. Arrows, single injection of bradykinin (Brad.) into or infiltration (Infiltr.) of the receptive field (RF) with the algesic agent. The force registration in the insert in (A) corresponds to the values in kp (kilopond) underneath the histogram. The receptor is insensitive to stimuli that are likely to occur during normal activity of the muscle.

Mechanical sensitivity

In the original studies by Paintal (1960) and Bessou and Laporte (1960) on group III and by Iggo (1961) on group IV muscle receptors, many units were found that could be activated by local pressure stimulation. Some of these had a high mechanical threshold and responded also to painful chemical stimuli. Paintal denoted these receptors 'pressure-pain receptors' and assumed that one of their functions was to elicit pain sensations from muscle. Most of the group IV and many of the group III units lack sensitivity to small degrees of muscle stretch (Iggo 1961; Franz and Mense 1975; Kumazawa and Mizumura 1977; Kaufman *et al.* 1982). Stretching a cat gastrocnemius muscle with forces exceeding 4 N resulted in an activation of a small proportion of group IV receptors, all of which did not respond to local pressure stimulation (Kniffki *et al.* 1978).

A very effective stimulus for activating muscle nociceptors in animal experiments is squeezing the muscle with a forceps with broadened tips. The force required for receptor activation is smilar to that needed to elicit pain from a muscle of similar size in humans (Paintal 1960; Iggo 1961; Franz and Mense 1975).

The size of the mechanosensitive receptive field (RF) of a muscle nociceptor can only be determined with limitations, particularly if it is located deep within the muscle. The reported sizes of superficially located fields or the projections of deep RFs on the muscle surface range from spotlike to several cm^2 in the gastrocnemius muscle of the cat and dog (Kumazawa and Mizumura 1977; Mense and Meyer 1985).

Generally, receptors with group IV afferent fibres have a higher threshold to local pressure stimulation than endings with group III fibres. All the units conducting at less than 1 m/s were of the high-threshold mechanosensitive (HTM) type or could not be excited with mechanical stimuli; among the units conducting at more than 5 m/s, HTM receptors were the minority (Mense 1978).

Some of the afferent units with endings in muscle and other deep tissues had two RFs, that is, they could be activated from two sites in the muscle that were separated by an insensitive region. Afferent units with two RFs were relatively frequent among low-threshold mechanosensitive (LTM) receptors (33 per cent in the GS muscle of the cat; Mense and Meyer 1985) and rare among nociceptive units. Among afferent fibres from the cat tail, units were found that had one HTM RF in deep tissues (muscle, joint, periosteum) and another one in the skin distal to the deep RF (Mense *et al.* 1981). The anatomical basis of this feature may be branching of the afferent fibre close to its area of termination.

Approximately one-third of all group IV units that were recorded from dorsal rootlets and could be activated by electrical stimulation of the GS nerve did not respond to mechanical probing of the muscle (Franz and Mense 1975). Many of these (44 per cent) could be excited by close intraarterial injection of the endogenous algesic agent bradykinin (BK). Under the conditions of an *in vivo* experiment it is difficult to tell whether an afferent unit really lacks mechanosensitivity or whether the mechanosensitive RF has not been found because of its small size and/or unfavourable location. The recently detected 'silent' or 'sleeping' nociceptors offer a new interpretation of this set of data. Silent nociceptors have been described in skin, joint capsule, and viscera (Grigg *et al.* 1986; Häbler *et al.* 1988; Meyer and Campbell 1988; Handwerker *et al.* 1991). In skeletal muscle such receptors have not yet been found.

Chemical excitability

Effective stimulants for free nerve endings in skeletal muscle are endogenous pain-producing substances such as BK, 5-hydroxytryptamine (5-HT), and potassium ions in concentrations of 60 mM or higher (Fock and Mense 1976; Kumazawa and Mizumura 1977; Kaufman *et al.* 1982). Hypertonic NaCl solutions (4.5–6.0 per cent) are also effective excitants of group III and IV muscle receptors. Similarly to the activation by potassium, the stimulating effects of hypertonic solutions are considered to be non-specific (that is, not mediated by pharmacological receptors), because all muscle receptors, including the primary endings of muscle spindles, are excited by this stimulus (Iggo 1961).

On a molar basis, the nonapeptide BK has been found to be the most effective stimulant for muscle nociceptors (Fock and Mense 1976). Unmyelinated afferent units from muscle respond in a well graded manner to increasing concentrations of BK (Kumazawa and Mizumura 1977). The action of BK on neurones has been shown to be mediated by pharmacological BK receptors (B_1 and B_2; Barabé *et al.* 1984). Under pathological conditions (lowering of pH, ischaemia, blood clotting, vascular damage), BK is cleaved from plàsma proteins and 5-HT is released from platelets. Large amounts of potassium are present in the sarcoplasm of each muscle cell. Thus, muscle lesions of any kind release endogenous substances that may excite free nerve endings. These substances belong to the so-called 'vasoneuroactive substances' (Sicuteri 1967).

The above substances, particularly BK, excite not only nociceptors but also non-nociceptive endings in muscle. Therefore, an excitability by BK cannot be taken as an indication of the nociceptive nature of a receptor. It is well known that slowly adapting mechanoreceptors of the skin also respond to BK (Fjällbrant and Iggo 1961; Beck and Handwerker 1974; but see Kress and Reeh, Chapter 11, this volume). However, BK activates almost exclusively the slowly conducting afferent units (group III and IV) and not the encapsulated stretch receptors (Mense 1977).

The doses of pain-producing substances required to excite muscle nociceptors in animal experiments are similar to those eliciting muscle pain in humans (Coffman 1966). The time course of the receptor activation (latency and duration)—at least in the case of BK injections—also resembles that of pain elicited by BK in humans.

The functional identification of a receptive ending ideally includes the administration of all possible stimuli that may act on the ending under physiological circumstances. If only mechanical stimuli are used, the majority of the units classified as HTM will be nociceptive, but some receptors will be included that actually are thermosensitive (see below).

Many muscle nociceptors respond to both noxious local pressure and injections of BK (close arterial or intramuscular), but there are also receptors that can be activated by only one type of noxious stimulation (mechanical or chemical). This finding may indicate that different types of nociceptors are present in skeletal muscle, similarly to the skin where mechano-, mechanoheat-, and polymodal nociceptors have been found (see Campbell and Meyer, Chapter 5, this volume).

Thermal sensitivity

Some of the muscle group IV receptors respond to small temperature changes in the innocuous range (20–40°C; Iggo 1961; Kumazawa and Mizumura 1977; Mense and Meyer 1985; Mense 1986). When tested with mechanical stimuli they have an extremely high threshold and do not encode the stimulus intensity well in their discharges. Therefore, the response to noxious pressure stimuli may reflect a mechanical damage and not a true mechanosensitivity.

There are also group IV muscle receptors that have a thermal threshold in the noxious range (above 43°C, below 20°C; Iggo 1961; Kumazawa and Mizumura 1977). In contrast to the endings classified as thermosensitive, most of these units also respond to noxious local pressure and endogenous algesic agents and thus behave like polymodal nociceptors in the skin.

Influence of hypoxia and adrenaline in vitro

In the rat hemidiaphragm–phrenic nerve preparation, LTM and HTM receptors with behaviours similar to those encountered in skeletal muscle *in vivo* can be distinguished (Kieschke *et al.* 1988). Experimental hypoxia of approximately 20 mmHg in the organ bath had an excitatory action on both LTM and HTM units. In some receptors the mechanical threshold determined with von Frey hairs was lowered during hypoxia. These data indicate that hypoxia may be an important factor in the control of the excitability of nociceptors in deep tissue.

Adrenaline at concentrations of 0.5–5 μM in the organ bath had a differential efect on LTM and HTM receptors. About half of the latter responded with an increase in discharge frequency, whereas the LTM units were not excited. A finding of probable clinical significance was that HTM receptors that initially were not responsive to adrenaline often developed a sensitivity to the catecholamine when their RFs were irritated by a constant mechanical stimulus of noxious intensity (Kieschke *et al.* 1988). This finding suggests that damaged nociceptors—for example, in pathologically altered tissue—are more sensitive to adrenaline than receptors in intact tissue.

Recordings of muscle nociceptors in man

The technique of microneurography has recently also been applied to muscle nerves in humans (see Ochoa *et al.*, Chapter 21, this volume). The results obtained from single group III and IV muscle afferent units show that the response behaviour of human muscle nociceptors is indistinguishable from that of nociceptors in the cat and rat.

Modulating factors at the nociceptive ending

Bradykinin

The mechanical sensitivity of muscle nociceptors can be increased by endogenous substances. This process of receptor sensitization probably accompanies all types of tissue lesion and is the best established peripheral mechanism explaining the clinical symptoms of tenderness and hyperalgesia. BK is one of the substances that has a sensitizing action on muscle nociceptors in addition to its excitatory effect. A nociceptor sensitized by BK has a lowered mechanical threshold and, therefore, can be activated by innocuous stimuli. The BK dose required for sensitizing muscle nociceptors was found to be lower than that required for activating the units. This means that a nociceptor can be sensitized without being activated (Mense and Meyer 1988).

The BK-induced sensitization appears to be a quite specific process because: (1) LTM (presumably non-nociceptive) group III and IV receptors were not sensitized; and (2) the sensitization did not affect all aspects of the nociceptor function. Some units were sensitized to stretch and contractions but not to local pressure stimuli, whereas others exhibited increased sensitivity predominantly to local pressure (Mense and Meyer 1988).

Interactions between endogenous substances

Prostaglandins of the E type (PG E) and 5-HT have been shown to sensitize slowly conducting muscle afferent units to BK, that is, following administration of these substances BK has a stronger excitatory action on the receptors (Fig. 7.2; Mense

1981). BK on the other hand is known to release PGE_2 from tissue cells (Jose *et al.* 1981) and also from sympathetic efferent fibres (Levine *et al.* 1986). By this mechanism, BK is capable of potentiating its own action. There is evidence indicating that the PG-induced sensitization of nociceptors is mediated by the cyclic adenosine monophosphate (cAMP) second messenger system (Taiwo *et al.* 1990; see Kress and Reeh, Chapter 11, this volume).

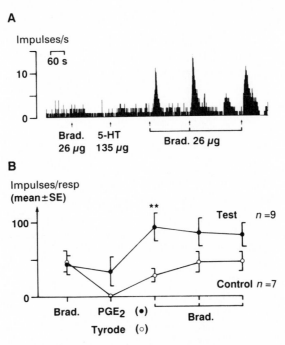

Fig. 7.2 Sensitization of group IV afferent units to bradykinin (Brad.) by serotonin (5-HT) and prostaglandin E_2 (PGE_2). (A) High-threshold mechanosensitive receptor; conduction velocity of afferent fibre 1.1 m/s. (B) Statistical evaluation of data obtained with Brad. and PGE_2 in series of injections as shown in (A). Open circles, control series in which, instead of PGE_2, the vehicle (tyrode solution) was injected. Filled circles, test series. resp, response. **, $p < 0.01$, U test, two-sided. From Mense (1981).

In accordance with the findings that BK releases PGs from tissue cells and that PGs potentiate the stimulating action of the kinin on muscle receptors, administration of acetylsalicylic acid (ASA)—a blocker of PG synthesis—was found to reduce the BK-induced activations of slowly conducting muscle afferent units (Mense 1982). This finding suggests that there is a PG component in the BK-induced excitation of muscle group IV receptors.

Leukotriene D4 as a desensitizing substance

Leukotrienes (LTs) are also released from tissue cells under pathological condtions, and some (for example, LTB_4) have been shown to promote inflammatory processes and induce hyperalgesia in behavioural experiments (Samuelsson 1983; Piper 1984). In contrast, LTD_4 has been found to have a desensitizing effect on HTM receptors in rat muscle (Hoheisel *et al.* 1994). Infiltration of the RFs with 100 ng–1 µg LTD_4 was followed by a significant reduction of the response magnitude to mechanical stimulation.

Neuropeptides

Results from receptors in the rat hemidiaphragm–phrenic nerve preparation *in vitro* have shown that HTM units increase their resting discharge in the presence of substance P (SP) (10–100 µM; Reinert *et al.* 1992). The responses of the receptors to local pressure stimulation were not altered by SP, however. The data suggest that SP may have a modulatory function in muscle pain, but does not sensitize muscle nociceptors to mechanical stimuli. The excitatory action of SP was restricted to HTM receptors, that is, the resting activity of LTM units was not influenced by SP.

Response behaviour of muscle nociceptors under pathophysiological and pathological conditions

Ischaemic contractions

Interruption of the blood supply to a resting extremity for 20 min does not cause pain, but, if the muscle is forced to contract under ischaemic conditions, pain develops within about 1 min (Lewis *et al.* 1931). The mechanisms underlying this type of ischaemic pain are still a matter of controversy. Accumulation of acidic metabolites including lactate (Moore *et al.* 1934), potassium ions (Harpuder and Stein 1943), or the lack of oxidation of metabolic products (Pickering and Wayne 1933–34) have all been proposed as causal factors.

A substance probably involved in ischaemic muscle pain is BK. The kinin is released from plasma proteins during ischaemia (Sicuteri *et al.* 1964; Nakahara 1971) and, because of its strong action on nociceptors, is likely to contribute to the pain of intermittent claudication. Lactate, phosphate, and potassium ions have been tested for their excitatory action on muscle group III and IV afferent units in the cat and have been found to be rather ineffective on a molar basis (Kniffki *et al.* 1978).

Ischaemia without contractions is not an effective stimulus for slowly conducting muscle afferent units unless it lasts for long periods of time. Ligation of an artery to resting muscle for 5 min in an anaesthetized cat did not activate muscle group III and IV units (Mense and Stahnke 1983). Following a longer-lasting complete interruption of the blood supply (experimentally induced by circulatory arrest), most of the slowly conducting muscle afferent units developed a bursting backgroud activity 15–60 min after the onset of ischaemia. The increase in activity lasted for periods of several minutes up to half an hour; then the units fell silent and could no longer be activated by electrical stimulation of the muscle nerve (Mense 1991). The latter finding indicates that the prolonged ischaemia affected not only the action potential-generating system at the receptive ending but also the electrical conduction of the afferent fibre.

In experiments using the antidromic collision technique, Bessou and Laporte (1958) found that during ischaemic contractions a large proportion of the muscle group IV afferent units are activated. Single-fibre recordings from group III and IV muscle receptors yielded a relatively small population of units (approximately 10 per cent) that reacted in a way that suggested an involvement in the mediation of ischaemic pain (see below; Mense and Stahnke 1983). The receptors specifically responding to ischaemic contractions were not or were only weakly activated during contractions without arterial occlusion but showed clear excitations when the contractions were repeated under ischaemic conditions. The time course of the activation was similar to that of the pain induced in human volunteers performing ischaemic contractions (Lewis *et al.* 1931) with the receptor activity to rise 30–60 s after the onset of the contractions (Fig. 7.3; Paintal 1960; Mense and Stahnke 1983; Kaufman *et al.* 1984). The receptors that showed strong reactions to ischaemic contractions were group IV units; group III receptors were only liminally affected. Most of the receptors tested with ischaemic contractions did not react at all, although the chemical changes induced by the ischaemic work were probably present in the entire muscle. This finding supports the notion that the free nerve endings in skeletal muscle comprise different functional types.

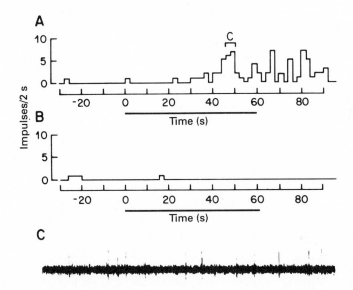

Fig. 7.3 Effect of ischaemia on the response to static contraction of a group IV afferent (conduction velocity 0.8 m/s) whose receptive field was in triceps surae. (A) Stimulation of afferent by ischaemic static contraction (represented by bar). Note maintained stimulation of afferent after end of contraction. (B) Non-ischaemic contraction (represented by bar) had no effect on afferent. (C) Recording of impulse activity of group IV afferent during period of time, depicted by bracket with 'c' over it in (A). From Kaufman *et al.* (1984).

As to the mechanisms of receptor activation during ischaemic contractions, a speculative interpretation is that the ischaemia-induced decrease in the partial pressure of O_2 (pO_2) or pH releases BK, PGE_2, and potassium ions (Harpuder and Stein 1943; Uchida and Ueda 1969; Jennische *et al.* 1982), which sensitize muscle nociceptors so that they respond to the force of contraction. During exhausting work the pH inside the muscle may drop to 6.0–6.6 (Caldwell 1956; Sahlin *et al.* 1976). As a low pH has been found to be a powerful sensitizing factor for cutaneous nociceptors (Steen *et al.* 1992), an ischaemia-induced increase in proton concentration may contribute to ischaemic pain. Calcitonin gene-related peptide (CGRP) may also be involved as the peptide has been shown to be released from ischaemic heart muscle with BK enhancing the release (Franco-Cereceda *et al.* 1989).

Inflammation

In experimental animals, a myositis can be induced by infiltrating a muscle with carrageenan, a sulfated polysaccharide. The carrageenan-induced myositis is thought to be a neurogenic inflammation, mediated by the release of SP and other agents from nociceptive afferent units (Lam and Ferrell 1990). Starting approximately 2 h after the carrageenan injection, the muscle exhibits signs of a myositis (hyperaemia, oedema, infiltration by polymorphonuclear leucocytes; Berberich *et al.* 1988). In the carrageenan-inflamed rat paw, these changes are known to be associated with the release of vasoneuroactive substances that are liberated in a temporal order, namely, 5-HT and histamine first, then BK, and finally PGs (DiRosa *et al. 1971*).

In cat and rat, the myositis-induced changes in the response behaviour of slowly conducting muscle afferent units were similar although quantitative differences exist. In both species, the resting activity of the receptors was increased. Both the proportion of units exhibiting resting discharge and the mean discharge frequency were higher in inflamed muscle (Berberich *1988; Diehl et al.* 1988).

The pattern of the resting discharge in fibres from inflamed muscle was irregular, often of intermittent nature, with phases of bursting activity alternating with long periods of silence. Bursting discharges are likely to be very effective at central synapses and may cause (spontaneous) pain if they occur in nociceptive afferent units. An increased resting discharge was not only present in HTM (presumably nociceptive) units but also in receptors responding to innocuous pressure (in inflamed muscle comprising true LTM receptors and sensitized HTM units).

As was to be expected from the data concerning sensitization, the proportion of receptors with a high mechanical threshold decreased in inflamed muscle. In normal muscle of the cat, aproximately 80 per cent of the group IV units are HTM; the proportion dropped significantly in inflamed muscle. Apparently, the tenderness is mainly due to a sensitization of group IV receptors as the mechanical threshold of group III units did not change significantly. In contrast, spontaneous pain and dysaesthesias may be predominantly caused by activity in group III units, since in the cat these were the ones that showed a significant increase in background activity in inflamed muscle (Berberich *et al.* 1988).

The inflammation-induced sensitization of muscle receptors is probably caused by a release of vasoneuroactive substances (BK, PGs, 5-HT) and neuropeptides from the inflamed tissue. As shown above, SP may increase the resulting activity of nociceptors and thus could contribute to spontaneous muscle pain. The neuropeptide is also known to release histamine from tissue mast cells, which, in turn, may influence blood vessels (Holzer 1988; Coderre *et al.* 1989) and nerve endings in muscle. The results of a recent study suggest that the local release of nitric oxide (NO) may be involved in the vasodilatation of a carrageenan-induced inflammation (Ialenti *et al.* 1992). The action of these latter substances on muscle nociceptors remains to be established.

Neuroanatomy of free nerve endings in skeletal muscle and tendon

Frequency of nociceptive fibres in a muscle nerve

The available experimental evidence indicates that small-diameter afferent fibres from muscle have to be activated in order to elicit pain. Histologically, these units are either thin myelinated (Aδ or group III fibres) or non-myelinated (C or group IV fibres). In this

chapter the afferent fibre types are classified in groups I–IV according to the nomenclature of Lloyd (1943), which was developed specifically for muscle afferent fibres and
uses the fibre diameter as a classification criterion.

The nerve to a mid-sized locomotor muscle in the cat, the lateral gastrocnemius–soleus
(LGS), contains approximately 4000 nerve fibres. One-third of the fibres are myelinated
and two-thirds non-myelinated (Stacey 1969; Mitchell and Schmidt 1983). Of the latter,
50 per cent are sensory and, of these, 43 have been found to be nociceptive (Mense and
Meyer 1985).

The proportion of nociceptors given above for the LGS nerve can probably not be
transferred to other muscles, because the reported differences in sensory innervation are
substantial (Richmond *et al.* 1976; Abrahams 1986).

Morphological features of the free nerve ending

Data on the morphology of functionally identified muscle nociceptors are lacking; from
indirect evidence it can be inferred that nociceptors in muscle and tendon are most
probably free nerve endings. Electron microscopic investigations have shown that this
type of ending is formed by small-diameter afferent fibres. Group IV afferent fibres
are assumed to terminate exclusively in free nerve endings, while group III fibres supply
both free nerve endings and other types of muscle receptor (for example, paciniform
corpuscles). The typical location of free nerve endings in skeletal muscle is the wall of
arterioles and the surrounding connective tissue (Stacey 1969).

Electron microscopic data demonstrate that the so-called free nerve endings in muscle
and tendon are almost completely ensheathed by Schwann cells. Only small areas of the
axonal membrane are directly exposed to the interstitial fluid (Andres *et al.* 1985; von
Düring and Andres 1990). The exposed membrane areas often form varicosities and are
supplied with mitrochondria and vesicles. These are structural specializations characteristic of receptive areas. The electron microscopic reconstruction of free endings in the
calcaneal tendon of the cat showed that different morphological types of ending
connected to group III and IV afferent fibres exist (Andres *et al.* 1985). At present,
it is not possible to correlate the morphological types with the functional ones classified
in electrophysiological experiments.

The existence of different morphological types in the tendon supports the notion that
the free nerve endings of deep tissues, including skeletal muscle, do not form a
homogeneous population of polymodal receptors but comprise functionally different
(for example, nociceptive and non-nociceptive) receptors. Electron microscopic reconstructions of free nerve endings in muscle have not been performed. Preliminary data
suggest that the main morphological features of these endings are similar in tendon and
muscle (Fig. 7.4; von Düring and Andres 1990).

Immunohistochemical properties of somata of nociceptive muscle afferents in the dorsal root ganglion

Neuropeptides are present predominantly in primary afferent units of small diameter
and can be released together with transmitter substances from afferent terminals in the
spinal cord (Hökfelt *et al.* 1980; Kow and Pfaff 1988). No neuropeptide has been found
that can be considered specific for nociceptive fibres from muscle. Dorsal root ganglion
(DRG) cells projecting in a muscle nerve have been reported to contain SP, CGRP, and

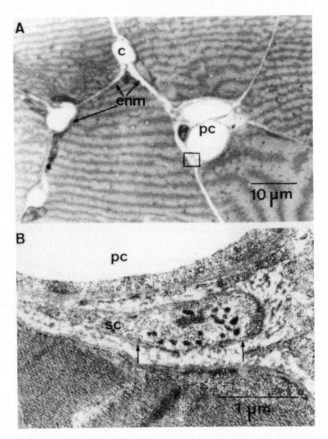

Fig. 7.4 Histological section through a free nerve ending formed by a group IV fibre in the soleus muscle of the cat. (A) The box in the wall of a precapillary segment (pc) of a blood vessel marks the area that is enlarged in (B). C, capillary; enm, endomysium. (B) The terminal axon contains numerous dense core and clear vesicles. The arrows mark regions of exposed axonal membrane. From von Düring and Andres (1990).

somatostatin (SOM) and thus present a peptide pattern similar to that of cutaneous nerves (Molander and Grant 1987; O'Brien *et al.* 1989).

Recent data from experiments in which single DRG cells with receptive endings in muscle were first functionally identified and then injected with a dye indicate that at least some cell bodies whose peripheral processes terminate in HTM (presumably nociceptive) receptors exhibit CGRP-like immunoreactivity (Fig. 7.5). CGRP-like immunoreactivity has not only been found in nociceptive units but also in other types of muscle receptors including LTM units. Most of the cutaneous and deep receptor types studied so far showed CGRP-like immunoreactivity in some of their cell bodies in the DRG (Hoheisel *et al.* 1994). The neuropeptide was present predominantly in perikarya of small size that had slowly conducting axons. These findings suggest that CGRP may exist in many thin myelinated and non-myelinated muscle afferent units irrespective of their function.

SP as a transmitter or modulator of pain sensations is still a subject of some controversy (Nicoll *et al.* 1980; Frenk *et al.* 1988; Kellstein *et al.* 1990). An important finding in this regard is that the great majority (10 of 12) of individually identified nociceptive DRG cells of the cat did not exhibit SP-like immunoreactivity (Leah *et al.* 1985). Recently, however, many HTM units in the DRG of the guinea-pig have been reported to contain SP-immunoreactive cells (Lawson *et al.* 1994).

HTM (C.V. 1,3m/s)

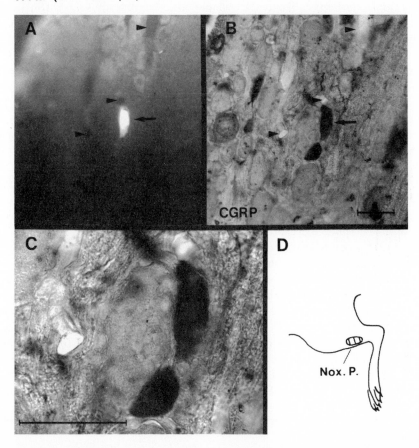

Fig. 7.5 Immunocytochemical data from a rat DRG cell that terminated in a HTM (presumably nociceptive) ending in skeletal muscle. (A) Fluorescent soma of the DRG cell (arrow) marked with intracellular iontophoresis of lucifer yellow. The arrowheads indicate histological landmarks (for example, blood vessels). (B) Same section as in (A) following incubation with antibodies to CGRP. Scale bar, 50 μm. (C) Enlargement of (B). Scale bar, 50 μm. (D) Location of the afferent unit's RF in the anterior tibial muscle. The receptor required noxious pressure stimulation (Nox. P.) for activation. Conduction velocity (C.V.) of afferent fibre, 1.3 m/s. From Mense (1991).

Neuropeptide content of free nerve endings in skeletal muscle

Immunohistochemical studies have shown that, in the GS muscle of the rat, free nerve endings are present that exhibit immunoreactivity to CGRP, SP, and vasoactive intestinal polypeptide (VIP; Reinert and Mense 1993). The majority of these fibres are located in the connective tissue around small arteries and arterioles. The numerical area density of CGRP-immunoreactive nerve endings was found to be 5–6 times higher than that of SP-immunoreactive endings, and VIP-immunoreactive fibres were much less numerous than SP-immunoreactive ones. As in the DRG (Lee *et al.* 1985; Ju *et al.* 1987), an extensive coexistence of CGRP and SP is present in free nerve endings in muscle.

In the calcaneal tendon of the rat, the bulk of immunoreactive fibres are present in the peritenonium externum, whereas the collagen fibre bundles are largely free from these endings. The overall innervation density of neuropeptide-immunoreactive endings in the Achilles tendon was 5–7 times higher in tendon than in muscle (Reinert and Mense 1994).

As to SP, muscle nerves have been reported to contain less SP than skin nerves (McMahon *et al.* 1984). This finding has been teleologically explained by assuming that—because of the tight muscle fascia—the oedema caused by the release of SP from muscle afferent fibres via the axon reflex would be deleterious for the tissue. Neuropeptides also influence imune cells and synoviocytes (Lotz *et al.* 1987). These latter actions may be of particular importance for the development and maintenance of chronic arthritis and other painful disorders of deep somatic tissues.

The mechanisms by which neuropeptides contribute to muscle pain may be complex; intramuscular injections of small amounts of CGRP or SP alone have been reported not to elicit pain in humans, whereas a combination of both, or of CGRP with neurokinin A, was painful (Pedersen-Bjergaard *et al.* 1991).

After a 12-day period of experimental myositis, the immunoreactive endings in the rat GS muscle were found to have an increased numerical area density. This effect was most prominent in SP-immunoreactive endings (Fig. 7.6; Reinert and Mense 1993). To what extent this increase in numerical area density also affects nociceptive fibres is unknown.

An increase in fibre density has also been reported following surgical and chemical sympathectomy (Cole *et al.* 1983; Aberdeen *et al.* 1992). These findings shed a new light on older results obtained in electron microscopic investigations of free nerve endings, most of which were performed in surgically sympathectomized animals. It is conceivable that the published results on the morphology of free endings are influenced by the sympathectomy and do not reflect the normal appearance of these structures.

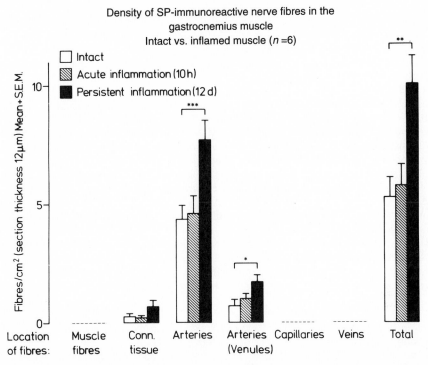

Fig. 7.6 Innervation density of SP-immunoreactive nerve endings in the various components of muscle tissue (medial head of gastrocnemius muscle of rat). On the ordinate, the numerical area density in cross-sections of the muscle is given as fibres per cm^2 tissue at a given section thickness of 12 μm. Open bars, Intact (non-injected muscle); hatched bars, acute inflammation of 10-h duration induced by injecting the muscle with carrageenan; filled bars, persistent (subacute) inflammation of 12-day duration induced by a single injection of complete Freund's adjuvant into the muscle. *, $p < 0.05$; **, $p < 0.01$; ***, $p < 0.001$; U test, two-sided. From Reinert and Mense (unpublished).

References

Aberdeen, J., Milner, P., Lincoln, J., and Burnstock, G. (1922). Guanethidine sympathectomy of mature rats leads to increases in calcitonin gene-related peptide and vasoactive intestinal polypeptide-containing nerves. *Neuroscience* **47**, 453–61.

Abrahams, V.C. (1986). Group III and IV receptors of skeletal muscle. *Can. J. Physiol. Pharmacol.* **64**, 509–14.

Andres, K.H., von Düring, M., and Schmidt, R.F. (1985). Sensory innervation of the Achilles tendon by group III and IV afferent fibers. *Anat. Embryol.* **172**, 145–56.

Barabé, J., Caranikas, S., D'Orléans-Juste, P., and Regoli, D. (1984). New agonist and antagonist analogues of bradykinin. *Can. J. Physiol. Pharmacol.* **62**, 627–9.

Beck, P.W. and Handwerker, H.O. (1974). Bradykinin and serotonin effects on various types of cutaneous nerve fibres. *Pflügers Arch.* **347**, 209–22.

Berberich, P., Hoheisel, U., and Mense, S. (1988). Effects of a carrageenan-induced myositis on the discharge properties of group III and IV muscle receptors in the cat. *J. Neurophysiol.* **59**, 1395–409.

Besson, J.M. and Chaouch, A. (1987). Peripheral and spinal mechanisms of nociception. *Physiol. Rev.* **67**, 67–186.

Bessou, P. and Laporte, Y. (1958). Activation des fibres afférentes amyéliniques d'origine musculaire. *C. R. Soc. Biol., Paris* **152**, 1587–90.

Bessou, P. and Laporte, Y. (1960). Activation des fibres afférentes myélinisées de petit calibre d'origine musculaire (fibres du groupe III). *J. Physiol., Paris* **52**, 19–20.

Caldwell, P.C. (1956). Intracellular pH. *Int. Rev. Cytol.* **5**, 229–77.

Coderre, T.J., Basbaum, A.I., and Levine, J.D. (1989). Neural control of vascular permeability: interactions between primary afferents, mast cells, and sympathetic efferents. *J. Neurophysiol.* **62**, 48–58.

Coffman, J.D. (1966). The effect of aspirin on pain and hand blood flow responses to intra-arterial injection of bradykinin in man. *Clin. Pharmacol. Ther.* **7**, 26–37.

Cole, D.F., Bloom, S.R., Burnstock, G., Butler, J.M., McGregor, G.P., Saffrey, M.J., Unger, W.G., and Zhang, S.Q. (1983). Increase in SP-like immunoreactivity in nerve fibres of rabbit iris and ciliary body one to four months following sympathetic denervation. *Exp. Eye Res.* **37**, 191–7.

Diehl, B., Hoheisel, U., and Mense, S. (1988). Histological and neurophysiological changes induced by carrageenan in skeletal muscle of cat and rat. *Agents Actions* **25**, 210–13.

DiRosa, M., Giroud, J.P., and Willoughby, D.A. (1971). Studies of the mediators of the acute inflammatory response induced in rats in different sites by carrageenan and turpentine. *J. Pathol.* **104**, 15–29.

Fjällbrant, N. and Iggo, A. (1961). The effect of histamine, 5-hydroxytryptamine and acetylcholine on cutaneous afferent fibres. *J. Physiol.* **156**, 578–90.

Fock, S. and Mense, S. (1976). Excitatory effects of 5-hydroxytryptamine, histamine, and potassium ions on muscular group IV afferent units: a comparison with bradykinin. *Brain Res.* **105**, 459–69.

Franco-Cereceda, A., Saria, A., and Lundberg, J.M. (1989). Differential release of calcitonin gene-related peptide and neuropeptide Y from the isolated heart by capsaicin, ischaemia, nicotine, bradykinin and ouabain. *Acta physiol. scand.* **135**, 173–87.

Franz, M. and Mense, S. (1975). Muscle receptors with group IV afferent fibres responding to application of bradykinin. *Brain Res.* **92**, 369–83.

Frenk, H., Bossut, D., Urca, G., and Mayer, D.J. (1988). Is substance P a primary afferent neurotransmitter for nociceptive input? I. Analysis of pain-related behaviors resulting from intrathecal administration of substance P and 6 excitatory compounds. *Brain Res.* **455**, 223–31.

Grigg, P., Schaible, H.-G., and Schmidt, R.F. (1986). Mechanical sensitivity of group III and IV afferents from posterior articular nerve in normal and inflamed cat knee. *J. Neurophysiol.* **55**, 635–43.

Häbler, H.J., Jänig, W., and Koltzenburg, M. (1988). A novel type of unmyelinated chemosensitive nociceptor in the acutely inflamed urinary bladder. *Agents Actions* **25**, 219–21.

Handwerker, H.O., Kilo, S., and Reeh, P.W. (1991). Unresponsive afferent nerve fibres in the sural nerve of the rat. *J. Physiol.* **435**, 229–42.

Harpuder, K. and Stein, I. (1943). Studies on the nature of pain arising from an ischemic limb. *Am. Heart J.* **25**, 429–48.

Hoheisel, U., Mense, S., and Scherotzke, R. (1994). Calcitonin gene-related peptide-immunoreactivity in functionally identified primary afferent neurones in the rat. *Anat. Embryol.* **189**, 41–9.

Hökfelt, T., Johansson, O., Ljungdahl, Å., Lundberg, J.M., and Schultzberg, M. (1980). Peptidergic neurones. *Nature* **284**, 515–21.

Holzer, P. (1988). Local effector functions of capsaicin-sensitive sensory nerve endings: involvement of tachykinins, calcitonin gene-related peptide and other neuropeptides. *Neuroscience* **24**, 739–68.

Ialenti, A., Ianaro, A., Moncada, S., and Di Rosa, M. (1992). Modulation of acute inflammation by endogenous nitric oxide. *Eur. J. Pharmacol.* **211**, 177–82.

Iggo, A. (1961). Non-myelinated afferent fibres from mammalian skeletal muscle. *J. Physiol.* **155**, 52–3.

Jennische, E., Hagberg, H., and Haljamäe, H. (1982). Extracellular potassium concentration and membrane potential in rabbit gastrocnemius muscle during tourniquet ischemia. *Pflügers Arch.* **392**, 335–9.

Jose, P.J., Page, D.A., Wolstenholme, B.E., Williams, T.J., and Dumonde, D.C. (1981). Bradykinin-stimulated prostaglandin E_2 production of endothelial cells and its modulation by antiinflammatory compounds. *Inflammation* **5**, 363–78.

Ju, G., Hökfelt, T., Brodin, E., Fahrenkrug, J., Fischer, J.A., and Frey, P. (1987). Primary sensory neurons of the rat showing calicitonin gene-related peptide immunoreactivity and their relation to substance P, somatostatin-, galanin-, vasoactive intestinal polypeptide- and cholecystokinin-immunoreactive ganglion cells. *Cell Tissue Res.* **247**, 417–31.

Kaufman, M.P., Iwamoto, G.A., Longhurst, J.C., and Mitchell, J.H. (1982). Effects of capsaicin and bradykinin on afferent fibers with endings in skeletal muscle. *Circ. Res.* **50**, 133–9.

Kaufman, M.P., Rybicki, K.J., Waldrop, T.G., and Ordway, G.A. (1984). Effect of ischemia on responses of group III and IV afferents to contraction. *J. appl. Physiol.* **57**, 644–50.

Kellstein, D.E., Price, D.D., Hayes, R.L., and Mayer, D.J. (1990). Evidence that substance P selectively modulates C-fiber-evoked discharges of dorsal horn nociceptive neurons. *Brain Res.* **526**, 291–8.

Kieschke, J., Mense, S., and Prabhakar, N.R. (1988). Influence of adrenaline and hypoxia on rat muscle receptors in vitro. *Progr. Brain Res.* **74**, 91–7.

Kniffki, K.-D., Mense, S., and Schmidt, R.F. (1978). Responses of group IV afferent units from skeletal muscle to stretch, contraction and chemical stimulation. *Exp. Brain Res.* **31**, 511–22.

Kow, L.-M. and Pfaff, D.W. (1988). Neuromodulatory actions of peptides. *Ann. Rev. Pharmacol. Toxicol.* **28**, 163–88.

Kumazawa, T. and Mizumura, K. (1977). Thin-fibre receptors responding to mechanical, chemical and thermal stimulation in the skeletal muscle of the dog. *J. Physiol.* **273**, 179–94.

Lam, F.Y. and Ferrell, W.R. (1990). Mediators of substance P-induced inflammation in the rat knee joint. *Agents Actions* **31**, 298–307.

Lawson, S.N., Crepps, B.A., Bao, J., Brighton, B.W., and Perl, E.R. (1994). Substance P-like immunoreactivity (SP-LI) in dorsal root ganglia (DRGs) of anaesthetized guinea-pigs is related to sensory receptor type in A- and C-fiber neurones. *J. Physiol.* **476**, 39.

Leah, J.D., Cameron, A.A., and Snow, P.J. (1985). Neuropeptides in physiologically identified mammalian sensory neurones. *Neurosci. Lett.* **56**, 257–63.

Lee, Y., Takami, K., Kawai, Y., Girgis, S., Hillyard, C.J., MacIntyre, I., Emson, P.C., and Tohyama, M. (1985). Distribution of calcitonin gene-related peptide in the rat peripheral nervous system with reference to its coexistence with substance P. *Neuroscience* **415**. 1227–37.

Levine, J.D., Taiwo, Y.O., Collins, S.D., and Tam, J.K.(1986). Noradrenaline hyperalgesia is mediated through interaction with sympathetic postganglionic neurone terminals rather than activation of primary afferent nociceptors. *Nature* **323**, 158–60.

Lewis, T., Pickering, G.W., and Rothschild, P. (1931). Observations upon muscular pain in intermittent claudication. *Heart* **15**, 359–83.

Lloyd, D.P.C. (1943). Neuron patterns controlling transmission of ipsilateral hind limb reflexes in cat. *J. Neurophysiol.* **6**, 293–315.

Lotz, M., Carson, D.A., and Vaughan, J.H. (1987). Substance P activation of rheumatoid synoviocytes: neural pathway in pathogenesis of arthritis. *Science* **235**, 893–5.

McMahon, S.B., Sykova, E., Wall, P.D., Woolf, C.J., and Gibson, S.J. (1984). Neurogenic extravasation and substance P levels are low in muscle as compared to skin in the rat hindlimb. *Neurosci. Lett.* **52**, 235–40.

Mense, S. (1977). Nervous outflow from skeletal muscle following chemical noxious stimulation. *J. Physiol.* **267**, 75–88.

Mense, S. (1978). Muskelreceptoren mit dünnen markhaltigen und marklosen Fasern: receptive Eigenschafen und mögliche Funktion. Habilitationsschrift, Fachbereich Medizin, Kiel University, Germany.

Mense, S. (1981). Sensitization of group IV muscle receptors to bradykinin by 5-hydroxytryptamine and prostaglandin E_2. *Brain Res.* **225**, 95–105.

Mense, S. (1982). Reduction of the bradykinin-induced activation of feline group III and IV muscle receptors by acetylsalicylic acid. *J. Physiol.* **326**, 269–83.

Mense, S. (1986). Slowly conducting afferent fibers from deep tissues: neurobiological properties and central nervous actions. *Progr. sensory Physiol.* **6**, 139–219.

Mense, S. (1991). Auslösende Faktoren des Muskelschmerzes unter besonderer Berücksichtigung der Ischämie. In *Schmerztherapie bei ischämischen Krankheiten*, Schmerzstudien 9 ed. Ch. Maier and J. Wawersik). pp. 45–56. Fischer, Stuttgart.

Mense, S. and Meyer, H. (1985). Different types of slowly conducting afferent units in cat skeletal muscle and tendon. *J. Physiol.* **363**, 403–17.

Mense, S. and Meyer, H. (1988). Bradykinin-induced modulation of the response behaviour of different types of feline group III and IV muscle receptors. *J. Physiol.***398**, 49–63.

Mense, S. and Stahnke, M. (1983). Responses in muscle afferent fibres of slow conduction velocity to contractions and ischaemia in the cat. *J. Physiol.* **342**, 383–97.

Mense, S., Light, A.R., and Perl, E.R. (1981). Spinal terminations of subcutaneous high-threshold mechanoreceptors. In *Spinal cord sensation* (ed. A.G. Brown and M. Réthelyi), pp. 79–86. Scottish Academic Press, Edinburgh.

Meyer, R.A. and Campbell, J.N. (1988). A novel electrophysiological technique for locating cutaneous nociceptive and chemospecific receptors. *Brain Res.* **441**, 81–6.

Mitchell, J.H. and Schmidt, R.F. (1983). Cardiovascular reflex control by afferent fibers from skeletal muscle receptors. In J.T. Shepherd, F.M. Abboud (Vol. Eds.), *Handbook of physiology*. Section 2. *The cardiovascular system*. Vol. III, *Peripheral circulation and organ blood flow,* Part 2 (ed. J.T. Shepherd and F.M. Abboud), pp. 623–58. American Physiological Society, Bethesda, Maryland.

Molander, C. and Grant, G. (1987). Spinal cord projections from hindlimb muscle nerves in the rat studied by transganglionic transport of horseradish peroxidase, wheat germ agglutinin conjugated horseradish peroxidase, or horseradish peroxidase with dimethylsulfoxide. *J. comp. Neurol.* **260**, 246–55.

Moore, R.M., Moore, R.E., and Singleton, A.O. (1934). Experiments on the chemical stimulation of pain-endings associated with small blood-vessels. *Am. J. Physiol.* **107**, 594–602.

Nakahara, M. (1971). The effect of a tourniquet on the kinin–kininogen system in blood and muscle. *Thromb. Diathes. Haemorrh.* **26**, 264–74.

Nicoll, R.A., Schenker, C., and Leeman, S.E. (1980). Substance P as a transmitter candidate. *Ann. Rev. Neurosci.* **3**, 227–68.

O'Brien, C., Woolf, C.J., Fitzgerald, M., Lindsay, R.M., and Molander, C. (1989). Differences in the chemical expression of rat primary afferent neurons which innervate skin, muscle or joint. *Neuroscience* **32**, 493–502.

Paintal, A.S. (1960). Functional analysis of group III afferent fibres of mammalian muscles. *J. Physiol.* **152**, 250–70.

Pedersen-Bjergaard, U., Bogeskov Nielsen, L., Jensen, K., Edvinsson, L., Jansen, I., and Olesen, J. (1991). Algesia and local responses induced by neurokinin A and substance P in human skin and temporal muscle. *Peptides* **10**, 1147–52.

Perl, E.R. (1984). Pain and nociception. In: *Handbook of physiology*. Section 1. *The nervous system*. Vol. III, Part 2 (ed. I. Darian-Smith), pp, 915–75. American Physiological Society, Bethesda, Maryland.

Pickering, G.W. and Wayne, E.J.(1933–34). Observations on angina pectoris and intermittent claudication in anaemia. *Clin. Sci.* **1**, 305–25.

Piper, P.J. (1984). Formation and actions of leukotrienes. *Physiol. Rev.* **64**, 744–61.

Reinert, A. and Mense, S. (1993). Inflammatory changes in the density of neuropeptide-containing nerve endings in skeletal muscle of the rat. *Pflügers Arch.* **422**, R62.

Reinert, A. and Mense, S. (1994). Dichte von SP- und CGRP-immunoreaktiven Nervenendigungen in der Achillessehne der Ratte. *Anat. Anz.* **176**(suppl.), 80.

Reinert, A., Vitek, M., and Mense, S. (1992). Effects of substance P on the activity of high- and low-threshold mechanosensitive receptors of the rat diaphragm in vitro. *Pflügers Arch.* **420**, R47.

Richmond, F.J.R., Anstee, G.C.B., Sherwin, E.A., and Abrahams, V.C. (1976). Motor and sensory fibres of neck muscle nerves in the cat. *Can. J. Physiol. Pharmacol.* **54**, 294–304.

Sahlin, K., Harris, R.C., Nylind, B., and Hultman, E. (1976). Lactate content and pH in muscle samples obtained after dynamic exercise, *Pflügers Arch.* **67**, 143–9.

Samuelsson, B. (1983). Leukotrienes: mediators of immediate hypersensitivity reactions and inflammation. *Science* **220**, 568–75.

Sicuteri, F. (1967). Vasoneuroactive substances and their implication in vascular pain. *Res. clin. Stud. Headache* **1**, 6–45.

Sicuteri, F., Franchi, G., and Fanciullacci, M. (1964). Bradichinina e dolore da ischemia. *Settim. Med.* **52**, 127–39.

Stacey, M.J. (1969). Free nerve endings in skeletal muscle of the cat. *J. Anat.* **105**, 231–54.

Steen, K.H., Reh, P.W., Anton, F., and Handwerker, H.O. (1992). Protons selectively induce lasting excitation and sensitization to mechanical stimulation of nociceptors in rat skin in vitro. *J. Neurosci.* **12**, 86–95.

Taiwo, Y.O., Bjerknes, L.K., Goetzl, E.J., and Levine, J.D. (1990). Mediation of primary afferent peripheral hyperalgesia by the cAMP second messenger system. *Neuroscience* **32**, 577–80.

Torebjörk, E. (1985). Nociceptor activation and pain. *Phil. Trans. R. Soc., London* **B308**, 227–34.

Uchida, Y. and Ueda, H. (1969). Kininogen and kinin activity during local ischemia in man. *Jap. Heart J.* **10**, 503–8.

von Düring, M. and Andres, K.H. (1990). Topography and ultrastructure of group III and IV nerve terminals of the cat's gastrocnemius–soleus muscle. In *The primary afferent neuron* (ed. W. Zenker and W.L. Neuhuber), pp. 35–41. Plenum Press, New York.

8 Neurobiology of articular nociceptors

HANS-GEORG SCHAIBLE AND ROBERT F. SCHMIDT

Morphology of articular nociceptors

The innervation of joints

Since the pioneering work of Gardner (1944) and Freeman and Wyke (1967) the innervation of the cat's knee joints has received more attention in the literature than that of other joints or in other species (for references see Heppelmann et al. 1995). The following review will, therefore, concentrate on the innervation of the knee joint of the cat which has been investigated in some detail in connection with the numerous functional studies of this joint under normal and pathophysiological conditions. This joint is mainly innervated by the medial (MAN) and the posterior articular nerves (PAN) (Freeman and Wyke 1967). According to Table 8.1, each nerve contains approximately 650 afferent fibres and about 500 unmyelinated sympathetic efferents (Langford and Schmidt 1983). Within the afferent fibres, the majority are thinly myelinated group III and unmyelinated group IV units (MAN, 91 per cent; PAN, 74 per cent). The small contribution of the group I fibres in the PAN is presumably due to stray fibres joining in from muscle spindles of the popliteus muscle (McIntyre et al. 1978). The maximum diameter within afferent group IV fibres is 0.3–0.4 µm; the maximum within the sympathetic efferent fibres is around 0.8–0.9 µm (Heppelmann et al. 1988).

Table 8.1 Composition of the cat's articular nerves

Fibres (group)	MAN*	PAN*
I	—	27 (4%)
II	59 (9%)	149 (22%)
III	131 (21%)	94 (14%)
IV	440 (70%)	410 (60%)
Afferents	630 (100%)	680 (100%)
Sympathetic	500	515

* MAN, Medial articular nerve; PAN, Posterior articular nerve.

Ultrastructure of articular nociceptors and other sensory 'free nerve terminals'

In electron microscope studies on the medial aspect of the knee joint, the fine nerve filaments were found to innervate mainly a thin superficial layer of the joint capsule, the inside and outside surface of the ligamentum patellae, and the ligamentum collaterale mediale. Barely any nerve fibres could be detected within the densely packed connective tissue of these areas.

The terminal portions of group III afferent fibres display three major areas (Fig. 8.1; Heppelmann et al. 1990, 1995): (1) the proximal portion of the afferent fibre is myelinated and runs within a perineural sheath; (2) more distally there is an intermediate portion that has lost its myelin but that is still running within the perineural sheath; (3) the distal portion starts at the end of the perineural sheath. It runs into the tissue, and forms the sensory terminal tree. This terminal tree consists usually of 2–4 branches with a length of about 80–200 μm. In addition, there are short side branches with a length of 10–20 μm. The branches innervate a predominantly two-dimensional area of tissue of about 150×200 μm (Heppelmann *et al.* 1990).

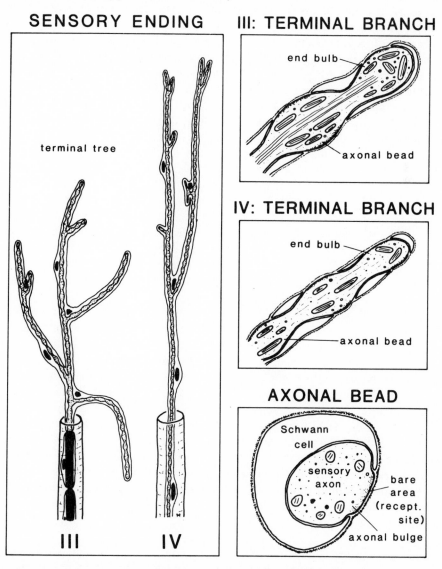

Fig. 8.1 Schematic drawings of group III and IV sensory endings in the knee joint capsule of the cat. A terminal tree is formed by several long and short branches of various orientations. The sensory axons consist of periodically arranged thick and thin segments forming spindle-shaped beads. The axolemma is not completely unsheathed by its accompanying Schwann cells; the bare areas presumably are the receptive sites.

The unmyelinated afferent group IV fibres have a proximal and a distal terminal portion. The proximal one is defined as that still running within the perineural sheath, the distal one as that outside (Fig. 8.1). The major branches of the distal portion are quite long, sometimes more than 300 μm. They have frequent short side branches with a length of less than 10 μm (Heppelmann *et al.* 1990). The fibres usually run parallel to vessels, but the distances to the vessel walls vary considerably.

In the terminal areas of both fibre types mast cells can be found. Some of them have a distance of less than 2 μm to the nerve fibres. The distal portions are covered by Schwann cells but this coverage is very incomplete. Altogether about one-third of the membrane surface is not being covered by these cells. These 'bare areas' are particularly frequent at the so-called axonal beads (Fig. 8.1; see also below). The areas not covered by Schwann cells show in the axoplasma below the fibre membrane a fine filamentous structure that is somewhat more electron-dense than the neighbouring areas. These areas look very similar to the receptor matrix described by Andres and von Düring (1973).

As just mentioned, the intermediate and final fibre sections display regular axonal thickenings that in three-dimensional reconstructions appear to be lined up like pearls on a string. These axonal beads contain numerous glycogen granules and vesicles (Heppelmann *et al.* 1990). In group III fibres there are about seven beads per 100 μm of fibre length, whereas with the group IV fibres there are 9–10 per 100 μm.

The group III fibre terminals have, in addition, in the centre of their axoplasma a neurofilament core consisting of numerous microfilaments. This finding is specific for group III fibres, which can be identified by this feature. The group III afferents end in terminal end bulbs, which in size and content are comparable to the axonal beads. The difference is that the organelles are irregularly distributed within the ending. Also, the neurofilament core is no longer visible. The group IV fibres do not have a terminal bulb but just taper out as a very thin ending.

Unfortunately, neither the shape nor the area of innervation by the terminal portions of the fine afferent nerve fibres give any clue as to their function. In regard to the cytoplasmic content of the afferents it was seen that the mitochondria are not regularly distributed in the terminal regions. They accumulate in the axonal beads of both fibre types and in the end bulbs of the group III afferents, whereas in the thin fibre portions between the axonal beads barely any mitochondria are present. In addition, the number of mitochondria, that is, their density, increases considerably in the intermediate and, particularly, in the distal portions of group III fibres relative to the proximal ones.

If it is agreed that the total volume of mitochondria is proportional to the production and storage of adenosine triphosphate (ATP) as a readily available pool of energy, then the results presented here point to considerable differences in the energy requirements between individual units of group III and group IV fibres, particularly in the group III range (for a discussion see Hanesch *et al.* 1992*b*). Functionally speaking, these results may indicate the following:

1. Since the saltatory conduction of action potentials in the proximal portions of group III afferents requires only a small amount of energy, the density of mitochondria is low in these portions whereas in the distal portions a much higher energy consumption requires the presence of larger numbers of mitochondria.

2. In the group IV fibres the differences in mitochondrial content between the proximal

and distal portions are small because both areas use approximately the same amount of energy (mainly because of the lack of a myelin sheath).
3. The large variations in mitochondrial content, respectively in energy consumption, of the terminal portions of various individual units most probably are related to differences in their sensory function, that is, high-threshold (nociceptive) fine afferents may contain fewer mitochondria per surface area than low-threshold mechanosensitive units, because the high-threshold units are activated much more rarely than the low-threshold ones.

Neuropeptides in articular afferents

Afferents in joint nerves of several species including humans contain neuropeptides. In order to identify the proportion of joint afferents containing particular neuropeptides, the dorsal root ganglion cells of knee joint afferents have been labelled with fast blue (this marker is retrogradely transported) and treated with antisera to several neuropeptides. In the rat, calcitonin gene-related peptide (CGRP)-like immunoreactivity (CGRP-li) was identified in 7 of 9 (78 per cent) RT97 negative (small dark) cells and in 37 of 53 (70 per cent) RT97 positive (large light) cells supplying the knee joint; substance P-(SP)-like immunoreactivity (SP-li) was contained in 12 of 18 (66 per cent) RT97 negative and in 10 of 59 (17 per cent) RT97 positive neurones. None of the labelled neurones contained somatostatin-li cells (O'Brien *et al.* 1989). In the MAN and PAN of cat's knee, about 16–17 per cent of the afferents contained SP-li cells, and about 32–35 per cent of the afferents showed CGRP-li cells. SP-li was found in the dorsal root ganglion (DRG) cells with the smallest diameters, whereas CGRP-li was identified in small- as well as in medium-sized somata (Hanesch *et al.* 1991). Neurokinin A-li was found in about 4.5 per cent of the MAN afferents (Hanesch *et al.* 1992a). The coexistence of neuropeptides in articular afferents has not been investigated in detail. It is also not known whether all joint afferents contain peptides or whether a proportion is non-peptidergic.

Other studies have identified peptide-containing nerve fibres in the different tissue layers of animal and human joints (for a review see Schaible and Grubb 1993). It has not been determined, however, whether these fibres were afferent or efferent. Evidence was provided for the presence of SP-li and CGRP-li. Fibres containing these peptides were considered as afferent and, interestingly, they were also described in the synovial layer where the presence of free nerve endings has been disputed in histological studies. Nerve fibres with neuropeptide Y-li (NPY-li) cells were predominantly found adjacent to and within blood vessels, and immunoreactivities of galanin and of Met-enkephalin and Leu-enkephalin have also been reported.

The neuropeptide content of dorsal root ganglia exhibits some plasticity during inflammation in the peripheral tissue. The synthesis of both SP-li and CGRP-li in the dorsal root ganglia was found to be increased (for reviews see Hanesch *et al.* 1993; Schaible and Grubb 1993). For somatostatin, increases (Ohno *et al.* 1990) as well as no changes (Smith *et al.* 1992) have been observed.

Response properties of articular afferents

Mechanosensitivity of medial articular nerve afferent fibres of the normal joint

Group II articular afferent units (conduction velocity 21–65 m/s) of the MAN in cats have no resting discharges (that is, they do not signal the angle or position of the joint). The vast majority of them is excited by gentle local mechanical stimulation (probing, touching, rubbing of the receptive field) and by movements in the working range of the knee joint. Although they may encode the intensity of pressure and a particular movement up to the noxious range, the magnitude of their overall responsiveness is more closely related to the direction of the movement than to its intensity. Comparable results have been obtained from other joints and in other species (for a review, see Schaible and Grubb 1993). Thus, group II articular afferent units are probably not involved in joint nociception and pain. Rather, they presumably subserve proprioceptive functions such as deep pressure sensation and kinaesthesia (Proske *et al.* 1988; Dorn *et al.* 1991; Schaible and Grubb 1993.)

In group III (conduction velocity, 2.5–20 m/s) and group IV (conduction velocity, < 2.5 m/s) afferent units of the cat MAN, resting discharges occur in about one-third of all fibres. The frequency of these irregular discharges is usually below 0.5 Hz (Schaible and Schmidt 1983*a*). Groups III and IV units exhibit different sensitivities to passive movements. Units are either readily (Fig. 8.2 (A)) or marginally activated by non-noxious events (Fig. 8.2 (B)), or they are only activated by noxious movements (Fig. 8.2 (C)), or they are not activated by any movements, even extremely noxious ones, although they have detectable receptive fields (Fig. 8.2 (D)). All in all, approximately 55 per cent of the group III and 70 per cent of the group IV units with detectable receptive fields either respond only to (potentially) noxious movements or fail to respond to movements completely (Schaible and Schmidt 1983*b*). The units that are excited while the joint is being moved through its normal working range cannot be considered nociceptive. Fibres that are only activated by noxious stimuli (movements outside the normal working range against tissue resistance) can be referred to as nociceptors as defined by the specificity theory.

Later, it had to be appreciated that a further category of fine afferent units exists in normal tissue that is completely insensitive to any mechanical stimulation (mechano-insensitive or silent nociceptors). Such units are very common in the cat PAN (Grigg *et al.* 1986). They may develop mechanosensitivity in the course of joint inflammation (see below; for a review on the development of the concept of silent or 'sleeping' nociceptors see Schaible and Grubb 1993; Schmidt and Schaible 1994).

The ankle joint of the rat is innervated by fine afferent units with conduction velocities ranging from 0.3 to 24 m/s (Guilbaud *et al.* 1985). These units do not have resting discharges in normal rats, and their response behaviour to local mechanical stimulation appears to be similar to that reported for the cat's knee joint (responses to movements were not studied and silent units were not observed). In the ankle joint of the chicken, fine sensory units have been described that again resemble those in the cat (Gentle 1992). The fine afferents had no resting activity; they could be activated by local probing of the capsular tissue to give slowly adapting responses graded in frequency according to the stimulus strength. Very few of these units responded to joint movement.

Mechanosensitivity of joint afferents from the inflamed joint

In our experimental model of an acute arthritis, the inflammation is induced by the injection of kaolin and carrageenan into the joint cavity. This procedure leads to a long-lasting inflammation with behavioural changes of the awake cat and histological signs of acute severe inflammation with cellular infiltration (Schaible and Grubb 1993). As a consequence of the inflammation, fine articular afferents show profound changes of their discharge properties (Coggeshall *et al.* 1983; Schaible and Schmidt 1985, 1985*a*). During inflammation, resting activity is observed in 75 per cent of Group III and 83 per cent of group IV units of the MAN. The discharges are irregular and sometimes of high frequency. Both the percentages of units with resting activity and the frequencies of their discharges are more than twice as high as in the control sample. This resting activity might represent the neural correlate of spontaneous pain, particularly in view of our observation that numerous nociceptors (usually silent in the normal joint) exhibit resting activity under these conditions.

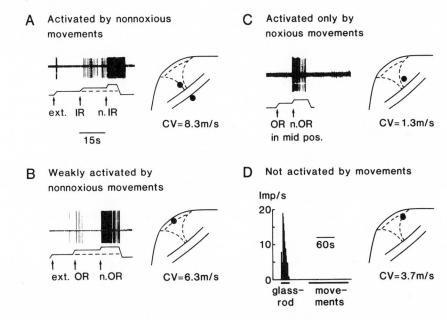

Fig. 8.2 Classification of fine articular afferents from the MAN according to their response during passive movements of the knee joint. The insets on the right of each record display the receptive fields on the medial aspect of the joint capsule and the conduction velocity (CV) of each unit. The time-scale in (A) also applies to (B) and (C). ext., Extension; IR and OR, innocuous inward and outward rotations, respectively (pronation and supination, respectively); n.IR and n.OR, noxious inward and outward rotations, respectively; mid pos., midposition (normal resting position of the joint between flexion and extension). The activity in (D) is displayed as a peristimulus–time histogram; the movement programme included noxious flexions, extensions, and rotations.

Nearly all fine afferent units from inflamed joints have low thresholds to movement, and most of them respond well to flexion and extension. The increase in the number of easily excitable afferents corresponds to the clear decrease in the number of units belonging to the other classes. The fibres that in the normal joint mainly or exclusively respond to noxious movements become very sensitive to movement when the joint is inflamed. The message 'noxious' is now sent to the central nervous system, even if movement takes place in the normally innocuous range (Schaible and Schmidt 1988*a*). The remaining fraction of fibres that do not respond to movement is only very small in the inflamed joint. It follows from this that most of the units must have become sensitive to movement as again confirmed in continuous observations. Obviously, units that do not respond to movements in the normal joint must also be regarded as nociceptors. Thus, they respond to movement only in the case of true tissue damage. This recruitment of a large population of fibres during the inflammatory process leads to a massive amplification of the afferent signals reaching the central nervous system (CNS) (Table 8.2).

Table 8.2   Influence of an acute inflammation

Medial articular nerve	Joint		Change
	Normal	Inflamed	
Resting activity (impulses/30 s)	1800	11 100	6.2 ×
Low-threshold units (no. of fibres)	240 fibres	550 fibres	2.3 ×
Movement (impulses/30 s)	4400	30 900	7.0 ×

Similar changes in the mechanical properties of fine articular units in the course of an experimental joint inflammation have been reported for the ankle joints of the rat (Guilbaud *et al.* 1985) and the chicken (Gentle and Thorp 1994). In both investigations the inflammation led to increases in the size of the receptive fields of the mechanosensitive units and further to decreases in the thresholds to local probing and to the appearance of resting discharges in a certain percentage of units. When tested, movements of the joint produced responses in a higher proportion of units from inflamed than from normal joints.

There are differences in the time course of sensitization of the various types of articular afferents (Schaible and Schmidt 1988*a*). Low-threshold units, mainly in the group II and III fibre range, developed increased reactions in the first hour after the injection of the inflammatory compounds, sometimes starting immediately after the injection (usually low-threshold group II units). In high-threshold afferents, including originally silent ones, the sensitization became evident within the second to third hour after induction of inflammation with a further increase later on.

As regards the latter category of silent units, different levels of unresponsiveness have been described (Schmidt and Schaible 1994; Schmidt *et al.* 1994). For instance, in Fig. 8.2 (D) a unit is shown that, despite being activated by local mechanical probing, could not be activated by joint movements, even very noxious ones. The unit shown in Fig. 8.3 did not even have a local receptive field under normal conditions but became sensitized in the course of inflammation to the point that it developed resting activity and vigorous responses to movements in the working range of the joint.

Chemosensitivity of articular afferents

Most group III and IV articular afferents exhibit sensitivity for chemical substances such as inflammatory mediators. This chemosensitivity is thought to be important for the activation and sensitization of articular afferents during inflammation. Several inflammatory mediators (prostaglandins, thromboxanes, leukotrienes, kinins, and others) have been identified in synovial fluid. They are either produced by tissues in the joints and/or released during joint inflammation in both human joint disease and in experimental arthritis (for a review, see Schaible and Grubb 1993). In order to investigate their putative pathogenic role in the production of the inflammation-evoked discharges, mediators have been administered locally to the joint tissues, for example, by close intraarterial injection, and their effects on the response properties of identified joint afferents have been analysed.

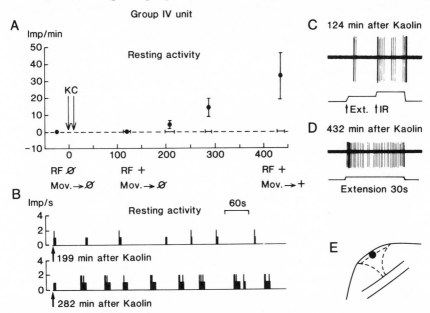

Fig. 8.3 Sensitization of a mechano-insensitive (silent) group IV afferent unit during the development of an experimental arthritis in the cat's knee joint. (A) Mean and standard deviation of resting discharges quantified during the indicated times (bars); (B) peristimulus time histograms; (C) and (D) responses to movements in the inflamed state. Ext., extension; IR, pronation; K, kaolin; C, carrageenan; Mov., movements; Ø, no response; +, response; (E) Receptive field (dot).

Some inflammatory mediators induced patterns of firing in afferent nerve fibres that are similar to those seen under inflammatory conditions. Single-unit recordings have revealed, however, that joint afferents are not homogeneous with regard to their chemosensitivity; that is, a mediator may only affect the discharge behaviour of subgroups of units. Moreover, the chemosensitivity is not clearly correlated with the mechanical threshold of the units. An inflammatory mediator may excite or sensitize subgroups of high-threshold (nociceptive) units as well as subgroups of non-nociceptive units. It should also be noted that there are still big gaps in our understanding as only some mediators and antagonists have been studied and as the interactions between individual mediators have not been adequately determined. The following paragraphs will briefly summarize the effects of those mediators that have been studied.

Bradykinin

Intraarterial bolus injections of bradykinin (0.026–26 μg) close to the joint excited the vast majority of the III and IV afferents in the MAN of the cat's knee (Kanaka *et al.*

1985). In the rat, similar doses (0.1–10 µg) excited approximately half of the units supplying the ankle (Grubb *et al.* 1991). The excitatory effect of bradykinin started 10–20 s after close arterial injection and usually lasted 30–60 s. Repeated application of bradykinin resulted in a pronounced tachyphylaxis. Bradykinin also sensitized 70 and 44 per cent of the group III and IV units in the cat and rat, respectively, to movements (Neugebauer *et al.* 1989; Grubb *et al.* 1991). This sensitization included a lowering of threshold in high-threshold group III and IV units (to become responsive to innocuous movements) or the induction of mechanosensitivity in initially mechanoinsensitive (silent) afferents (Neugebauer *et al.* 1989). A typical example of a sensitization is shown in Fig. 8.4 (A). In some units the sensitization appeared to be long-lasting, whereas in others it lasted only a few minutes. It usually outlasted the excitatory effect (Neugebauer *et al.* 1989).

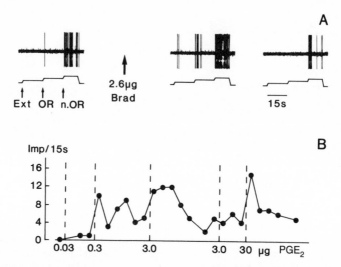

Fig. 8.4 Sensitization of joint afferents to mechanical stimuli by inflammatory mediators. (A) Group III unit, which responded initially mainly to noxious outward rotation (n.OR). Two minutes after the close intraarterial injection of bradykinin, the unit showed an enhanced response to n.OR and, in addition, responses to extension (Ext) and innocuous outward rotation (OR). The effects of bradykinin (Brad.) were reversible (specimen on the right). (B) Sensitization of a group III unit by intraarterial injections of PGE$_2$. The graph shows the responses to innocuous outward rotation before and after injections of PGE$_2$. Before PGE$_2$ the unit responded only to noxious movements.

Bradykinin sensitivity (excitation or sensitization) in group III and IV does not seem to be related to the mechanical threshold of fibres since high- and low-threshold fibres (and some initially mechanoinsensitive afferents) appeared to be affected (Kanaka *et al.* 1985; Neugebauer *et al.* 1989). In contrast, bradykinin rarely excited low-threshold group II mechanoreceptors in the knee joint of the cat (Kanaka *et al.* 1985).

Prostaglandins

Prostaglandins (PGs), PGE$_2$ and PGI$_2$, seem to be particularly important mediators of inflammatory joint disease since, in comparison to other prostaglandins, they are present in high concentrations in inflamed tissue (for a review, see Schaible and Grubb 1993).

Bolus injections of PGE_2 administered intraarterially to the normal knee joint were shown to excite and sensitize group III and IV articular units in the cat (Schaible and Schmidt 1988*b*). In the MAN about 60 per cent of the group III and IV units could be excited by PGE_2 (0.03–30 μg), and 64 and 25 per cent of group III and IV units, respectively, were found to be sensitized to movements. The excitatory effects started approximately 30 s after close arterial injection of PGE_2. Recovery was typically seen within 4 min, but some fibres continued to discharge at an enhanced rate throughout the recording period. The sensitizing effect was generally seen within 1–2 min after close arterial injection of PGE_2 and lasted > 10 min. A typical example is displayed in Fig. 8.4 (B). Excitation was seen in both low- and high-mechanical-threshold group III and IV fibres. Interestingly, the sensitizing effect to mechanical stimulation was observed in low- and high-threshold group III units but only, however, in those group IV units that had low thresholds and not in those with high thresholds.

In the rat, only 18 per cent of group III and IV mechanoreceptors of the ankle joint were excited by PGE_2, and only 20 per cent were sensitized to movements (Grubb *et al.* 1991). In contrast, both PGI_2 and cicaprost, a more stable and potent agonist at the I type prostaglandin receptor, were found to excite and sensitize the majority of group III/ IV mechanoreceptors. Thus, in the rat PGI_2 may play a more important role than PGE_2 (Birrell *et al.* 1991). In the cat, PGI_2 (0.3–30 μg) also had an excitatory and/or sensitizing effect (for mechanical stimuli) in a higher proportion of articular groups III and IV units than PGE_2 (Schepelmann *et al.* 1992). The duration of the effects of PGI_2 was shorter than that of PGE_2 (Schepelmann *et al.* 1992).

There are interactions between bradykinin and prostaglandins. Both PGE_1 and PGE_2 have been shown to enhance the reflex rise in blood pressure produced by injecting bradykinin into the joint cavity (Moncada *et al.* 1975). In single-unit recordings, PGE_2 was shown to enhance the excitatory effects of bradykinin in 50 per cent of group III fibres and in 75 per cent of group IV fibres in the MAN of cat's knee (Schaible and Schmidt 1988*b*) and in 90 per cent of group III and IV fibres in the rat ankle (Grubb *et al.* 1991). In about 50 per cent of the cat knee joint afferents (low and high threshold) and in some initially mechanoinsensitive afferents, the combined application of PGE_2 and bradykinin was found to have stronger sensitizing effects on the responses to movements (change of threshold or size of response) than the application of bradykinin or PGE_2 alone. These findings demonstrate the power of the combination of inflammatory compounds. The interaction of bradykinin with PGI_2 was similar to that with PGE_2 (Schepelmann *et al.* 1992).

Serotonin

Serotonin (5-HT) was a potent excitant of approximately two-thirds of group III/IV mechanoreceptors in the ankle joint of normal and arthritic rats (Birrell *et al.* 1990). The response to 5-HT consisted of a rapid transient excitatory component that was particularly prone to tachyphylaxis and a delayed excitation that started after 15–30 s and lasted for up to 5 min. The initial transient burst was inhibited by $5-HT_3$ receptor antagonists, for example, ketanserin. In the cat, group III (43 per cent) and group IV fibres (73 per cent) of the MAN of the knee joint were excited by 5-HT; in the group III fibres this excitation was more pronounced (longer duration, less tachyplaxis) when the joint was inflamed (Herbert and Schmidt 1992). Spontaneous activity, a marked characteristic of sensitized articular afferents in arthritic joints, was reduced by both 5-HT$_2$ and 5-HT$_3$ antagonists in fibres supplying the rat ankle joint, indicating that 5-HT may be involved in the sensitization of mechanoreceptors in adjuvant-induced monoarthritis (Birrell *et al.* 1990). In the MAN of the inflamed knee joint of the cat, 5-HT sensitized a proportion of group III and group IV units to movements for short periods (Herbert and Schmidt 1992).

Cellular mechanisms in the sensory endings

Using methods currently employed, it is impossible to study the molecular aspects of the activation and/or sensitization of the receptive endings themselves. Recordings from the afferent axons have shown, however, that phorbol esters activated some articular afferents suggesting that the activation of intracellular second messengers may be important (for details see Schepelmann *et al.* 1993).

Inhibitory influences on joint afferents

While joint afferents are excited and sensitized by inflammatory mediators, their activity may be inhibited by other compounds. *Non-steroidal anti-inflammatory drugs (NSAIDs)* have been found to reduce both spontaneous and mechanically evoked activity in group III and IV fibres in both acute (Heppelmann *et al.* 1986) and chronic models of joint inflammation (Guilbaud and Iggo 1985; Grubb *et al.* 1991) in the cat and rat, respectively. The reductions of activity were seen within 10–20 min of application of these NSAIDs. Possibly these NSAIDs exerted their effect by inhibiting prostaglandin synthesis, but other mechanisms are also discussed (see McCormack and Brune 1991). In the cat with acute inflammation, but not in the rat with chronic ankle inflammation, PGE$_2$ rapidly reversed the inhibitory effects of both indomethacin and acetysalicylic acid on group III and IV afferents in a dose-dependent manner (Heppelmann *et al.* 1986; Grubb *et al.* 1991).

Close arterial injections of *capsaicin* (10^{-4}–10^{-6} M) were shown to induce a brief discharge in both group III and IV afferents. This was followed by a rapid loss of mechano- and chemosensitivity of the afferents. In some cases recovery was seen within a few minutes. Excitation and subsequent desensitization by bradykinin were mainly found in 'nociceptive' group III and IV fibres having high thresholds or not being activated by movements (He *et al.* 1990). The mechanisms underlying these desensitizing effects are not yet clear.

Afferent fibres seem to be equipped with *opioid receptors* (for a review see Stein 1994). In recordings from knee joint afferents in the cat, ongoing activity in most group III and IV fibres from the inflamed joint was reduced in a naloxone reversible manner by κ opioid receptor agonists (U50,488H and ethylketocyclazocine) and/or, to a lesser extent, by μ receptor agonists (Russell *et al.* 1987). The effects of δ receptor agonists have not been studied. The release of substance P into the knee joint was also reduced after the administrations of μ and δ opioid receptor agonists, but not after κ opioid receptor agonists (Yaksh 1988). Thus, the importance of specific opioid receptor types does not seem to be entirely settled. In humans the intraarticular application of morphine (μ receptor agonist) produced pain relief following knee arthroscopy without obvious systemic effects (for a review see Stein 1994).

It was suggested that during inflammation 'endogenous antinociception' can be mediated by opioid peptides released locally from immune cells involved in the inflammatory process (see Stein 1994). It is possible, however, that this effect is only present under more chronic conditions. During acute inflammation of the knee joint of the cat, naloxone did not alter the afferent discharges; thus a tonic opioidergic suppression of the inflammation-evoked afferent activity was not evident in this situation (Schepelmann *et al.* 1995).

Peptidergic functions of articular afferents

Neuropeptides may be released from the peripheral and/or the intraspinal terminations of peptidergic joint afferents. While the release from peripheral terminations is thought to mediate a 'neurogenic inflammation' in the joint, the release from the central terminals is thought to be involved in the nociceptive processing in the spinal cord and its functional plasticity. The following sections will address studies that have described the role of the neuropeptides.

The efferent effects of neuropeptides in the joint

The electrical stimulation of C fibres in PAN of cat's knee evoked a plasma extravasation in the joint. This was reduced by the application of neurokinin (NK) receptor antagonists (Ferrell and Russell 1985) suggesting the involvement of SP (see also Yaksh 1988). Subsequent studies showed that mainly NK_1 receptors and the endogenous NK_1 receptor agonist SP seem to be responsible for the neurogenic extravasation in the knee (Lam and Ferrell 1989*a*, *b*, 1990, 1991). While no synergistic effect of SP and CGRP has been found in this study (Lam and Ferrell 1991), a synergistic action of SP and CGRP on plasma extravasation has been described by others. When the rat knee joint was co-perfused with SP and CGRP in such low concentrations that neither SP nor CGRP alone caused an effect, synergistic effects of both peptides were detected (Green *et al.* 1992). SP also has other actions in joint such as an increase in the production of prostaglandins (Lotz *et al.* 1987).

Several studies have suggested that afferent fibres and neuropeptides contribute to the expression of chronic inflammation in the joint. Inflammatory signs were attenuated after impairment of afferent fibres, for example by capsaicin (Colpaert *et al.* 1983; Levine *et al.* 1986; Inman *et al.* 1989; Lam and Ferrell 1989*a*; but see Hara *et al.* 1984; Cervero and Plenderleith 1987). The effects of both SP (see above) and CGRP (Louis *et al.* 1989) could be important.

Some studies on human synovial tissue seem to support the experimental evidence that neuropeptides are released during joint disease (Devillier *et al.* 1986; Lygren *et al.* 1986; Larsson *et al.* 1989; Marshall *et al.* 1990). In synovial tissue of rheumatoid arthritis patients, a reduction in the contents of neuropeptides such as immunoreactive SP and immunoreactive CGRP was found (Grönblad *et al.* 1988; Mapp *et al.* 1990; Pereira da Silva and Carmo-Fonseca 1990). This depletion of neuropeptides was postulated to result from previous release of the peptides. The picture emerging from clinical studies is, however, not totally clear. More data are necessary to provide definitive evidence linking different neuropeptides to human pathologies and to determine the role of each of these neuropeptides in the development and maintenance of human joint disease.

The effects of neuropeptides in the spinal cord (afferent functions)

During acute and chronic inflammation of the joint, the response properties of spinal neurones show pronounced alterations. These changes form a functional plasticity that is important for the generation of joint pain under inflammatory conditions (see Schaible and Grubb 1993). The cellular mechanisms of this functional plasticity are now under investigation. It is apparent that excitatory amino acids and their receptors play an important role in the generation and maintenance of inflammation-evoked hyperexcitability (for a review see Neugebauer *et al.* 1994*a*). The following sections will briefly summarize studies that also suggest an involvement of neuropeptides in the generation and maintenance of hyperexcitability in spinal cord neurones.

Tachykinins

In studies using antibody-coated microprobes in cat and rat, immunoreactive SP was found to be intraspinally released during the application of noxious pressure to the joint but not during the application of innocuous mechanical stimuli such as innocuous pressure and movements within the working range (Neugebauer *et al.* 1994*b*; Schaible *et al.* 1990). In recordings from spinal cord neurones with afferent input from the knee, the NK$_1$ receptor antagonist CP96,345 reduced the responses of the neurones to noxious pressure but not the responses to innocuous pressure applied to the normal knee (Neugebauer *et al.* 1994*b*). Both sets of data show that SP and NK$_1$ receptors contribute to the intraspinal processing of nociceptive information from the normal joint.

After development of inflammation, release of immunoreactive SP was also found during the application of innocuous mechanical stimuli to the joint in the cat (Schaible *et al.* 1990). The application of the antagonist CP96,345 at this stage reduced the responses to innocuous and noxious pressure (Neugebauer *et al.* 1995). Thus the NK$_1$ system seems to be more activated under inflammatory conditions and may then contribute to typical signs of joint inflammation, namely, the painfulness during innocuous mechanical stimulation (see also Sluka *et al.* 1992). Most probably, immunoreactive SP was released from high-threshold afferents that were sensitized (Schaible and Schmidt 1985, 1988*a*) and then responded to innocuous mechanical stimuli. The blockade of NK$_1$ receptors by CP96,345 during the induction of inflammation and in the first period of inflammation (about 90 min postinduction) attenuated the further development of hyperexcitability (Neugebauer *et al.* 1995). Using an *in situ* spinal cord perfusion method, Oku *et al.* (1987) found an increased basal release of immunoreactive SP in polyarthritic rats and significant release over baseline during forced movements of the ankle joint (considered as innocuous in normal animals). In contrast, forced movements did not evoke release of immunoreactive SP in the normal rat whereas noxious pinching of the skin did. These data suggest the persistence of the release of immunoreactive SP during chronic inflammation. Neurokinin A was also released during acute inflammation but not during innocuous stimulation of the normal joint (Hope *et al.* 1990).

Calcitonin gene-related peptide (CGRP)

In cat and rat, there was substantial basal release of immunoreactive CGRP in the spinal cord under normal conditions, and release of immunoreactive CGRP could be enhanced over baseline by electrical stimulation of unmyelinated afferent nerve fibres and by application of noxious pressure to the joint. No consistent change of release was noted during the application of innocuous mechanical stimuli such as light pressure and flexion of the joint (Schaible *et al.* 1994). During development of inflammation in the joint induced by kaolin and carrageenan, basal release was found to be enhanced in the cat (spinalized) but not in the rat (not spinalized). In contrast, in the rat release of immunoreactive CGRP was enhanced over baseline during innocuous pressure applied to the inflamed knee joint (this stimulus did not evoke additional release when applied to the normal joint), whereas in the cat this stimulus did not cause increased release of immunoreactive CGRP. Thus, in both species, the release of immunoreactive CGRP was significantly altered at an early stage of inflammation, although the differences in the pattern were noted. Release of immunoreactive CGRP was also suggested for the monkey spinal cord (Sluka *et al.* 1992). The effects of CGRP on spinal cord neurones are now being studied.

References

Andres, K.-H. and von Düring, M. (1973). Morphology of cutaneous receptors. In *Handbook of sensory physiology*, Vol. II (ed. A. Iggo), pp. 3–28. Springer, Berlin.

Birrell, G.J., McQueen, D.S., Iggo, A., and Grubb, B.D. (1990). The effect of 5-HT on articular sensory receptors in normal and arthritic rats. *Br. J. Pharmacol.*, **101**, 715–21.

Birrell, G.J., McQueen, D.S., Iggo, A., Coleman, R.A., and Grubb, B.D. (1991). PGI$_2$-induced activation and sensitization of articular mechanonociceptors. *Neurosci. Lett.*, **124**, 5–8.

Cervero, F. and Plenderleith, M.B. (1987). Adjuvant arthritis in adult rats treated at birth with capsaicin. *Acta Physiol. Hungarica* **69**, 497–500.

Coggeshall, R.E., Hong, K.A.P., Langford, L.A., Schaible, H.-G., and Schmidt, R.F. (1983). Discharge characteristics of fine medial articular afferents at rest and during passive movements of inflamed knee joints. *Brain Res.* **272**, 185–8.

Colpaert, F.C., Donnerer, J., and Lembeck, F. (1983). Effects of capsaicin on inflammation and on the substance P content of nervous tissues in rats with adjuvant arthritis. *Life Sci.* **32**, 1827–34.

Devillier, P., Weill, B., Renoux, M., Menkes, C., and Pradelles, P. (1986). Elevated levels of tachykinin-like immunoreactivity in joint fluids from patients with rheumatic inflammatory diseases. *N. Engl. J. Med.* **314**, 1323.

Dorn, T., Schaible, H.-G., and Schmidt, R.F. (1991). Response properties of thick myelinated group II afferents in the medial articular nerve of normal and inflamed knee joints of the cat. *Somatosens. Motor Res.* **8**, 127–36.

Ferrell, W.R. and Russell, N.J.W. (1985). Plasma extravasation in the cat knee joint induced by antidromic articular nerve stimulation. *Pflügers Arch.* **404**, 91–3.

Freeman, M.A.R. and Wyke, B. (1967). The innervation of the knee joint. An anatomical and histological study in the cat. *J. Anat.* **101**, 505–32.

Gardner, E. (1944). The distribution and termination of nerves in the knee joint of the cat. *J. Comp. Neurol.* **80**, 11–32.

Gentle, M.J. (1992). Ankle joint (artc. intertarsalis) receptors in the domestic fowl. *Neuroscience* **49**, 991–1000.

Gentle, M.J. and Thorp, B.H. (1944). Sensory properties of ankle joint capsule mechanoreceptors in acute monoarthritic chickens. *Pain* **57**, 361–74.

Green, P.G., Basbaum, A.I., and Levine, J.D. (1992). Sensory neuropeptide interactions in the production of plasma extravasation in the rat. *Neuroscience* **50**, 745–9.

Grigg, P., Schaible, H.-G., and Schmidt, R.F. (1986). Mechanical sensitivity of group III and IV afferents from posterior articular nerve in normal and inflamed cat knee. *J. Neurophysiol.* **55**, 635–43.

Grönblad, M., Konttinen, Y. T., Korkola, O., Liesi, P., Hukkanen, M., and Polak, J.M. (1988). Neuropeptides in synovium of patients with rheumatoid arthritis and osteoarthritis. *J. Rheumatol.* **15**, 1807–10.

Grönblad, M., Korkala, O., Konttinen, Y., Nederström, A., Hukkanen, M., Tolvanen, E., and Polak, J.M. (1991). Silver impregnation and immunohistochemical study of nerves in lumbar facet joint plical tissue. *Spine* **16**, 34–8.

Grubb, B.D., Birrell, J., McQueen, D.S., and Iggo, A. (1991). The role of PGE$_2$ in the sensitization of mechanoreceptors in normal and inflamed ankle joints of the rat. *Exp. Brain Res.* **84**, 383–92.

Guilbaud, G. and Iggo, A. (1985). The effect of acetylsalicylate on joint mechanoreceptors in rats with polyarthritis. *Exp. Brain Res.* **611**, 164–8.

Guilbaud, G., Iggo, A., and Tegner, R. (1985). Sensory receptors in ankle joint capsules of normal and arthritic rats. *Exp. Brain Res.* **58**, 29–40.

Hanesch, U., Heppelmann, B., and Schmidt, R.F. (1991). Substance P- and calcitonin gene-related peptide-immunoreactivity in primary afferent neurons of the cat's knee joint. *Neuroscience* **45**, 185–93.

Hanesch, U., Heppelmann, B., and Schmidt, R.F. (1992*a*). Neurokinin A-like immunoreactivity in articular afferents of the cat. *Brain Res.* **586**, 332–5.

Hanesch, U., Heppelmann, B., Messlinger, K., and Schmidt, R.F. (1992*b*). Nociception in normal and arthritic joints: structural and functional aspects. In *Hyperalgesia and allodynia* (ed. W.D. Willis), pp. 1–400. Raven Press, New York.

Hanesch, U., Pfrommer, U., Grubb, B.D., and Schaible, H.-G. (1993). Acute and chronic phases of unilateral inflammation in rat's ankle are associated with an increase in the proportion of calcitonin gene-related peptide-immunoreactive dorsal root ganglion cells. *Eur. J. Neurosci.* **5**, 1154–61.

Hara, A., Sakurada, T., Sakurada, S., Matsumura, H., and Kisara, K. (1984). Antinociceptive effects of neonatal capsaicin in rats with adjuvant arthritis. *Naunyn-Schmiedebergs Arch. Pharmacol.* **326**, 248–53.

He, X., Schepelmann, K., Schaible, H.-G., and Schmidt, R.F. (1990). Capsaicin inhibits responses of fine afferents from the knee joint of the cat to mechanical and chemical stimuli. *Brain Res.* **530**, 147–50.

Heppelmann, B., Pfeffer, A., Schaible, H.-G., and Schmidt, R.F. (1986). Effects of acetylsalicylic acid and indomethacin on single groups III and IV sensory units from acutely inflamed joints. *Pain* **26**, 337–51.

Heppelmann, B., Heuss, C., and Schmidt, R.F. (1988). Fiber size distribution of myelinated and unmyelinated axons in the medial and posterior articular nerves of the cat's knee joint. *Somatosens. Res.* **5**, 267–75.

Heppelmann, B., Messlinger, K., Neiss, W.F., and Schmidt, R.F. (1990). Ultrastructural three-dimensional reconstruction of group III and group IV sensory nerve endings ('free nerve endings') in the knee joint capsule of the cat: evidence for multiple receptive sites. *J. Comp. Neurol.* **292**, 103–16.

Heppelmann, B., Messlinger, K., Neiss, W.F., and Schmidt, R.F. (1995). Fine sensory innervation of the knee joint capsule by group III and group IV nerve fibers in the cat. *J. Comp. Neurol.* **351**, 415–28.

Herbert, M.K. and Schmidt, R.F. (1992). Activation of normal and inflamed fine articular afferent units by serotonin. *Pain* **50**, 79–88.

Hope, P.J., Jarrott, B., Schaible, H.-G., Clarke, R.W., and Duggan, A.W. (1990). Release and spread of immunoreactive neurokinin A in the cat spinal cord in a model of acute arthritis. *Brain Res.* **533**, 292–9.

Inman, R.D., Chiu, B., Rabinovich, S., and Marshall, W. (1989). Neuromodulation of synovitis: capsaicin effect on severity of experimental arthritis. *J. Neuroimmunol.* **24**, 17–22.

Kanaka, R., Schaible, H.-G., and Schmidt, R.F. (1985). Activation of fine articular afferent units by bradykinin. *Brain Res.* **327**, 81–90.

Lam, F.Y. and Ferrell, W.R. (1989*a*). Inhibition of carrageenan-induced joint inflammation by substance P antagonist. *Ann. Rheumat. Dis.* **48**, 928–32.

Lam, F.Y. and Ferrell, W.R. (1989*b*). Capsaicin suppresses substance P-induced joint inflammation in the rat. *Neurosci. Lett.* **105**, 155–8.

Lam, F.Y. and Ferrell, W.R. (1990). Mediators of substance P-induced inflammation in the rat knee joint. *Agents Actions* **31**, 298–307.

Lam, F.Y. and Ferrell, W.R. (1991). Specific neurokinin receptors mediate plasma extravasation in the rat knee joint. *Br. J. Pharmacol.* **103**, 1263–7.

Langford, L.A. and Schmidt, R.F. (1983). Afferent and efferent axons in the medial and posterior articular nerves of the cat. *Anat. Rec.* **206**, 71–8.

Larsson, J., Ekblom, A., Henriksson, K., Lundberg, T., and Theodorsson, E. (1989). Immunoreactive tachykinins, calcitonin gene-related peptide and neuropeptide Y in human synovial fluid from inflamed knee joints. *Neurosci. Lett.* **100**, 326–30.

Levine, J.D., Dardick, S.J., Roizen, M.F., Helms, C., and Basbaum, A.I. (1986). Contributions of sensory afferents and sympathetic efferents to joint injury in experimental arthritis. *J. Neurosci.* **6**, 3423–9.

Lotz, M., Carson, D.A., and Vaughyn, J.H. (1987). Substance P activation of rheumatoid synoviocytes: neural pathway in pathogenesis of arthritis. *Science* **235**, 893–5.

Louis, S.M., Jamieson, A., Russell, N.J.W., and Dockray, G.J. (1989). The role of substance P and calcitonin gene-related peptide in neurogenic plasma extravasation and vasodilatation in the rat. *Neuroscience* **32**, 581–6.

Lygren, I., Ostensen, M., Burhol, P.G., and Husby, G. (1986). Gastrointestinal peptides in serum and synovial fluid from patients with inflammatory joint disease. *Ann. Rheumat. Dis.* **45**, 637–40.

McCormack, K. and Brune, K. (1991). Dissociation between the antinociceptive and anti-inflammatory effects of the nonsteroidal anti-inflammatory drugs. A survey of their analgesic efficacy. *Drugs* **41**, 533–47.

McIntyre, A.K., Proske, U., and Tracey, D.J. (1978). Afferent fibers from muscle receptors in the posterior nerve of the cat's knee joint. *Exp. Brain Res.* **33**, 415–24.

Mapp, P.I., Kidd, B.L., Gibson, S.J., Terry, J.M., Revell, P.A., Ibrahim, N.B.N., Blake, D.R., and Polak, J.M. (1990). Substance P-, calcitonin gene-related peptide- and C-flanking peptide of neuropeptide Y-immunoreactive fibres are present in normal synovium but depleted in patients with rheumatoid arthritis. *Neuroscience* **17**, 143–53.

Marshall, K.W., Chiu, B., and Inman, R.D. (1990). Substance P and arthritis: analysis of plasma and synovial fluid levels. *Arthritis Rheumatism* **33**, 87–90.

Moncada, S., Ferreira, S.H., and Vane, J.R. (1975). Inhibition of prostaglandin biosynthesis as the mechanism of analgesia of aspirin-like drugs in the dog knee joint. *Eur. J. Pharmacol.* **31**, 250–60.

Neugebauer, V., Schaible, H.-G., and Schmidt, R.F. (1989). Sensitization of articular afferents to mechanical stimuli by bradykinin. *Pflügers Arch.* **415**, 330–5.

Neugebauer, V., Lücke, T., and Schaible, H.-G. (1994*a*). Requirement of metabotropic glutamate receptors for the generation of inflammation-evoked hyperexcitability in rat spinal cord neurons. *Eur. J. Neurosci.* **6**, 1179–86.

Neugebauer, V., Schaible, H.-G., Weiretter, F., and Freudenberger, U. (1994*b*). The involvement of substance P and neurokinin-1 receptors in the responses of rat dorsal horn neurons to noxious but not to innocuous mechanical stimuli applied to the knee joint. *Brain Res.* **666**, 207–15.

Neugebauer, V., Weiretter, F., and Schaible, H.-G. (1995). The involvement of substance P and neurokinin-1 receptors in the hyperexcitability of dorsal horn neurons during development of acute arthritis in rat's knee joint. *J. Neurophysiol.* **73**, 1574–83.

O'Brien, C., Woolf, C.J., Fitzgerald, M., Lindsay, R.M., and Molander, C. (1989). Differences in the chemical expression of rat primary afferent neurons which innervate skin, muscle or joint. *Neuroscience* **32**, 493–502.

Ohno, H., Kuraishi, Y., Nanayama, T., Minami, M., Kawamura, M., and Satoh, M. (1990). Somatostain is increased in the dorsal root ganglia of adjuvant-inflamed rat. *Neurosci. Res.* **8**, 179–88.

Oku, R., Satoh, M., and Tagaki, H. (1987). Release of substance P from the spinal dorsal horn is enhanced in polyarthritic rats. *Neurosci. Lett.* **74**, 315–19.

Pereira da Silva, J.A. and Carmo-Fonseca, M. (1990). Peptide containing nerves in human synovium: immunohistochemical evidence for decreased innervation in rheumatoid arthritis. *J. Rheumatol.* **17**, 1592–9.

Proske, U., Schaible, H.-G., and Schmidt, R.F. (1988). Joint receptors and kinaesthesia. *Exp. Brain Res.* **72**, 219–24.

Russell, N.J.W., Schaible, H.-G., and Schmidt, R.F. (1987). Opiates inhibit the discharges of fine afferent units from inflamed knee joint of the cat. *Neurosci. Lett.* **76**, 107–12.

Schaible, H.-G. and Grubb, B.D. (1993). Afferent and spinal mechanisms of joint pain. *Pain* **55**, 5–54.

Schaible, H.-G. and Schmidt, R.F. (1983*a*). Activation of groups III and IV sensory units in medial articular nerve by local mechanical stimulation of knee joint. *J. Neurophysiol.* **49**, 35–44.

Schaible, H.-G. and Schmidt, R.F. (1983*b*). Responses of fine medial articular nerve afferents to passive movements of knee joint. *J. Neurophysiol.* **49**, 1118–26.

Schaible, H.-G. and Schmidt, R.F. (1985). Effects of an experimental arthritis on the sensory properties of fine articular afferent units. *J. Neurophysiol.* **54**, 1109–22.

Schaible, H.-G. and Schmidt, R.F. (1988*a*). Time course of mechanosensitivity changes in articular afferents during a developing experimental arthritis. *J. Neurophysiol.* **60**, 2180–95.

Schaible, H.-G. and Schmidt, R.F. (1988*b*). Excitation and sensitization of fine articular afferents from cat's knee joint by prostaglandin E_2. *J. Physiol.* **403**, 91–104.

Schaible, H.-G., Jarrott, B., Hope, P.J., and Duggan, A.W. (1990). Release of immunoreactive substance P in the cat spinal cord during development of acute arthritis in cat's knee: a study with antibody bearing microprobes. *Brain Res.* **529**, 214–23.

Schaible, H.-G., Freudenberger, U., Neugebauer, V., and Stiller, U. (1994). Intraspinal release of immunoreactive calcitonin gene-related peptide during development of inflammation in the joint in vivo—a study with antibody microprobes in cat and rat. *Neuroscience* **62**, 1293–305.

Schepelmann, K., Messlinger, K., Schaible, H.-G., and Schmidt, R.F. (1992). Inflammatory mediators and nociception in the joint: excitation and sensitization of slowly conducting afferent fibers of cat's knee by prostaglandin I2. *Neuroscience* **50**, 237–47.

Schepelmann, K., Messlinger, K., and Schmidt, R.F. (1993). The effects of phorbol ester on slowly conducting afferents of the cat's knee joint. *Exp. Brain Res.* **92**, 391–8.

Schepelmann, K., Messlinger, K., Schaible, H.-G., and Schmidt, R.F. (1995). The opioid antagonist naloxone does not alter discharges of nociceptive afferents from the acutely inflamed knee joint of the cat. *Neurosci. Lett.* **187**, 212–14.

Schmidt, R.F. and Schaible, H.-G. (1994). Silent primary afferents. In *Cellular mechanisms of sensory processing*, Nato ASI Series, Series H, Vol. 79 (ed. L. Urban), pp. 289–96. Springer, Berlin.

Schmidt, R.F., Schaible, H.-G., Messlinger, K., Heppelmann, B., Hanesch, U., and Pawlak, M. (1994). Silent and active nociceptors: structure, functions and clinical implications. *Proceedings of 7th World Congress on Pain. Vol. 2. Progress in pain research and management* (ed. G.F. Gebhart, D.L. Hammond, and T.S. Jensen, pp. 213–50. IASP Press, Seattle.

Sluka, K.A., Dougherty, P.M., Sorkin, L.S., Willis, W.D., and Westlund, K.N. (1992). Neural changes in acute arthritis in monkeys. III. Changes in substance P, calcitonin gene-related peptide and glutamate in the dorsal horn of the spinal cord. *Brain Res. Rev.* **17**, 29–38.

Smith, G.D., Harmar, A.J., McQueen, D.S., and Seckl, J.R. (1992). Increase in substance P and CGRP, but not somatostatin content of innervating dorsal root ganglia in adjuvant mono-arthritis in the rat. *Neurosci. Lett.* **137**, 257–60.

Stein, C. (1994). Interaction of immune-competent cells and nociceptors. In *Proceedings of the 7th World Congress on Pain. Vol. 2. Progress in pain research and management* (ed. G.F. Gebhart, D.L. Hammond, and T.S. Jensen, pp. 285–97. IASP Press, Seattle.

Yaksh, T.L. (1988). Substance P release from knee joint afferent terminals; modulation by opioids. *Brain Res.* **458**, 319–24.

9 Visceral nociceptors

FERNANDO CERVERO

Introduction

The observations that led Sherrington to propose the concept of the nociceptor were made in experimental studies of spinal reflexes evoked by cutaneous stimulation (Sherrington 1906). Since then, much of the evidence in favour of the existence of a category of sensory receptor concerned with the processing of noxious stimuli has come from studies of the innervation of the skin in both animals and man. To a large extent what we know today about nociceptors in general is the result of studies restricted to the analysis of cutaneous sensation (see Perl, Chapter 1, this volume). It is only more recently that studies of nociceptors from subcutaneous tissues, including muscles, joints, tendons, and ligaments, have been carried out and published (see Mense, Chapter 7, this volume; Schaible and Schmidt, Chapter 8, this volume).

The Cinderella of this field is undoubtedly the sensory innervation of internal organs. The accessibility of the skin and the easier experimental protocols involving somatic reflexes and sensations, including those in man, have been responsible for a general lack of information about the functional properties of visceral sensory afferents.

It is also true that the more we know about the mechanisms of cutaneous and visceral sensation the more we realize that these two processes, while having many common features, also have important differences. The skin is the source of a large range of complex sensory experiences, including tactile recognition, temperature sensation, pain, and related phenomena like itch and prickle. The innervation of the skin includes many different types of sensory receptor whose activities relate to the various forms of sensation. On the other hand, we seldom have any sensory experiences from our internal organs other than pain and discomfort (Bonica 1990) and, even when other sensations such as bladder or stomach fullness are felt, these can easily evolve towards pain if the stimulus persists. This particular observation has been responsible for the notion that all internal organs are innervated by a single class of sensory receptor whose main function is to participate in the autonomic regulation of the organ (motility, secretion, control of blood flow, etc.) but which, when excited by intense stimuli, will also contribute to the triggering of unpleasant and aversive sensations.

The scientific interpretation of the mechanisms of visceral sensation and visceral pain has therefore included from the beginning two different and opposing ideas: that the viscera are innervated by separate classes of sensory receptors, some concerned with autonomic regulation and some concerned with sensation, including pain; or that internal organs are innervated by a single and homogeneous class of sensory receptors that at low frequencies of activation send normal regulatory signals and at high frequencies, induced by intense stimuli, signal pain (Fig. 9.1). The first interpretation extends the concept of nociceptor to the visceral domain and the second applies a strict 'pattern' theory to the peripheral encoding of sensory events in the viscera (Cervero and Jänig 1992).

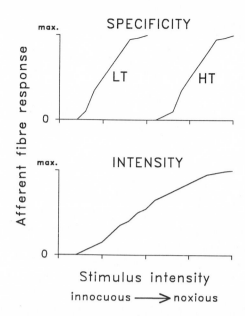

Fig. 9.1 Schematic diagram portraying the two classical theories for the encoding of noxious stimuli by peripheral afferent fibres. The specificity theory postulates the existence of two different classes of primary afferent fibres (low-threshold (LT) and high-threshold (HT)) responsible for the separate encoding of innocuous and noxious events. The intensity theory proposes that all peripheral stimuli are encoded by a single and homogeneous population of afferent fibres capable of encoding stimulus intensities ranging from innocuous to noxious. From Cervero and Jänig (1992) with permission.

It is an indication of how little work has been done in the field of visceral sensation that this conflict has lasted for a long time (but see Cervero and Jänig 1992). Therefore, a review of visceral nociceptors, such as the present one, still needs to address the question of whether or not nociceptors exist in the viscera, since the afferent innervation of internal organs has become the last line of defence of those who still adhere to theories of sensation based on patterns of impulses in non-specific sensory receptors.

In this chapter three questions will be addressed to approach this central point of disagreement: (1) the evidence in favour of the existence of separate classes of sensory receptor in the viscera, particularly the results that show the presence of high-threshold sensory receptors in internal organs; (2) the evidence in favour of the existence of a single and homogeneous class of sensory receptor in the viscera and the results that show that these receptors can encode a wide range of stimulus intensities; and (3) a discussion of the properties of the so-called 'silent' nociceptors in internal organs and their possible functional roles. These three questions will be addressed with the aim of discussing the roles of the various types of visceral sensory receptors in the signalling of visceral pain. A more detailed account of the sensory innervation of the viscera in general and of the ranges and types of sensations that can be evoked from all internal organs has been published recently (Cervero 1994).

High-threshold receptors in the viscera

The presence of groups of sensory receptors with a high threshold to natural stimuli (mainly mechanical) and an encoding function contained entirely within the noxious range of stimulation has been documented in many of the internal organs whose afferent innervation has been studied in detail. A description of the functional properties of these receptors is outlined below.

Heart

The existence of specific cardiac nociceptors was suggested by the findings of Uchida and co-workers (Uchida and Murao 1974a–c, 1975) and was proposed by the Coleridges' laboratory (Baker et al. 1980; Coleridge and Coleridge 1980). These authors claim that there is a distinct group of pure chemoreceptors connected to unmyelinated sympathetic afferents and specifically activated by stimuli capable of evoking cardiac pain. They described a small population of chemosensitive receptors whose endings were mostly in the ventricles. The majority had unmyelinated fibres and a few were connected to small myelinated afferents. They were insensitive to light touch and virtually none of them fired in phase with the cardiac rhythm. Even large increases in ventricular pressure had little effect on impulse frequency. However, they were all very sensitive to bradykinin applied locally or injected into the left atrium.

Baker et al. (1980) have also reported that the responses of low-threshold mechanoreceptors connected to sympathetic afferents were also greatly increased by the administration of bradykinin. They accepted the possibility that this increased responsiveness could contribute to the sensation of cardiac pain and conceded that their cardiac nociceptors may not have an exclusive role in the signalling of ischaemic pain.

Veins

A recent report (Michaelis et al. 1994) describes the properties of a population of afferent fibres in the cat with receptive fields in the saphenous vein. These authors show that most of these afferents could be activated by intense mechanical stimuli and/or by the application of algesic chemicals such as bradykinin, capsaicin, or hypertonic saline. They concluded that these afferents could be involved in the signalling of pain from the veins, especially under pathological conditions.

Lungs and airways

Two kinds of sensory receptor in the airways could be regarded as part of the nociceptive innervation of the respiratory system:

1. *Rapidly adapting stretch receptors.* These receptors are also known as 'deflation receptors', 'cough receptors', and, most commonly, as 'irritant receptors'. They are located in the lung parenchyma, in the bronchioles, and in the distal bronchi and are connected to small myelinated afferent fibres (Widdicombe 1974, 1986; Paintal 1977a, b, 1986; Sant'Ambrogio 1982, 1987). They are mechanoreceptors that respond with irregular and rapidly adapting discharges to lung deflation, to large deformations of the airways, to gentle touch of the inner surface of the bronchi, and, in particular, to the inhalation of dusts and irritants. These properties suggest that they may be located in the

mucosa of the airways. Irritant receptors are also excited by a number of chemical mediators such as serotonin, histamine, prostaglandins, and acetylcholine administered either as aerosols or intravenously (Paintal 1977b). Irritant receptors are involved in the triggering of the cough reflex and of reflexes associated with coughing, including bronchoconstriction and mucus secretion. In addition, they may play a role in the signalling of bronchopulmonary pain.

2. *J-receptors*. These receptors are connected to unmyelinated afferent fibres and are often described as C-fibre receptors (Widdicombe 1974, 1986; Sant'Ambrogio 1982, 1987). They are mainly chemosensitive, although they can also be activated by mechanical stimuli. They respond to large inflations or deflations of the lungs and to a variety of chemicals such as bradykinin, prostaglandins, serotonin, histamine, acetylcholine, CO_2, phenyl diguanide, capsaicin, nicotine, lobeline, and others (Widdicombe 1974, 1986; Paintal 1977b, 1986). They are also sensitive to pulmonary congestion and oedema, presumably as a consequence of the increase in interstitial volume produced by increased pulmonary capillary pressure (Paintal 1986). C-fibre receptors are also involved in the triggering of the cough reflex and of a number of reflexes associated with defensive respiratory responses such as bronchoconstriction and mucus secretion (Widdicombe 1986). In addition, it has been suggested that they play an important role in the generation of dyspnoeic sensations during pulmonary oedema (Paintal 1977a, 1986).

Oesophagus

A comprehensive examination of oesophageal mechanosensitive afferents running in the thoracic sympathetic nerves of the opossum has been published by Sengupta *et al.* (1990). This study describes two types of mechanoreceptor connected to small myelinated and unmyelinated afferent fibres: (1) 'wide-dynamic-range' mechanonociceptors (see below); and (2) 'high-threshold' mechanonociceptors.

This second group of receptors has a high threshold to distension (about 30 mmHg) and encodes pressure stimuli of up to 120 mmHg. The receptors do not respond to normal peristalsis of the oesophagus but their maximum discharges at saturation pressure are similar to those of the previous group. In a separate study, Sengupta *et al.* (1992) have also shown that both types of mechanonociceptor are activated by the systemic administration of bradykinin and that the mechanism of action involves a direct effect of the peptide on a B_2 receptor subtype on the fibre endings.

Biliary system

Cervero (1982) carried out a study of the afferent innervation of the biliary system of the ferret in order to identify the types of afferent fibre that could be involved in the signalling of biliary pain. In this study a technique for the natural stimulation of the biliary system that permitted the distinction between noxious and innocuous intensities of stimulation was developed. It involved the application of controlled distensions of the gall bladder and ducts while recording their effects on the systemic blood pressure of the animals. Raising the biliary pressure above physiological levels induced transient blood pressure increases that were not affected by bilateral vagotomy but were often abolished by bilateral section of the splanchnic nerves. This cardiovascular reflex, which since Sherrington (1906) has been regarded as a nociceptive reaction, was used to assess the level of biliary pressure that could be interpreted as noxious.

Cervero (1982, 1983) reported that biliary afferents recorded from either the splanchnic nerve or the biliary plexus could be classified into two distinct groups according to their thresholds and their encoding ranges. About two-thirds of the afferents had low thresholds to biliary distension and encoded changes of biliary pressure within the physiological range. These afferents are probably involved in local or systemic reflexes related to gastrointestinal function. The other third were receptors with a high threshold to biliary distension and encoded mechanical stimuli in the noxious range only (Fig. 9.2). They had mechanically sensitive receptive fields in the gall bladder and ducts, showed no background activity, and did not respond to physiological changes of biliary pressure. Because of these properties they were classified as visceral nociceptors concerned with the signalling of events that could lead to pain perception.

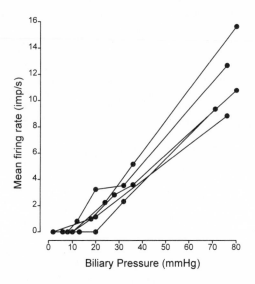

Fig. 9.2 Stimulus–response functions of five high-threshold afferents from the biliary system of the ferret. These fibres show thresholds above the maximum physiological level of biliary pressure and an encoding range contained within noxious intensities of biliary pressure. Data from Cervero (1982); redrawn from Cervero (1983).

Small intestine

Recordings from intestinal afferents in sympathetic nerves were first reported by Gernandt and Zotterman (1947). They described responses to low-intensity mechanical stimulation of the mesenteries, which they attributed to the activation of mesenteric Pacinian corpuscles. In addition, they reported that noxious stimulation of the intestine, such as pinching the enteric wall, evoked activity in small-diameter afferent fibres, which they interpreted as being related to the signalling of intestinal pain.

A series of studies by Longhurst and co-workers have described the functional properties of a group of splanchnic afferent fibres that are thought to be mainly concerned with nociception (Longhurst *et al.* 1984, 1991; Lew and Longhurst 1986; Longhurst and Dittman 1987; Stahl and Longhurst 1992). These are sympathetic afferents that innervate the small intestine, the stomach, the liver, the pancreas, and the biliary system. Each individual afferent innervates only one of these organs and, very rarely, two of them. The afferents are either small myelinated or unmyelinated with the former being mainly mechanosensitive and the latter either insensitive to mechanical stimulation or activated only by very intense mechanical probing of their receptive fields.

The main characteristic of many of these afferents is their sensitivity to algesic chemicals such as bradykinin and capsaicin as well as to pain-producing stimuli like ischaemia and hypoxia (Longhurst *et al.* 1984; Lew and Longhurst 1986). Chemical stimulation sensitizes these afferents to subsequent stimuli, a process that involves the local release of prostaglandins and perhaps lactic acid (Longhurst and Dittman 1987; Longhurst *et al.* 1991; Stahl and Longhurst 1992). Because of all these properties these afferents are thought to mediate the intestinal pain evoked by ischaemia and irritation of the alimentary canal.

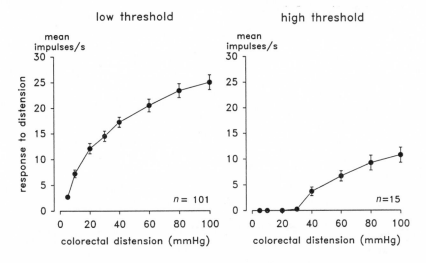

Fig. 9.3 Stimulus–response functions of low- and high-threshold pelvic nerve afferents innervating the colon of the rat. The *x*-axis represents graded (0–100 mmHg) distending pressure and the *y*-axis represents the mean increase in impulses/s of the fibres to graded colorectal distension. Data from Sengupta and Gebhart (1994*a*) and unpublished observations from these authors who have kindly supplied the figure.

Colon

The functional properties of colonic afferents projecting to the sacral spinal cord of the rat via the pelvic nerve have been reported (Sengupta and Gebhart 1994*a*). About three-quarters of the afferents had low thresholds to colonic distension, whereas the remaining showed high thresholds to this mechanical stimulus. High-threshold fibres responded at colonic intensities higher than 30 mmHg and encoded the stimulus intensity up to 100 mmHg (Figs 9.3 and 9.4). These sensory fibres constitute a distinct and separate class of mechan-osensitive afferent innervating the colon with encoding functions similar to those of high-threshold fibres in other viscera. However, Sengupta and Gebhart (1994*a*) reported that these afferents may not be the only ones responsible for colonic pain. Contributions from low-threshold afferents and from the so-called 'silent' nociceptors may also be important.

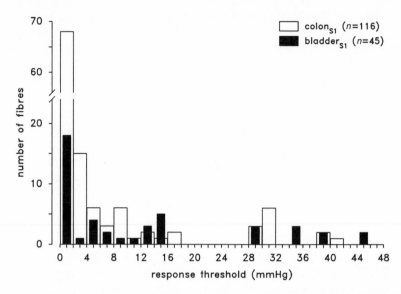

Fig. 9.4 Frequency histograms of thresholds for response of pelvic nerve afferents in the sacral (S1) dorsal root to distension of the colon or urinary bladder of the rat. '*n*' indicates the number of afferent fibres. Data from Sengupta and Gebhart (1994*a, b*) and unpublished observations from these authors who have kindly supplied the figure.

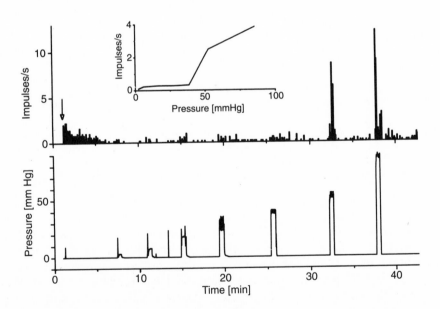

Fig. 9.5 A high-threshold mechanosensitive unit from the guinea-pig's ureter. This fibre did not respond to peristaltic contractions of the ureter, gave a long-lasting discharge after probing the receptive field (arrow), and responded to imposed distensions with a high threshold. The stimulus–response function of this fibre is shown in the inset. From Cervero and Sann (1989) with permission.

Ureter

A comprehensive study of the afferent innervation of the ureter was carried out by Cervero and Sann (1989). They studied the electrophysiological responses of 67 afferent fibres from the guinea-pig's ureter using an *in-vitro* preparation of ureter and associated nerves. All recordings were from mechanosensitive units with unmyelinated afferent fibres, which were then classified into two distinct groups according to their ability to respond to contractions of the ureter. The first group (called U-1) contained only 9 per cent of the units, all of which were sensitive to peristaltic contractions of the ureter. They responded to imposed distensions with a short latency and a low threshold (mean = 8 mmHg) and did not show spontaneous activity or afterdischarges. The second group (called U-2) contained the vast majority of the units. None of them were sensitive to peristaltic contractions of the ureter and all responded to imposed distensions with a latency greater than 3 s and a high threshold (mean = 34 mmHg) (Fig. 9.5). These units had spontaneous activity of up to 2.4 Hz and showed afterdischarges to mechanical stimuli lasting up to several minutes. Units of the U-2 type were also sensitive to strong local distensions imposed with an artificial kidney stone, to hypoxia of the ureteric mucosa, and to intraluminal application of bradykinin, capsaicin, and potassium. Similar groups of low- (U-1) and high-threshold (U-2) units have been found in the ureter of the chicken, though the proportions in this species are closer to 50/50 (Hammer *et al.* 1993).

On the basis of these results Sann and Cervero (1988) and Cervero and Sann (1989) concluded that U-1 units were low-threshold mechanoreceptors concerned with the regulation of ureteric motility and that U-2 units were ureteric nociceptors. They proposed that U-2 units could mediate the intense pain sensations and pseudoaffective reactions that follow acute distension of the ureter and localized stretch of its wall.

Semenenko and Cervero (1992) have shown that the proportion of visceral afferent fibres from the guinea-pig ureter that contain substance P, calcitonin gene-related peptide (CGRP), or both peptides is virtually identical to the proportion of high-threshold mechanosensitive afferent fibres from the same internal organ (Cervero and Sann 1989). It is tempting to suggest that the presence of these peptides in ureteric afferents determines the functional properties of the afferent even though this is only supported by indirect evidence. Further studies are needed to identify any possible correlation between the neurochemical contents and the functional roles of visceral afferent fibres.

Urinary bladder

In the cat, all mechanosensitive pelvic afferents with unmyelinated axons have high thresholds (above 40 to 50 mmHg) to distension of the bladder and respond only to clearly noxious levels of distension or to very intense contractions of the bladder (Clifton *et al.* 1976; Coggeshall and Ito 1977; Häbler *et al.* 1990). These units form a small but distinct population of high-threshold afferents responding exclusively to noxious mechanical events in the normal bladder.

The proportion of high-threshold mechanosensitive afferents from the bladder has been estimated at only 2.4 per cent by Häbler *et al.* (1990) but this is a substantial underestimate. These authors recorded from unmyelinated dorsal root fibres in the S2 segment of the cat and identified them as pelvic nerve afferents by electrical stimulation of this nerve. They recorded from 297 such afferents and found only seven that were sensitive to distensions and contractions of the bladder. Since all of them were high-threshold fibres they calculated that 2.4 per cent (that is, 7 of 297) were high-threshold mechanosensitive afferents from the bladder. However, they did not take into account that the failure of pelvic afferents to respond to mechanical stimulation of the bladder could have been due to the fact that two-thirds of the afferents in the pelvic nerve innervate pelvic viscera other than the bladder (Bahns *et al.* 1987).

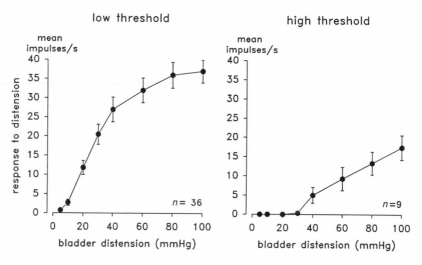

Fig. 9.6 Stimulus–response functions of low- and high-threshold pelvic nerve afferents innervating the urinary bladder of the rat. The *x*-axis represents graded (0–100 mmHg) distending pressures and the *y*-axis represents mean increase in impulses/s of the fibres to graded urinary bladder distension. Data from Sengupta and Gebhart (1994*b*) and unpublished observations from these authors who have kindly supplied the figure.

The functional properties of bladder afferents projecting to the sacral spinal cord of the rat via the pelvic nerve have been reported (Sengupta and Gebhart 1994*b*). About 80 per cent of the afferents had low thresholds to bladder distension, whereas the remaining showed high thresholds to this mechanical stimulus. High-threshold fibres responded at bladder intensities higher than 30 mmHg and encoded the stimulus intensity up to 100 mmHg (Figs 9.4 and 9.6). These authors also showed that high-threshold bladder afferents could be desensitized after instillation of acetic acid into the bladder.

Uterus

In electrophysiological studies of uterine afferent fibres Abrahams and Teare (1969) reported the presence of mechanically sensitive uterine afferents in the hypogastric nerves of the cat. These mechanoreceptors responded to manual compression of the uterus and to intense uterine and vaginal distension sometimes requiring up to 100 mmHg of pressure.

Comprehensive electrophysiological studies of uterine afferent fibres in the rat using *in vivo* and *in vitro* preparations have been reported by Berkley and colleagues (Berkley *et al.* 1987, 1988, 1990, 1993; Robbins *et al.* 1990). They studied afferent discharges in the hypogastric and pelvic nerves evoked by mechanical and chemical stimulation of the uterus.

Afferents in the hypogastric nerve responded to intense mechanical stimuli of the uterus and of the broad ligament and more rarely to uterine contractions. The stimulation intensities required for the activation of these afferents always produced transient ischaemia around the site of stimulation or contracted area (Berkley *et al.* 1987, 1988). These afferent fibres were shown to have lower thresholds to mechanical stimulation of the uterus when the rats were in oestrus than when they were in metoestrus (Berkley *et al.* 1988; Robbins *et al.* 1990). Hypogastric afferent fibres responded also to the application of algesic chemicals such as bradykinin, 5-HT, and KCl, as well as to high doses of CO_2 and sodium cyanide. Because of their responsiveness, Berkley *et al.* (1988, 1993) suggested that these afferent fibres could be involved in the signalling of noxious events from the uterus particularly during uterine irritation.

On the other hand, afferents in the pelvic nerve responded to a variety of mechanical stimuli applied to the uterus and vagina. Those with vaginal receptive fields responded best to the movement of probes inside the vagina and were observed more frequently during the proestrus stage of the cycle (Berkley *et al.* 1990). Pelvic afferents with receptive fields in the cervix and the body of the uterus were observed less frequently and responded to distension of the uterus and to intraarterial injection of algesic chemicals. Overall, pelvic afferents were shown to have a wider range of responsiveness to uterine mechanical and chemical stimuli than hypogastric afferents. Therefore Berkley *et al.* (1990, 1993) concluded that they were likely to subserve physiological reproductive functions during mating, conception, and parturition, in addition to playing some role in nociception.

A report by Hong *et al.* (1993) describes the properties of hypogastric afferent fibres with receptive sites in the uterus of the cat. Most of the afferents were unmyelinated with the remaining being small myelinated. Two populations of sensory receptor were found: low-threshold mechanoreceptors and polymodal nociceptors. The latter responded only to intense mechanical stimuli of the uterus and to the intraarterial injection of algesic chemicals and were thought to be specifically concerned with the signalling of nociceptive events.

Intensity-encoding receptors in the viscera

A number of reports have described sensory receptors in internal organs with a low threshold to natural stimuli (mainly mechanical) and an encoding function that spans innocuous and noxious intensities of stimulation. It has been suggested that these receptors constitute a single and homogeneous category of sensory receptors that encode the stimulus intensity in the magnitude of their discharges (intensity-encoding). A description of the properties of these receptors is outlined below.

Heart

The existence of specific cardiac nociceptors has been vigorously denied by Malliani and co-workers (Casati *et al.* 1979; Malliani 1982, 1986; Malliani and Lombardi 1982; Malliani *et al.* 1986). Casati *et al.* (1979) recorded from cardiac receptors connected to sympathetic unmyelinated afferent fibres and concluded that they were all mechanosensitive and capable of responding to normal mechanical events in the ventrices. On the basis of these observations and the sensitivity of the same endings to bradykinin (Lombardi *et al.* 1981), they concluded that this group of receptors were not specific nociceptors but non-specific sensory endings that could respond to a variety of stimulus intensities ranging from innocuous to noxious. They proposed an 'intensity' mechanism for the encoding of cardiac pain so that 'when sufficient levels of afferent impulses are reached and an appropriate activation of the central ascending pathways is established, a breakthrough may occur giving rise to the conscious perception of pain' (Malliani and Lombardi 1982).

Oesophagus

As mentioned above, Sengupta *et al.* (1990) have described, in the opossum, two types of mechanoreceptor connected to small myelinated and unmyelinated afferent fibres running in sympathetic thoracic nerves: (1) 'wide-dynamic-range' mechanoreceptors and (2) high-threshold mechanonociceptors (see above).

The first group of tension receptors have low thresholds to oesophageal distension (about 3 mmHg) and encode pressure stimuli monotonically in the range 3–120 mmHg. Their maximum discharges at saturation pressure are of around 20 impulses per second. These receptors also respond to normal oesophageal peristaltic contractions.

One possible role for the intensity-encoding mechanonociceptors would be the triggering of sensations of oesophageal distension that are not painful at low pressure levels but that become progressively uncomfortable at higher intensities. A central summation mechanism would operate to add an unpleasant character to sensations of oesophageal distension of increasing intensities.

Colon

Several laboratories have reported the functional properties of sympathetic afferent fibres with receptive fields in the colon. One of the groups (Floyd and Morrison 1974; Floyd *et al.* 1976) described the properties of colonic afferents with axons in the hypogastric and splanchnic nerves in dogs and cats. These afferents were reported to have up to six punctate mechanosensitive sites located along the blood vessels of the colon, particularly at branching points. The afferent fibres were mostly small myelinated and the mechanical thresholds were low.

The laboratory of W. Jänig has also carried out a comprehensive examination of the sympathetic afferent innervation of the colon in cats (Blumberg *et al.* 1983; Haupt *et al.* 1983). They recorded afferent fibres in the inferior splanchnic nerves and in the upper lumbar rami and studied their responses to controlled distensions of the colon and to the application of algesic chemicals. Two-thirds of the fibres were unmyelinated and the remaining third were small myelinated. Most fibres had low levels of background activity of between 0.5 and 3 Hz.

Four types of mechanosensitive colonic afferents were distinguished according to the presence or absence of phasic components in their responses to a 60-s sustained distension of the colon. Groups I and II had only phasic responses to distension and formed just over 10 per cent of the total sample. Groups III and IV showed, in addition or exclusively, a steady tonic discharge that lasted for the duration of the stimulus. Mechanosensitive sites were identified as punctate receptive fields along the vessels of the colon. Their mechanical thresholds formed a continuum spanning the innocuous and noxious ranges: all of the type I and II fibres and most of the type III fibres had thresholds below 25 mmHg, whereas 45 per cent of the type IV fibres had mechanical thresholds above 25 mmHg. In addition to their mechanical sensitivity, most sympathetic colonic afferents responded to ischaemia of the colon and to the administration of algesic chemicals such as bradykinin and KCl.

A separate study examined the functional properties of sacral dorsal root afferent with axons in the pelvic nerve and mechanical receptive fields in the colon (Jänig and Koltzenburg 1991). Thirty-six mechanosensitive colonic afferents were studied and were classified according to their adaptation characteristics into two groups of roughly equal sizes. One group of mostly unmyelinated afferents responded tonically to increasing distensions of the colon and the other group of mostly small myelinated afferents responded phasically. Both groups of fibres were described as being part of a homogeneous population of afferents with low thresholds to distension and monotonic stimulus–response functions ranging from innocuous to noxious levels. Data on the individual mechanical thresholds or on the range of thresholds of the fibres were not supplied in this study but the average of the population was given as 21 ± 12 (SD) mmHg.

As described above, Sengupta and Gebhart (1994*a*) have examined the functional properties of colonic afferents projecting to the sacral spinal cord of the rat via the pelvic nerve. About three-quarters of the afferents had low thresholds to colonic distension (less than 10 mmHg) and encoded the stimulus intensity up to 100 mmHg (Figs 9.3 and 9.4). Many of these sensory fibres responded to bradykinin. The low threshold of these afferent fibres and their wide encoding range make them similar to the intensity-encoding fibres described in other locations and in other animal species.

Bladder

Mechanosensitive afferents in the hypogastric and lumbar splanchnic nerves of the cat respond to passive distension of the bladder with a wide range of thresholds (4–30 mmHg) (Floyd *et al.* 1976; Bahns *et al.* 1986) and are able to encode bladder distensions below and above noxious levels (up to 80–100 mmHg). Their threshold to bladder contractions is also in the range 4–25 mmHg (Bahns *et al.* 1986). The receptive fields of these afferents have been described as one to six punctate sites on the surface of the bladder and along blood vessels (Floyd *et al.* 1976) or as single mechanosensitive spots on the bladder serosa (Bahns *et al.* 1986). Three-quarters of these afferents have conduction velocities above 2 m/s with the remainder being C-fibres. Low levels of background activity below 1 impulse per second have been observed in some of these afferents (Bahns *et al.* 1986).

Mechanosensitive bladder afferents in the pelvic nerve of the cat are more numerous than those in sympathetic nerves (Jänig and Koltzenburg 1992). They have normally no background activity and fall into two distinct categories depending on whether they are myelinated or unmyelinated.

The first group of afferents have small myelinated axons and respond to distensions and contractions of the bladder with a wide range of thresholds from 4 to 25 mmHg (Clifton *et al.* 1976; Coggeshall and Ito 1977; Bahns *et al.* 1987; Häbler *et al.* 1993). They do not show background activity when the bladder is empty, respond to mechanical stimuli in a monotonic fashion, and encode a range of intensities from innocuous to noxious (Bahns *et al.* 1987; Häbler *et al.* 1993). A small proportion of myelinated sacral afferents (6 per cent) have thresholds to bladder distension above 30 mmHg and respond only to intravesical pressures in the range 50–100 mmHg (Häbler *et al.* 1993). On the other hand, all unmyelinated mechanosensitive afferents have high thresholds to distension (see above).

In the rat, there is a large population of low-threshold bladder afferents projecting to the sacral spinal cord via the pelvic nerve (Sengupta and Gebhart 1994*b*). About 80 per cent of all mechanosensitive afferents have low thresholds to bladder distension (less than 10 mmHg) and encode the stimulus intensity in an intensity-like manner up to 100 mmHg (Figs 9.4 and 9.6). These low-threshold bladder afferents can be desensitized after instillation of acetic acid into the bladder.

Testes

The laboratory of T. Kumazawa has carried out extensive investigations on the functional properties of testicular receptors in the dog using both *in vivo* and *in vitro* preparations (see Kumazawa, Chapter 13, this volume). The vast majority of the recordings have been made from small myelinated fibres, some of which lose their myelin sheaths as they approach their receptive fields. Two types of afferents have been described: a very small group of low-threshold rapidly adapting mechanoreceptors, which form less than 3 per cent of the total number of fibres studied; and a much larger group of afferents connected to 'polymodal receptors'.

These are receptors that respond to a variety of stimuli, including mechanical, chemical, and thermal ones. They have little or no background activity and have several receptive sites on the surface of the testes. They respond to a wide range of intensities of mechanical stimulation and show also a very wide range of thresholds from 0.9 to 270 g/mm^2. Receptors connected to unmyelinated afferents have higher thresholds than those with myelinated axons, but the depth of the receptive sites within the testes also contributes to the differences in threshold. They are claimed to respond to innocuous intensities of mechanical stimulation on the grounds that their threshold stimuli are not felt as painful when applied to the skin of the experimenters.

Polymodal receptors are also sensitive to heat stimuli, with thresholds at around 45°C, and to algesic chemicals such as bradykinin, hypertonic saline, and potassium but show little sensitivity to acetylcholine, substance P, serotonin, or prostaglandins. Repeated stimulation at frequent intervals leads to desensitization of the receptors, whereas sensitization is observed when the repetition interval is longer than 20 min. Equally, sensitization of their responses to bradykinin and other algesic chemicals occurs following the application of prostaglandins and serotonin, an effect antagonized by indomethacin.

Kumazawa and colleagues have argued that 'polymodal receptors' are similar to the polymodal nociceptors of the skin with the difference that their mechanical sensitivity extends into the innocuous range (Kumazawa 1986). Because of this they suggest that 'polymodal receptors' encode noxious mechanical events in the testes by the intensity of their discharges (Kumazawa and Mizumura 1984; Kumazawa 1986). Otherwise, their thermal and chemical sensitivities are consistent with a functional role as nociceptors, although it must be pointed out that the circumstances during which their sensitivity to noxious heat could normally come into play are obscure. As for the issue of their mechanical sensitivity it is questionable that low-intensity punctate stimulation of the tunica vaginalis is a non-painful stimulus since it has been reported that this serosa is extremely sensitive to pain in humans (MacKenzie 1909).

'Silent' nociceptors in the viscera

The presence of 'silent' nociceptors in the viscera and their possible role in the signalling of visceral pain states have been discussed at length by Jänig and Koltzenburg (1990, 1992). Essentially the argument is similar to that put forward by McMahon and Koltzenburg (1990*a, b*), namely, that a large and previously unidentified component of the afferent innervation of internal organs consists of unresponsive afferent fibres that become active after inflammation of the peripheral organ. These afferents are function-ally different from the rest of visceral afferent fibres and are mainly concerned with stimuli such as tissue injury and inflammation. Jänig and Koltzenburg (1990, 1992) propose that this new type of sensory receptor is present in most viscera and contributes to the signalling of chronic visceral pain, to long-term alterations of spinal reflexes, and to abnormal autonomic regulation of internal organs. However, the experimental data on which these proposals are based are remarkable for their scarcity and deserve careful evaluation.

The published data on 'silent' visceral nociceptors is contained in a study of the afferent innervation of the cat's urinary bladder (Häbler *et al.* 1988, 1990). These authors studied the responses to mechanical and chemical stimuli of pelvic nerve afferents with sensory endings in the urinary bladder. An experimental cystitis was induced in the animals by the instillation into the bladder of mustard oil or turpentine. Häbler *et al.* (1988, 1990) described the existence of some non-mechanosensitive afferents that were excited by the application of mustard oil to the bladder mucosa. Following the induction of an inflammation with either mustard oil or turpentine, three afferent fibres were found that began to respond to mechanical stimulation of the bladder.

Häbler *et al.* state that these fibres were not responsive to bladder distensions in the normal state. However, examination of the units illustrated in the paper shows that they were indeed activated, albeit with low rates of firing, by distensions or contractions of the normal bladder over 40 mmHg. Also, these units were not challenged prior to inflammation with bladder distensions above 50 mmHg, a level that is very close to the threshold of the high-threshold afferents present in the bladder. Serious doubts must therefore be raised about the unresponsiveness to mechanical stimuli in the normal state of these three 'silent' nociceptors.

Whereas the data of Häbler *et al.* clearly demonstrate that bladder afferents can be sensitized by stimuli that produce local inflammation of the mucosa, it is arguable whether these three afferents really represent a new class of nociceptor present in all internal organs. An alternative explanation is that these afferents were connected to mechanosensitive endings with high thresholds to distension or contraction and that they became sensitized by the inflammatory process.

Functional considerations

Are there visceral nociceptors?

In view of the differences of opinion about the functional properties of visceral afferents it seems necessary to address, first of all, the question of the existence or otherwise of a category of visceral sensory receptor akin to the well identified nociceptors of the skin and other somatic structures. So, are there visceral nociceptors?

To a large extent the answer to this question depends on personal preferences, qualified by the conditions required for the identification of a sensory receptor as a nociceptor. If the nociceptor label can be attached to a well defined population of sensory receptors with a high threshold for activation and an encoding range contained entirely within noxious levels, then there is plenty of evidence in the literature for the existence of such a category of visceral afferent fibre. As reviewed above, there are separate groups of high-threshold sensory receptors in virtually all the internal organs examined so far, where they constitute a population of some 30 per cent of the total afferent innervation (with the exception of the ureter where the proportion is much higher). The thresholds of these sensory receptors fall into a relatively narrow range and do not overlap with those of the low-threshold afferents. Therefore, it is not unreasonable to attribute to these sensory receptors a function in the encoding of nociceptive events and, as such, they are visceral nociceptors.

There are, however, a number of problems. For instance, there is insufficient evidence regarding the potential sensitivities of these receptors to non-mechanical stimulation, particularly to the application of chemicals. It could be that their high mechanical thresholds are not matched with an equally selective sensitivity to noxious chemicals. This is particularly important in the viscera, where the chemistry of the receptor environment and the chemical changes that are constantly occurring in organs such as those of the gut and urinary system are quite considerable. It has been argued that the adequate stimulus for these receptors has not been fully identified and that they could be highly sensitive to so far untried forms of non-mechanical stimulation (Gebhart and Sengupta 1994; Sengupta and Gebhart 1994c). If this is the case, then these high-threshold mechanoreceptors could participate in regulatory activities of the organ and/ or in the signalling of non-noxious events, a role that would disqualify them from being, strictly speaking, nociceptors.

The heart of the problem is whether or not there is a conceptual requirement for a direct and selective relationship between the activation of putative nociceptors and the triggering of nociceptive reactions, including pain sensation. It is interesting to note that this argument is the same as that put forward 20 or 30 years ago for cutaneous nociceptors, and that this issue was only resolved with the use of microneurography in conscious human beings (see Torebjörk *et al.*, Chapter 14, and Ochoa *et al.*, Chapter 21, this volume). The difficulty of applying similar techniques to the innervation of internal organs may mean that we are still some way away from fulfilling the 'sensory' requirement of putative visceral nociceptors. However, in the absence of clear evidence to the contrary, it is reasonable to assume that high-threshold mechanoreceptors in the viscera are concerned with the signalling and encoding of mechanical noxious events in internal organs. The term visceral nociceptor looks like a convenient shorthand to refer, for the time being, to these sensory receptors, in the same way that it has been applied to high-threshold mechanoreceptors in muscles and in joints.

There is also the possibility that visceral afferents, both low- and high-threshold, could participate in pain states not immediately related to visceral dysfunction. Such an argument has been put forward recently by Schott (1994) in a thought-provoking paper where a possible link between activity in visceral afferent fibres and sympathetically maintained pain states is proposed and discussed.

What are the roles of 'silent' and of intensity-encoding afferents in viscera pain?

In addition to high-threshold mechanoreceptors, there are two other populations of sensory receptors in the viscera responding to noxious stimuli: 'silent' nociceptors and intensity-encoding receptors. It is very likely that their activity contributes or even determines certain forms of visceral sensation, including visceral pain, in addition to or even instead of, that of high-threshold receptors.

The main question about 'silent' nociceptors is whether or not these sensory receptors are qualitatively, and not just quantitatively, different from classical nociceptors. 'Silent' nociceptors could be simply very-high-threshold nociceptors whose sensitization by intense noxious stimuli brings their thresholds down and into the innocuous range. As such, the difference with classical nociceptors is only one of degree and not of substance. However, in so far as intense noxious stimuli lead to longer-lasting processes such as tissue injury and inflammation, it could also be argued that these receptors play a different functional role to classical nociceptors, particularly in acute and chronic inflammatory states or in situations of visceral hypersensitivity, such as irritable bowel syndrome.

In any case, the numerical relevance of 'silent' nociceptors has clearly been over-estimated. According to Gebhart and Sengupta (1994), 'silent' visceral afferents in the colon and bladder amount to not more than 40–45 per cent of the total afferent innervation instead of the 80–90 per cent quoted by other authors (Jänig and Koltzen-burg 1990, 1992). Also, the process of sensitization does not necessarily imply a nociceptive role, least of all in the viscera where heightened sensitivity to internal stimuli is required for the correct adaptation of many homeostatic processes. More experimental studies are needed in order to establish the precise function of this group of sensory receptors and their relevance in visceral pain states.

The population of intensity-encoding visceral afferents represents a unique group of sensory receptors without clear parallels in somatic locations. These are sensory receptors that encode a wide range of stimulus intensities, from innocuous to noxious. Their low thresholds indicate that they are active during the normal regulatory activity of the organs and their wide encoding range shows that they can also contribute a considerable amount of afferent activity during intense stimulation.

It is very interesting that these receptors have been found mainly in the gut and urinary bladder. These are organs from which sensations other than pain can be elicited, particularly during mild distension. There is a close parallel between the activity of intensity-encoding afferents in the oesophagus, the colon, and the bladder and the sensations of fullness that can be evoked from these organs, which, if unrelieved, can lead to intense pain sensations. These afferents could therefore be involved in regulatory activities of the organs (swallowing, micturition, defecation), in the signalling of the initial phases of distension during these activities and contribute, in addition to the high-threshold populations, to the pain sensations produced by intense or prolonged distensions.

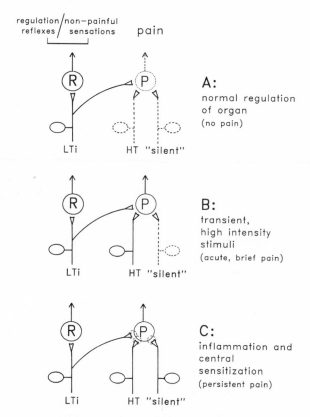

Fig. 9.7 Diagrammatic representation of speculative functional roles for the different types of visceral sensory receptor. Visceral afferents are shown to activate two central mechanisms, one responsible for regulatory reflexes and non-painful sensations (R) and the other for the triggering of pain (P). (A) During normal organ regulation low-threshold intensity-encoding afferents (LTi) are active but these low levels of activity are not sufficient to trigger the central pain mechanism. (B) Transient high-intensity stimuli will evoke greater responses in the LTi fibres as well as activate high-threshold afferents (HT). These two groups of fibres can now trigger acute, brief visceral pain. (C) During more prolonged forms of stimulation, including those leading to inflammation, 'silent' nociceptors are sensitized, and their afferent barrages, added to discharges in the HT afferents, can sensitize central neurones to their LT inputs. As a result, some normal regulatory activity in the viscera could now be perceived as painful. From Cervero and Jänig (1992) with permission.

Cervero and Jänig (1992) have discussed the contributions of the different populations of visceral sensory afferent to the triggering of visceral pain by reference to a series of simple and speculative models that suggest some possible mechanisms for the initial central processing of visceral nociceptive information (Fig. 9.7). Their starting point is the acceptance that the peripheral encoding of noxious events in viscera is mediated by several categories of visceral receptors that include high-threshold receptors, 'silent' nociceptors, and 'intensity-encoding' receptors. They suggest that different forms of visceral pain may be subserved by different mechanisms so that the roles of the various types of visceral receptor may be cumulative and diverse rather than exclusive and unique.

The suggestion is that at some point in the central nervous system (CNS), regulatory visceral reflexes and visceral pain are mediated by separate central mechanisms. This could already happen in the spinal cord, since experimental evidence indicates that some spinal neurones are only activated by noxious stimulation of viscera whereas others can be excited by innocuous intensities of stimulation. Neurones concerned with regulatory reflexes are driven by activity in low-threshold visceral receptors, including 'intensity-encoding' afferents (LTi). These fibres also project to neurones concerned with the processing of noxious stimuli but, at most physiological levels of stimulation, their action are subliminal.

In the diagram of Fig. 9.7 it is also proposed that brief, acute visceral pain, such as acute colic pain or the pain produced by an intense contraction of a hollow organ, could be triggered initially by the activation of high-threshold (HT) afferents and by the brief, high-frequency bursts that such stimuli evoke in LTi afferents. Increased activity in LTi afferents can now drive nociceptive pathways, added to the excitation mediated by HT fibres. In the colon, bladder or oesophagus, where the proportion of HT receptors is lower, this leads to a range of sensations as more and more activity is recruited from LTi afferents. In the biliary system or the ureter, where the nociceptive afferent innervation is exclusively mediated by HT receptors, pain appears as the only sensory experience.

More prolonged forms of visceral stimulation, including those leading to hypoxia and inflammation of the tissue, result in the sensitization of HT receptors and the bringing into play of the previously unresponsive 'silent' nociceptors. This in turn triggers central mechanisms that enhance and sustain the peripheral input and evoke persistent pain even if the afferent barrage decreases. Pain is now enhanced by a central mechanism brought into action by a peripheral barrage (Fig. 9.7). Prolonged activity in visceral high-threshold receptors and in 'silent' nociceptors evoked by persistent visceral injury induces profound changes in the central processing of these signals. As a result, activation of low-threshold visceral receptors, normally leading to regulatory activity of some internal organs or to non-painful sensations, evokes now pain of visceral origin and contributes to hyperalgesic states that includes both visceral tissues and their superficial and deep somatic reference zones.

References

Abrahams, V.V. and Teare, J.I. (1969). Peripheral pathways and properties of uterine afferents in the cat. *Can. J. Physiol. Pharmacol.* **47**, 576–7.

Bahns, E., Ernberger, U., Jänig, W., and Nelke, A. (1986). Functional characteristics of lumbar visceral afferent fibres from urinary bladder and the urethra in the cat. *Pflügers Arch.* **407**, 510–18.

Bahns, E., Halsband, U., and Jänig, W. (1987). Responses of sacral visceral afferents from the lower urinary tract, colon and anus to mechanical stimulation. *Pflügers Arch.* **410**, 296–303.

Baker, D.G., Coleridge, H.M., Coleridge, J.C.G., and Nerdrum, T. (1980). Search for a cardiac nociceptor: stimulation by bradykinin of sympathetic afferent nerve endings in the heart of the cat. *J. Physiol., London* **306**, 519–36.

Berkley, K.J., Robbins, A., and Sato, Y. (1987). Uterine afferent fibers in the rat. In *Fine afferent nerve fibers and pain* (ed. R.F. Schmidt, H.-G. Schaible, and C. Vahle-Hinz), pp. 129–36. VCH Verlagsgesellschaft mbH, Weinheim.

Berkley, K.J., Robbins, A., and Sato, Y. (1988). Afferent fibers supplying the uterus in the rat. *J. Neurophysiol.* **59**, 142–63.

Berkley, K.J., Hotta, H., Robbins, A., and Sato, Y. (1990). Functional properties of afferent fibers supplying reproductive and other pelvic organs in pelvic nerve of female rat. *J. Neurophysiol.* **63**, 256–72.

Berkley, K.J., Robbins, A., and Sato, Y. (1993). Functional differences between afferent fibers in the hypogastric and pelvic nerves innervating female reproductive organs in the rat. *J. Neurophysiol.* **69**, 533–44.

Blumberg, H., Haupt, P., Jänig, W., and Kohler, W. (1983). Encoding of visceral noxious stimuli in the discharge patterns of visceral afferent fibres from the colon. *Pflügers Arch.* **398**, 33–40.

Bonica, J.J. (1990). *The management of pain.* Lea & Febiger, Philadelphia.

Casati, R., Lombardi, F., and Malliani, A. (1979). Afferent sympathetic unmyelinated fibres with left ventricular endings in cats. *J. Physiol., London* **292**, 135–48.

Cervero, F. (1982). Afferent activity evoked by natural stimulation of the biliary system in the ferret. *Pain* **13**, 137–51.

Cervero, F. (1983). Mechanisms of visceral pain. In *Persistent pain*, Vol. 4 (ed. S. Lipton and J. Miles), pp. 1–19. Grune & Stratton, London.

Cervero, F. (1994). Sensory innervation of the viscera: peripheral basis of visceral pain. *Physiol. Rev.* **74**, 95–138.

Cervero, F. and Jänig, W. (1992). Visceral nociceptors: a new world order? *Trends Neurosci.* **15**, 374–8.

Cervero, F. and Sann, H. (1989). Mechanically evoked responses of afferent fibres innervating the guinea-pig's ureter: an *in vitro* study. *J. Physiol., London* **412**, 245–66.

Clifton, G.L., Coggeshall, R.E., Vance, W.H., and Willis, W.D., Jr (1976). Receptive fields of unmyelinated ventral root afferent fibres in the cat. *J. Physiol., London* **256**, 573–600.

Coggeshall, R.E. and Ito, H. (1977). Sensory fibres in ventral roots L7 and S1 in the cat. *J. Physiol., London* **267**, 215–35.

Coleridge, H.M. and Coleridge, J.C.G. (1980). Cardiovascular afferents involved in regulation of peripheral vessels. *Ann. Rev. Physiol.* **42**, 413–27.

Floyd, K. and Morrison, J.F.B. (1974). Splanchnic mechanoreceptors in the dog. *Quart. J. exp. Physiol.* **59**, 361–6.

Floyd, K., Hick, V.E., and Morrison, J.F.B. (1976). Mechanosensitive afferent units in the hypogastric nerve of the cat. *J. Physiol., London* **259**, 457–71.

Gebhart, G.F. and Sengupta, J.N. (1994). On visceral nociceptors. In *Peripheral neurons in nociception: physio-pharmacological aspects* (ed. J.M. Besson, G. Guilbaud, and H. Ollat), pp. 23–37. John Libbey Eurotext, Paris.

Gernandt, B. and Zotterman, Y. (1947). Intestinal pain: an electrophysiological investigation on mesenteric nerves. *Acta physiol. scand.* **12**, 56–72.

Häbler, H.-J., Jänig, W., and Koltzenburg, M. (1988). A novel type of unmyelinated chemo-sensitive nociceptor in the acutely inflamed urinary bladder. *Agents Actions* **25**, 219–21.

Häbler, H.-J., Jänig, W., and Koltzenburg, M. (1990). Activation of unmyelinated afferent fibres by mechanical stimuli and inflammation of the urinary bladder in the cat. *J. Physiol., London* **425**, 545–62.

Häbler, H.-J., Jänig, W., and Koltzenburg, M. (1993). Myelinated primary afferents of the sacral spinal cord responding to slow filling and distension of the urinary bladder. *J. Physiol., London* **463**, 449–60.

Hammer, K., Sann, H., and Pierau, F.-K. (1993). Functional properties of mechanosensitive units from the chicken ureter in vitro. *Pflügers Arch.* **425**, 353–61.

Haupt, P., Jänig, W., and Kohler, W. (1983). Response pattern of visceral afferent fibres supplying the colon upon chemical and mechanical stimuli. *Pflügers Arch.* **398**, 41–7.

Hong, S.K., Han, H.C., Yoon, Y.W., and Chung, J.M. (1993). Response properties of hypogastric afferent fibres supplying the uterus in the cat. *Brain Res.* **622**, 215–25.

Jänig, W. and and Koltzenburg, M. (1990). On the function of spinal primary afferent fibres supplying colon and urinary bladder. *J. auton. nerv. Syst.* **30** (Suppl.), S89–S96.

Jänig, W. and Koltzenburg, M. (1991). Receptive properties of sacral primary afferent neurons supplying the colon. *J. Neurophysiol.* **65**, 1067–77.

Jänig, W. and Koltzenburg, M. (1992). Pain arising from the urogenital tract. In *The autonomic nervous system.* Vol. 2: *Nervous control of the urogenital system* (ed. C.A. Maggi), pp. 523–76. Harwood Academic Publishers, Chur, Switzerland.

Kumazawa, T. (1986). Sensory innervation of reproductive organs. In *Visceral sensation*, Progress in Brain Research, Vol. 67 (ed. F. Cervero and J.F.B. Morrison). Elsevier, Amsterdam.

Kumazawa, T. and Mizumura, K. (1984). Functional properties of the polymodal receptors in the deep tissues. In *Sensory receptor mechanisms* (ed. W. Hamann and A. Iggo), pp. 1193–202.

Lew, W.Y.W. and Longhurst, J.C. (1986). Substance P, 5-hydroxytriptamine and bradykinin stimulate abdominal visceral afferents. *Am. J. Physiol., Regul. integr. comp. Physiol.* **250**, R465–R473.

Lombardi, R., Della Bella, P., Casati, R., and Malliani, A. (1981). Effects of intracoronary administration of bradykinin on the impulse activity of afferent sympathetic unmyelinated fibers with left ventricular endings in the cat. *Circ. Res.* **48**, 69–75.

Longhurst, J.C. and Dittman, L.E. (1987). Hypoxia, bradykinin and prostaglandins stimulate ischemically sensitive visceral afferents. *Am. J. Physiol., Heart Circ. Physiol.* **253**, H556–H567.

Longhurst, J.C., Kaufman, M.P., Ordway, G.A., and Musch, T.I. (1984). Effects of bradykinin and capsaicin on endings of afferent fibers from abdominal visceral organs. *Am. J. Physiol., Regul. integr. comp. Physiol.* **247**, R552–R559.

Longhurst, J.C., Rotto, D.M., Kaufman, M.P., and Stahl, G.L. (1991). Ischemically sensitive abdominal visceral afferents: response to cyclooxygenase blockade. *Am. J. Physiol., Heart circ. Physiol* **261**, H2075–H2081.

MacKenzie, J. (1909). *Symptoms and their interpretation.* Shaw and Sons, London.

McMahon, S.B. and Koltzenburg, M. (1990*a*). Novel classes of nociceptors: beyond Sherrington. *Trends Neurosci.* **13**, 199–201.

McMahon, S.B. and Koltzenburg, M. (1990*b*). The changing role of primary afferent neurones in pain. *Pain* **43**, 269–72.

Malliani, A. (1982). Cardiovascular sympathetic afferent fibers. *Rev. Physiol. Biochem. Pharmacol.* **94**, 11–74.

Malliani, A. and Lombardi, F. (1982). Consideration of the fundamental mechanisms eliciting cardiac pain. *Am. Heart J.* **103**, 575–578.

Malliani A. (1986). The elusive link between transient myocardial ischaemia and pain. *Circulation* **73**, 201–4.

Malliani, A., Lombardi, F., and Pagani, M. (1986). Sensory innervation of the heart. In *Visceral sensation, Progress in Brain Research*, Vol. 67 (ed. F. Cervero and J.F.B. Morrison), pp. 39–48. Elsevier, Amsterdam.

Michaelis, M., Göder, Häbler, H.-J., and Jänig, W. (1944). Proerties of afferent nerve fibres supplying the saphenous vein in the cat. *J. Physiol., London* **474**, 233–43.

Paintal, A.S. (1977*a*). Thoracic receptors connected with sensation. *Br. med. Bull.* **33**, 169–74.

Paintal, A.S. (1977*b*). Effects of drugs on chemoreceptors, pulmonary and cardiovascular receptors, *Pharmacol. Ther.* **3**, 41–63.

Paintal, A.S. (1986). The visceral sensations: some basic mechanisms. In: *Visceral sensation. Progress in brain research.* (ed. F. Cervero and J.F.B. Morrison). Vol. 67, pp. 3–19. Amsterdam, Elsevier.

Robbins, A., Sato, Y., Hotta, H., and Berkley, K.J. (1990). Responses of hypogastric nerve afferent fibers to uterine distension in estrous or metestrous rats. *Neurosci. Lett.* **110**, 82–5.

240   *Visceral nociceptors*

Sann, H. and Cervero, F. (1988). Afferent innervation of the guinea-pig's ureter. *Agents Actions*
    25, 243–5.
Sant'Ambrogio, G. (1982). Information arising from the tracheobronchial tree of mammals.
    Physiol. Rev. **62**, 531–69.
Sant'Ambrogio, G. (1987). Nervous receptors of the tracheobronchial tree. *Ann. Rev. Physiol.* **49**,
    611–27.
Schott, G.D. (1994). Visceral afferents: their contribution to 'sympathetic dependent' pain. *Brain*
    117, 397–413.
Semenenko, F.M. and Cervero, F. (1992). Afferent fibres from the guinea-pig ureter: size and
    peptide content of the dorsal root ganglion cells of origin. *Neuroscience* **47**, 1197–2011.
Sengupta, J.N. and Gebhart, G.F. (1994*a*). Characterization of mechanosensitive pelvic nerve
    afferent fibers innervating the colon of the rat. *J. Neurophysiol.* **71**, 2046–60.
Sengupta, J.N. and Gebhart, G.F. (1994*b*). Mechanosensitive properties of pelvic nerve afferent
    fibers innervating the urinary bladder of the rat. *J. Neurophysiol.* **72**, 2420–30.
Sengupta, J.N. and Gebhart, G.F. (1994*c*). Gastrointestinal afferent fibers and sensation. In
    Physiology of the gastrointestinal tract, Vol. 3 (ed. L.R. Johnson), pp. 483–519. Raven Press,
    New York.
Sengupta, J.N., Saha, J.K., and Goyal, R.K. (1992). Differential sensitivity to bradykinin of
    esophageal distension-sensitive mechanoreceptors in vagal and sympathetic afferents of the
    opossum. *J. Neurophysiol.* **68**, 1053–67.
Sengupta, J.N., Saha, J.K., and Goyal, R.K. (1990). Stimulus–Response function studies of
    esophageal mechanosensitive nociceptors in sympathetic afferents of opossum. *J. Neurophysiol.*
    64, 796–812.
Sherrington, C.S. (1906). *The integrative action of the nervous system.* Scribner, New York.
Stahl, G.L. and Longhurst, J.C. (1992). Ischemically sensitive visceral afferents. Importance of H^+
    derived from lactic acid and hypercapnia. *Am. J. Physiol., Heart circ. Physiol.* **262**, H748–H753.
Uchida, Y. and Murao, S. (1974*a*). Bradykinin-induced excitation of afferent cardiac sympathetic
    nerve fibers, *Jap. Heart J.* **15**, 84–91.
Uchida, Y. and Murao, S. (1974*b*). Potassium-induced excitation of afferent cardiac sympathetic
    nerve fibers, *Am. J. Physiol.* **226**, 603–7.
Uchida, Y. and Murao, S. (1974*c*). Excitation of afferent cardiac sympathetic nerve fibers during
    coronary occlusion. *Am. J. Physiol.* **226**, 1094–9.
Uchida, Y. and Murao, S. (1975). Acid-induced excitation of afferent cardiac sympathetic nerve
    fibers. *Am. J. Physiol.* **228**, 27–33.
Widdicombe, J.G. (1974). Enteroceptors. In *The peripheral nervous system* (ed. J.I. Hubbard), pp.
    455–85. Plenum Press, New York.
Widdicombe, J.G. (1986). Sensory innervation of the lungs and airways. In *Visceral sensation*,
    Progress in Brain Research, Vol. 67 (ed. F. Cervero and J.F.B. Morrison), pp. 49–64. Elsevier,
    Amsterdam.

PART 3
Transduction mechanisms and sensitization

10 Signal transduction in nociceptors: general principles

CARLOS BELMONTE

Basic principles in sensory transduction

Sensory transduction is the mechanism by which external physical changes are transformed into internal biochemical and/or electrical signals. Such electrical signals are propagated and processed through different levels of the central nervous system to elicit a sensation. Sensory transduction takes place in specialized portions of sensory receptor cells (sensory receptors), which differ from each other in their ability to respond preferentially to a particular form of energy. In turn, sensory receptors of the same class are connected to the brain through specific sensory pathways, whose selective excitation leads to a given modality of sensation. However, the relationship between activation of peripheral nociceptors and conscious sensations is complex. Modulation and plasticity occurring at every level of the transmission pathway are responsible for the final characteristics of the evoked conscious sensation.

In strict terms, receptor cells found in living organisms detect the manifestations of just two of the four fundamental forces of the universe: the gravitational force and the electromagnetic force (Block 1992). However, different classes of sensory receptor cells can be differentiated because each of them respond preferentially to a limited portion of the infinite range of one of these forms of energy. Therefore, the type of energy to which sensory cells are specifically tuned has been used as a criterion for their classification: chemoreceptors are excited by molecules of various types; temperature changes excite thermoreceptors; photons are selectively detected by photoreceptors while mechanoreceptors respond to mechanical energy (Table 10.1). Receptor cells belonging to one of these general classes may elicit more than one modality of sensation. This is the case, for instance, of chemoreceptor cells, which evoke sensations such as smell or taste, depending on their location, individual properties, selectivity for certain molecules, and sensory circuits and pathways which connect them to the brain.

Nociceptors cannot be classified as a separate entity among sensory receptor cells on the basis of their transducing specificity for a particular type of energy. The parameter used to distinguish this population within the general group of sensory receptors is the intensity of the stimulating energy rather than its form. Nociceptors may be sensitive to chemical, thermal, and/or mechanical stimuli, provided that these reach an intensity level that causes (or threatens to cause) detectable cellular injury in their surroundings. Moreover, subclasses of nociceptors are often distinguished, on the basis of properties other than biophysical transducing characteristics (conduction velocity, target tissue).

Nevertheless, there is increasing evidence that the cellular and molecular processes involved in sensory transduction by the various types of receptor cells have common basic principles (Shepherd 1994). These principles are apparently applicable also to nociceptors, in spite of their limited specificity for the type of stimulating energy.

Table 10.1 Main forms of energy that are detected by sensory receptors in mammals. Modified from Mountcastle (1980)

Examples of receptor types and function served in response to various incident stimuli

---

Mechanical force

Mechanoreceptors serving:

(1) touch-pressure in skin and subcutaneous tissues (both organized and free nerve endings)

(2) position sense and kinaesthesia (mechanoreceptors of joints and vestibular receptors of inner ear)

(3) hearing (mechanoreceptors of cochlea)

(4) stretch receptors of muscle and tendon

(5) visceral pressure receptors (carotid and right atrium)

Light

Photoreceptors of eye, serving vision

Heat

Thermoreceptors, separately for:

(1) warmth

(2) cold

Substances in solution

Chemoreceptors, separately for:

(1) taste

(2) smell

Osmoreceptors

Carotid body receptors

Extremes of mechanical force; heat or its absence; presence of certain chemicals

Nociceptors, serving pain

Transduction steps

The similarity of membrane mechanisms for each class of sensory receptor, despite their apparent diversity among living organisms, allows the representation of the peripheral operation of sensory systems as a unified scheme, such as the one outlined in Fig. 10.1 (Block 1992).

The primary transducer or detector (upper box) is the place where *detection* of the stimulus takes place and corresponds to a molecular entity located in the cell membrane that is modified by the stimulus (mechanoelectrical transduction channels, photoreceptor or odorant receptor molecules, etc.). The detector is usually linked to *perireceptor structures* that may act to convey the stimulus to the detector or to modify some of its characteristics; examples include light-transmitting structures in the eye, accessory cells in encapsulated cutaneous receptors, mucus or odorant binding proteins in olfactory cells. At the detector, the energy of the stimulus is transduced to another form of

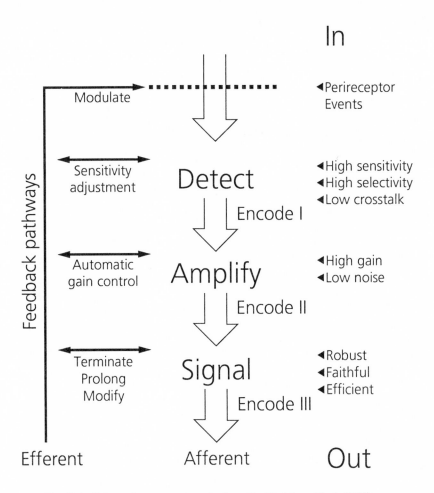

Fig. 10.1 Scheme for sensory transduction. Modified from Block (1992).

energy, either chemical or electrical, and the information becomes encoded (Encode I). This signal, usually very weak, is amplified in a next *amplification* step at which filtering can be added again (Encode II). Finally, the amplified signal is transmitted to its destination by a *signalling* stage, at which further filtering may occur (Encode III). There are feedback pathways that allow the modulation of the response characteristics of each of the stages of the sensory transduction process. The response can be moulded by changing the input signal itself, the sensitivity of the detector, the gain or bandpass characteristic of the amplifier, or the encoding process.

Although this general scheme for the operation of all categories of receptors is generally accepted (Shepherd 1991, 1994), our present knowledge of the information-processing steps and basic operations for each type of sensory receptor is uneven. Cellular and molecular mechanisms of transduction in photoreceptors or in olfactory and cochlea receptor cells are relatively well identified in comparison with those in nociceptors, where most details of the transduction steps are still unknown. This is

Table 10.2 Transduction steps in visual, olfactory, gustatory, and mechanoreceptive cells as proposed by Shepherd (1991, 1994). On the right side of the table, possible steps for nociceptive cells have been added in parallel.

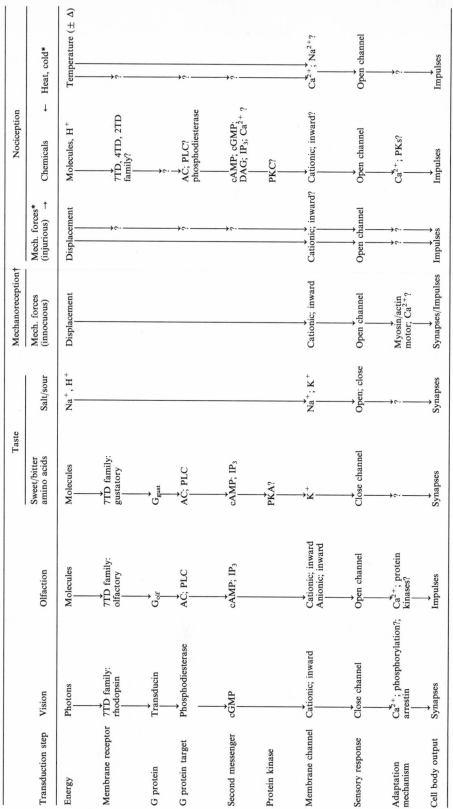

Transduction step	Vision	Olfaction	Taste: Sweet/bitter amino acids	Taste: Salt/sour	Mechanoreception† Mech. forces (innocuous) Displacement	Nociception Mech. forces* (injurious) → Displacement	Nociception Chemicals ↓	Nociception Heat, cold* ← Temperature (± Δ)
Energy	Photons	Molecules	Molecules	Na^+, H^+	Displacement	Displacement	Molecules, H^+	Temperature (± Δ)
Membrane receptor	7TD family: rhodopsin	7TD family: olfactory	7TD family: gustatory			? ?	7TD, 4TD, 2TD family?	?
G protein	Transducin	G_{olf}	G_{gust}				?	
G protein target	Phosphodiesterase	AC; PLC	AC; PLC			? ?	AC; PLC? phosphodiesterase	?
Second messenger	cGMP	cAMP; IP_3	cAMP; IP_3			? ?	cAMP; cGMP; DAG; IP_3; Ca^{2+}; ?	?
Protein kinase			PKA?				PKC?	
Membrane channel	Cationic; inward	Cationic; inward / Anionic; inward	K^+	Na^+; K^+	Cationic; inward	Cationic; inward? / Cationic; inward?	Cationic; inward?	Ca^{2+}; Na^{2+}?
Sensory response	Close channel	Open channel	Close channel	Open; close	Open channel	Open channel / Open channel	Open channel	Open channel
Adaptation mechanism	Ca^{2+}; phosphorylation?; arrestin	Ca^{2+}; protein kinases?	?	?	Myosin/actin motor; Ca^{2+}?	? ? / ? ?	Ca^{2+}; PKs?	?
Cell body output	Synapses	Impulses	Synapses	Synapses	Synapses/Impulses	Impulses	Impulses	Impulses

cAMP, Cyclic adenosine monophosphate; cGMP, cyclic guanosine monophosphate; IP_3, inositol 1,4,5-trisphosphate; PLC, phospholipase C; AC, Adenylate cyclase; DAG, diacylglycerol.
† Mechanosensory fibres and hair cells. TD, transducing domains; PK, protein kinase; * noxious mechanical and thermal stimuli may act through the release of endogenous chemical agents by injured cells.

illustrated in Table 10.2, in which information on nociceptors has been presented in parallel with the data available for other types of sensory receptors (Shepherd 1994).

Perireceptor events

The influence of perireceptor events in the transmission and modulation of the stimulus to nociceptive endings is largely ignored. Nociceptors are naked nerve terminals embedded in an intercellular matrix that contains collagen fibrils and proteoglycans (see Kruger and Halata, Chapter 2, this volume). They are devoid of specialized structures that would act as filters for the transmission of mechanical forces to the receptive sites, as occurs with many types of low-threshold mechanoreceptors (Zelená 1994). Receptor sites in nociceptive terminals appear to be discontinuous patches of bare axolemma, which are separated from the adjacent tissue only by the basal lamina of the nerve fibre. (Heppelmann *et al.* 1990). Thus, the receptive plasma membrane appears to be particularly exposed to the direct action of stimuli. However, the role played by collagenous fibrils and viscous intercellular matrix surrounding nociceptive nerve endings in the modulation of chemical, mechanical, and thermal noxious stimuli is still undefined.

In joints, hyaluronic acid, a glycosaminoglycan that fills the intercellular space within the collagen fibrillar network surrounding the cells, vessels, and neural elements of the solid tissues of the joint, has been proposed to act as a elastoviscous buffer, reducing the transmission of mechanical stretch to the transducing membrane of nerve endings (Balazs 1982). In favour of this possibility is the observation that spontaneous and movement-evoked impulse activity of joint nociceptors decreases in normal and inflamed joints after intraarticular injection of an elastoviscous solution of sodium hyaluronan (Pozo *et al.* 1996). The same inhibition was obtained with this substance in osteoarthritic pain in humans (Balazs and Denlinger 1984). In contrast, injection of non-elastoviscous solutions of low-molecular-mass hyaluronan did not cause a decrease of joint nociceptor activity in the cat or of joint pain in humans (Pozo *et al.* 1996). Whether this filtering mechanism is present also in nociceptive endings of other tissues and contributes to determining the high mechanical threshold of nociceptors remain to be established.

In addition to a buffering effect on mechanical forces, glycosaminoglycans and proteoglycans that are bound to the plasma membrane of nerve terminals and extend into the extracellular space may modify the surface charge and limit by electrostatic binding the diffusion of molecules to the nerve ending. Moreover, because of their ability to bind significant amounts of Ca^{2+} (Comper and Laurent 1978), glycosaminoglycans may also act as an ionic buffer for this ion (Fukami 1986).

Thus, the nature and influence of accessory factors in nociceptor transduction are still undefined. However, the possibility that they play a significant role in conditioning the stimulating signal reaching the primary transducer, as occurs in other receptor structures (Fukami 1986; Carr *et al.* 1990; Kinnamon and Getchell 1991), deserves experimental consideration.

Detection and amplification of the stimulus

Nociceptors may respond to one or to various forms of energy and this property has determined the distinction between mechanonociceptors, mechanoheat nociceptors, polymodal nociceptors, cold nociceptors, or mechano-insensitive nociceptors (see Campbell and Meyer, Chapter 5, this volume). This diversity suggests that the various types of nociceptive neurones are equipped with different transduction mechanisms for each of the forms of stimulating energy to which they are sensitive. The extreme example is that of polymodal nociceptors, which respond to strong mechanical forces, to a large variety of exogenous and endogenous chemicals, and to heat or cold (Fig. 10.2). In spite of the apparent diversity of their adequate stimulus, nociceptors seem to possess detection mechanisms based on 'an adaptation of a superfamily of membrane signalling mechanisms which converts the stimulus energy into an allosteric molecular change, leading to the gating of ionic current in a membrane channel' (Shepherd 1994), as do other modalities of sensory receptors responding to stimuli of different nature.

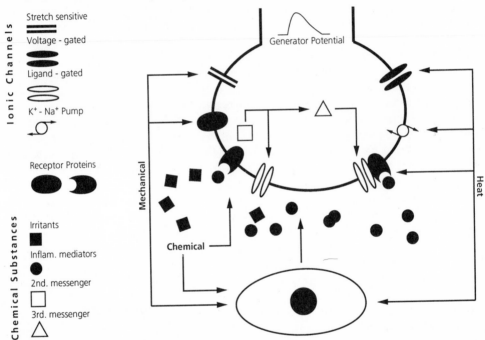

Fig. 10.2   Diagram of a polymodal nociceptive ending. The hypothetical mechanisms for the action of the various forms of incident energy have been represented schematically. Mechanical forces may act directly on mechanosensitive channels and/or membrane proteins or indirectly, through endogenous mediators released by cells damaged by the stimulus. Release of endogenous agents by injured cells would also be caused by irritant chemicals, which can additionally interact with the membrane of the nerve ending, and by noxious heat. Temperature changes may also affect directly ionic channel conductances or the sodium–potassium pump. Ionic currents generated by these mechanisms will cause a generator potential at the non-regenerative portion of the nociceptive terminal, leading finally to a firing of nerve impulses.

Biophysical and biochemical methods used in other types of receptor cells to gather information on their transduction characteristics are not applicable to nociceptive terminals, because of the technical difficulties imposed by their very small size. Therefore, the available information on transduction processes in nociceptors has been obtained indirectly by recording electrical activity from the soma of primary sensory neurones presumed to be nociceptive, or nerve impulses from sensory afferents, in preparations where the extracellular milieu of nociceptive terminals can be controlled experimentally (see Belmonte *et al.* 1994).

Mechanical forces

Nociceptors respond to mechanical stimulation with a discharge of nerve impulses. Some nociceptive neurones are exclusively sensitive to this type of stimulus; other are additionally activated by chemical or thermal stimuli, and/or change their mechanically evoked response when these other stimuli are also applied (Perl 1992).

Mechanical distortion produces a change in the ion permeability in patch-clamped membranes. This appears to be due to the opening by stretch of mechanically sensitive channels (MSCs) (Guharay and Sachs 1984; Sachs 1986). MSCs are a heterogeneous population of channels with differences in sensitivity (from random thermal fluctuations to tissue-damaging forces), in the type of response (stretch-activated or stretch-inactivated), and in biophysical properties (ion selectivity, conductance). MSCs are present in a great number of cells and, in addition to stimulus detection, they participate in a variety of other cell functions, such as volume regulation or contraction (Morris 1992). The mechanisms that confer mechanosensitivity to a channel have been categorized in two main groups: direct mechanisms, involving tension exerted directly on the channel proteins; and indirect mechanisms, involving second messengers controlled by mechanosensitive enzymes (Hudspeth and Gillespie 1994).

Mechanosensitive ionic channels have been envisaged as a deformable cylinder embedded in the membrane and stretched by membrane tension. The external force field opens the channel by increasing the tension, including the contribution of the elastic energy stored in the channel (Sachs 1992). In some structures, such as the hair cells, the machinery of transduction lies on top of the hair bundle, near the stereociliary tips (Hudspeth 1982), where a few transduction channels are located. The molecular gate of these channels is attached to an elastic element, the gating spring, the tension in which favours channel opening (Howard *et al.* 1988; Hudspeth and Gillespie 1994). In other cells, it has been suggested that MSCs are linked to the cytoskeleton, being in series with some of its component(s) (Guharay and Sachs 1984; Sokabe *et al.* 1991).

Extracellular matrix attachments may also be sites at which forces are transmitted to the cell. It has been proposed that transmembrane integrins act as a molecular path to transmit the mechanical signal to the cytoskeleton, because they bind actin-associated proteins and therefore link physically the extracellular matrix with the microfilaments. The alteration of the cytoskeleton organization by mechanical forces will induce biochemical changes in the cell (Wang *et al.* 1993). Other structures in a cell are directly sensitive to stress and may additionally act as transducers; these include voltage-activated channels or cellular enzymes such as adenylate cyclase or protein kinase C (Sachs 1992). However, the sensitivity and slow time course of the responses evoked by these structures make their direct responsibility in sensory mechanotransduction doubtful.

In nociceptors, the presence of a selective channel for mechanotransduction has not been proved directly. Capsaicin blocks the response of single Aδ nociceptive fibres of the cornea to acid and heat but not to mechanical stimulation (Belmonte *et al.* 1991). Furthermore, diltiazem, a calcium channel antagonist that at high doses blocks the cyclic nucleotide-gated channels of photoreceptors, reduced the responsiveness of corneal polymodal nociceptors to chemicals, without apparently affecting their mechanosensitivity (Pozo *et al.* 1992, but see Kress and Reeh, Chapter 11, this volume). This suggests that mechanotransduction and chemotransduction in nociceptors may take place through different mechanisms, but does not prove the existence of MSCs in nociceptive terminals. White and Levine (1991) reported that gentamycin suppresses the initial, high-frequency discharge evoked by sustained mechanical stimulation of C mechanoheat nociceptors of the skin, but not the tonic component of the response. The latency of this tonic discharge was attenuated by potassium channel blockers and by agents that interfere with protein kinase activity. The interpretation was that different transduction mechanisms are involved in the early and late mechanically evoked impulse responses of nociceptors; however, the data from these experiments are too indirect to conclude that they reflect a separate blockade of two types of MSCs. Similarly, in the cornea, topical application of gentamycin, gadolinium (Gd^{3+}), and amiloride, blockers of MSCs in other types of mechanoreceptors, do not suppress selectively the response of polymodal nociceptors to mechanical stimulation and, at high doses, affect equally the response to mechanical and to acidic stimulation (Chen and Belmonte, unpublished observations).

Thus, it is unknown what mechanism(s) mediate transduction of mechanical forces in nociceptors, to what degree MSCs are involved, and how they are gated by stress. Activation of mechanotransduction causes depolarization, presumably mediated through the entrance of sodium because the permeability of MSCs to calcium is not very high (Yang and Sachs 1990). Differences in density of MSCs in the transducing areas between low-threshold mechanoreceptors and nociceptors may explain in a simple way their different mechanical threshold. However, other factors such as cytoskeleton organization (Heppelmann *et al.* 1990) and/or second messenger pathways may be the cause of the various threshold and adaptation characteristics of these populations of mechanoreceptive terminals.

Chemical stimuli

A great variety of molecules may act on nociceptive terminals, leading to a change in membrane potential and eventually to a discharge of nerve impulses. Substances acting as chemical stimuli for nociceptors may have an external origin or be produced endogenously.

Exogenous compounds are in many cases chemicals that injure directly epithelial tissue and nerve endings. There is a wide variety of chemicals that can stimulate nociceptors. Sensory irritants have been classified into three main groups: chemicals that react with nucleophilic groups (HO, HN, SH groups); agents that break disulfide bonds; and others forming a third, heterogeneous group that does not fit into these two classes and includes compounds such as ethanol (Alarie 1973; Silver 1990).

Endogenous compounds include ions, arachidonic acid metabolites, kinins, amines, cytokines, acetylcholine, amino acids, nitric oxide (NO), neuropeptides, opioids, adenosine triphosphate (ATP), and adenosine (Handwerker and Reeh 1991; Rang *et al.* 1991). These substances are released as a part of the injury/inflammatory response caused by noxious stimuli and will act on nociceptive terminals, triggering the transduction process (see Kress and Reeh, Chapter 11, Bevan, Chapter 12, and Kumazawa, Chapter 13, this volume).

Considering the widely divergent physicochemical properties of exogenous irritants, it is doubtful that they act through a specific receptor molecule placed in the membrane of nociceptive nerve endings. The existence of such a receptor protein in the lipid bilayer of nociceptive terminals was proposed by Nielson and colleagues (Nielson *et al.* 1984; Nielson and Babko 1985), who suggested that the receptor protein possesses a site for each one of the chemical irritant groups (neutrophilic and disulfide linkage groups) as well as a site with hydrogen donor ability, for physical absorption. It is more likely that many of the compounds stimulating nociceptive nerve endings dissolve in the membrane, depending on their liposolubility, and alter membrane and cellular properties, including surface charge, ionic channels, and the metabolic state of the cell (Price 1984). The net result of these actions is a depolarization of the nerve terminals and a discharge of nerve impulses, whose firing frequency is proportional within certain limits to the concentration of the irritant substance (Silver 1990). However, some exogenous compounds interact with a specific membrane receptor. This is the case for capsaicin, a substance that acts selectively on nociceptive neurones, apparently on the same channel as protons (Bevan and Geppetti 1994), thus resembling endogenous mediators.

The membrane mechanisms used by the endogenous compounds to acutely activate nociceptive terminals are presumably similar to those described in chemoreceptor cells of other sensory systems (Shepherd 1994). There, stimulating molecules initiate their effects by binding to a specific receptor molecule on the membrane surface of the nerve ending.

The receptor protein may be an ion channel itself, whose gating depends on the binding of the stimulating molecule, so that permeant ions flow through the channel when this is open. These ligand-gated channels, which usually contain four membrane-spanning domains, are suspected to mediate at least the effects of serotonin (5-HT), protons, and capsaicin on nociceptive neurones (see Bevan, Chapter 12, this volume).

Many other endogenous noxious agents do not couple directly to the ion channel whose activity they regulate, but bind to a receptor with seven membrane-spanning domains, which is coupled to a protein of the guanyl-nucleotide-binding (G) protein family. Receptors of this type are differentiated to respond to a range of different neurotransmitters and neuropeptides and have also been identified in primary sensory neurones for bradykinin, prostaglandins, 5-HT, adenosine, or histamine. Their general operating mechanism is the well known G-protein-coupled receptor system (see Levitan and Kaczmarek 1991). Occupation of the receptor by an agonist molecule causes it to associate with the membrane-bound G protein, a trimeric complex of α, β and γ subunits. This interaction allows GTP to displace GDP from the guanyl nucleotide-binding site in the G protein, causing a dissociation of the α subunit from the $\beta\gamma$ complex. In most cases, it appears that the free α subunit interacts with the effector in the next stage of the transduction pathway, though, in some instances, the $\beta\gamma$ complex is believed to play this role. The effector can be an ion channel located in the plane of the membrane or an enzyme, whose activity catalyses the formation of a second messenger. This in turn triggers a sequence of events that ultimately modulates an ion channel. Several second messenger systems have been identified, some of them with important roles in the modulation of neuronal excitability. These include: (1) the adenylate cyclase/cyclic AMP-dependent protein kinase system; (2) the guanylate cyclase/cyclic GPM protein kinase system; (3) the phospholipase-mediated production of inositol trisphosphate (IP_3), diacylglycerol (DAG), and arachidonic acid; and (4) the calcium-activated systems. All of these have been implicated in sensory transduction (Shepherd 1994).

In this general scheme, it becomes evident that amplification of the signal can be obtained at each step of the process, so that a reduced number of stimulating molecules may activate finally a large number of ion channels of different type. Furthermore, the duration and characteristics of the effect are also susceptible to modulation, so that long-lasting effects on other cellular processes can be triggered by the second messenger-coupled receptor system.

Information about the participation of second and third messengers formed by these systems in the activation and sensitization of nociceptors is fragmentary. Dorsal root ganglion cells have been often used as a model to analyse the contribution of the various messenger systems to nociceptor transduction. In this volume (Chapter 12) Bevan analyses in detail the available information on signalling pathways for the principal endogenous mediators involved in the excitation and sensitization of nociceptors. Nevertheless, there is no direct proof that mechanisms identified in the soma of primary sensory neurones are also present at their peripheral terminals where transduction takes place. In fact, there is experimental evidence suggesting that this may not be the case (Kirchoff *et al.* 1992). Electrophysiological recording experiments in nociceptive fibres of several tissues as well as behavioural experiments have also been performed, using drugs that interfere at various levels of the second messenger systems to elucidate their participation in the activation and sensitization of peripheral nociceptors by endogenous agents (Taiwo and Levine 1991). Chapters 11 by Kress and Reeh and 13 by Kumazawa offer an extensive review of our present knowledge in this field.

The final targets of intracellular messengers are ion channels, whose gating and modulation will change the conductance of the membrane. Different types of ion channels (voltage-sensitive, ligand-sensitive, and mechanically sensitive) are present in primary sensory neurones (Hille 1992; Koerber and Mendell 1992; Nowycky 1992); they can be phosphorylated by protein kinases activated by second messengers, many of them at multiple sites and by diverse types of protein kinases. This will determine differences in the probability of opening, open time, or voltage dependence and, as a consequence, will serve as a means of modulating the amplitude and time course of the membrane potential changes elicited by the stimulus and the ensuing discharge of impulses. Again, ion channels specifically involved in the response of nociceptors to chemicals have not yet been identified (see below).

Temperature changes

A proportion of the population of mechanosensitive nociceptors are also excited by temperatures approaching noxious levels (over 40–42°C in the skin). Transduction mechanisms in cutaneous thermal receptors have been poorly studied. Several hypotheses have been advanced to explain the specific temperature sensitivity of neurones (Spray 1974). The classical view is that a temperature-dependent electrogenic pump, the sodium–potassium pump, is affected by temperature changes, so that temperature decrease causes a reduction in the pump activity and, consequently, a depolarization (Bade *et al.* 1978; Braun *et al.* 1980; Carpenter 1981), resulting partly from a decrease in the hyperpolarizing current generated by the pump and partly from a depolarizing shift in potassium equilibrium potential, E_K, as a result of changes in the ionic gradient of

Na$^+$ and K$^+$ ions. However, cold receptors have a cyclic pattern of impulse activity with increasing frequency and amplitude at higher temperatures, suggestive of an underlying oscillating generator potential that seems to be strongly controlled by calcium (Schäfer *et al.* 1982, 1988). This ion does not contribute greatly to the receptor potential as current carrier. However, inflow of calcium produces a hyperpolarization and a concomitant reduction of the discharge rate, possibly through the stimulation of a calcium-stimulated outward conductance, and vice versa for reduced calcium entry. Calcium movements would be temperature-dependent and not associated to depolarization caused by action potentials. They are blocked by menthol but not by verapamil or 1,4-dihydropyridine type channel modulators, which suggests that they occur mainly through low-voltage-activated calcium channels (Schäfer *et al.* 1982, 1988; Schäfer 1987).

Unlike thermal receptors, polymodal nociceptors do not have an static discharge closely tuned by temperature values. They respond to temperature variations only when values causing injury are approached; heating is often more effective than cold (Kumazawa and Mizumura 1980; Belmonte and Giraldez 1981). Temperature elevations possibly influence ionic pumps and conductances in nociceptive terminals (Kumazawa *et al.* 1988; Nobile *et al.* 1990). However, there is no proof that their thermosensitivity is based on the same mechanisms as those of low-threshold warm and cold receptors. Changes in the responsiveness of polymodal nociceptive terminals to heat often go in parallel with a modified chemosensitivity (Kumazawa *et al.* 1987, 1988). Thermo- and chemosensitivity are simultaneously affected by drugs like capsaicin and present cross-sensitization (Kumazawa *et al.* 1988; Mizumura *et al.* 1988; Szolcsanyi *et al.* 1988; Lang *et al.* 1990; Belmonte *et al.* 1991). Moreover, in the monkey skin, some polymodal units respond to heat with a short latency but others respond only after several seconds, thus suggesting that they were secondarily activated by local release of chemical agents (Treede *et al.* 1995). Thus, the possibility exists that a part and perhaps in some cases all of the firing response to heat was due to the release by damaged cells of algesic substances, which will contribute to or cause the excitation of polymodal nociceptive terminals.

Signalling mechanisms in nociceptors

Generator potentials associated to the activation of nociceptive terminals have never been recorded due to technical limitations. Nevertheless, they are expected to occur at the non-regenerative portion of the nerve ending, consecutively to the activation of the transducing process. As mentioned above, it is unknown which ions may carry generator currents and what type of channel(s) are involved for each modality of stimulus. They could be non-selective cationic channels, in analogy with other sensory cells (see Hille 1992), but this possibility is still speculative. Increases or decreases of extracellular potassium concentration in testicular polymodal nociceptors augmented or reduced, respectively, the response to chemicals (bradykinin and hypertonic NaCl). These are the expected changes in excitability consequent on passive depolarization or hyperpolarization of the membrane of the nerve ending caused by potassium. Ouabain or long-term perfusion with zero potassium (which suppress the electrogenic Na$^+$–K$^+$ pump) increased spontaneous firing and responsiveness to chemical stimuli (Kumazawa *et al.* 1988). In the *in vitro* skin-nerve preparation of the rat, addition of the potassium channel blockers 4-aminopyridine (4-AP) and tetraethylammonium (TEA) did not modify the responsiveness to physical stimuli (mechanical and thermal) of C nociceptive fibres, although they developed a continuous discharge, possibly due to the interference of 4-AP and TEA, respectively, with voltage-sensitive and calcium-dependent potassium channels at the level of the action potential generator region (Kirchoff *et al.* 1992). In the testis *in vitro* and in the cornea *in situ* removal of calcium from the perfusion solution evoked the development of spontaneous activity in polymodal nociceptors. Also, responses to mechanical or to chemical excitation with hypertonic saline or acid were unaffected or enhanced, probably due in this last case to non-specific change of the membrane's surface charge. In contrast, the excitatory effects of bradykinin in testis or of sensitization to repeated heating in the cornea were eliminated in zero calcium conditions (Kumazawa *et al.* 1987; Belmonte *et al.* 1994). Thus, calcium does not appear to be critical for primary transduction, but seems to play a role in second-messenger mediated sensitization. This evidence is still indirect, and more experimental data are needed to produce a coherent picture of the ionic mechanisms involved in the activation and sensitization of nociceptors by chemical agents.

Concluding remarks

On the basis of indirect electrophysiological and pharmacological evidence obtained from primary sensory neurones and nociceptive fibres, it can be hypothesized that nociceptive terminals possess multiple mechanisms for detection, amplification, and filtering of input signals (Fig. 10.2). These mechanisms will mediate transduction of the various forms of stimulating energy and also the modulation of the input signal at the successive steps of the transduction process. Different types of stimuli may interact at threshold or subthreshold levels to produce propagated responses. Such interactions are still poorly understood. Sensitization to one type of stimulus (mechanical, for instance) may not be accompanied by a parallel sensitization to another form of energy (namely, thermal). Thus, summation of membrane potential changes caused by activation of separate transduction mechanisms is not sufficient to explain the interplay of the different types of stimuli in nociceptive terminals. It appears more probable that the different amplification and modulation mechanisms that are present at sensory terminals interact to produce a discharge of nerve impulses of a given frequency, time course, and firing pattern. Such interaction would also define other characteristics of the impulse response such as ongoing activity, postdischarge, sensitization, or inactivation.

From the perspective that several molecular mechanisms may exist in nociceptive endings for the transduction and amplification of the various forms of stimulating energy, a definite categorization of nociceptors based on the propagated responses elicited by one or more of these stimuli could be somewhat simplistic. These nociceptor types may, in fact, represent cases where the transducer mechanism for a given form of energy is so prevalent over the others, that only this form of stimuli will elicit a propagated response under normal circumstances. When summation of various subthreshold stimuli occurs, as presumably occurs during inflammation, responsiveness to other types of stimuli will become evident.

However, these speculations still lack direct experimental support. New data are needed to produce a coherent picture on how stimuli are transduced and how nerve impulses are generated at nociceptive terminals. Until then, the molecular and cellular basis of transduction in nociceptors will remain an unexplored field, open to future research.

Acknowledgements

I wish to express my appreciation to Humphrey P. Rang and Gordon M. Shepherd for their comments and suggestions, and to Jennifer Laird and Fernando Cervero for their help with the presentation of the manuscript. This work was supported by SAF-93-0267 of the Comisión Interministerial de Ciencia y Tecnología, Spain.

References

Alarie, Y. (1973). Sensory irritation by airborne chemicals. *CRC Crit. Rev. Toxicol.* **2**, 299–363.

Bade, H., Braun, H.A., Hensel, H., and Schäfer, K. (1978). Discharge pattern of cold fibres related to hypothetical receptor mechanisms. *J. Physiol.* **284**, 83P.

Balazs, E.A. (1982). The physical properties of synovial fluid and the special role of hyaluronic acid. In *Disorders of the knee* (ed. A.J. Helfet), pp. 61–74. Lippincott Co, Philadelphia.

Balazs, E.A. and Denlinger, J.L. (1984). The role of hyaluronic acid in arthritis and its therapeutic use. In *Osteoarthritis: current clinical and fundamental problems* (ed. J.C. Peyron), pp. 165–74. Ciba Geigy, Paris.

Belmonte, C. and Giraldez, F. (1981). Responses of cat corneal sensory receptors to mechanical and thermal stimulation. *J. Physiol.* **321**, 355–68.

Belmonte, C., Gallar, J., Pozo, M.A., and Rebollo, I. (1991). Excitation by irritant chemical substances of sensory afferent units in the cat's cornea. *J. Physiol.* **437**, 709–25.

Belmonte, C., Gallar, J., Lopez-Briones, L.G., and Pozo, M.A. (1994). Polymodality in nociceptive neurons: Experimental models of chemotransduction. In *Cellular mechanisms of sensory processing*, NATO Series, Vol. H 79 (ed. L. Urban), pp. 87–117. Springer-Verlag, Berlin.

Bevan, S. and Geppetti, P. (1994). Protons: small stimulants of capsaicin-sensitive sensory nerves. *Trends Neurosci.* **17**, 509–12.

Block, S.M. (1992). Biophysical principles of sensory transduction. In *Sensory transduction* (ed. D.P. Corey and S.D. Roper), pp. 1–17. Rockefeller University Press, New York.

Braun, H.A., Bade, H., and Hensel, H. (1980). Static and dynamic discharge patterns of bursting cold fibers related to hypothetical receptor mechanisms. *Pflügers Arch.* **386**, 1–9.

Carpenter, D.O. (1981). Ionic and metabolic bases of neuronal thermosensitivity. *Fed. Proc.* **40**, 2808–13.

Carr, W.E.S., Gleeson, R.A., and Trapido-Rosenthal, H.G. (1990). The role of perireceptor events in chemosensory processes. *Trends Neurosci.* **13**, 212–15.

Comper, W.D. and Laurent, T.C. (1978). Physiological function of connective tissue polysaccharides. *Physiol. Rev.* **58**, 255–315.

Fukami, Y. (1986). Studies of capsule and capsular space of cat muscle spindles. *J. Physiol.* **376**, 281–97.

Guharay, F. and Sachs, F. (1984). Stretch-activated single ion channel currents in tissue-cultured embryonic chick skeletal muscle. *J. Physiol.* **352**, 685–701.

Handwerker, H.O. and Reeh, P.W. (1991). Pain and inflammation. In *Pain research and clinical management*, Vol. 4 (ed. M.R. Bond, J.E. Charlton, and C.J. Woolf), pp. 59–70. Elsevier, Amsterdam.

Heppelmann, B., Messlinger, K., Neiss, W.F., and Schmidt, R.F. (1990). Ultrastructural three-dimensional reconstruction of group III and group IV sensory nerve endings ("free nerve endings") in the knee joint capsule of the cat: evidence for multiple receptor sites. *J. comp. Neurol.* **292**, 103–16.

Hille, B. (1992). *Ionic channels of excitable membranes.* Sinauer Associates Inc, Sunderland, Massachusetts.

Howard, J., Roberts, W.M., and Hudspeth, A.J. (1988). Mechanoelectrical transduction by hair cells. *Ann. Rev. Biophys. Chem.* **17**, 99–124.

Hudspeth, A.J. (1982). Extracellular current flow and the site of transduction by vertebrate hair cells. *J. Neurosci.* **2**, 1–10.

Hudspeth, A.J. and Gillespie, P.G. (1994). Pulling springs to tune transduction: adaptation by hair cells. *Neuron* **12**, 1–9.

Kinnamon, S.C. and Getchell, T.V. (1991). Sensory transduction in olfactory receptor neurons and gustatory receptor cells. In *Smell and taste in health and disease* (ed. T.V. Getchell, R.L. Doty, L.M. Bartoshuk, and J.B. Snow, Jr.), pp. 145–72.

Kirchhoff, C., Leah, J.D., Jung, S., and Reeh, P.W. (1992). Excitation of cutaneous sensory nerve endings in the rat by 4-aminopyridine and tetraethylammonium. *J. Neurophysiol.* **67**, 125–31.

Koerber, H.R. and Mendell, L.M. (1992). Functional heterogeneity of dorsal root ganglion cells. In *Sensory neurons. Diversity, development, plasticity* (ed. S.A. Scott), pp. 77–96. Oxford University Press, New York.

Kumazawa, T. and Mizumura, K. (1980). Mechanical and thermal responses of polymodal receptors recorded from the superior spermatic nerve of the dog. *J. Physiol.* **299**, 233–45.

Kumazawa, T., Mizumura, K., and Sato, J. (1987). Thermally potentiated responses to algesic substances of visceral nociceptors. *Pain* **28**, 255–64.

Kumazawa, T., Mizumura, K., and Sato, J. (1988). Modulation of testicular polymodal receptor activities. *Prog. Brain Res.* **74**, 325–35.

Lang, E., Novak, A., Reeh, P.W., and Handwerker, H.O. (1990). Chemosensitivity of fine afferents from rat skin in vitro. *J. Neurophysiol.* **63**, 887–901.

Levitan, I.B. and Kaczmarek, L.K. (1991). *The neuron. Cell and molecular biology.* Oxford University Press, New York.

Mizumura, K., Sato, J., and Kumazawa, T. (1988). Appearance of cold sensitivity in testicular polymodal receptors after treatment with clioquinol. In *Fine afferent nerve fibers and pain* (ed. R.F. Schmidt, H.-G. Schaible, and C. Vahle-Hinz, pp. 158–64. VCH, Weinheim.

Morris, C.E. (1992). Are stretch-sensitive channels in molluscan cells and elsewhere physiological mechanotransducers? *Experientia* **48**, 852–8.

Mountcastle, V.B. (1980). *Medical physiology.* C.V. Mosby Co, St Louis, Missouri.

Nielson, G.D., Babko, J.C., and Holst, E. (1984). Sensory irritation and pulmonary irritation by airborne allyl acetate, allyl alcohol, and allyl ether compared to acrolein. *Acta Pharmacol. Toxicol.* **54**, 292–8.

Nielson, G.D. and Babko, J.C. (1985). Exposure limits for irritants. *Ann. Am. Conf. indust. Hyg.* **12**, 119–33.

Nobile, M., Carbone, E., Lux, H.D., and Zucker, H. (1990). Temperature sensitivity of Ca currents in chick sensory neurons. *Pflügers Arch.* **415**, 658–63.

Nowycky, M.C. (1992). Voltage-gated ion channels in dorsal root ganglion neurons. In *Sensory neurons. Diversity, development, plasticity* (ed. S.A. Scott), pp. 97–115. Oxford University Press, New York.

Perl, E.R. (1992). Alterations in the responsiveness of cutaneous nociceptors. In *Hyperalgesia and allodynia* (ed. W.D. Willis, Jr.), pp. 59–79. Raven Press, Ltd, New York.

Pozo, M.A., Gallego, R., Gallar, J., and Belmonte, C. (1992). Blockade by calcium antagonists of chemical excitation and sensitization of polymodal nociceptors in the cat's cornea. *J. Physiol.* **450**, 179–89.

Pozo, M.A., Balazs, E.A., and Belmonte, C. (1996). Reduction of sensory responses to passive movements of inflamed knee joints by hylan, a hyaluronan derivative. Osteoarthritis and cartilage (submitted).

Price, S. (1984). Mechanisms of stimulation of olfactory neurons: an essay. *Chem. Senses* **8**, 341–54.

Rang, H.P., Bevan, S., and Dray, A. (1991). Chemical activation of nociceptive peripheral neurones. *Br. Med. Bull.* **47**, 534–48.

Sachs, F. (1986). Biophysics of mechanoreception. *Membrane Biochem.* **6**, 173–95.

Sachs, F. (1992). Stretch-sensitive ion channels: an update. In *Sensory transduction* (ed. D.P. Corey and S.D. Roper), pp. 241–60. Rockefeller University Press, New York.

Schäfer, K. (1987). A quantitative study of the dependence of feline cold receptor activity on the calcium concentration. *Pflügers Arch.* **409**, 208–13.

Schäfer, K., Braun, H.A., and Hensel, H. (1982). Static and dynamic activity of cold receptors at various calcium levels. *J. Neurophysiol.* **47**, 1017–28.

Schäfer, K., Braun, H.A., and Rempe, L. (1988). Classification of a calcium conductance in cold receptors. *Prog. Brain Res.* **74**, 29–36.

Shepherd, G.M. (1991). Sensory transduction. Entering the mainstream of membrane signalling. *Cell* **67**, 845–51.

Shepherd, G.M. (1994). *Neurobiology*. Oxford University Press, New York.

Silver, W.L. (1990). Physiological factors in nasal trigeminal chemoreception. In *Chemical senses*. Vol. 2. *Irritation* (ed. B.G. Green, J.R. Mason, and M.R. Kare), pp. 21–37. Marcel Dekker, New York.

Sokabe, M., Sachs, F., and Jing, Z. (1991). Quantitative video microscopy of patch clamped membranes: stress, strain, capacitance and stretch channel activation. *Biophys. J.* **59**, 722–8.

Spray, D.C. (1974). Metabolic dependence of frog cold receptor sensitivity. *Brain Res.* **72**, 354–9.

Szolcsanyi, J., Anton, F., Reeh, P., and Handwerker, H.O. (1988). Selective excitation by capsaicin of mechano-heat sensitive nociceptors in rat skin. *Brain Res.* **446**, 262–8.

Taiwo, Y.O. and Levine, J.D. (1991) Further confirmation of the role of adenyl cyclase and of cAMP-dependent protein kinase in primary afferent hyperalgesia. *Neuroscience* **44**, 131–5.

Treede, R.-D., Meyer, R.A., Raja, S.N., and Campbell J.N. (1995). Evidence for two different heat transduction mechanisms in nociceptive primary afferents innervating monkey skin. *J. Physiol.* **483**, 747–58.

Wang, N., Butler, J.P., and Ingber, D.E. (1993). Mechanotransduction across cell surface and through the cytoskeleton. *Science* **260**, 1124–7.

White, D.M. and Levine, J.D. (1991). Different mechanical transduction mechanisms for the immediate and delayed responses of rat C-fiber nociceptors. *J. Neurophysiol.* **66**, 363–8.

Yang, X.-C. and Sachs, F. (1990). Characterization of stretch-activated ion channels in *Xenopus* oocytes. *J. Physiol.* **431**, 103–22.

Zelená, J. (1994). *Nerves and mechanoreceptors*. Chapman & Hall, London.

11 Chemical excitation and sensitization in nociceptors

MICHAELA KRESS AND PETER W. REEH

Introduction

From early psychophysical studies a variety of exogenous and endogenous substances have been found to induce pain and hyperalgesia, that is, to be algogenic. To study the underlying mechanisms several behavioural and reflex models have been developed in animals. However, the main obstacle that the investigator encountered in both psychophysical and whole animal models was the complexity of the organism. Thus it was difficult to differentiate between peripheral and central mechanisms. Single-fibre recordings provided a tool to isolate the contributions of primary afferents. However, to approach cellular mechanisms, a further reduction of the complexity was needed and achieved with the development of *in vitro* models. Controlled application of defined mediator concentrations became feasible allowing the investigation of the direct effects on nociceptive nerve endings. These sensory terminals, however, comprise receptive membrane sections, action potential generator region(s), and conductive zones of the axon, each of which could be the target of a chemical mediator. To differentiate these would require intracellular recording of the membrane potential or currents; this is not achievable due to the submicroscopic size of nociceptive nerve endings and their embedding in the tissue. Considering the cell soma in dissociated sensory ganglion cultures to be a model of its receptive ending, valuable information can be obtained from patch-clamp recordings of chemically mediated membrane effects. Each of these models has its restrictions, but by taking the information from all of them together the confusing array of inflammatory mediators and of their primary, secondary, and subsequent actions may become clearer.

Endogenous compounds

Mediators

Bradykinin

The nonapeptide bradykinin (BK) and closely related compounds such as kallidin or T-kinin are enzymatically generated from high and low molecular weight kininogen precursors circulating in plasma and also present in interstitial fluid. Similarly to the coagulation system, activation of the contact-sensitive Hageman factor (F. XII) is the initial step of plasma kallikrein activation while a confusing array of control mechanisms regulates the cellular secretion of tissue kallikrein (Proud and Kaplan 1988). Finally, the active compounds result from cleavage of kininogens through the action of kallikrein. Kinin production becomes upregulated in inflammation, for example by bacterial endotoxins, uric acid, and other salt crystals via F. XII activation and by depletion of a C1 esterase inhibitor of kallikrein during antigen–antibody reactions. Furthermore, degranulating mast cells release proteases that exert kallikrein-like activity (Proud and Kaplan 1988). Kinins have a half-life of 15 s which is due to the ubiquitous activity of kininases including angiotensin-converting enzyme (kininase II; Goodman *et al.* 1991). Kininase activity, however, is strongly inhibited in an acidic environment, such as is present in inflamed and ischaemic tissue which contributes to increased bradykinin levels under such conditions (Edery and Lewis 1962).

BK, apart from its other physiological roles, for example, in regulation of vascular tension and permeability, has long been known as an 'algogenic', that is, a pain-producing substance (Keele and Armstrong 1964), effective in concentrations of 10^{-7} to 10^{-4} M. In addition, hyperalgesia to heat stimulation resulted from intradermal injections (Manning *et al.* 1991). A variety of nocifensive reflexes and reactions at different levels of processing in the central nervous system (CNS) have been obtained in response to BK application in several animal models (see, for example, Bauer *et al.* 1992; Dray *et al.* 1992*b*; Holzer-Petsche 1992; Schuligoi *et al.* 1994); BK-induced hypersensitivity to noxious mechanical stimulation, as observed in behavioural tests in rats (Levine *et al.* 1986*b*; Steranka *et al.* 1988), has not been reported from human psychophysical studies (Manning *et al.* 1991). In primary nociceptive afferents of the cat knee joint, a corresponding increase in mechanical excitability has been observed following close arterial injection of BK, while exposure of cutaneous nerve endings, *in vitro*, to BK and even to an ample combination of inflammatory mediators did not yield sensitization to punctate pressure stimulation (Neugebauer *et al.* 1989; Lang *et al.* 1990; Kessler *et al.* 1992). In contrast, the excitatory effects and the sensitization to heat stimulation evoked by BK were readily corroborated *in vitro* although they were transient and prone to tachyphylaxis (Lang *et al.* 1990; Kumazawa *et al.* 1991; Koltzenburg *et al.* 1992; Fox *et al.* 1993; Rueff and Dray 1993*b*).

Among cutaneous polymodal nociceptors, that is, mechanoheat-sensitive unmyelinated (CMH) and thinly myelinated afferents (AMH), about half of the population was excited by a 1-min exposure of the receptive fields to 10^{-5} M BK (Lang *et al.* 1990). In 'deep' tissue, the proportion of C-fibres sensitive to BK seems to be much higher than in skin; values between 73 and 93 per cent have been reported in the literature (see Lang *et al.* 1990 for discussion). In the skin, units not sensitive to heat but sensitive to mechanical and cold stimulation were less frequently responsive to BK (Lang *et al.* 1990). BK's sensitizing effect on heat stimulation appears to be independent of its excitatory actions, since some cat cutaneous nociceptors could not be driven by close arterial injection of BK but became sensitized nonetheless (Beck and Handwerker 1974). However, due to its vasodilatory effect, BK may have increased skin temperature and thus the efficacy of heat stimulation. Actually, chemical and heat responsiveness seem to be functionally interrelated in some respects. Heat thresholds of units sensitive to combined inflammatory mediators including BK (as well as serotonin (5-HT), histamine (HA), and prostaglandin E_2 (PGE_2)) have been found to be significantly lower, by 2.6°C on average, as compared to chemically insensitive CMH fibres (see Fig. 11.1). In addition, preceding heat stimulation reliably facilitated subsequent neuronal responses to BK even when a pronounced tachyphylaxis to BK had already developed (Lang *et al.* 1990). This finding is not due to the well established temperature dependence of the BK response in nociceptors (Kumazawa and Mizumura 1984). The conditioning effect of heat stimulation was absent when the combination of inflammatory mediators (see above) was used as a test stimulus, suggesting that noxious heat may mobilize substances synergistic to BK that are contained in the above combination anyway, for example, 5-HT or HA (Kessler *et al.* 1992). Alternatively, heat and inflammatory mediators may have triggered common intracellular signals whose levels cannot possibly be further increased once having reached a certain activity (occlusion).

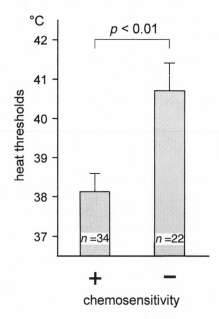

Fig. 11.1 Lower heat thresholds of chemosensitive polymodal nociceptors. Ramp-shaped radiant heat stimuli (32 to 45°C intracutaneous, 20-s duration) were applied to epidermal receptive fields of 56 CMH single fibres in a rat skin-nerve preparation *in vitro*. The spike trains induced by this stimulation were analysed off-line and the temperature at discharge of the first spike was taken as the heat threshold. Chemosensitivity was subsequently tested superfusing the receptive fields at the corium side with a mixture of BK, 5-HT, HA, and PGE2 (10^{-5} M, 5 min). Units exhibiting no ongoing activity previously were regarded as chemosensitive if they delivered more than 50 spikes (within 15 min) in a coherent train starting during the chemical stimulation. The Mann–Whitney U-test was used for statistical comparison (Reischl and Reeh, unpublished).

In line with a synergism of inflammatory factors in exciting nociceptive afferents was the finding that a larger than normal proportion of unmyelinated units was sensitive to BK after induction of an experimental inflammation with carrageenan (Kirchhoff *et al.* 1990). Exogenously added BK seemed to synergize with endogenous mediators sensitizing nociceptors. Similarly, more than 80 per cent (instead of 50 per cent) of units responded to BK if this was combined with the other mediators, 5-HT, HA, and PGE_2 (Kessler *et al.* 1992). Recently, however, nociceptor responses not only to BK but also to combined inflammatory agents turned out to be facilitated in inflamed skin *in vitro* 1 day after a freeze lesion had been made. This was not likely to be due to a synergism of exogenous and endogenous mediators since all relevant factors seemed to be contained in the chemical stimulus. Indeed, the finding had a more trivial cause: it resulted from an increased level of background activity, as generally seen in inflamed tissue, which added to the chemical responses of nociceptive primary afferents (Brehm and Reeh, unpublished). This indicates that the chemical responsiveness, which is probably determined by the number and potency of membrane receptors and by second messenger levels, is not altered during the first day of inflammation.

Upon BK application in cellular models, two principal intracellular transients have been reported. First, Ca^{2+} activity increases in a dose-dependent manner with a half-maximal effect at 10^{-8} M BK (Burgess *et al.* 1989; Reiser *et al.* 1990). Second, and probably secondarily, intracellular cyclic guanosine monophosphate (cGMP) levels rise upon BK stimulation of neuronal cell lines (Reiser *et al.* 1984; Burgess *et al.* 1989). In sensory dorsal root ganglion cells (DRG) both transients seem to be triggered by a sodium influx causing depolarization and possibly excitation (Burgess *et al.* 1989; Kano *et al.* 1994). Neuronal BK effects seem to be mediated by the receptor subtype B_2, which, via G-proteins, activates phospholipase C (PLC) resulting in inositol 1, 4, 5-triphosphate/diacylglycerol (IP_3 DAG) production; DAG in turn activates protein kinase C (PKC; Brown and Higashida 1988; Burgess *et al.* 1989; Dray *et al.* 1992a). Since phorbolesters are known to activate the same enzyme and thus to mimic the BK action, the BK-induced Na^+-conductance seems to depend on PKC activation (Burgess *et al.* 1989). Being slower in onset and longer in duration, the Ca^{2+}-uptake induced by BK and phorbolesters appears to result mainly from a voltage-sensitive Ca^{2+}-conductance and is secondary to depolarization (Burgess *et al.* 1989). DAG, in addition, acts on phospholipase A_2 (PLA_2) releasing arachidonic acid and increasing eicosanoid production in DRG cells (Portilla *et al.* 1988). Whether this pathway is of importance in the BK-induced depolarization of DRG sensory neurones is still unclear. Recent behavioural evidence also suggests a contribution of the B_1 receptor subtype in the maintenance of inflammatory mechanical hyperalgesia following Freud's complete adjuvant arthritis (Davis and Perkins 1994). This BK receptor also acts via the IP_3/DAG pathway. An electrophysiological correlate for the finding has not yet been found.

Serotonin (5-hydroxytryptamine)

Serotonin (5-HT) is synthesized from tryptophan by hydroxylation and consecutive decarboxylation in enterochromaffin cells of the gastrointestinal tract. Platelets actively incorporate 5-HT when passing through gastrointestinal capillaries (Goodman *et al.* 1991). In haemorrhage but also in inflammation, platelets accumulate in the affected tissue (Farr *et al.* 1983). Upon activation, for example, by collagen or 'platelet-activating factor' (PAF) from inflammatory cells, thrombocytes mobilize 5-HT from storage granules, together with adenosine diphosphate (ADP) thus autocatalysing their activation and aggregation. In addition, cutaneous mast cells of several species, although not of humans, contain 5-HT. Once released from any of these cells, 5-HT is broken down within seconds. Following desamination by monoamine oxidase, serotonin is further degraded by enzymes present in most tissues.

5-HT plays a potential role in inflammatory vasodilatation by triggering nitric oxide release from endothelial cells (Furchgott and Vanhoute 1989). Also, early psychophysical investigations have shown that 5-HT produces pain, that is, it may act as an alogen. Applied to the blister base, pain occurred with a delay of 10 to 45 s; the threshold concentration was 10^{-6} M. With repeated application at 10-min intervals a pronounced tachyphylaxis was observed (Keele and Armstrong 1964; Richardson *et al.* 1985). A cross-tachyphylaxis was found when the supernatant of clotted blood was applied, which points to 5-HT as a pain-producing constituent of the serum when platelets have aggregated and released 5-HT (Keele and Armstrong 1964). Unfortunately, no information on a possible capacity to induce mechanical or thermal hyperalgesia is available from human psychophysical studies.

In rat behavioural models, a dose-dependent development of mechanical hyperalgesia has been reported from intracutaneous injections of 5-HT at doses greater than 10 ng. Withdrawal thresholds appeared transiently decreased for 20 min following injections (Taiwo and Levine 1992). No information about changes in responsiveness to thermal stimuli is available from this study.

Most information about 5-HT effects within the nociceptive system comes from electrophysiological studies. Very similarly to the results in human pain reports, the responses of all types of neurones showed a profound tachyphylaxis. In recordings from single cutaneous afferents of the cat, a large proportion of nociceptive afferents, that is, 90 per cent of CMH units and 60 per cent of Aδ-high-threshold mechanosensitive (HTM) units, were excited by close-arterially applied 5-HT. However, about 30 per cent of C-low-threshold mechanosensitive (LTM) fibres and 40 per cent of slowly adapting (SA) Aβ-fibres also responded, both being non-nociceptive (Beck and Handwerker 1974). In contrast, later *in vitro* recordings from rat skin in which SA units did not respond to 5-HT (see below) indicated that close arterial injections overestimated the magnitude and prevalence of 5-HT responsiveness, probably as a result of vascular effects. Using this application technique in the cat, other workers found about half of unmyelinated afferents from muscle to be excited by 5-HT. However, responses were less pronounced and showed a higher degree of tachyphylaxis than that shown by responses to BK (Mense and Schmidt 1974; Fock and Mense 1976). These findings were corroborated by recordings from cardiac afferents and visceral units from the walls of abdominal and pelvic organs (Nishi *et al.* 1977; Jänig and Morrison 1986).

Recordings performed in various isolated organ models are not fully in line with the *in vivo* studies; 10^{-5} M 5-HT excited a smaller proportion (25 per cent) of exclusively nociceptive afferents. All 5-HT-sensitive units were also excited by BK (Kumazawa and Mizumura 1984; Lang *et al.* 1990). The sensitizing action of 5-HT is more pronounced than its excitatory effect (Rueff and Dray 1993*a*). A facilitating action of 5-HT on nociceptor responses to BK occurred even in those units that were initially not excited by the kinin or by 5-HT itself (Hiss and Mense 1976; Lang *et al.* 1990). Thus, a common cellular basis could be assumed for chemosensitive units. However, a cross-tachyphylaxis of BK and 5-HT responses was never observed indicating at least partially independent actions of the two mediators (Beck and Handwerker 1974; Lang *et al.* 1990). Combining BK and 5-HT into one chemical stimulus (together with PGE_2 and HA) clearly attenuated the tachyphylaxis but did not fully prevent it (Kessler *et al.* 1992; see also Fig. 11.4). In addition to BK-induced reflex responses, those to heat were also facilitated upon 5-HT administration to the spinal cord–tail preparation (Rueff and Dray 1993*a*). A sensitization to punctate mechanical stimuli with von Frey hairs, as reported from behavioural experiments using the paw pressure test, was not observed with 5-HT *in vitro* (Taiwo and Levine 1992; Lang *et al.* 1990).

Similarly to peripheral nerve endings, sensory ganglion cells from cat and rabbit were depolarized and excited by 5-HT (Sampson and Jaffe 1974; Simonds and DeGroat 1980; Higashi and Nishi 1982). Concentrations of 10^{-5} M were needed to induce a transient fast inactivating current in C but not A cells of the nodose ganglion but only at rapid onset of the chemical stimulation (Higashi and Nishi 1982). In 1-day-old dissociated cultures from DRGs of the adult rat a transient inward current was, however, observed in only 3 of 17 capsaicin-sensitive neurones (Kress, Vyklicky, and Reeh, unpublished). This lack of effect could be due to a rapid elimination of 5-HT binding sites from the cell membrane within 1 day after dissociation (Mulderry 1994). However, in the isolated intact DRG, intracellular recordings revealed no significant effect of 5-HT on membrane potential and resistance (Tegeder and Reeh 1991).

In recent studies emphasis has been laid on clarifying the transduction mechanism for the excitatory and sensitizing effects of serotonin. According to recent classifications seven classes of 5-HT receptors exist (for a review see Hoyer *et al.* 1994). Receptor subclasses 5-HT_1, 5-HT_2, and 5-HT_3 have been located in peripheral neurones. A potent 5-HT_3 receptor antagonist prevented hyperalgesia to paw pressure in the carrageenan model of the rat when co-administered with the inflammatory agent (Escalier *et al.* 1989). Metoclopramide, which antagonizes 5-HT_3-receptor-mediated effects, reversibly suppressed responses of polymodal nociceptive afferents to a mixture of inflammatory mediators containing 5-HT, BK, HA, and PGE_2 (Fig. 11.2). This indicates that nociceptor excitation by an artificial inflammatory exudate depends considerably on a contribution of 5-HT, via 5-HT_3 receptor binding, since ketanserin, which blocks 5-HT_2 receptors, was ineffective in most cases (Handwerker *et al.* 1990). Though this mechanism is in accord with 5-HT_3 effects on the human blister base, recent evidence has been presented from the neonatal rat spinal cord with attached tail *in vitro* that 5-HT_2 receptors might mediate sensitization to chemical and heat stimulation, whereas 5-HT_1-like receptors may account for the excitatory effects (Rueff and Dray 1993*a*). The 5-HT_3 receptor, which is exclusively present in neurones, represents the only ion channel among 5-HT receptors. This receptor subtype seems to convey 5-HT effects in nodose ganglion cells where ($+$)-tubocurarin attenuated the depolarization (Higashi and Nishi 1982; see Hoyer *et al.* 1994). A contribution of other receptor sybtypes cannot be excluded, but still awaits experimental evidence.

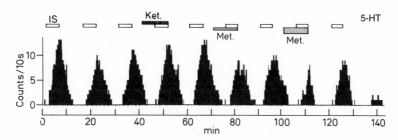

Fig. 11.2 Nociceptor responses to a combination of inflammatory mediators blocked by metoclopramide but not ketanserin. In the rat skin-nerve preparation, a CMH fibre's receptive field was stimulated with a superfusion of 'inflammatory soup' (IS) containing BK, 5-HT, HA, and PGE2 in a 10^{-5} M concentration. Ketanserin (Ket.; 10^{-5} M), a 5-HT_2 receptor blocker did not modulate the chemical response, whereas metoclopramide (Met.; 10^{-5}, 3×10^{-5} M), a 5-HT_3 receptor antagonist, dose-dependently reduced it. 5-HT itself evoked only a small response by the end of the protocol (Britting, Steen, and Reeh, unpublished).

Histamine

The major sources of histamine (HA) in mammalian tissue are the storage granules of mast cells and of basophilic leucocytes infiltrating from the blood. Other tissues containing HA include the gastric mucosa, neurones in the CNS, and cells in regenerating or rapidly growing tissue. These cells are capable of synthesizing HA from the amino acid L-histidine via decarboxylation. In man there are two major pathways of inactivation, namely, methylation and further conversion by monoamine oxidase (MAO), or, alternatively, HA can undergo oxidative deamination, which again yields imidazole acetic acid and its ribose excreted in the urine (Goodman *et al.* 1991).

Apart from its function as a neurotransmitter in the CNS and as a regulating agent of gastric secretion, HA's important role in allergic responses and immediate hypersensitivity has long been known. The most prominent sensation occurring with the local introduction of HA into superficial layers of the intact skin is itching which develops 20 to 50 s after application (Keele and Armstrong 1964). In addition, a wheal and a local reddening develop that are due to vasoactive effects inducing plasma extravasation and vasodilatation. Surrounding these local signs, HA is particularly effective in inducing a widespread flare response, which is interpreted as an 'axon reflex' and as a correlate of 'neurogenic inflammation' (see Lynn, Chapter 17, this volume). Also, in an area surrounding the wheal, an 'itchy' sensation could be evoked with slight stroking. Upon injection of higher doses (about 1 mM concentration) burning or pricking pain sensations rather than itching could be evoked (Keele and Armstrong 1964). Similarly, pain but not itching was induced when injecting HA into deeper layers of the skin (Keele and Armstrong 1964). This is in contrast to more recent findings when a non-invasive technique, iontophoresis, was used for HA administration and no pain sensation was induced (Magerl *et al.* 1990*b*). The discrepancy suggests an interaction of HA with compounds released with even minimal tissue damage.

Both painful and itching stimuli are apparently detected by unmyelinated afferents since itch can no longer be induced after desensitizing the skin nociceptors with capsaicin or after C-fibre block by sustained pressure to the nerve (Simone *et al.* 1991; LaMotte 1992). However, HA itself at 10^{-5} M concentration induced a weak activation only in 15 per cent of cutaneous nociceptors, and only those responded that were also excited by BK or mustard oil. Discharge increased when a higher concentration was applied (10^{-4} M; Lang *et al.* 1990; Handwerker *et al.* 1991). Responses were clearly weaker than those to BK. Pretreatment with BK, however, resulted in increased HA responses and additional recruitment of CMH-fibres (Lang *et al.* 1990; Koppert *et al.* 1993). In a correlative psychophysical study, this interaction was reflected by a suppression of HA-induced itching, which was replaced by burning pain after pretreatment with BK (Koppert *et al.* 1993). This interaction, however, was not reciprocal. In respect to inflammatory pain, HA can probably be excluded as an algogen since histamine effects did not add to or facilitate nociceptor responses to other inflammatory mediators, for example BK, as has been reported for cutaneous as well as visceral afferents *in vitro* (Mizumura *et al.* 1990; Koppert *et al.* 1993). In contrast, a certain sensitization to heat due to histamine was observed in visceral polymodal nociceptors only (Mizumura *et al.* 1994).

Three membrane receptor subtypes are known for HA. In sensory ganglion neurones, the H_1 receptor has functionally been demonstrated, acting via an increase of IP_3 and DAG that results in intracellular Ca^{2+} release (Ninkovic and Hunt 1985; Tani *et al.* 1990). The interaction with the BK transduction may take place within this second messenger pathway (see above). However, in none of 10 capsaicin-sensitive DRG cells did 10^{-5} M HA yield an inward current or a depolarization upon a 10-s HA application (Kress, Vyklicky, and Reeh, unpublished).

Eicosanoids

Eicosanoids are ubiquitous 'tissue hormones' that derive mainly from arachidonic acid, an essentially fatty acid constituent of every cell membrane. This precursor is released by the hydrolytic activity of phospholipase A_2 (PLA_2) which is the rate-limiting step in eicosanoid production. The enzyme is under the control of cytosolic calcium and of many hormones that interact through membrane receptors and G-proteins. Free arachidonic acid is rapidly processed either by the ubiquitous cyclooxygenase (COX), leading to prostaglandins and thromboxanes, or by the competing lipoxigenases which, in different tissues, start the synthesis of leukotrienes and hydroxyeicosatetraenoic acids (HETEs). As unsaturated fatty acid derivatives the eicosanoids are very sensitive to spontaneous and enzymatic oxidation, which results in rapid loss of biological activity.

Prostaglandins (PG) E_2 and I_2 (prostacyclin) and some of the lipoxigenase products play a major role as inflammatory mediators, the latter as chemotactic agents attracting and activating leucocytes and monocytes, the former as potent vasodilators and by increasing the permeability of vascular walls. The particular potency of the inflammatory prostaglandins and the fact that they cannot be stored lend importance to a group of compounds, aspirin and the 'non-steroidal anti-inflammatory drugs' (NSAIDs), that block the COX. One enzymatic step higher, the glucocorticoids indirectly inhibit the phospholipase and, by that means, reduce all eicosanoid synthesis. Not yet of clinical relevance, inhibitors of the lipoxygenases and of both eicosanoid pathways are only in experimental use. Some of the anti-inflammatory COX-blockers, for example, ibuprofen, show general analgesic properties suitable for treating pain of apparently non-inflammatory origin, for example, headache. This has promoted the widespread idea that the prostaglandins could be algesic substances directly exciting or, at least, sensitizing nociceptors in many tissues. Since 1971 (Vane 1971) a large amount of evidence has accumulated that apparently supports this assumption (see Levine *et al.* 1993). However, most of this evidence is indirect, resulting from psychophysiological, behavioural, and electrophysiological experiments in which the prostaglandins were injected in high concentration into the complex environment of the tissue or of blood supplying the tissue under investigation. This opens the possibility of secondary effects from the multitude of biological actions attributed to the prostaglandins. Examples are plasma-extravasation conveying BK, degranulation of mast cells releasing HA and 5-HT and, in some non-human species, even activation of blood platelets that excite nociceptors directly (Macintyre and Gordon 1975; Wallengren and Hakanson 1992; Ringkamp *et al.* 1994). Thus, injection of vehicle solution cannot possibly be an adequate control for prostaglandins and other pleiotropic substances.

Tissue preparations, *ex vivo*, by reducing the number of possible secondary interactions, have recently provided more differentiated insight into prostaglandin actions on nociceptors. These models unanimously show that the prostaglandins are unable to evoke nociceptor discharge and related reflex responses (Mizumura *et al.* 1987; Lang *et al.* 1990; Fox *et al.* 1993; Rueff and Dray *et al.* 1993*b*). This is also true for corneal nociceptors *in vivo*, which innervate a tissue free of blood vessels (Belmonte *et al.* 1994).

Sensitization of nociceptive primary afferents can separately alter their sensitivity to heat, mechanical and chemical stimulation, and to BK in particular. In the neonatal rat tail–spinal cord preparation (after Otsuka) with the epidermal barrier removed, a 20–40 per cent increase in reflex responses to heat was found after superfusion of the tail with various prostaglandins (Rueff and Dray 1993*b*). In the dog-testis preparation *in vitro*, in a concentration (10^{-5} M) 1000 times higher than actually found in inflammatory exudates, PGE_2 induced a significant increase in heat-evoked nociceptor discharge by 1 spike/s, on average, and this effect was prone to tachyphylaxis (Mizumura *et al.* 1993*b*). Using the same preparation and concentration of PGE_2 (Mizumura *et al.* 1987), a response to twice isotonic saline was found to be augmented, which indicates a non-specific effect, since this stimulus is excitatory to primary afferents of all sensory categories (see below). In the skin-nerve preparation, an ample mixture of inflammatory mediators, including PGE_2 (and BK, 5-HT, HA: 10^{-5} M), did not induce a more pronounced or prolonged heat sensitization as was to be expected from the strong but transient sensitizing effect of BK (Kessler *et al.* 1992; Koltzenburg *et al.* 1992).

Many of the hyperalgesic actions of intradermally injected prostaglandins have previously been verified using paw pressure testing in the rat (see, for example, Khasar *et al.* 1993). *In vitro*, the threshold to punctate (von Frey) pressure stimulation of the nocireceptive fields has been tested and showed no change upon repeated application of PGE_2 (10^{-5} M; Mizumura *et al.* 1987; Lang *et al.* 1990; Kessler *et al.* 1992). Even prolonged cutaneous superfusion (30 min, see Fig. 11.4) using the combined inflammatory mediators did not alter the von Frey thresholds (Reischl and Reeh, unpublished). The cat knee joint is the only preparation where prostaglandins, intraarterially injected, show an excitatory action on nociceptive afferents; in addition, PGE_2 induces sensitization to joint movements (Schaible and Schmidt 1988). Attempts to reproduce these findings in the rat ankle joint failed; PGE_2 did not excite nor sensitize the mechanonociceptors (Grubb *et al.* 1991). Moreover, this preparation, when inflamed after injection of Freund's adjuvant, provided an indication of the anti-nociceptive effects of aspirin independently of cyclooxygenase blockade: Spontaneous activity and mechanical hypersensitivity of fibres from the arthritic joint were reduced by the drug but close-arterial PGE_2 was unable to restore these typical symptoms of articular inflammation (Grubb *et al.* 1991). A very similar drug effect on nociceptors in normal skin *in vitro* has recently been seen with flurbiprofen, an NSAID that significantly reduced the responses to controlled electromechanical stimulation. Substitution of PGE_2 did not counteract the mechanical desensitization (Brehm and Reeh 1994). Flurbiprofen is being used in this ongoing study, since both its R- and S-enantiomeres have proven effective in the paw pressure test, although only S-flurbiprofen prevents prostaglandin synthesis by COX-blockade (Brune *et al.* 1992).

More consistently but again not free of contradiction, prostaglandins are reported to enhance the excitatory effect of BK on nociceptors. Studying this interaction is complicated by the fact that BK belongs to the agents that stimulate PLA_2 and, by that means, release endogenous eicosanoids. In this context, COX-blocking experiments using NSAIDs gain particular significance. Thus, the writhing response in mice, evoked by intraperitoneal injection of BK, is presensitized with PGE_2 but hardly affected by a number of NSAIDs (Walter *et al.* 1989). These findings were confirmed *in vitro*, using the rat tail–spinal cord preparation, but it was only the effects of higher BK concentrations that were unaffected by indomethacine and aspirin (Rueff and Dray 1993*b*). In the dog-testis preparation, PGE_2 and PGI_2 were effective at very low concentration (10^{-7} M), but their sensitizing effect showed pronounced tachyphylaxis (Mizumura *et al.* 1991). Aspirin was effective in this preparation and the suppression of BK responses thus induced could be counteracted with PGE_2 (Mizumura *et al.* 1987). In open contrast and in another visceral organ, the newly developed trachea–vagus nerve preparation of guinea-pig, BK effects on chemosensitive afferents were not influenced by ibuprofen (Fox *et al.* 1993).

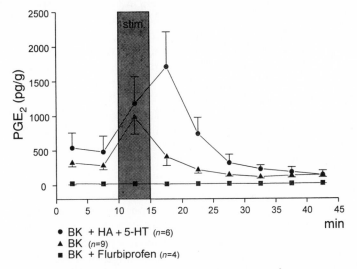

Fig. 11.3 Stimulated release of PGE_2 from skin preparations of the rat. The hairy skin of the rat hindpaw was subcutaneously excised and rinsed for 30 min. The skin flap was then repeatedly incubated in oxygenated physiological solution (SIF, 5 ml for 5 min each) contained in nine consecutive test tubes that were mounted in a shaking bath at 32°C. The third tube contained the inflammatory mediator(s) in 10^{-5} M concentration and, in four cases, additional flurbiprofen (10^{-6} M), which was also administered to the animal (25 mg/kg intraperitoneally) prior to skin dissection. The peak levels of PGE_2 were significantly different from baseline and from each other (Mann-Whitney U-test; Brehm, Schäfer, Bänkler, and Reeh, unpublished).

The nociceptor domain least sensitive to prostaglandins under *in vitro* conditions appears to be the skin of the rat, since PGE_2 pretreatment (10^{-5} M) had no effect on the prevalence and magnitude of BK responses in contrast to other inflammatory mediators (Lang *et al.* 1990; Brehm and Reeh 1994), that showed prominent synergistic interactions (Kessler *et al.* 1992; Koppert *et al.* 1993). This could have been due to occlusion with endogenously released prostaglandin. Therefore, flurbiprofen was again employed and the skin deprived of prostanoids (see Fig. 11.3). Under this condition, the nociceptor responses to combined inflammatory mediators (BK, 5-HT, HA$\pm PGE_2$: 10^{-6} or 10^{-5} M at pH 6.1) were not significantly different from those in normal skin. Furthermore, in cross-over experiments ($\pm PGE_2$), there was no significant difference in response magnitude whether or not PGE_2 was included (Reeh and Brehm 1993).

A diversity of mediator actions in different preparations, tissues, and species is usually taken as an indication for the existence of different receptor subtypes heterogeneously distributed. An EP_3 receptor for PGE_2 is reported responsible for the transient enhancement of BK responses in the dog-testis preparation (Kumazawa *et al.* 1993). This receptor is linked to the cyclic adenosine monophosphate (cAMP) second messenger system downregulating adenylyl cyclase activity. Such a linkage would separate sensitization to BK from sensitization to heat, which, in the same preparation and in the skin *in vitro* appears to be mediated by increasing cAMP levels. For the latter effect, however, high concentrations (10^{-4} M, respectively 10^{-3} M) of stable, membrane-permeable cAMP analogues were needed (Mizumura *et al.* 1993a; Kress *et al.* 1995b). On the other hand, PGI_2 (prostacyclin) also increases BK responses in the dog-testis preparation, but the IP receptor for PGI_2 causes an elevation in intracellular cAMP levels (Mizumura *et al.* 1991). This would be in line with an assumed cellular model for prostaglandin actions, nodose ganglion cells, which show a cAMP-mediated inhibition of K^+-conductance with an accompanying increase in excitability. The channel responsible is normally gated by Ca^{2+}-ions and contributes to the after-hyperpolarization following spike discharge that restricts the firing rate of neurones (Fowler *et al.* 1985). Release of this restriction, if present in nociceptors, would explain an increase in suprathreshold response without alteration of the threshold, exactly what was seen with ramp-shaped heat stimulation after superfusion of receptive fields in the skin with dibutyryl-cAMP (Kress *et al.* 1996).

The alternative pathway in arachidonic acid metabolism, which leads, via lipoxygenation to leukotrienes and HETEs, has also been implicated in the theory of inflammatory pain (Levine *et al.* 1993). Behavioural evidence from paw pressure testing suggests a hyperalgesic action of leukotriene B_4 (LTB_4) and of the (8R,15S)-di HETE enantiomer, the latter being the final mediator released from leucocytes that are attracted and activated by LTB_4 (Levine *et al.* 1984, 1985, 1986a). Single-fibre recordings *in vivo* with intracutaneous injections appear to support these conclusions (Martin 1990; White *et al.* 1990). In an isolated model, however, the perfused rabbit ear, the major leukotrienes (B_4, C_4, and D_4) exhibited a potent suppression of BK—and 5-HT—but not of acetylcholine (ACh)-evoked nocifensive reflex responses (Schweizer *et al.* 1984). This finding promoted the idea that part of the analgesic actions of NSAIDs might be due to increased leukotriene synthesis because of the increased availability of the arachidonic acid substrate during COX-blockade. The controversial picture of the lipoxygenase products cannot yet be clarified by findings from *in vitro* experiments. To our knowledge, the only piece of evidence available is that superfusion of nocireceptive fields with LTD_4 (in oxygen free-solution) for up to 30 min ($n = 6$) did not change the responses of polymodal C-fibres to combined inflammatory mediators in the skin (Kirchhoff and Reeh, unpublished).

(Nor)adrenaline

Adrenaline and noradrenaline (NA) are released from postganglionic terminals of the peripheral sympathetic system. They are synthesized from the amino acid thyrosin by hydroxylation and further decarboxylation. While peripheral sympathetic fibres generate NA in the adrenal gland further processing via *N*-methyltransferase yields adrenaline secreted into the blood. Both substances can be released from storage vesicles and their activity is limited within seconds by re-uptake and enzymatic degradation (Goodman *et al.* 1991).

Sympathetic efferents comprise roughly 20 per cent of unmyelinated fibres in peripheral nerves (Baron *et al.* 1994). On the basis of the beneficial effects of sympathetic blocks in certain patients, a contribution of the sympathetic nervous system and with it of adrenergic transmission had been anticipated for the development of syndromes of chronic pain and hyperalgesia; this has been discussed since (Jänig and Koltzenburg 1991; Koltzenburg and McMahon 1991; Ochoa 1992). Early blister base studies on volunteers showed that, if at all, adrenaline was effective in inducing acute pain only at very high doses (1 mM; Keele and Armstrong 1964). However, in patients with causalgia, the application of local NA or sympathetic stimulation was observed to provoke intense pain inside the affected area (Wallin *et al.* 1976). In line with these observations behavioural experiments reported decreased tolerance to paw pressure after intradermal injection of 10 µg NA in rats made hyperalgesic with topical chloroform (Levine *et al.* 1986*b*). Interestingly, tail-flick latencies were increased after eliminating sympathetic efferents (Coderre *et al.* 1984). Another study, in contrast, reported a lowered thermal nocifensive threshold from 30 days after neonatal chemical ablation of the sympathetic nervous system, which could be due to a regenerative overgrowth of non-sympathetic neurones (Abelli *et al.* 1993), However, alterations of the skin temperature regulation due to loss of vasoconstrictor function may contribute to the controversial findings. Some of the findings were corroborated by single-fibre recordings *in vivo*, where stimulation of sympathetic efferents resulted in a facilitation of sustained nociceptor responses to a combination of 5-HT, HA, KCl, and HCl injected into the skin (Sanjue and Jun 1989; see also Koltzenburg and McMahon 1991). In contrast, enhanced heat responses following a conditioning heat stimulus were not affected by simultaneous sympathetic stimulation (Shea and Perl 1985). Similarly, NA had no excitatory nor sensitizing effects on nociceptive afferents from normal skin *in vitro* nor were BK responses facilitated by exposure of the receptive fields to NA at a 10^{-6} M concentration. Only unphysiological concentrations of NA (10^{-5} to 10^{-4} M) induced an enhancement of BK responses (Lang *et al.* 1990).

As far as the mechanism of action of NA is concerned, there is still no consensus. Obviously, nociceptors are not responsive to NA under normal conditions, but sensitivity seems to evolve from some kind of tissue injury, and the resulting excitation can be reduced by yohimbine or rauwolscine indicating an involvement of α_2-receptors (Sato and Perl 1991). This is puzzling since this receptor subtype is supposed to decrease cAMP levels, whereas an increase of cAMP has been reported to result from many other substances effective in exciting or sensitizing nociceptors (see Bevan, Chapter 12, this volume). One may speculate that, upon inflammation, membrane receptors may become accessible in nociceptors that transduce the noradrenaline signal via an as yet unknown mechanism such as has been observed in DRG cells following nerve ligation (McLachlan *et al.* 1993). Recently, evidence has been presented that cytokines might play a role in sympathetically maintained pain (Cunha *et al.* 1991; see below).

Other endogenous compounds

Acetylcholine   The parasympathetic and sudomotor transmitter substance acetylcholine (ACh) is generally accepted as an algogenic agent (see below). Nevertheless, ACh has hardly ever been implicated in a theory of physiological pain mechanisms, since a histological relationship between possible sources of ACh and nociceptive nerve endings was not apparent and since extrajunctional ACh is barely detectable because of the ubiquitous activity of the choline esterases. It is still not known whether ACh appears in inflammatory exudates or in other painful conditions, but possible sources of ACh in the close vicinity of primary afferent terminals have been identified. Thus, in corneal epithelial cells high concentrations of ACh have been found, which may be released by injury, and ACh has been shown to excite corneal nerve endings (Pesin and Candia 1982; Tanellian 1991). Regarding skin, it has recently been demonstrated that human keratinocytes synthesize, store, and secrete ACh, which plays a role in regulating cell–cell attachment but may well, in addition, be released in larger amounts upon cutaneous injury (Grando *et al.* 1993).

ACh produces burning pain when applied to a blister base or iontophoresed into human skin; relatively high concentrations (around 10^{-4} M) are needed for this effect (Keele and Armstrong 1964; Magerl *et al.* 1990*a*). Such topical treatments leave the skin with a certain numbness and with a refractoriness to reapplication of ACh at intervals shorter than 9 min (Keele and Armstrong 1964; Magerl *et al.* 1990*a*). Intraperitoneal ACh induces pain-related behaviour as measured in the 'writhing test' in mice in which the ACh effect appears to be particularly sensitive to the action of NSAIDs (Bently *et al.* 1981; Amanuma *et al.* 1984). In the isolated rabbit ear preparation, ACh, like other algesic substances, induces a reflex drop in blood pressure assumed to result from the excitation of 'perivascular', probably deep cutaneous nociceptors. Nicotinic ACh receptors appear to mediate the responses, although the muscarinic antagonist, atropine, showed suppressive effects at relatively high concentrations (around 10^{-4} M) that were, however, discarded as a possibly local anaesthetic action (Keele and Armstrong 1964; Juan 1982).

A great deal of work on ACh effects in single-nerve-fibre recordings was performed between 1948 and 1975 (see Akoev 1981). Very widespread excitatory effects of ACh were reported from many categories of nerve endings and even of axons. Since almost all of the work had been done *in vivo* and using close-arterial injection, it was postulated that many of the apparently non-specific sensory actions of ACh may be due to the pressure of the injection fluids, to the abrupt vasodilatation induced by ACh, and to possible excitation of epineurial nerve endings that were mistaken for fibres of passage (Diamond 1959). Later it was shown that, in a desheathed nerve preparation, no excitatory effect of ACh on sensory axons of any conduction velocity can be evoked (Zimmermann and Sanders 1982).

In the skin-nerve preparation *in vitro* and in the cornea, only unmyelinated C-fibre endings were excited by ACh and its analogue, carbachol (Tanellian 1991; Steen and Reeh 1993*a*). About half of the polymodal C-units and a third of the mechanocold sensitive and high-threshold mechanosensitive C nociceptors were activated in a dose-dependent manner (10^{-7} to 10^{-4} M; Steen and Reeh 1993*a*). These concentrations were not different from the effective concentrations of BK (Lang *et al.* 1990). Using selective agonists and antagonists to muscarinic as well as nicotinic receptors, an involvement of both receptor subtypes could be shown, although the study was not extended to allow a quantitative comparison. A major finding was that repeated carbachol treatment of polymodal nociceptors left almost all fibres with a marked and sustained desensitization to mechanical (von Frey) stimulation, whereas the heat responsiveness appeared unchanged (Steen and Reeh 1993*a*). This may help to explain the antinociceptive effect of epibatidine, a newly identified nicotinic agonist of extreme potency (Bradley 1993).

Nicotinic and muscarinic ACh receptor subtypes show an enormous diversity of distinct molecular, pharmacological, and functional properties. This diversity links ACh to ligand-gated ion channels as well as to any known second messenger system, in addition to eicosanoid synthesis and to mast cell degranulation (Mei *et al.* 1989; Sokolovsky 1989; Deneris *et al.* 1991). Any evidence specifically relating to nociception is lacking.

Glutamate   The excitatory amino acid L-glutamate is one of the important compounds in synaptic transmission. However, L-glutamate can also be released from activated macrophages, at least in the central nervous system (Piani *et al.* 1991). Intracutaneous injection of L-glutamate has been reported to induce pain and also to excite peripheral nociceptors in the isolated spinal cord–tail preparation of the neonatal rat, albeit at a very high threshold concentration of more than 10^{-4} M (Follenfant and Nakamura-Craig 1992). None of the other amino acids tested were effective in exciting nociceptors (Ault and Hildebrand 1993). The excitatory action of glutamate was stereoselective for the L-isomer and probably conveyed by kainate receptor subtypes (Agrawal and Evans 1988). It cannot be decided whether sensory terminals or axons respond to L-glutamate.

GABA   γ-aminobutyric acid (GABA), an inhibitory transmitter in the central nervous system, has also been reported to cause excitation of unmyelinated afferents in the rat spinal cord–tail preparation via $GABA_A$-receptors (Ault and Hildebrand 1994). Similarly, $GABA_A$-induced depolarizing membrane currents are known to exist in sensory ganglion neurones (Gallagher *et al.* 1983; Vyklicky *et al.* 1993). However, nothing is known about its presence in peripheral tissue or its liberation upon inflammation.

ATP   All cells contain ATP as a source of energy in high, that is, millimolar concentration and, upon cell damage, it is set free together with the cytosol. ATP itself has been shown to induce pain and hyperalgesia when applied to the blister base, albeit at a high concentration (about 2×10^{-4} M; Keele and Armstrong 1964). Double-blind intradermal injections of ATP, ADP, AHP, adenosine and of several adenosine dinucleotides induced no sensations that subjects could distinguish from those to buffered saline injection; only millimolar ATP concentrations caused some itching (Zeilhofer and Reeh 1991, unpublished). Excitatory effects of extracellular ATP may relate to a direct action on a cation conductance associated with the P_2 receptor subtype, in sensory DRG cells (Krishtal *et al.* 1988; Rang *et al.* 1994). Upon breakdown, adenosine appears which produced neither pain nor flare reactions when applied to the human blister base (Keele and Armstrong 1964). Findings from central neurones indicate a general decrease of neuronal excitability due to an increase in potassium conductances (Greene and Haas 1991). However, it has been reported that hyperalgesia in the paw pressure test resulted from intradermal injection of adenosine and that pain in humans resulted from intravenous injections (Taiwo and Levine

1990). These findings were not corroborated in electrophysiological experiments where adenosine did not affect C- or Aδ-mechanoreceptor discharge in either normal or inflamed ankle joints of the rat (Ashgar *et al.* 1992).

Neuropeptides

A variety of neuropeptides is synthesized in ganglion cells and preferentially transported through the axons of predominantly C-fibres into the peripheral nerve endings from which they are released upon depolarization, spike discharge, or upon a hormonal signal, for example from PGE_2 (Geppetti 1993; Hua and Yaksh 1993; Regoli *et al.* 1994). A multitude of potent biological actions is attributed to the neuropeptides, including the phenomenon of neurogenic inflammation (Chahl 1988; Levine *et al.* 1993; see Lynn, Chapter 17, this volume). The best known neuropeptides in primary afferents are substance P (SP), neurokinin A (NKA), and calcitonin gene-related peptide (CGRP). Their actions are partly direct, such as the relaxing effect of CGRP on vascular smooth muscles, and partly indirect through release of secondary mediators, as in the case of SP which stimulates nitric oxide secretion from endothelial cells, mast cell degranulation, and prostaglandin synthesis (Regoli *et al.* 1994). The latter seems to be particularly relevant in the skin *in vitro*, since ongoing work in our laboratory shows that SP (10^{-5} M) provokes an increase in PGE_2 production to almost the same extent as does BK (see Fig. 11.3). Even more significantly, after capsaicin treatment to the innervating nerves (sural and saphenous), a considerable part of the BK-induced PGE_2-release is lost suggesting a partially indirect effect of BK via nociceptor excitation and SP release. Capsaicin is well known to induce a lasting depletion of SP in cutaneous nerves (Lynn and Shakhanbeh 1988).

Intradermal injection of SP is reported to be painful or pruritogenic because of secondary HA release (Heyer *et al.* 1991; Pedersen-Bjergaard *et al.* 1991). CGRP and NKA do not lead to any sensation in the skin, but combinations of CGRP with SP or NKA become painful when injected into muscle (Pedersen-Bjergaard *et al.* 1991). NKA and SP, but not CGRP injected into the rat paw, induce hyperalgesia as measured using a paw pressure test (Nakamura-Craig and Gill 1991). In several *in vitro* preparations SP did not exhibit any excitatory effects in respect to nocifension and nociception (Mizumura *et al.* 1987; Cohen and Perl 1990; Kessler *et al.* 1992; Ault and Hildebrand 1993). Therefore, the pain from SP injection has been interpreted as a sensitizing action of the neuropeptide increasing the effect of the mild needle injury and of the mediators released by that. Compatible with this idea, enhanced responsiveness to BK and to combined inflammatory mediators following SP pretreatment has been described and found significant in the skin-nerve preparation *in vitro* (Mizumura *et al.* 1987; Kessler *et al.* 1992). Although the SP concentration needed to induce the sensitizing effect was rather high (10^{-5} M), it could not be attributed to HA release, since HA was already contained in the test solution of inflammatory mediators (Kessler *et al.* 1992). This study was later extended to CGRP, NKA, and combinations with SP. However, no sensitizing effect was encountered when, in this investigation, the neuropeptides were applied during 10 min of a sustained (30-min) stimulation with combined inflammatory mediators (Fig. 11.4). From these findings, we suggested a conditioning effect of SP on the chemosensitivity of cutaneous nociceptors that undergoes occlusion when the chemical response has fully developed. The sensitizing action of SP also did not extend to heat and mechanical responsiveness (Mizumura *et al.* 1987; Cohen and Perl 1990; Kessler *et al.* 1992).

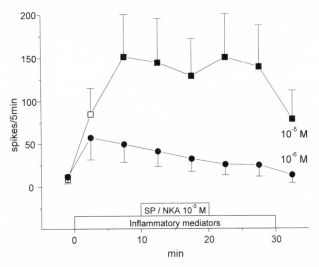

Fig. 11.4 Sustained application of inflammatory mediators to cutaneous nociceptors. In the rat skin-nerve preparation, a combination of inflammatory mediators (BK + 5-HT + HA + PGE$_2$) at concentrations of either 10^{-6} M or 10^{-5} M was superfused over the receptive fields of CMH fibres ($n = 15$ and 10). Only the higher concentration was able to induce sustained discharge which, in addition, was significantly (black square symbols; $p < 0.05$, U-test) higher in magnitude than with 10^{-6} M concentration. During the central 10 min, substance P (SP, $n = 6$) or neurokinin A (NKA, $n = 9$) was added to the superfusate but showed no modulatory effect. In other experiments (not shown) CGRP and combinations of SP + CGRP and SP + NKA also remained ineffective (Reischl, Steen, and Reeh, unpublished).

In cellular models using different sensory ganglion cells, there is converging evidence that SP (and NKA) induce sodium influx and blockade of several K$^+$ channels, which causes only transient depolarization because of rapid desensitization (Spigelman and Puil 1988; Ishimatsu 1994). In non-sensory neurones and in mast cells, SP effects are finally mediated through adenylyl cyclase activation and cAMP (Church *et al.* 1991; Shen and Suprenant 1993).

Cytokines: interleukins 1,6,8; tumour necrosis factor α

The cytokines, that is interleukins (IL) and tumour necrosis factor α (TNFα), are a family of proteins that are released mainly from monocytes/macrophages when activated in inflammation. They promote inflammation by mobilizing and stimulating other inflammatory cells and inducing fever (Goodman *et al.* 1991). In addition, IL-1β, IL-6, IL-8, and TNFα have been shown to induce the development of ipsi- and contralateral behavioural hyperalgesia following intraplantar injections in the rat. The effect was greatly reduced after pretreatment with indomethacin (Ferreira *et al.* 1988; Cunha *et al.* 1991, 1992). Evidence has been presented that PGE$_2$ levels in the perfusate are enhanced after infusion of 20 ng/ml IL-1β into the isolated rabbit ear. PGE$_2$ levels remained elevated for more than 3 hours after IL-1β cessation. PGE$_2$ liberation was antagonized with the cyclooxygenase inhibitor diclofenac as was the accompanying pain reflex by IL-1β infusion. These findings suggest secondary effects of the interleukins as a mechanism of action (Schweizer *et al.* 1988). Another secondary mechanism might be the stimulation of nerve growth factor (NGF) synthesis, which can induce mechanical hyperalgesia in which the sympathetic nervous system seems to be involved (Gadient *et al.* 1990; McMahon 1991; Yoshida and Gage 1992). NGF again exerts secondary effects through degranulation of mast cells thus liberating HA and, probably, 5-HT (Horigome *et al.* 1993).

Physicochemical stimuli

pH

Corrosive acids have long been known to produce severe pain when contacting skin or mucous membrane (for a review see Keele and Armstrong 1964). However, under pathological conditions increases of interstitial proton concentration have been observed yielding a local pH as low as 5.4 in inflammation and 5.7 in cardiac ischaemia (Häbler 1929; Jacobus *et al.* 1977). An intracellular pH value of 6.2 is reached within 2 min in human quadriceps muscle during exhausting and painful isometric contraction (Pan *et al.* 1988). Two mechanisms contribute to the inflammatory acidification. First, though local perfusion is increased in inflamed tissue, cells switch to anaerobic glycolysis due to a relative ischaemia caused by imbalance of perfusion and massive increase in local metabolism. Second, pumps exist, for example, in leucocytes that actively transport lactic acid into the interstitial space (McCarty *et al.* 1966). In psychophysical experiments, buffer solutions of pH 6.2 were found to be painful when injected intracutaneously or applied to blister base (Keele and Armstrong 1964). However, pain appeared transient which is probably due to the high buffering capacity of the tissue and the removal of protons from the injection site via the bloodstream. Similarly, pain sensations have been reported from CO_2 pulses applied to the nasal mucosa resulting in low pH by hydration (Kobal and Hummel 1990; Anton *et al.* 1992). In recent work, an intracutaneous pressure infusion of pH 5.2 buffer was found to produce sustained pain that increased with flow rate. In addition, hyperalgesia in response to punctate pressure stimulation occurred (Steen and Reeh, 1993*b*).

The psychophysical model of sustained pain from acidic buffer infusion has meanwhile been used to study the interaction between tissue acidosis and inflammatory mediators (BK, 5-HT, HA, PGE_2). The combined mediators, painful by themselves when injected into the skin, greatly enhanced the acidotic pain in a more than additive and dose-dependent way. Even small, hardly perceivable doses of the inflammatory mediators left the skin of volunteers with a sustained sensitization to subsequent pH-stimulation (Steen *et al.* 1996). The psychophysical model was also used to follow up previous indications that salicylic acid might antagonize mechanisms of pH-sensitivity (Barker and Levitan 1972). Indeed, salicylic acid but also acetysalicylic acid (aspirin), indomethacin and ibuprofen potently reduced the acidotic pain when topically applied to the painful skin area in different formulations. The drug effects were competitive (with the intensity of pH-stimulation), dose-dependent, and local, that is, independent of systemic absorption. In addition, a local anaesthetic action, as shown for benzocaine cream, could be excluded for the NSAIDs (Steen *et al.* 1995, 1996).

PH-effects on nociceptors and nocifensive reflexes were discovered relatively late, since *in vitro* techniques or recording from the non-vascularized cornea were required to gain control over the chemical environment of nociceptors (Steen *et al.* 1990). Corneal nociceptors were shown to be driven by acetic acid, and cutaneous nociceptors *in vitro* begin to discharge at pH values between 6.1 and 6.9 (Belmonte *et al.* 1991; Steen *et al.* 1992). The C-fibre activity increases with lower pH values down to pH 5.2 and continues for half an hour and longer without adaptation at constant superfusion. Lower pH values than 5.2 elicit smaller nociceptor responses, probably due to a developing conduction block at sodium channel sites (Hille 1992). The excitatory effect probably depends on intracellular acidification, since solutions of the membrane-permeant CO_2 are more effective than phosphate-buffered solutions of the same pH 6.1. In addition, the carboanhydrase blocker acetazolamide reversibly reduced the excitatory effect of CO_2 (Steen *et al.* 1992). The latter finding has recently been corroborated with lingual nerve recordings from chemosensory units responding to CO_2 superfusion of the rat tongue (Komai and Bryant 1993; Bryant and Moore 1995).

The pH-sensitivity in the skin-nerve preparation *in vitro* has been further investigated by searching for possible blockers of the mechanism. In a preparation of the urinary bladder, ruthenium red had been found to block a pH-induced release of neuropeptides from capsaicin-sensitive nerve endings (Maggi *et al.* 1988; Geppetti *et al.* 1991). In cutaneous nociceptors, however, ruthenium red did not affect the pH-responsiveness, even at concentrations that effectively reduced the excitotoxicity of capsaicin. Moreover, the compound (10^{-5} M) was found to induce bursting discharge in nociceptors in a concentration-dependent way (St. Pierre and Reeh, unpublished). This finding agreed with a neurogenic inflammation reported from topical application of ruthenium red to the rabbit eye (Anderssen and Legreves 1991). A calcium channel blocker, diltiazem, at 10^{-3} M concentration was reported to selectively block the pH-sensitivity of corneal nociceptors (Pozo *et al.* 1992). This effect could dose-dependently be confirmed in cutaneous nociceptors; it was, however, accompanied by a concomitant loss of the mechanical and heat responsiveness and of the electrical excitability of the nerve endings. A use-dependent conduction block by diltiazem, similar to the action of local anaesthetics, had to be concluded (Wegner *et al.* 1996).

Two of the above psychophysical findings on pH-induced pain found support from *in vitro* studies: Acetylsalicylic acid caused a reduction of pH-dependent sustained discharge in nociceptors at a concentration of 10^{-4} M which is in the range of plasma levels in rheumatic patients under aspirin treatment. A similar effect of salicylic acid seemed to be obscured by an intrinsic excitatory action of the drug at higher concentrations (Stefanidis *et al.* 1994). The second finding supported *in vitro* was the synergism of low pH with inflammatory mediators in exciting nociceptors. The acidification of the inflammatory combination (BK, 5-HT, HA, PGE_2 10^{-6} M, pH 6.1) recruited a considerably larger population of polymodal nociceptors than either pH alone or inflammatory mediators. In addition, the chemical responses were markedly enhanced, and the tachyphylaxis of the inflammatory mediators was counteracted by acidification (Steen *et al.*, 1995). In spite of the actions of aspirin, PGE_2 does not seem to play a major role in this synergistic interaction (see 'Eicosanoids', this chapter).

As far as the mechanism of pH-induced excitation is concerned, essential information has come from biophysical studies on DRG cells. Intracellular voltage recording from the intact DRG *in vitro* has consistently shown a pH-dependent sustained depolarization without firing independently of the conduction velocity of the peripheral axon. In parallel, the excitability and the action potential amplitude decreased (Tegeder and Reeh 1993). Thus, these 'sensory' cells did not behave like a model of their own peripheral nerve endings upon pH challenge. This seems to change, to a certain extent, when DRG cells are dissociated, cultivated, and recorded using the patch-clamp technique in the whole-cell mode. Two different types of inward current have been described for such conditions. Protons, in most cells, induce a fast sodium inward current that inactivates at a time constant of 0.5 s and is due to a proton-gated and -transformed calcium channel with activation starting at pH 7.0 and a maximum flux at around pH 6.0 (Krishtal and Pidoplichko 1980; Konnerth *et al.* 1987; Davies *et al.* 1988; Morad and Gallewaert 1989). A second pH-induced cation conductance was found to exist only in the subpopulation of DRG neurones that is sensitive to capsaicin which is generally taken as a criterion for nociceptive properties (Bevan and Yeats 1991). Acidic solutions of a pH below 6.2 induce this sustained depolarizing current that inactivates slowly and increases in amplitude with increasing proton concentration (Bevan and Yeats 1991). The current was enhanced significantly when a solution of low pH (6.1) was applied together with a combination of inflammatory mediators that by itself hardly evoked any conductance change (BK, 5-HT, HIS, and PGE_2; Fig. 11.5). Similarly, protons were observed to dose-dependently facilitate the capsaicin-induced inward current (Petersen and LaMotte 1993). However, no corresponding findings yet exist on primary afferents. In addition to excitatory effects, protons have long been known to inhibit voltage-dependent sodium channels and, thus, to exert local anaesthetic effects (Hille 1992). Since in primary afferents the excitatory effects have been demonstrated to predominate at pathophysiological pH levels, the molecular transduction mechanism in the nerve endings should be further elucidated as well.

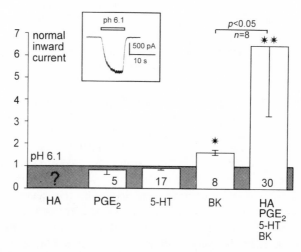

Fig. 11.5 Normalized inward currents of capsaicin-sensitive DRG neurones from 1-day-old dissociated cultures from the rat. The grey base represents the normalized amplitude of the pH-induced current (see also inset). Columns represent normalized peak currents induced by inflammatory mediators (all at 10^{-5} M) at pH 6.1 with PGE_2 and 5-HT having no modulatory effect. BK significantly enhances the pH response (*$p < 0.05$). The sensitizing effect of the mediator combination is significant as compared to pH 6.1 (**$p < 0.001$) and significantly greater than that of BK alone ($p < 0.05$). No data are yet available for HA (?). Numbers give the totals of cells investigated with the whole-cell patch-clamp technique (Kress, Vylicky, and Reeh, unpublished).

Nitric oxide

Only recently, the endothelial-derived relaxation factor (EDRF) turned out to be the radical gas nitric oxide (NO˙) produced in many different kinds of cells. NO˙ is generated from L-arginine by nitric oxide synthase (NOS) for which several subtypes exist. A constituent form of NOS has been found in the central nervous system whereas primary afferent neurones in the DRG express the inducible form under conditions of peripheral inflammation. In the periphery, NO˙ is released from endothelium and from activated white blood cells, for example, macrophages, during inflammation (for a review see Moncada and Higgs 1991). It therefore must be considered as a constituent of the inflammatory environment. Once generated, NO˙ is rapidly inactivated by non-enzy-matic oxidation when oxygen is present. It therefore has a half-life of seconds only. However, it is lipid-soluble and can rapidly permeate membranes. Since NO˙ is unstable in aqueous solutions containing oxygen, experimental use is restricted to NO˙ donors, such as SIN-1 (3-morpholino-sydnone imine), or to NOS antagonists, such as *N*-monomethyl-L-arginine (L-NMMA) (Feelisch 1991).

From behavioural models indirect evidence was presented for analgesic NO˙ effects when the analgesic action of myrcene and dipyrone was abolished with the NOS inhibitor L-NMMA (Duarte *et al.* 1990, 1992). However, in psychophysical experiments, NO˙ solutions injected intradermally produced pain, dose-dependently with a threshold of 12 nM, and reached a maximum pain rating at 50 nM (Holthusen and Arndt 1994). This was corroborated by single-fibre recordings *in vitro*, when NO˙ gas 0.126 per cent in nitrogen was directly applied to the fluid over cutaneous receptive fields that evoked nociceptor-discharge and induced mechanical sensitization, although both effects were not very prominent (Kress *et al.* 1994).

Several secondary pathways have been reported that can be activated by NO˙. As a radical it can attack membrane lipids, proteins, or nucleic acids and thus induce long-term modifications. Well established is the activation of soluble guanylyl cyclase forming cGMP, which in turn can open or inhibit ion channels directly or by phosphorylation via protein kinases. Second, cAMP levels can be decreased by stimulation of phosphodies-terases through cGMP (for reviews see Garthwaite 1991; Meller and Gebhart 1993). Nociceptor excitation and sensitization, however, presumably do not depend on cGMP since stable analogues of the nucleotide did not excite nor sensitize cutaneous afferents *in vitro* (Kress, M., Rödl, J., and Reeh, P.W., submitted for publication).

Potassium ions

Potassium is the predominant intracellular cation (around 140 mM), and the extra-cellular concentration can rise rapidly following cell damage. Because of its depolarizing action, potassium was expected to produce pain. Isotonic concentrations of potassium salts caused burning pain in human subjects when applied close to skin cuts or to a blister base and when injected into muscle. Dose-dependency of the potassium-induced pain was observed with a threshold at 55 mM. After a short delay, a burning pain was recorded with accompanying hyperalgesia that subsided and left the site of application anaesthetized (Keele and Armstrong 1964). Though potassium ions non-specifically excited all classes of afferents, close-arterial injections of twice isotonic KCl solution could be used to separate sympathetic efferents from unmyelinated afferent units in nerve branches innervating the cat knee joint. However, the effects of potassium on nociceptive afferents have not been studied in detail (Kanaka *et al.* 1985; Schaible and Schmidt 1988).

Increasing the extracellular potassium concentration in the tissue blocks potassium outflow in the nerve endings. This can also be achieved using pharmacological tools, 4-aminopyridine (4-AP) and tetraethylammonium (TEA), which induce sustained bursting activity in all cutaneous fibre classes when applied to receptive fields *in vitro* (Kirchhoff *et al.* 1992). This is in contrast to a relatively minor depolarization upon 4-AP application in neurones of the isolated spinal ganglion (Waddell *et al.* 1989). On the other hand, if the ongoing discharge in fibres were due to a major depolarization, one would expect a conduction block to develop by sodium channel inactivation. This is probably the case with depolarization and excitation enforced by high extracellular potassium concentration and accounts for the transient pain and subsequent anaesthesia in the blister base experiments.

C nociceptors, however, may be the least sensitive of all fibre classes to conduction block by depolarization. A proportion of unmyelinated nerve endings in the rat (25 per cent: mechanoheat-sensitive, mechanocold-sensitive, and high-threshold mechanoreceptor C-fibres) is definitely insensitive to the blocking action of tetrododoxin (TTX) which means that they generate and conduct action potentials by means of a TTX-resistant sodium channel (Kirchhoff *et al.* 1989). This channel, however, is known to need stronger depolarization in order to become inactivated than does the TTX-sensitive sodium channel in all other peripheral nerve endings (Hille 1992). Partial TTX-resistance of C-fibres in peripheral nerve has recently been confirmed using grease-gap recording from rat dorsal roots (Grafe, personal communication).

Free radicals

Hydrogen peroxide and the oxygen radicals, superoxide anion and hydroxyl radical, are generated in high quantities upon inflammation, for example from activated leucocytes (Halliwell and Gutteridge 1989). For example, millimolar concentrations have been measured in the supernatant of leucocytes during oxidative burst (Cochrane *et al.* 1988). They are synthesized by various sets of enzymes or released from electron transport chains in mitochondria. Drugs eliminating the action of radicals, for example, superoxide dismutase or selenoenzymes, have been used to treat arthritic pain with limited success (Parnham and Graf 1987). Superoxide dismutase reduced oedema formation in Freud's adjuvant arthritis or following carrageenan injection by 20 per cent only (Hirschelmann and Bekemeier 1981). This is in line with recent findings *in vitro* that oxygen radicals excited nociceptors only occasionally and non-specifically, and that only a mild facilitation of their chemical responses occurred with superfusion of 1 mM hydrogen peroxide (Kress *et al.* 1995a). Extreme concentrations of hydrogen peroxide (300 mM), however, activated cardiac vagal afferents in the rat (Ustinova and Schultz 1994). Reactive oxygen species probably contribute to the development and maintenance of inflammation by chemotactic effects and by activating thrombocytes rather than by having direct excitatory effects (Salvemini *et al.* 1989).

Due to their aggressive chemistry, oxygen radicals can achieve a variety of biological effects. Enzymes, for example, guanylyl-cyclase, become activated while others like Ca^{2+}- and Na^+-K^+-ATPase and glutamine synthase have been found to be inactivated

(Weiss 1986). Furthermore, prostacyclin release and thromboxane synthesis are stimulated (Polgar and Taylor 1980; Marshall *et al.* 1984). Which mechanisms are active in nociceptors, if any, is unclear at present.

Exogenous compounds

Capsaicin

Capsaicin (8-methyl-vanillyl-6-nonenamide) is the pungent compound in hot peppers. Its topical application to skin and mucous membranes has long been known to cause an intense burning sensation and flare reaction, initially, while repeated or prolonged application leads to desensitization (Keele and Armstrong 1964; Maggi and Meli 1988). Capsaicin can be detected by tasting at 10^{-7} M, whereas the threshold concentration for evoking pain on the tongue was reported to be 10^{-6} M (Keele and Armstrong 1964). Upon single intradermal injection, the lowest concentration of capsaicin to produce a burning pain sensation was in the micromolar range (0.1 µg in 100 µl vehicle; Simone *et al.* 1989). Also, injection into paravenous tissue and occluded small finger veins (but not perfusion of larger hand-vein segments) was reported to be painful (Arndt *et al.* 1993). In addition, mechanical and heat hyperalgesia occurred within seconds following intradermal injection and, with higher doses, the hyperalgesia reached a maximum within 7 min and decreased later on (Culp *et al.* 1989; Simone *et al.* 1989; Simone and Ochoa 1991). Recently evidence was presented that different qualities of hyperalgesia appear in three zones around the injection site with the largest one being hyperalgesic to normally painful mechanical stimulation, the medium-sized zone exhibiting tenderness to gentle stroking of the skin, and the smallest area being hyperalgesic to heat. All changes returned to normal within 24 hours (LaMotte *et al.* 1991). With four times a day total application for 6 weeks, 0.075 per cent capsaicin at first induced burning pain which decreased in magnitude and duration with time. Pain thresholds with heat stimulation were initially lowered but became elevated by the end of the chronic treatment. Simultaneously, suprathreshold pain ratings decreased. In contrast, mechanical pain thresholds and ratings were not affected. All changes recovered within 2 weeks after capsaicin discontinuation (Simone and Ochoa 1991).

A correlative study in humans investigated single nociceptive afferents that responded to topical capsaicin application to the skin or intracutaneous injection and that were, in addition, sensitized to heat but not to mechanical stimulation (LaMotte *et al.* 1992). Only mechanoheat-responsive C and Aδ fibres responded in rat skin to topical application or intracutaneous and close arterial injections, and heat sensitization could be observed (Szolcsányi *et al.* 1988; Baumann *et al.* 1991). No changes in mechanical responsiveness were found in nociceptive afferents that could account for the hyperalgesic effects of capsaicin in humans or for the sensitization of dorsal horn neurones and the expansion of their receptive fields after intradermal capsaicin in the monkey. With superfusion of cutaneous receptive fields by controlled concentrations of capsaicin *in vitro*, 87 per cent of C-fibres, including mechanoheat- and mechanocold-sensitive units were found to be affected by the agent. However, even at threshold concentration (10^{-7}, 10^{-6}, or 10^{-5} M), one-third of the nerve endings exhibited desensitization to mechanical stimulation as a first sign of the capsaicin action, without discharging a single spike (St. Pierre and Reeh, unpublished). Thus, excitatory (in the other two-thirds of the sample) and neurotoxic effects of capsaicin are difficult to separate on the basis of concentration. After capsaicin, responsiveness to heat stimulation of single unmyelinated cutaneous and corneal afferents *in vivo* was sometimes lost completely but recovered within 1 day. In parallel, mechanical responsiveness in the cat cornea was strongly depressed at 0.3 or 3.3 mM concentration and the SP content of the rat skin was decreased for up to 4 days following 33 mM topical capsaicin application (Belmonte *et al.* 1991; Lynn *et al.* 1992). Even more neurotoxic, capsaicin applied to a peripheral nerve leads to a permanent and selective block in a large population of primary afferent C fibres (Petsche *et al.* 1983; Waddell and Lawson 1989).

Capsaicin causes a depolarization in small sensory DRG neurones, and, simultaneously, an unspecific cation current can be recorded that is carried by calcium and sodium ions (Baccaglini and Hogan 1983; Bevan and Forbes 1988; Wood *et al.* 1988; Petersen *et al.* 1989; Vlachová and Vyklicky 1993). In addition, potassium permeability may be reduced (Petersen *et al.* 1987). The cation conductance is not abolished by conventional calcium and sodium blockers, such as nifedipine, ω-conotoxin, and tetrodotoxin, but the toxic calcium influx is greatly reduced by ruthenium red (Wood *et al.* 1988; Dray *et al.* 1990). This dye also attenuated activation of nociceptors and the release of neuropeptides (Maggi *et al.* 1988; Amann 1990; Dray *et al.* 1990; St. Pierre and Reeh, unpublished). Other intracellular actions comprise an increase in cGMP levels and DAG, IP_3, and arachidonic acid release, which, probably, are secondary to calcium influx (Wood *et al.* 1989; Dray 1992). To account for the activation of nociceptors a specific receptor has been postulated that binds capsaicin and related compounds such as the partial antagonist capsazepine and the potent agonist resiniferatoxin (for reviews see Dray 1992; Szallasi 1994). As a possible endogenous mechanism operating at the capsaicin receptor site, the action of hydrogen ions, that is intracellular acidosis, has been suggested because large similarities exist between capsaicin- and pH-induced cellular effects and a positive interaction of the two stimuli has been reported (Bevan and Geppetti 1994; Petersen and LaMotte 1993).

Formalin

Formalin, as used in the popular formalin test (after Dubuisson and Dennis 1977), is a rather badly defined chemical irritant. The commercially available solution contains 35–40 per cent paraformaldehyde (usually 37 per cent) but, in addition, 10 per cent methanol to prevent formic acid development. When diluted to a '2.5 per cent' solution, as mostly used, the final concentration is about 0.9 per cent paraformaldehyde (308 mM) and 0.25 per cent methanol. However, the dilution is usually done using isotonic saline and thus results in a twice hypertonic final solution, which may become irritant by its osmotic pressure (see below). Quantitative comparisons with pure and fresh solutions of paraformaldehyde in water are lacking, but preliminary results (unpublished) from our laboratory suggest a similar excitatory potency and time course of action for both sorts of formalin solutions. Also, methanol (0.25 per cent) did not excite a number of cutaneous nociceptors *in vitro*. Even so, the active irritant principle of formalin is actually unknown, since formaldehyde in water becomes hydrated to form methylene glycol, a detergent and cryoprotectant. The equilibrium between both chemicals is greatly in favour of the glycol, which is the substance penetrating rapidly while the small proportion of 'carbonylformaldehyde' fixes the tissue by cross-linking macromolecules (see Fox *et al.* 1985).

The formalin pain model has recently been extensively reviewed (Porro and Cavazzutti 1993). This thorough survey shows that formalin responses have been extensively studied on various levels of the CNS, but only preliminary reports are available on primary afferent responses to formalin (Russell *et al.* 1987; Saade' *et al.* 1988; Klemm *et al.* 1989; Puig and Sorkin 1994). Much of the concurrent interest in formalin pain has focused on the distinct biphasic pain-related behaviour that occurs after formalin injection in rodents, but not in other species including humans who experience a prolonged, monophasically declining pain sensation (Porro and Cavazzutti 1993). In particular, the second phase of formalin pain has stimulated much experimental work and a number of explanatory hypotheses that fall into two major groups: (1) formalin causes a chemical injury with transient nociceptor discharge followed by an acute inflammation, which, through its mediators, induces a prolonged second phase of primary afferent activity (for example, Hunskaar *et al.* 1986); (2) the injury discharge triggers spinal mechanisms of sensitization that amplify the decreasing input from the periphery in such a way that a second phase of neuronal discharge in the dorsal horn and pain-related behaviour result (Dickenson and Sullivan 1987). Crucial for a decision between both theses is obviously the question as to how much primary afferent input is present during the second as compared to the first phase of the formalin response. All available evidence from primary afferent recording indicates a prominent second phase of peripheral input through nociceptive C and Aδ fibres (Saade' *et al.* 1988; Klemm *et al.* 1989; Puig and Sorkin 1994). However, the studies do not permit a quantitative conclusion, since formalin was applied more or less directly to the receptive field of each individual fibre or fibre bundle, and it is unknown how a large population of nociceptors would respond to the 'blind' injection of formalin into the innervation territory of a cutaneous nerve. Therefore, extrapolations from single-fibre to population responses are needed.

Previous and recent work, both *in vivo* and *in vitro*, has confirmed that formalin excites almost every single nerve ending of any sensory category and fibre class (Klemm *et al.* 1989; Puig and Sorkin 1994). Sufficient concentration (100–308 mM) and exposure time (3 min) lead to a complete desensitization of all sensory endings to physical and repeated formalin stimulation; occasional recovery (within 1 hour) only occurred among nociceptors. Lower concentrations (1–10–30 mM) can induce nociceptor sensitization to heat but not mechanical stimulation (Klemm *et al.* 1989). *In vivo* as *in vitro*, a late phase of activity, following injury discharge and a subsequent silent period, only developed in Aδ and C fibres, but in almost every single case, and it reached the initial discharge rate, on average, when near-threshold concentrations (1–30 mM) of formalin had been applied *in vitro* (see fig. 3 in Klemm *et al.* 1989; Porro and Cavazzutti 1993; Puig and Sorkin 1994). The *in vitro* study has recently been extended to include a number of polymodal nociceptors ($n = 15$ C fibres) that were all incubated with 308 mM formalin for 3 min: 12 units developed a second phase of discharge reaching a peak rate, on average per minute, that was markedly higher than during the initial injury response (Riedl and Reeh, unpublished). Even the instantaneous firing frequencies were, at the very least, not lower since spikes tended to occur in bursts or clusters during the second phase of formalin-induced discharge. By the time of this sustained activity, the electrical excitability of the nerve endings was lost, but maintained in the axons passing through saphenous nerve branches *in vitro* (Riedl and Reeh, unpublished). Thus, we assume that the axon stump, severed by the formalin injury, becomes an ectopic generator of spikes just as cut, strangled, or otherwise impaired axons in other models (of neuropathy) can become generators of discharge (see Linsney, Chapter 20, this volume). Explanatory support for this assumption comes from voltage-clamp studies on muscle fibres, in which formalin (40 mM) inhibits the sodium channel inactivation (Nonner *et al.* 1980). Following an eventual action potential, this produces a sustained afterdepolarization that, in close vicinity to intact membrane sections, could well act as a spike generator.

The temporal profiles reported for formalin-induced primary afferent discharge in the rat closely resemble the time course of pain-related behaviour in rodents (Russell *et al.* 1987; Saade' *et al.* 1988; Klemm *et al.* 1989; Porro and Cavazzutti 1993; Puig and Sorkin 1994). Onset and duration of the second phase discharge seem to be exactly the same *in vivo* as *in vitro* in the superfused skin-nerve preparation, where blood-borne mediators, platelets, and inflammatory cells are absent (Klemm *et al.* 1989; Puig and Sorkin 1994). This is an argument against the undoubted inflammatory response being essential for the second phase of formalin-induced pain. A selective reduction of this particular response phase by NSAIDs would, therefore, argue for a more direct antinociceptive rather than anti-inflammatory action (Hunskaar *et al.* 1986).

'Blind' injection of formalin into the cutaneous tissue will expose nociceptive nerve endings to high concentrations of the irritant which will result in a more prominent second as compared to first phase of induced discharge, according to the above findings *in vitro*. In addition, in the border zone of the injection bleb, formalin will slowly infiltrate adjacent nocireceptive fields, which again will predominantly induce a dominant second-phase response, according to recent single-fibre recordings from rat sural nerve (Puig and Sorkin 1994). The first phase of the sensory population response from formalin-injected skin will obviously be accentuated by the violent injury discharge of dying Aβ-mechanoreceptors (Klemm *et al.* 1989; Puig and Sorkin 1994). However, Aβ-fibre activity does not essentially contribute to spinal sensitization, which primarily depends on C-fibre input (for a review see Woolf 1994). Thus, at present, not much room seems to be left for spinal mechanisms to explain the biphasic pain-related behaviour of formalin-injected rodents.

Osmolarity and ionic environment

Exudates gained from inflamed pleural cavities or joints or from abscesses frequently exhibit an increased osmotic pressure. Elevations of up to threefold isotonic pressure have been found (Schade 1924; Häbler 1929). Secretory activity of inflammatory cells, extravasation of plasma proteins, and enzymatic breakdown of macromolecules are the probable reasons. Apart from the increased potassium and hydrogen ion concentrations, the compositions of the other electrolytes, in particular sodium chloride, are not consistently altered (Schade 1924; Häbler 1929). In spite of this fact, 'osmotic' effects in respect to pain have always been tested using hypertonic saline solutions. Sodium, however, being membrane-permeant may exert other than just osmotic actions. Injections of hypertonic saline or of distilled water into skin and muscle produce a sharp, burning pain that is typically followed by a period of anaesthesia lasting for at least half an hour (Keele and Armstrong 1964). The pain intensity depends on the saline concentration; the threshold corresponds to about twice hypertonic conditions (0.6 osm/l). The first report of pure non-ionic hypertonic solutions evoking pain comes from a new model in which isolated hand vein segments are perfused (Arndt and Klement 1991). Saline as well as glucose solutions of, at least, 1 osm/kg produced about equal intensities of aching pain. This is in contrast to intra- and subcutaneous injections, which are painless if fourfold hypertonic sucrose (with electrolytes at physiological concentration) is used, but which become very painful if the same concentration of saline is administered (Wedekind and Reeh, unpublished). The discrepancy may indicate the involvement of secondary mediators released from elements of the venous wall which is well known to respond to osmotic stress.

Hypertonic saline (5–10-fold isotonic) has also been used in respective single-fibre studies to excite 80–100 per cent of the slowly conducting primary afferents tested in cat skeletal muscle, dog scrotal contents, and cat colon (Iggo 1961; Kumazawa and Mizumura 1980; Haupt *et al.* 1983). In agreement with the excitatory effects of hypertonic saline, neuropeptide release has been reported from ocular and urinary bladder preparations (Mandahl *et al.* 1984; Maggi *et al.* 1990). An investigation, evaluating osmotic effects in more detail *in vitro*, has not yet been fully published (Wedekind and Reeh 1992; Reeh 1994). Isolated receptive fields of rat cutaneous mechanosensitive afferents were exposed to various hypertonic concentrations of sodium chloride and sucrose in a physiological electrolyte solution, to a half isotonic solution, and to distilled water. Hypertonic saline strongly excited about 85 per cent of the nociceptors and a third of the low-threshold mechanoreceptors with Aβ and C fibres; the effect was dose-dependent and started to occur at twice isotonic saline concentration. In striking contrast, hypertonic sucrose and distilled water induced only low–frequent ongoing activity, apparently unrelated to the actual stimulus concentration and to its on- and offset, in about half of the nociceptors tested; almost no discharge was induced in low-threshold mechanoreceptors. Half isotonic solutions were completely ineffective. The action of distilled water may be underestimated in the *in vitro* model, since sodium ions, essential for transduction and spiking, may be lacking to a greater extent than if distilled water was injected into the cutaneous tissue. Non-ionic hyperosmolarity, however, does not seem to be a strong stimulant to cutaneous nociceptors. Indicative for an excitatory role of the sodium ion itself was the observation that all nociceptive units superfused with distilled water (for 3 min) developed a violent *decrescendo* discharge for minutes when the superfusion was switched to isotonic electrolyte solution again. We assume that sensory nerve endings possess a relatively high resting conductance for sodium, possibly further challenged by distilled water, and that drastic elevations of the extracellular sodium concentration lead to sodium influx and depolarization.

A major consequence of strong hypertonic solutions (of any composition) and of distilled water, superfused over receptive fields for 3 min, was drastic or total desensitization to mechanical and partly to electrical stimulation of. the nerve endings. This desensitization occurred in about half of all units tested irrespective of receptor type and fibre class. Some of the units showed a recovery within 30 min or more, but only one desensitized unit recovered from superfusion of distilled water. Desensitization was not obviously correlated with previous excitation. These findings are in accord with the 'anaesthesia' reported from the psychophysical experiments (see above).

Osmotic stimuli were assumed to be ideal for challenging putative 'stretch (in)activated channels'. However, our study could not shed much light on this hypothetical concept of mechanical transduction. The effectiveness of osmotic gradient on cell volume depends entirely on membrane permeability, in particular to water. If this is very low, as is possibly the case with nerve endings, neither hyper- nor hypotonic environments can produce much shrinkage or swelling of the fibre terminal.

Mustard oil and other irritants

Mustard oil, as contained in mustard seeds and horseradish, is subsumed among a very heterogeneous group of organic chemicals named irritants. The only common principle of these agents is that they, more or less rapidly, induce irritant sensations without overtly damaging the tissue to which they are applied. The temporal spectrum of the actions runs from acute transdermal excitation of nociceptors, as with methylene chloride (paint remover), to slow induction of inflammation resulting in hyperalgesia within hours, as with topically applied arachidonic acid (Adriaensen *et al.* 1980; Young *et al.* 1984). Transitions from acute to chronic effects, however, are continuous, since, for example, mustard oil can excite nociceptors acutely as well as induce inflammation, depending on the concentration applied and the duration of exposure (Reeh *et al.* 1986; Heyer *et al.* 1991). A necessarily incomplete list of further irritants would contain the 'tear gases' (chloroacetophenon and 2-chlorobencylidene malononitrile), phenylbenzoquinon (as used in writhing tests in mice), and a number of solvents (xylene, acetone, chloroform, turpentine) that disrupt the epidermal barrier function and probably attack lipid nerve membranes (Woolf 1983; Szolcsányi 1984; Levine *et al.* 1986*b*). Irritants are known or assumed to act through toxic effects, while other chemicals used to induce inflammation and hyperalgesia, such as yeast, carrageenan, and Freud's complete adjuvant, depend entirely on the immunological response of the organism (Kocher *et al.* 1987; Russell *et al.* 1987; Bartho *et al.* 1990).

Mustard oil (allyl-iso-thiocyanate) appears to be the most frequently used irritant in research; one reason is that it easily penetrates the epidermis of hairy skin when topically applied. Diluted in ethanol or paraffin oil, mustard oil (10, 20, 30 per cent up to 100 per cent) induces a concentration-dependent burning pain sensation that fades away only after wash-off or complete evaporation (Magerl *et al.* 1990*a*; Heyer *et al.* 1991). Prolonged applications of higher concentration, in particular under an occlusive dressing, produce a burn-like, blistering lesion in human skin (Magerl *et al.* 1994). In human microneurography recordings, pain sensation was related to excitation of polymodal cutaneous C fibres, every single one of which was driven by the strong irritants methylene chloride and mustard oil (Adriaensen *et al.* 1980; Handwerker *et al.* 1991). Temporal, and probably spatial summation of C-fibre discharge was needed; low-frequency activity did not provoke any sensation (Adriaensen *et al.* 1980). In rat skin *in vivo*, minute amounts of dilute mustard oil (3 μl, 10 per cent) excited every polymodal C unit tested and, in addition, low-threshold C mechanoreceptors (Reeh *et al.* 1986). Transient sensitization to heat stimulation was most prominent after mustard oil treatment both in rat and human nociceptors. A lowering of the thresholds to punctate (von Frey) mechanical stimulation was not found in rats and inconsistent in humans (Reeh *et al.* 1986; Handwerker *et al.* 1991). Recordings from dorsal horn neurones in the rat spinal cord, however, revealed a sensitization to mechanical stimulation and an expansion of the mechanoreceptive 'firing zones' in the skin after (adjacent) mustard oil application (Woolf and King 1990). As a possible correlate in human psychophysics, mechanical hyperalgesia has been found to exceed an area of topical application of capsaicin which acts similarly to mustard oil in many respects (Szolcsányi 1984; Kilo *et al.* 1994).

The lack of peripheral, in contrast to spinal signs of mechanical sensitization has been interpreted as a central increase in neuronal excitability due to postsynaptic effects of neurotransmitters/neuromodulators released from spinal C-fibre terminals and triggered by the irritant-induced input (Woolf and King 1990). Even more sustained consequences of mustard oil treatment (to the nasal mucosa) could be visualized using immunocy-tochemical staining for the c-fos nuclear protein in trigeminal second-order neurones (Anton *et al.* 1991). The induced expression of c-fos was interpreted in terms of central plasticity challenged by the noxious chemical stimulation. Nonetheless, a final decision about a possible primary afferent contribution to mechanical sensitization from mustard oil (and other stimulants of nociceptors) appears premature for several reasons. Instillation of mustard oil into the urinary bladder of the cat not only induced intense discharges of sacral unmyelinated afferents but also enhanced their responsiveness to alterations of the intravesical pressure (Häbler *et al.* 1990). Even in skin a new aspect of nociceptor sensitization to mechanical stimulation has been described using mustard oil as an irritant (Schmelz *et al.* 1994). Employing transcutaneous electrical stimulation and microneurography recording in humans, receptive fields of polymodal C fibres have been shown to possess 'silent' extensions or spots where the units could hardly be driven by mechanical stimuli. After topical application of mustard oil, these sites became sensitive to noxious or even innocuous probing with von Frey hairs. Last but not least, there is a class of thinly myelinated nociceptors, high-threshold mechanoreceptors, that regularly exhibit a wide-range mechanical sensitization in rat skin in response to mechanical injury (Reeh *et al.* 1986). This type of fibre, with large receptive fields and high discharge rates, has not yet been systematically investigated using irritants or other chemical stimulants of nociceptors.

Conclusion

Exogeneous algogenic substances (irritants) have not contributed much to understand-ing the transduction mechanisms in nociceptive nerve endings that lead to sustained or chronic neural discharge and sensitization. Only capsaicin seems to partly act through a physiological mechanism involved in the nociceptor response to tissue acidosis. En-dogeneous mediators and related second messenger effects are generally held to explain the painful symptoms accompanying inflammatory and other diseases. Indeed, BK and 5-HT co-operate in exciting nociceptors, but this effect is prone to tachyphylaxis and adaptation. HA and PGE_2 do not, or only transiently, prevent this loss of excitatory action. In addition to exciting, BK induces a sensitization to heat that can lower the nociceptor thresholds into the temperature range of the body or of inflamed tissue. It is not known whether this sensitization is maintained during continuous presence of BK or other mediators.

Hyperosmolarity, reactive oxygen species, and transiently increased extracellular potassium levels, as found in inflamed tissues, cannot explain significant ongoing discharge in nociceptors nor sensitization. However, the tissue acidosis present in many painful conditions has specific excitatory and algogenic effects that are facilitated by the inflammatory mediators and vice versa. pH-induced pain and nociceptor discharge are non-adapting and sustained; aspirin and related compounds act as competitive antagonists. Unfortunately, no recent clinical data are available relating the time course of local pH to pain and hyperalgesia. The nociceptive nerve ending not only performs transduction but also spike train encoding, spike propagation, and, in addition, neurosecretion. Each of these properties may be the target of chemical mediators. The differentiation deserves more attention, in future studies.

References

Abelli, L., Geppetti, P., and Maggi, C.A. (1993). Relative contribution of sympathetic and sensory nerves to thermal nociception and tissue trophism in rats. *Neuroscience* **57**, 739–45.

Adriaensen, H., Gybels, J., Handwerker, H.O., and Van Hees, J. (1980). Latencies of chemically evoked discharges in human cutaneous nociceptors and of the concurrent subjective sensations. *Neurosci. Lett.* **20**, 55–9.

Agrawal, S.G. and Evans, R.H. (1988). The primary afferent depolarizing action of kainate in the rat. *Br. J. Pharmacol.* **87**, 345–55.

Akoev, G.N. (1981). Catecholamines, acetylcholine and excitability of mechanoreceptors. *Prog. Neurobiol.* **15**, 269–94.

Amann, R. (1990). Desensitization of capsaicin-evoked neuropeptide release—influence of Ca^{2+} and temperature. *Naunyn-Schmiedebergs Arch. Pharmacol.* **342**, 67–6.

Amanuma, F., Wakaumi, C., Tanaka, M., Muramatsu, M., and Aihara, H. (1984). The analgesic effects of non-steroidal anti-inflammatory drugs on acetylcholine-induced writhing in mice. *Folia Pharmacol. Jap.* **84**, 543–51.

Anderssen, S.E. and Legreves, P. (1991). Ruthenium red and capsaicin induce a neurogenic inflammatory response in the rabbit eye—effects of omega-conotoxin, GIVA and tetrodotoxin. *Eur. J. Pharmacol.* **209**, 175–83.

Anton, F., Herdegen, T., Peppel, P., and Leah, J.D. (1991). c-Fos-like immunoreactivity in rat brain stem neurons following noxious chemical stimulation of the nasal mucosa. *Neuroscience* **41**: 629–41.

Anton, F., Euchner, I., and Handwerker, H.O. (1992). Psychophysical examination of pain induced by defined CO_2 pulses applied to the nasal-mucosa. *Pain* **49**, 53–60.

Arndt, J.O. and Klement, W. (1991). Pain evoked by polymodal stimulation of hand veins in humans. *J. Physiol., London* **440**, 467–78.

Arndt, J.O., Kingden-Milles, D., and Klement, W. (1993). Capsaicin did not evoke pain from human hand vein segments but did so after injection into the paravascular tissue. *J. Physiol., London* **463**, 491–9.

Ashgar, A.U.R., McQueen, D.S., and MacDonald, A.E. (1992). Absence of effect of adenosine on the discharge of articular mechanoreceptors in normal and arthritic rats. *Br. J. Pharmacol.* **105**, 309.

Ault, B. and Hildebrand, L.M. (1993). L-glutamate activates peripheral nociceptors. *Agents Actions* **39**, C142–4.

Ault, B. and Hildebrand, L.M. (1994). $GABA_A$ receptor-mediated excitation of nociceptive afferents in the rat isolated spinal cord–tail preparation. *Neuropharmacology* **33**, 109–14.

Baccaglini, P.I. and Hogan, P.G. (1983). Some rat sensory neurons in cultures express characteristics of differential pain sensory cells. *Proc. natl Acad. Sci., USA* **80**, 594–8.

Barker, J.L. and Levitan, H. (1972). The antagonism between salicylate-induced and pH-induced changes in the membrane conductance of molluscan neurons. *Biochim. Biophys. Acta* **274**, 638–43.

Baron, R., Jänig, W., and Kollman, W. (1994). Sympathetic and afferent somata projecting in hindlimb nerves and the anatomical organization of the lumbar sympathetic nervous system of the rat. *J. comp. Neurol.* **275**, 460–8.

Bartho, L., Stein, C., and Herz, A. (1990). Involvement of capsaicin-sensitive neurones in hyperalgesia and enhanced opioid antinociception in inflammation. *Naunyn-Schmiedebergs Arch. Pharmacol.* **342**, 666–70.

Bauer, M.B., Meller, S.T., and Gebhart, G.F. (1992). Bradykinin modulation of a spinal nociceptive reflex in the rat. *Brain Res.* **578**, 186–96.

Baumann, T.K., Simone, D.A., Shain, C.N., and LaMotte, R.H. (1991). Neurogenic hyperalgesia: the search for the primary cutaneous afferent fibers that contribute to capsaicin-induced pain and hyperalgesia. *J. Neurophysiol.* **66**, 212–27.

Beck, P.W. and Handwerker, H.O. (1974). Bradykinin and serotonin effects on various types of cutaneous nerve fibers. *Pflügers Arch.* **347**, 209–22.

Belmonte, C., Gallar, J., Pozo, M.A., and Rebollo, I. (1991). Excitation by irritant chemical substances of sensory afferent units in the cat's cornea. *J. Physiol., London* **437**, 709–25.

Belmonte, C., Gallar, J., Lopez-Briones, L.G., and Pozo, M.A. (1994). Polymodality in nociceptive neurons: experimental models of chemotransduction. In *Cellular mechanisms of sensory processing* (ed. L. Urban), pp. 87–117. Springer, Berlin.

Bentley, G.A., Newton, S.H., and Starr, J. (1981). Evidence for an action of morphine and the enkephalins on sensory nerve endings in the mouse peritoneum. *Br. J. Pharmacol.* **73**, 325–32.

Bevan, S.J. and Forbes, C.A. (1988). Membrane effects of capsaicin on rat dorsal root ganglion neurones in cell culture. *J. Physiol., London* **433**, 145–61.

Bevan, S. and Geppetti, P. (1994). Protons: small stimulants of capsaicin-sensitive sensory nerves. *Trends Neurosci.* **17**, 509–12.

Bevan, S. and Yeats, J. (1991). Protons activate a cation conduuctance in a subpopulation of rat dorsal root ganglion neurones. *J. Physiol., London* **433**, 145–61.

Bradley, D. (1993). Frog venom cocktail yields a one-handed painkiller. *Science* **261**, 1117.

Brehm, S. and Reeh, P.W. (1994). Responsiveness of polymodal nociceptors to defined mechanical stimulation—effects of combined inflammatory mediators, additional PGE2 and of antipyretic analgesics. *Pflügers Arch.—Eur. J. Physiol.* **426**, R54.

Brown, D.A. and Higashida, H. (1988). Inositol 1,4,5 triphosphate and diacylglycerol mimic bradykinin effects on mouse neuroblastoma × rat gioma hybrid cells. *J. Physiol., London* **397**, 185–207.

Brune, K., Geisslinger, G., and Menzel-Soglowek, S. (1992). Pure enantionmers of 2-arylpropionic acids: tools in pain research and improved drugs in rheumatology. *J. Clin. Pharmacol.* **32**, 944–52.

Bryant, B.P. and Moore, P.A. (1995). Factors affecting the sensitivity of the lingual trigeminal nerve to acids. *Am. J. Physiol.* **268**, R58–R65.

Burgess, G.M., Mullaney, I., McNeill, M., Dunn, P.M., and Rang, H.P. (1989). Second messengers involved in the mechanism of action of bradykinin in sensory neurons in culture. *J. Neurosci.* **9**, 3314–25.

Chahl, L.A. (1988). Antidromic vasodilatation and neurogenic inflammation. *Pharmacol. Ther.* **37**, 275–300.

Church, M.K., Ellati, S., and Caulfield, J.P. (1991). Neuropeptide-induced secretion from human skin mast cells. *Int. Arch. Allergy appl. Immunol.* **94**, 310–18.

Cochrane, C.G., Schrauffstatter, I.U., Hyslop, P., and Jackson, I. (1988). Cellular and biochemical events in oxidant injury. In *Oxygen radicals in tissue injury* (ed. B. Halliwell), pp. 49–54. American Society for Experimental Biology, Bethesda, Maryland.

Coderre, T.J., Abbott, F.V., and Melzack, R. (1984). Effects of peripheral antisympathetic treatments on the tail-flick, formalin and autonomy-tests. *Pain* **18**, 13–23.

Cohen, R.H. and Perl, E.R. (1990). Contributions of arachidonic acid derivatives and substance P to the sensitization of cutaneous nociceptors. *J. Neurophysiol.* **64**, 457–64.

Culp, W.J., Ochoa, J., Cline, M., and Dotson, R. (1989). Heat and mechanical hyperalgesia induced by capsaicin. *Brain* **112**, 1317–31.

Cunha, F.Q., Lorenzetti, B.B., Poole, S., and Ferreira, S.H. (1991). Interleukin-8 as a mediator of sympathetic pain. *Br. J. Pharmacol.* **104**, 765–7.

Cunha, F.Q., Poole, S., Lorenzetti, B.B. and Ferreira, S.H. (1992). The pivotal role of tumour necrosis factor alpha in the development of inflammatory hyperalgesia. *Br. J. Pharmacol.* **107**, 660–4.

Davies, N.W., Lux, H.D., and Morad, M. (1988). Site and activation of proton-induced sodium current in chick dorsal root ganglion neurones. *J. Physiol., London* **400**, 159–87.

Davis, A.J. and Perkins, M.N. (1994). Induction of B1 receptors in vivo in a model of persistent inflammatory mechanical hyperalgesia in the rat. *Neuropharmacology* **33**, 127–33.

Deneris, E.S., Connolly, J., Rogers, S.W., and Duvoisin, R. (1991). Pharmacological and functional diversity of neuronal nicotinic acetylcholine receptors. *Trends Pharmacol. Sci.* **12**, 34–40.

Diamond, J. (1959). The effects of injecting acetylcholine into normal and regenerating nerves. *J. Physiol., London* **145**, 611–29.

Dickenson, A.H. and Sullivan, A.F. (1987). Peripheral origins and central modulation of subcutaneous formalin-induced activity of rat dorsal horn neurons. *Neurosci. Lett.* **83**, 207–11.

Dray, A. (1992). Therapeutic potential of casaicin-like molecules. Mechanism of action of capsaicin-like molecules on sensory neurons. *Life Sci.* **51**, 1759–65.

Dray, A., Forbes, C.A., and Burgess, G.M. (1990). Ruthenium red blocks the capsaicin-induced increase in intracellular calcium and activation of membrane currents in sensory neurones as well as the activation of peripheral nociceptors in vitro. *Neurosci. Lett.* **110**, 52–9.

Dray, A., Patel, I.A., Perkins, M.N., and Rueff, A. (1992*a*). Bradykinin-induced activation of nociceptors: receptor and mechanistic studies on the neonatal rat spinal cord–tail preparation in vitro. *Br. J. Pharmacol.* **107**, 1129–34.

Dray, A., Patel, I.A., Perkins, M.N., Rueff, A., and Urban, L. (1992*b*). Desensitization of bradykinin-induced activation of peripheral nociceptors. *Agents Actions* **38** (suppl.), 93–7.

Duarte, I.D.G., Lorenzetti, B.B., and Ferreira, S.H. (1990). Peripheral analgesia and activation of the nitric oxide–cyclic GMP pathway. *Eur. J. Pharmacol.* **186**, 289–93.

Duarte, I.D., dos Santos, I.R., Lorenzetti, B.B., and Ferreira, S.H. (1992). Analgesia by direct antagonism of nociceptor sensitization involves the arginine–nitric oxide–cGMP pathway. *Eur. J. Pharmacol.* **217**, 225–7.

Dubuisson, D. and Dennis, S.G. (1977). The formalin test: a quantitative study of the analgesic effects of morphine, mepyridine and brain stem stimulation in rats and cats. *Pain* **4**, 161–74.

Edery, H. and Lewis, G.P. (1962). Inhibition of plasma kininase activity at slightly acid pH. *Br. J. Pharmacol.* **19**, 299–305.

Escalier, A., Kayser, V., and Guilbaud, G. (1989). Influence of a specific 5-HT3 antagonist on carrageenan-induced hyperalgesia in rats. *Pain* **36**, 249–55.

Farr, M., Scott, D.L., Constable, T.J., Hawker, R.J., Hawkings, C.F., and Stuart, J. (1983). Thrombocytosis of active rheumatoid disease. *Ann. Rheum. Dis.* **42**, 545–9.

Feelisch, M. (1991). The biochemical pathways of nitric oxide formation from nitrovasodilators: appropriate choice of exogenous NO donors and aspects of preparation and handling of aqueous NO solutions. *J. Cardiovasc. Pharmacol.* **17**, S25–S33.

Ferreira, S.H., Lorenzetti, B.B., Bristow, A.F., and Poole, S. (1988). Interleukin-1b as a potent hyperalgesic agent antagonized by a tripeptide analogue. *Nature* **334**, 698–700.

Fock, S. and Mense, S. (1976). Excitatory effects of 5-hydroxytryptamine, histamine and potassium ions on muscular group IV afferent units: a comparison with bradykinin. *Brain Res.* **105**, 459–69.

Follenfant, R.L. and Nakamura-Craig, M. (1992). Glutamate induces hyperalgesia in the rat paw. *Br. J. Pharmacol.* **106**, 49P.

Fowler, J.C., Wonderlin, W.F., and Weinreich, D. (1985). Prostaglandins block a calcium-dependent afterhyperpolarization independent of effects on Ca^{2+} influx in visceral afferent neurones. *Brain Res.* **345**, 345–9.

Fox, A.J., Barnes, P.J., Urban, L., and Dray, A. (1993). An in-vitro study of the properties of single vagal afferents innervating guinea pigs airways. *J. Physiol., London* **469**, 21–35.

Fox, C.H., Johnson, F.B., Whiting, J., and Roller, P.P. (1985). Formaldehyde fixation. *J. Histochem. Cytochem.* **33**, 845–53.

Furchgott, R.F. and Vanhoute, P.M. (1989). Endothelium-derived relaxing and contracting factors. *FASEB* **3**, 2007–18.

Gadient, R.A., Cron, K.C., and Otten, U. (1990). Interleukin 1b and tumor necrosis factor-a synergistically stimulate nerve growth factor (NGF) release from cultured rat astrocytes. *Neurosci. Lett.* **117**, 335–40.

Gallagher, J.P., Nakamura, J., and Shinnick-Gallagher, P. (1983). The effects of temperature, pH and Cl^- pump inhibitors on GABA responses from cat dorsal root ganglia, *Brain Res.* **267**, 249–59.

Garthwaite, J. (1991). Glutamate, nitric oxide and cell–cell signalling in the nervous system. *Trends Neurosci.* **14**, 60–7.

Geppetti, P. (1993). Sensory neuropeptide release by bradykinin—mechanisms and pathophysiological implications. *Regulat. Peptides* **47**, 1–23.

Geppetti, P., DelBianco, E., Patacchini, R., Santicioli, P., Maggi, C.A., and Tramontana, M. (1991). Low pH-induced release of calcitonin gene-related peptide from capsaicin-sensitive sensory nerves—mechanisms of action and biological response. *Neuroscience* **41**, 295–30.

Goodman, A.G., Rall, T.W., Nies, A.S., Taylor, P. (ed.) (1991). *Goodman and Gilman's The pharmacological basis of therapeutics* (8th edn). Pergamon Press, New York.

Grando, S.A., Kist, D.A., Qi, M., and Dahl, M.V. (1993). Human keratinocytes synthesize, secrete and degrade acetylcholine. *J. Invest. Dermatol.* **101**, 32–6.

Greene, R.W. and Haas, H.L. (1991). The electrophysiology of adenosine in the mammalian central nervous system. *Prog. Neurobiol.* **36**, 329–41.

Grubb, B.D., Birrell, G.J., McQueen, D.S., and Iggo, A. (1991). The role of PGE2 in the sensitization of mechanoreceptors in normal and inflamed ankle joints of the rat. *Exp. Brain Res.* **84**, 383–92.

Häbler, C. (1929). Über den K- und Ca-Gehalt von Eiter und Exsudaten und seine Beziehungen zum Entzündungsschmerz. *Klin. Wochensch.* **8**, 1569–72.

Häbler, H.-J., Jänig, W., and Koltzenburg, M. (1990). Activation of unmyelinated afferent fibres by mechanical stimuli and inflammation of the urinary bladder in the cat. *J. Physiol., London* **425**, 545–62.

Halliwell, B. and Gutteridge, J.M.C. (1989). *Free radicals in biology and medicine* (2nd edn). Clarendon Press, Oxford.

Handwerker, H.O., Reeh, P.W., and Steen, K.H. (1990). Effects of 5HT on nociceptors. In *Serotonin and pain* (ed. J.-M. Besson), pp. 1–15. Elsevier Science, Amsterdam.

Handwerker, H.O., Forster, C., and Kirchhoff, C. (1991). Discharge patterns of human C-fibers induced by itching and burning stimuli. *J. Neurophysiol.* **66**, 307–15.

Haupt, P., Jänig, W., and Kohler, W. (1983). Response pattern of visceral afferent fibres, supplying the colon upon chemical and mechanical stimuli. *Pflügers Arch.—Eur. J. Physiol.* **398**, 41–7.

Heyer, G., Hornstein, O.P., and Handwerker, H.O. (1991). Reactions to intradermally injected substance P and topically applied mustard oil in atopic dermatitis patients. *Acta dermatovenerol., Stockholm* **71**, 291–5.

Higashi, H. and Nishi, S. (1982). 5-hydroxytryptamine receptors of visceral primary afferent neurones on rabbit nodose ganglia. *J. Physiol., London* **323**, 543–67.

Hille, B. (1992). *Ionic channels of excitable membranes.* Sinauer, Sunderland, Massachusetts.

Hirschelmann, R. and Bekemeier, H. (1981). Effects of catalase, peroxidase, superoxide dismutase and 10 scavengers of oxygen radicals in carrageenin edema arthritis of rats. *Experientia* **37**, 11313–114.

Hiss, E. and Mense, S. (1976). Evidence for the existence of different receptor sites for algesic agents at the endings of muscular group IV afferent units. *Pflügers Arch.—Eur. J. Physiol.* **362**, 141–6.

Holthusen, H. and Arndt, J.O. (1994). Nitric-oxide evokes pain in humans on intracutaneous injection. *Neurosci. Lett.* **165**, 71–4.

Holzer-Petsche, U. (1992). Blood pressure and gastric motor responses to bradykinin and hydrochloric acid injected into somatic or visceral tissues. *Naunyn-Schmiedebergs Arch. Pharmacol.* **346**, 219–25.

Horigome, K., Pryor, J.C., Bullock, E.D., and Johnson, E.M. (1993). Mediator release from mast-cells by nerve growth factor—neurotrophin specificity and receptor mediation. *J. biol. Chem.* **268**, 14881–7.

Hoyer, D., Clark, D.E., Fozard, J.R., Hartig, P.R., Martin, G.R., Mylecharane, E.J., Saxena, O.R., and Humphrey, P.P.A. (1994). VII. International Union of Pharmacology classification of receptors for 5-hydroxytryptamine (serotonin). *Pharmacol. Rev.* **46**, 157–203.

Hua, X.Y. and Yaksh, T.L. (1993). Pharmacology of the effects of bradykinin, serotonin, and histamine on the release of calcitonin gene-related peptide from C-fiber terminals in the rat trachea. *J. Neurosc.* **13**, 1947–53.

Hunskaar, S., Berge, O.-B., and Hole, K. (1986). Dissociation between antinociceptive and anti-inflammatory effects of acetylsalicylic acid and indomethacin in the formalin test. *Pain* **25**, 125–32.

Iggo, A. (1961). Non-myelinated afferent fibres from mammalian skeletal muscle. *J. Physiol., London* **155**, 52P–53P.

Ishimatsu, M. (1994). Substance-P produces an inward current by suppressing voltage-dependent and voltage-independent K^+ currents in bullfrog primary afferent neurons. *Neurosci. Res.* **19**, 9–20.

Jacobus, W.E., Taylor, G.J., Hollis, D.P., and Nunnally, R.L. (1977). Phosphorus nuclear magnetic resonance of perfused working rat hearts. *Nature* **265**, 756–8.

Jänig, W. and Morrison, J.F.B. (1986). Functional properties of spinal visceral afferents supplying abdominal and pelvic organs, with special emphasis on visceral nociception. *Progr. Brain Res.* **67**, 87–114.

Jänig, W. and Koltzenburg, M. (1991). Sympathetic reflex activity and neuroeffector transmission change after chronic nerve lesions. In *Proceedings of the VIth World Congress on Pain* (ed. M.R. Bond, J.E. Charlton, and C.J. Woolf), pp. 365–71. Elsevier, Amsterdam.

Juan, H. (1982). Nicotinic receptors on perivascular sensory nerve endings. *Pain* **12**, 259–64.

Kanaka, R., Schaible, H.-G., and Schmidt, R.F. (1985). Activation of fine articular afferent units by bradykinin. *Brain Res.* **327**, 81–90.

Kano, M., Kawakami, T., Hikawa, N., Hori, H., Takenaka, T., and Gotoh, H. (1994). Bradykinin-responsive cells of dorsal root ganglia in culture: cell size, firing, cytosolic calcium, and substance P. *Cell. Mol. Neurobiol.* **14**, 49–57.

Keele, C.A. and Armstrong, D. (1964). *Substances producing pain and itch.* Edward Arnold, London.

Kessler, W., Kirchhoff, C., Reeh, P.W., and Handwerker, H.O. (1992). Excitation of cutaneous afferent nerve-endings in vitro by a combination of inflammatory mediators and conditioning effect of substance-P. *Exp. Brain Res.* **91**, 467–76.

Khasar, S.G., Green, P.G., and Levine, J.D. (1993). Comparison of intradermal and subcutaneous hyperalgesic effects of inflammatory mediators in the rat. *Neurosci. Lett.* **153**, 215–18.

Kilo, S., Schmelz, M., Koltzenburg, M., and Handwerker, H.O. (1994). Different patterns of hyperalgesia induced by experimental inflammations in human skin. *Brain* **117**, 385–96.

Kirchhoff, C.G., Reeh, P.W., and Waddell, P.J. (1989). Sensory endings of C- and A-fibres are differentially sensitive to tetrodotoxin in the rat skin, in vitro. *J. Physiol., London* **418**, 116P.

Kirchhoff, C., Jung, S., Reeh, P.W., and Handwerker, H.O. (11990). Carrageenan inflammation increases bradykinin sensitivity of rat cutaneous nociceptors. *Neurosci. Lett.* **111**, 206–10.

Kirchhoff, C., Leah, J., Jung, S., and Reeh, P.W. (1992). Excitation of cutaneous sensory nerve endings in the rat by 4-aminopyridine and tetraethylammonium. *J. Neurosc.* **67**, 125–31.

Klemm, F., Carli, G., and Reeh, P.W. (1989). Peripheral neural correlates of the formalin test in the rat. *Pflügers Arch.—Eur. J. Physiol.* **414**, S42.

Kobal, G. and Hummel, T. (1990). Brain responses to chemical stimulation of the trigeminal nerve in man. In *Chemical senses* (ed. B.G. Green, J.R. Mason, and M.R. Kare), pp. 123–39. Dekker, Basel.

Kocher, L., Anton, F., Reeh, P.W., and Handwerker, H.O. (1987). The effect of carrageenan-induced inflammation on the sensitivity of unmyelinated skin nociceptors in the rat. *Pain* **29**, 363–73.

Koltzenburg, M. and McMahon, S.B. (1991). The enigmatic role of the sympathetic nervous system in chronic pain. *Trends pharmacol. Sci.* **12**, 399–402.

Koltzenburg, M., Kress, M., and Reeh, P.W. (1992). The nociceptor sensitization by bradykinin does not depend on sympathetic neurons. *Neuroscience* **46**, 465–73.

Komai, M. and Bryant, B.P. (1993). Acetazolamide specifically inhibits lingual trigeminal nerve responses to carbon dioxide. *Brain Res.* **612**, 122–9.

Konnerth, A., Lux, H.D., and Morad, M. (1987). Proton-induced transformation of calcium channel in chick dorsal root ganglion cells. *J. Physiol., London* **386**, 603–33.

Koppert, W., Reeh, P.W., and Handwerker, H.O. (1993). Conditioning of histamine by bradykinin alters responses of rat nociceptor and human itch sensation. *Neurosci. Lett.* **152**, 117–20.

Kress, M., Riedl, B., Rödl, J., and Reeh, P.W. (1994). Effects of nitric oxide, methylene blue and cyclic nucleotides on nociceptive nerve endings in rat skin *in vitro*. In *The biology of nitric acid*, Vol. 3. *Physiology and clinical aspects* (ed. S. Moncada, M. Feelisch, R. Busse, and E.A. Higgs), pp. 319–23. Portland Press, London.

Kress, M., Riedl, B., and Reeh, P.W. (1995). Effects of oxygen radicals on nociceptive afferents in the rat skin, in vitro. *Pain* **62**, 87–94.

Krishtal, O.A. and Pidoplichko, V.I. (1980). A receptor for protons in the nerve cell membrane. *Neuroscience* **5**, 2325–7.

Krishtal, O.A., Marchenko, S.M., and Obukhov, A.G. (1988). Cationic channels activated by extracellular ATP in rat sensory neurons. *Neuroscience* **27**, 995–1000.

Kumazawa, T., Mizumura, K., Minagawa, M., and Tsujii, Y. (1991). Sensitizing effects of bradykinin on the heat responses of the visceral nociceptor. *J. Neurophysiol.* **66**, 1819–24.

Kumazawa, T., Mizumura, K., and Koda, H. (1993). Involvement of EP3 subtype of prostaglandin E receptors in PGE2-induced enhancement of the bradykinin response of nociceptors. *Brain Res.* **632**, 321–4.

Kumazawa, T. and Mizumura, K. (1980). Chemical responses of polymodal receptors of the scrotal contents in dogs. *J. Physiol., London* **299**, 219–311.

Kumazawa, T. and Mizumura, K. (1984). Functional properties of the polymodal receptors in the deep tissues. In *Sensory receptor mechanisms* (ed. W. Hamann and A. Iggo), pp. 193–202. Singapore.

LaMotte, R. (1992). Subpopulations of 'nocifensor neurons' contributing to pain and allodynia, itch and alloknesis. *Am. Pain Soc. J.* **1**, 115–26.

LaMotte, R.H., Shain, C.N., Simone, D.A., and Tsai, E.-F. P. (1991). Neurogenic hyperalgesia: psychophysical studies of underlying mechanisms. *J. Neurophysiol.* **66**, 190–211.

LaMotte, R.H., Lundberg, L.E.,, and Torebjörk, H.E. (1992). Pain, hyperalgesia and activity in nociceptive C units in humans after intradermal injection of capsaicin. *J. Physiol., London* **448**, 749–64.

Lang, E., Novak, A., Reeh, P.W., and Handwerker, H.O. (1990). Chemosensitivity of fine afferents from rat skin in vitro. *J. Neurophysiol.* **63**, 887–901.

Levine, J.D., Lau, W., Kwiat, G., and Goetzl, E.J. (1984). Leukotriene B4 produces hyperalgesia that is dependent on polymorphonuclear leukocytes. *Science* **225**, 743–5.

Levine, J.D., Gooding, J., Donatoni, P., Borden, L., and Goetzl, E.J. (1985). The role of the polymorphonuclear leukocyte in hyperalgesia. *J. Neurosci.* **5**, 3025–9.

Levine, J.D., Lam, D., Taiwo, Y.O., Donatoni, P., and Goetzl, E.J. (1986a). Hyperalgesic properties of 15-lipoxygenase products of arachidonic acid. *Proc. natl Acad. Sci., USA* **83**, 5331–4.

Levine, J.D., Taiwo, Y.O., Collins, S.D., and Tam, J.K. (1986b). Noradrenaline hyperalgesia is mediated through interaction with sympathetic postganglionic neurone terminals rather than activation of primary afferent nociceptors. *Nature* **323**, 158–60.

Levine, J.D., Fields, H.L., and Basbaum, A.I. (1993). Peptides and the primary afferent nociceptor. [Review.] *J. Neurosci.* **13**, 2273–86.

Lynn, B., Ye, W., and Cotsell, B. (1992). The actions of capsaicin applied topically to the skin of the rat on C-fibre afferents, antidromic vasodilatation and substance P levels. *Br. J. Pharmacol.* **107**, 400–6.

Lynn, B. and Shakhanbeh, J. (1985). Substance P content of the skin, neurogenic inflammation and numbers of C-fibres following capsaicin application to a cutaneous nerve in the rabbit. *Neuroscience* **24**, 769–75.

McCarty, D.J., Phelps, P., and Pyenson, J. (1966). Crystal-induced inflammation in canine joints. *J. exp. Med.* **124**, 99–114.

MacIntyre, D.E. and Gordon, J.L. (1975). Calcium-dependent stimulation of platelet aggregation by PGE2. *Nature* **258**, 337–9.

McLachlan, E.M., Jänig, W., Devor, M., and Michaelis, M. (1993). Peripheral nerve injury triggers noradrenergic sprouting within dorsal root ganglia. *Nature* **363**, 543–6.

McMahon, S.B. (1991). Mechanisms of sympathetic pain. *Br. med. Bull.* **47**, 584–60.

Magerl, W., Grämer, G., and Handwerker, H.O. (1990a). Sensations and local inflammatory responses induced by application of carbachol dopamine, 5-HT, histamine and mustard oil to the skin in humans. *Pflügers Arch.—Eur. J. Physiol.* **415**, R107.

Magerl, W., Westerman, R.A., Mohner, B., and Handwerker, H.O. (1990b). Properties of transdermal histamine iontophoresis: differential effects of season, gender, and body region. *J. Invest Dermatol.* **94**, 347–52.

Magerl, W., Koltzenburg, M., Meyer-Jürgens, D., and Handwerker, H.O. (1994). The somatotopic organization of nociceptor-induced vascular response pattern reflects central nociceptive processing in humans. In *Proceedings of the 7th World Congress on Pain*, Vol. 2. *Progress in pain research and management* (ed. G.F. Gebhart, D.L. Hammond, and T.S. Jensen), pp. 843–56. IASP Press, Seattle.

Maggi, C.A. and Meli, A. (1988). The sensory-efferent function of capsaicin-sensitive sensory neurons. *Gen. Pharmacol.* **9**, 1–43.

Maggi, C.A., Santicolli, P., Geppetti, P., Parlani, M., Astolfi, M., Pradelles, P., Patacchini, R., and Meli, A. (1988). The antagonism induced by ruthenium red on the actions of capsaicin on the peripheral terminals of sensory neurons: further studies. *Eur. J. Pharmacol.* **154**, 1–10.

Maggi, C.A., Abelli, L., Giulani, S., Somma, V., Furio, M., Patacchini, R., and Meli, A. (1990). Motor and inflammatory effect of hyperosmolar solutions on the rat urinary bladder in relation to capsaicin-sensitive sensory nerves. *Gen. Pharmacol.* **21**, 97–103.

Mandahl, A., Brodin, E., and Bill, A. (1984). Hypertonic KCl, NaCl and capsaicin intracamerally cause release of substance P-like immunoreactive material into the aqueous humor in rabbits. *Acta Physiolog. Scand.* **120**, 579–84.

Manning, D.C., Raja, S.N., Meyer, R.A., and Campbell, J.N. (1991). Pain and hyperalgesia after intradermal injection of bradykinin in humans. *Clin. Pharmacol. Therapeut.* **50**, 721–9.

Marshall, P.J., Kulmacz, R.J., and Lands, W.E.M. (1984). Hydroperoxides, free radicals and prostaglandin synthesis in *Oxygen radicals in chemistry and biology*, pp. 299–307. Walter de Gruyter, Berlin.

Martin, H.A. (1990). Leukotriene B4 induced decrease in mechanical and thermal thresholds of C-fiber mechanonociceptors in rat hairy skin. *Brain Res.* **509**, 273–9.

Mei, L., Roeske, W.R., and Yamamura, H.I. (1989). Molecular pharmacology of muscarinic receptor heterogeneity. *Life Sci.* **45**, 1831–51.

Meller, S.T. and Gebhart, G.F. (1993). Nitric oxide (NO) and nociceptive processing in the spinal cord. *Pain* **52**, 127–36.

Mense, S. and Schmidt, R.F. (1974). Activation of group IV afferent units from muscle by algesic agents. *Brain Res.* **72**, 305–10.

Mizumura, K., Sato, J., and Kumazawa, T. (1987). Effects of prostaglandins and other putative chemical intermediaries on the activity of canine testicular polymodal receptors studied in vitro. *Pflügers Arch.* **408**, 565–72.

Mizumura, K., Minagawa, M., Tsujii, Y., Sato, J., and Kumazawa, T. (1990). Differences in augmenting effects of various sensitizing agents on heat and bradykinin responses of the testicular polymodal receptor. In *Proceedings of the VIth World Congress on Pain* (ed. M.R. Bond, J.E. Charlton, and C.J. Woolf), pp. 77–82. Elsevier, Amsterdam.

Mizumura, K., Sato, J., and Kumazawa, T. (1991). Comparison of the effects of prostaglandins E2 and I2 on testicular nociceptor activities studied in vitro. *Naunyn-Schmiedebergs Arch. Pharmacol.* **344**, 368–76.

Mizumura, K., Koda, H., and Kumazawa, T. (1993*a*). Augmenting effects of cyclic AMP on the heat response of canine testicular polymodal receptors. *Neurosci. Lett.* **162**, 75–7.

Mizumura, K., Minagawa, M., Tsujii, Y., and Kumazawa, T. (1993*b*). Prostaglandin E2-induced sensitization of the heat response of canine visceral polymodal receptors in vitro. *Neurosci. Lett.* **161**, 117–19.

Mizumura, K., Minagawa, M., Koda, H., and Kumazawa, T. (1994). Histamine-induced sensitization of the heat response of canine visceral polymodal receptors. *Neurosci. Lett.* **168**, 93–6.

Moncada, S. and Higgs, E.A. (1991). Endogenous nitric oxide: physiology, pathology and clinical relevance. *Eur. J. Clin. Invest.* **21**, 3611–74.

Morad, M. and Gallewaert, G. (1989). Proton-induced transformation of Ca^{2+} channel: possible mechanism and physiological role. 71–80.

Mulderry, P.K. (1994). Neuropeptide expression by newborn and adult rat sensory neurons in culture: effects of nerve growth factor and other neurotrophic factors. *Neuroscience* **59**, 673–88.

Nakamura-Craig, M. and Gill, B.K. (1991). Effect of neurokinin A, substance P and calcitonin gene related peptide in peripheral hyperalgesia in the rat paw. *Neurosci. Lett.* **124**, 49–51.

Neugebauer, V., Schaible, H.-G., and Schmidt, R.F. (1989). Sensitization of articular afferents to mechanical stimuli by bradykinin. *Pflügers Arch.* **415**, 330–5.

Ninkovic, M. and Hunt, S. (1985). Opiate and histamine H_1 receptors are present on some substance-P containing dorsal root ganglion cells. *Neurosci. Lett.* **53**, 133–7.

Nishi, K., Sakanashi, M., and Takenaka, F. (1977). Activation of afferent cardiac sympathetic nerve fibers of the cat by pain producing substances and by noxious heat. *Pflügers Arch.* **372**, 53–61.

Nonner, W., Spalding, B.C., and Hille, B. (1980). Low intracellular pH and chemical agents slow inactivation gating in sodium channels of muscle. *Nature* **284**, 360–3.

Ochoa, J.L. (1992). Reflex sympathetic dystrophy: a disease of medical understanding. *Clin. J. Pain* **8**, 363–6.

Pan, J.W., Hamm, J.R., Rothman, D.S., and Shulman, R.G. (1988). Intracellular pH in human skeletal muscle by ^1H NMR. *Proc. natl. Acad. Sci., USA* **85**, 7836–9.

Parnham, M.J. and Graf, E. (1987). Seleno-organic compounds and the therapy of hydroperoxide-linked pathological conditions. *Biochem. Pharmacol.* **36**, 3095–102.

Pedersen-Bjergaard, U., Nielsen, L.B., Jensen, K., Edvinsson, L., Jansen, I., and Olesen, J. (1991). Calcitonin gene-related peptide, neurokinin A and substance P: effects on nociception and neurogenic inflammation in human skin and temporal muscle. *Peptides* **12**, 333–7.

Pesin, S.R. and Candia, O. (1982). Acetylcholine concentration and its role in ionic transport by the cornea! epithelium. *Invest. Ophthalmol. vis. Sci.* **22**, 651–9.

Petersen, M. and LaMotte, R.H. (1993). Effect of protons on the inward current evoked by capsaicin in isolated dorsal root ganglion cells. *Pain* **54**, 37–42.

Petersen, M., Pierau, F.-K., and Weyrich, M. (1987). The influence of capsaicin on membrane currents in dorsal root ganglion neurones of guinea-pig and chicken. *Pflügers Arch.* **409**, 403–10.

Petersen, M., Wagner, G., and Pierau, F.-K. (1989). Modulation of calcium currents by capsaicin in a subpopulation of sensory neurones of guinea pig. *Naunyn-Schmiedebergs Arch. Pharmacol.* **339**, 184–91.

294

Petsche, U., Fleischer, E., Lembreck, F., and Handwerker, H.O. (1983). The effect of capsaicin application to a peripheral nerve on impulse conduction in functionally identified afferent nerve fibres. *Brain Res.* **265**, 233–40.

Piani, D., Frei, K., Do, K.Q., Cuénod, M., and Fontana, A. (1991). Murine brain macrophages induce NMDA receptor mediated neurotoxicity in vitro by secreting glutamate. *Neurosci. Lett.* **133**, 159–62.

Polgar, P. and Taylor, L. (1980). Stimulation of prostaglandin synthesis by ascorbic acid via hydrogen peroxide formation. *Prostaglandins* **19**, 693–700.

Porro, C.A. and Cavazzutti, M. (1993). Spatial and temporal aspects of spinal cord and brainstem activation in the formalin pain model. *Prog. Neurobiol.* **41**, 565–607.

Portilla, D., Mordhorst, M., Bertrand, W., and Morrison, A.R. (1988). Protein kinase C modulates phospholipase C and increases arachidonic acid release in bradykinin stimulated MDCK cells. *Biochem. biophys. Res. Communi.* **153**, 454–62.

Pozo, M.A., Gallego, R., Gallar, J., and Belmonte, C. (1992). Blockade by calcium antagonists of chemical excitation and sensitization of polymodal nociceptors in the cat's cornea. *J. Physiol., London* **450**, 1179–89.

Proud, D. and Kaplan, A.P. (1988). Kinin formation: mechanisms and role in inflammatory disorders. *Ann. Rev. Immunol.* **6**, 49–83.

Puig, S. and Sorkin, L.S. (1994). Subcutaneous formalin evoked activity in single fibers of rat sural nerve. *Soc. Neurosci. Abstr.* **20**, 760.

Rang, H.P., Bevan, S., and Dray, A. (1994). Nociceptive peripheral neurons: cellular properties. In *Textbook of pain* (ed. P.D. Wall and R. Melzack), pp. 57–78. Churchill Livingstone, London.

Reeh, P.W. (1994). Chemical excitation and sensitization of nociceptors. In *Cellular mechanisms of sensory processing* (ed. L. Urban), pp. 119–31. Springer, Berlin.

Reeh, P.W. and Brehm. S. (1993). Nociceptor excitation by inflammatory mediators and by mechanical stimulation in rat skin is neither enhanced by PGE$_2$ nor suppressed by flurbiprofen. *Soc. Neurosci. Abstr.* **19**, 234.

Reeh, P.W., Kocher, L., and Jung, S. (1986). Does neurogenic inflammation alter the sensitivity of unmyelinated nociceptors in the rat? *Brain Res.* **384**, 42–50.

Regoli, D., Boudon, A., and Fauchère, J.-L. (1994). Receptors and antagonists for substance P and related peptides. *Pharmacol. Rev.* **46**, 551–9.

Reiser, G., Walter, U., and Hamprecht, B. (1984). Bradykinin regulates the level of guanosine 3′,5′-cyclic monophosphate (cyclic GMP) in neural cell lines. *Brain Res.* **290**, 367–71.

Reiser, G., Binmöller, F.-J., and Donié, F. (1990). Mechanisms for activation and subsequent removal of cytosolic Ca^{2+} in bradykinin-stimulated neuronal and glial cell lines. *Exp. Cell Res.* **186**, 47–53.

Richardson, B.P., Engel, G., Donatsch, P., and Stadler, P. (1985). Identification of serotonin M-receptor subtypes and their specific blockade by a new class of drugs. *Nature* **316**, 126–31.

Ringkamp, M., Schmelz, M., Kress, M., Allwang, M., Ogilvie, A., and Reeh, P.W. (1994). Activated human platelets in plasma excite nociceptors in rat skin, in vitro. *Neurosci. Lett.* **170**, 103–6.

Rueff, A. and Dray, A. (1993a). Pharmacological characterization of the effects of 5-hydroxytryptamine and different prostaglandins on peripheral sensory neurons in vitro. *Agents Actions* **38**, C13–C15.

Rueff, A. and Dray, A. (1993b). Sensitization of peripheral afferent fibers in the in vitro neonatal rat spinal-cord tail by bradykinin and prostaglandins. *Neuroscience* **54**, 527–35.

Russell, N.J.W., Heapy, C.G., and Jamieson, A. (1987). Afferent activity in models of inflammation. *Pain* **4** (suppl.), S255.

Saade', N.E., Tabbara, M., Atweh, S.F., and Jabbur, S.J. (1988). Discharges in small and large myelinated peripheral fibers evoked by formaldehyde injected in their cutaneous receptive fields. *Soc. Neurosci. Abstr.* **14**, 563.

Salvemini, D., deNucci, G., Sneddon, J.M., and Vane, J.R. (1989). Superoxide anions enhance platelet adhesion and aggregation. *Br. J. Pharmacol.* **97**, 1145–50.

Sampson, S.R. and Jaffe, R.A. (1974). Excitatory effects of 5-hydroxytryptamine, veratridine and phenyldiguanide on sensory ganglion cells of the nodose ganglion of the cat. *Life Sci.* **15**, 2157–65.

Sanjue, H. and Jun, Z. (1989). Sympathetic facilitation of sustained discharges of polymodal receptors. *Pain* **38**, 85–90.

Sato, J. and Perl, E.R. (1991). Adrenergic excitation of cutaneous pain receptors induced by peripheral nerve injury. *Science* **251**, 1608–10.

Schade, H. (1924). Die Molekularpathologie in ihrem Verhältnis zur Zellularpathologie und zum klinischen Krankheitsbild am Beispiel der Entzündung. *Münchner Med. Wochenschr.* **71**, 1–4.

Schaible, H.-G. and Schmidt, R.F. (1988). Time course of mechanosensitivity changes in particular afferents during a developing experimental arthritis. *J. Neurophysiol.* **60**, 2180–95.

Schmelz, M., Schmidt, R., Ringkamp, M., Handwerker, H.O., and Torebjörk, H.E. (1994). Sensitization of insensitive branches of C nociceptors in human skin. *J. Physiol., London* **480**, 389–94.

Schuligoi, R., Donnerer, J., and Amann, R. (1994). Bradykinin-induced sensitization of afferent neurons in the rat paw. *Neuroscience* **59**, 211–15.

Schweizer, A., Brom, R., Glatt, M., and Bray, M.A. (1984). Leukotrienes reduce nociceptive responses to bradykinin. *Eur. J. Pharmacol.* **105**, 105–12.

Schweizer, A., Feige, U., Fontana, A., Müller, K., and Dinarello, C.A. (1988). Interleukin-1 enhances pain reflexes. Mediation through increased prostaglandin E_2 levels. *Agents Actions* **25**, 246–51.

Shea, V.K. and Perl, E.R. (1985). Failure of sympathetic stimulation to affect responsiveness of rabbit polymodal nociceptors. *J. Neurophysiol.* **54**, 513–19.

Shen, K.Z. and Suprenant, A. (1993). Common ionic mechanisms of excitation by substance-P and other transmitters in guinea-pig submucosal neurons. *J. Physiol., London* **462**, 483–501.

Simonds, W.F. and DeGroat, W.C. (1980). Antagonism by picrotoxin of 5-hydroxytryptamine-induced excitation of primary afferent neurons. *Brain Res.* **192**, 592–7.

Simone, D.A. and Ochoa, J. (1991). Early and late effects of prolonged topical capsaicin on cutaneous sensibility and nerogenic vasodilatation in humans. *Pain* **47**, 285–94.

Simone, D.A., Baumann, T.K., and LaMotte, R.H. (1989). Dose-dependent pain and mechanical hyperalgesia in humans after intradermal injection of capsaicin. *Pain* **38**, 99–107.

Simone, D..A., Alreja, M., and LaMotte, R.H. (1991). Psychophysical studies of the itch sensation and itchy skin (alloknesis) produced by intracutaneous injection of histamine. *Somatosens. Motor Res.* **8**, 271–9.

Sokolovsky, M. (1989). Muscarinic cholinergic receptors and their interactions with drugs. *Adv. Drug Res.* **18**, 431–509.

Spigelman, I. and Puil, E. (1988). Excitatory responses of trigeminal neurons to substance P suggest involvement in sensory transmission. *Can. J. Physiol. Pharmacol.* **66**, 845–8.

Steen, K.H. and Reeh, P.W. (1993*a*). Actions of cholinergic agonists and antagonists on sensory nerve endings in rat skin, in vitro. *J. Neurophysiol.* **70**, 397–405.

Steen, K.H. and Reeh, P.W. (1993*b*). Sustained graded pain and hyperalgesia from harmless experimental tissue acidosis in human skin. *Neurosci. Lett.* **154**, 113–16.

Steen, K.H., Anton, F., and Reeh, P.W. (1990). Sensitization and selective excitation by protons of nociceptive nerve endings in rat skin, in vitro. *Pflügers Arch.—Eur. J. Physiol.* **415**, R106.

Steen, K.H., Reeh, P.W., Anton, F., and Handwerker, H.O. (1992). Protons selectively induce lasting excitation and sensitization to mechanical stimulation of nociceptors in rat skin, in vitro. *J. Neurosci.* **12**, 86–95.

Steen, K.H., Reeh, P.W., and Kreysel, H.W. (1995*a*). Topical acetylsalicylic, salicylic acid and indomethacin suppress pain from experimental tissue acidosis in human skin. *Pain,* **62**, 339–47.

Steen, K.H., Reeh, P.W., and Kreysel, H.W. (1995*b*). Dose-dependent competitive block by topical acetylsalicylic and salicylic acid of low pH-induced cutaneous pain. *Pain,* **64**, 71–82.

Stefanidis, D., Reeh, P.W., Kreysel, H.W., and Steen, K.H. (1994). Acetylsalicylic and salicylic acid suppress pH induced excitation of rat nociceptors. *Soc. Neurosci. Abstr.* **20**, 15.

Steranka, L.R., Manning, D.C., DeHaas, C.J., Ferkany, J.W., Borosky, S.A., Connor, J.R., Vavrek, R.J., Stewart, J.M., and Snyder, S.H. Bradykinin as a pain mediator: receptors are localized to sensory neurons, and antagonists have analgesic actions. *Proc. natl Acad. Sci., USA.* **85**, 3245–9.

Szallasi, A. (1994). The vanilloid (capsaicin) receptor: receptor types and species difference. *Life Sci.* **25**, 223–43.

Szolcsányi, J. (1984). Capsaicin and neurogenic inflammation: history and early findings. In *Antidromic vasodilatation and neurogenic inflammation* (ed. L.A. Chahl, J. Szolcsányi, and F. Lembeck), pp. 7–25. Hungarian Academy of Science, Budapest.

Szolcsányi, J., Anton, F., Reeh, P.W., and Handwerker, H.O. (1988). Selective excitation by capsaicin of mechano-heat sensitive nociceptors in rat skin. *Brain Res.* **446**, 262–8.

Taiwo, Y.O. and Levine, J.D. (1990). Direct cutaneous hyperalgesia induced by adenosine. *Neuroscience* **38**, 757–62.

Taiwo, Y.O. and Levine, J.D. (1992). Serotonin is a directly-acting hyperalgesic agent in the rat. *Neuroscience* **48**, 485–90.

Tanellian, D.L. (1991). Cholinergic activation of a population of corneal afferent nerves. *Exp. Brain Res.* **86**, 414–20.

Tani, E., Shiosaka, S., Ishiwaka, T., and Tohyama, M. (1990). Histamine acts directly on calcitonin gene-related peptide and substance P-containing trigeminal ganglion neurons as assessed by calcium influx and immunocytochemistry. *Neurosci. Lett.* **115**, 171–6.

Tegeder, C. and Reeh, P.W. (1991). Visualization of DRG neurons improves yield and stability of intracellular recordings from small cells. *Pflügers Arch.—Eur. J. Physiol.* **420** (suppl. 1), R45.

Tegeder, C. and Reeh, P.W. (1993). Protons induce sustained depolarization but no excitation in all cell types of the intact rat spinal ganglion. *Pflügers Arch.—Eur. J. Physiol.* **422**, R5.

Ustinova, E.E. and Schultz, H.D. (1994). Activation of cardiac vagal afferents by oxygen-derived free radicals in rats. *Circulation Res.* **74**, 895–903.

Vane, J.R. (1971). Inhibition of prostaglandin synthesis as a mechanism of action for aspirin-like drugs. *Nature* **231**, 232–5.

Vlachová, V. and Vyklicky, L. (1993). Capsaicin-induced membrane currents in cultured sensory neurons of the rat. *Physiol. Res.* **42**, 301–11.

Vyklicky, L., Philipp, M., Kuffler, D.P., and Orkland, R.K. (1993). $GABA_A$ membrane currents are insensitive to extracellular acidification in cultured sensory neurons of the frog. *Physiol. Res.* **42**, 313–17.

Waddell, P.J. and Lawson, S.N. (1989). The C-fibre conduction block caused by capsaicin on rat vagus nerve in vitro. *Pain* **39**, 237–42.

Waddell, P.J., McCarthy, P.W., and Reeh, P.W. (1989). The effect of 4-aminopyridine on action potential shape and firing pattern of rat dorsal root ganglion neurones. *Pflügers Arch.—Eur. J. Physiol.* **414**, 131–2.

Wallengren, J. and Hakanson, R. (1992). Effects of capsaicin, bradykinin and prostaglandin E_2 in the human skin. *Br. J. Dermat.* **126**, 111–17.

Wallin, B.G., Torebjörk, and Hallin, R.G. (1976). Preliminary observations on the pathophysiology of hyperalgesia in the causalgic pain syndrome. In *Sensory functions of the skin in primates* (ed. Y. Zotterman), pp. 489–99. Pergamon, Oxford.

Walter, T., Chau, T.T., and Weichmann, B.M. (1989). Effects of analgesics on bradykinin-induced writhing in mice presented with PGE_2. *Agents Actions* **27**, 375–7.

Wedekind, C. and Reeh, P.W. (1992). The effects of osmotically anisotonic solutions on sensory nerve endings in rat skin, in vitro. *Pflügers Arch.—Eur. J. Physiol.* **420**, R52.

Weiss, J.S. (1986). Oxygen, ischemia and inflammation. *Acta physiol. scand.* **548**, 9–37.

White, D.M., Basbaum, A.I., Goetzl, E.J., and Levine, J.D. (1990). The 15-lipoxygenase product, 8R,15S-diHETE, stereoscopically sensitizes C-fiber mechanoheat nociceptors in hairy skin of rat. *J. Neurophysiol.* **63**, 966–70.

Wood, J.N, Winter, J., James, I.F., Rang, H.P., Yeats, J., and Bevan, S. (1988). Capsaicin-induced ion fluxes in dorsal root ganglion cells in culture. *J. Neurosci.* **8**, 3208–20.

Wood, J.N., Coote, P.R., Minhas, A., Mullaney, I., McNeill, M., and Burgess, G.M. (1989). Capsaicin-induced ion influxes increase cGMP but not cAMP levels in rat sensory neurones in culture. *J. Neurochem.* **53**, 1203–11.

Woolf, C.J. (1983). Evidence for a central component of post-injury pain hypersensitivity. *Nature* **306**, 686–8.

Woolf, C.J. (1994). The dorsal horn: state-dependent sensory processing and the generation of pain. In *Textbook of pain* (ed. P.D. Wall and R. Melzack), pp. 101–12. Churchill Livingstone, Edinburgh.

Woolf, C.J. and King, A.E. (1990). Dynamic alterations in the cutaneous mechanoreceptive fields of dorsal horn neurons in the rat spinal cord. *J. Neurosci.* **10**, 2717–26.

Yoshida, K. and Gage, F.H. (1992). Cooperative regulation of nerve growth factor synthesis and secretion in fibroblasts and astrocytes by fibroblast growth factor and other cytokines. *Brain Res.* **569**, 14–25.

Young, J.M., Spires, D.A., Bedford, C.J., Wagner, B., Ballaron, S.J., and DeYoung, L.M. (1984). The mouse ear inflammatory response to topical arachidonic acid. *J. Invest. Dermatol.* **82**, 367–71.

Zimmermann, M. and Sanders, K. (1982). Responses of nerve axons and receptor endings to heat, ischaemia, and algesic substances. Abnormal excitability of regenerating nerve endings. In *Abnormal nerves and muscles as impulse operators* (ed. W.J. Culp and J. Ochoa), pp. 513–32. Plenum Press, New York.

12 Intracellular messengers and signal transduction in nociceptors

STUART BEVAN

Introduction

Signal transduction in nociceptive sensory neurones involves a wide range of underlying mechanisms. In undamaged tissues, noxious external stimuli (thermal or mechanical) act rapidly to evoke a train of action potentials, perhaps by acting directly on the nerve. Nociception is more complex in pathophysiological conditions of tissue injury or trauma where there may be chemical interactions between the nociceptive sensory nerves and the surrounding non-neuronal cells. Some non-neuronal cells express receptors for the neuropeptides (substance P and calcitonin gene-related peptide) released from small-diameter sensory nerves, and these cells respond by modifying their own production of chemical mediators. For this reason, a full understanding of sensory transduction in nociceptors often requires knowledge of the response of non-neuronal cells to chemical stimuli. Some chemical mediators do not evoke action potentials in the nociceptive neurones and so cannot be considered noxious stimuli *per se*; nevertheless they do exert a profound effect on nociception by modulating the transduction process for other stimuli. A well known example of such an indirect action is the sensitization of nociceptive afferent neurones by prostaglandins.

The neuronal responses noted above generally have a duration that follows the time course of the noxious stimuli and can be considered relatively rapid transduction events. Another type of longer-term signal transduction process also operates in nociceptive neurones. Recent experiments have shown that agents such as nerve growth factor (NGF), which is produced in increased amounts in chronic inflammatory conditions, can influence the properties of primary afferent neurones by acting at the level of gene transcription. The resultant changes in neuronal properties occur over a period of hours or days and can be a significant factor in the development of hyperalgesia and allodynia.

Despite the wealth of experimental studies on primary afferent neurones, many details of the transduction processes are poorly understood. The pathways are quite well known for some stimuli, while little or nothing is known about the transduction mechanisms for other stimuli (heat and mechanical transduction and some chemical activators). Furthermore, the processes that underlie sensitization and the molecular mechanisms by which NGF influences sensory neurone properties have to be fully elucidated. This chapter will review sensory transduction mechanisms and the role of intracellular mediators by focusing on the diverse actions of a few chemical agents that act either directly or indirectly on nociceptive neurones.

General mechanisms of receptor activation

Transduction of an excitatory signal in nociceptive afferent neurones requires that the membrane be depolarized to the threshold potential for action potential initiation. This can be achieved by increasing the relative membrane permeability for ions (for example, sodium) that have an electrochemical equilibrium potential more positive than the threshold potential. Typically, two mechanisms are employed. First, the membrane permeability to ions such as sodium or calcium is increased; second, the permeability of the 'resting' membrane to potassium is decreased, thereby raising the relative sodium permeability.

Some noxious chemical agents bind to specific receptor/ion channel complexes in the plasma membrane of the peripheral nerve terminals and gate channel activity directly. For an excitatory agent the usual effect is to depolarize the neurone by opening ion channels that have a high permeability to sodium and, in some cases, calcium ions.

Many substances produced upon tissue injury or during inflammation act via G-protein-coupled receptors. This group includes bradykinin, serotonin (5-HT), histamine, adenosine, formed from the breakdown of adenosine triphosphate (ATP), and the prostaglandins. These receptors have seven transmembrane domains and a cytoplasmic segment that interacts specifically with a subtype of G protein when the agonist binds to the receptor. The biochemical response depends on the type of G protein that is activated. Although many types of heterotrimeric G proteins have been described, they can be grouped into three main functional categories based on their α subunit composition. G_q is positively linked to activation of phospholipase enzymes, notably phospholipase C. G_s stimulates adenylate cyclase activity while G_i members of the $G_{i/o}$ family inhibit this enzyme. Other members of the $G_{i/o}$ family (transducins in photoreceptors) couple to inhibit phosphodiesterases (cGMP PDE). Typical excitatory membrane responses to G protein-coupled receptor activation are the opening of sodium-permeable ion channels or the closing of potassium channels. Some G proteins can also interact directly with ion channels to modify their function, and this type of G-protein interaction is thought to underlie the regulation of some, but not all, voltage-gated channels in neurones and heart cells (see Hille 1994). The full extent to which such direct G protein–ion channel regulation occurs in sensory neurones remains to be explored, but it is clear that various transmitter substances can inhibit voltage-activated calcium currents in a manner that is consistent with such a mechanism.

Neurotrophic factors, such as NGF, act via another class of receptors, which have a tyrosine kinase activity associated with their cytoplasmic domain.

Types of intracellular messengers

Calcium-mobilizing agents (inositol trisphosphate, IP_3) and calcium ions, diacylglycerol (DAG), the cyclic nucleotides cAMP (cyclic AMP) and cGMP (cyclic GMP), nitric oxide (NO), and the cyclooxygenase and lipoxygenase products of arachidonic acid have all been implicated in intracellular signalling in nociceptors. Phosphorylation or dephosphorylation is often a key step in transduction processes and many of these second messengers regulate the phosphorylation (via protein kinases) or dephosphorylation (via protein phosphates) of cellular components, including membrane-bound receptors, ion channels, and enzymes. NGF receptors also phosphorylate other proteins but do so directly via their intrinsic tyrosine kinase domain, which enables them to phosphorylate associated proteins. The roles of protein phosphatases in nociceptors have not been the focus of many studies. These enzymes are potentially as important as protein kinases for the regulation of cell functions, and there is already some evidence that they may have important effects in sensory neurones.

In addition to phosphorylation, some of the mediators that act on nociceptors can stimulate other biochemical processes (such as methylation, lipid modification of proteins, and production of the lipid derivative, ceramide) in other cell types, and these alternative pathways may well operate in nociceptive nerves.

Ligand-gated ion channels

The simplest transduction mechanism in nociceptive neurones involves a ligand binding to and gating a combined receptor/ion channel complex. Capsaicin, protons, 5-hydroxy-tryptamine (5-HT, via the $5\text{-}HT_3$ receptor), ATP (via the P_{2x} receptors), acetylcholine, and glutamate (via a kainate-type receptor) all operate in this way. The ion channels opened by these agents are all permeable to monovalent cations (notably sodium) and the cation influx is responsible for the depolarizing current and excitation. In general, the noxious effects can be ascribed to the depolarization and consequent generation of action potentials. Some of these agents can also induce hyperalgesia and some possible underlying mechanisms are discussed later in this chapter.

One of the best studied ligands in this class is 5-HT. 5-HT excites nociceptors by activating $5\text{-}HT_3$ receptors found on small-diameter afferent neurones (Robertson and Bevan 1991; Peters *et al.* 1992). These receptors are linked to ion channels that are permeable to sodium and calcium ions. 5-HT evokes pain when applied to a blister base and this is mimicked by the $5\text{-}HT_3$-selective agonist phenylbiguanide and antagonized by $5\text{-}HT_3$ receptor blockers with a potency that suggests antagonism at $5\text{-}HT_3$ receptors (Richardson *et al.* 1985; Fozard 1994). Application of $5\text{-}HT_3$ antagonists is ineffective against acute noxious stimuli in normal animals but is effective against inflammatory pain where 5-HT is likely to be produced (Fozard 1994).

Capsaicin is well known for its ability to stimulate nociceptive neurones. Capsaicin, like 5-HT, acts by opening a cation-permeable (sodium, potassium, calcium) ion channel (Bevan and Szolcsányi 1990), and there is good evidence that protons activate the same ion channels (Bevan and Docherty 1993; Bevan and Geppetti 1994). ATP also activates sensory neurones, including nociceptors, and application of ATP to a human blister base evokes the sensation of pain (Bleehan and Keele 1977). Although several types of purinergic receptors are present on sensory nerves, the stimulatory effects appear to be due to activation of cation channel-linked P_{2x} receptors. Recent molecular cloning experiments have shown that these receptor/ion channel complexes are constructed of protein subunits with only two transmembrane domains (Brake *et al.* 1994; Valera *et al.* 1994) and thus are structurally unlike the other known types of agonist-activated ion channels in nociceptors which are constructed of subunits with four transmembrane domains. Despite this structural difference, the functional properties of P_{2x}-operated channels are broadly similar to those found for $5\text{-}HT_3$ receptor- and capsaicin receptor-linked ion channels and they are permeable to both monovalent (sodium) and divalent (calcium) ions (see Bean 1992).

Phospholipase-linked G-protein-coupled receptors

Bradykinin

Bradykinin and the related peptide kallidin (Lys[0]-bradykinin) and their degradation products, des-Arg[9] bradykinin and des-Arg[10]-kallidin, are biologically active and act at two different types of kinin receptors (see Farmer and Burch 1992). Bradykinin and kallidin act preferentially at the B_2 receptor, while des-Arg[9] bradykinin and des-Arg[10]-kallidin act with much higher affinity at the B_1 than at the B_2 receptor. Both types of receptors are seven-transmembrane, G-protein-linked receptors (McEachern *et al.* 1991; Hess *et al.* 1985, 1992; McIntyre *et al.* 1993; Menke *et al.* 1994). B_2 receptors are expressed constitutively on a wide range of cell types, including nociceptive sensory nerves, and bradykinin can act directly on the nerve or indirectly via the release of other mediators from adjacent cells. In contrast, B_1 receptors are not normally expressed at significant levels in normal tissues, except some vascular tissue, but their expression is induced by tissue injury and infection (see Marceau and Regoli 1991; Hall 1992; Dray and Perkins 1993). This upregulation of B_1 receptors requires *de novo* protein synthesis (Regoli *et al.* 1978; Bouthillier *et al.* 1987; DeBlois *et al.* 1991), and there is strong evidence that the induction is stimulated by the release of cytokines, interleukin-1 and interleukin-2 (IL-1 and IL-2), from immunocompetent cells in the damaged tissue (Bouthillier *et al.* 1987; DeBlois *et al.* 1988, 1991; Perkins and Kelly 1994). The acute and some of the long-term effects of bradykinin are mediated via the B_2 receptor and bradykinin makes a major contribution to inflammatory pain and hyperalgesia (see Dray and Perkins 1993). In conditions of persistent inflammation, the induced B_1 receptors make an additional contribution to the hyperalgesia (Perkins *et al.* 1993; Dray and Perkins 1993; Davis and Perkins 1994).

Signalling via B_2 receptors

The intracellular events that are stimulated by bradykinin acting via B_2 receptors are illustrated in Fig. 12.1. The function of the B_2 receptor in dorsal root ganglion (DRG) neurones is dependent on pertussis-insensitive G proteins and can be inhibited when the neurones are dialysed with the inhibitory GTP analogue, GDPβS, and stimulated by stable GTP analogues (McGehee and Oxford 1991; McQuirk and Dolphin 1992). Bradykinin excites sensory neurones mainly through the G-protein-mediated activation of a phosphatidylinositol-specific phospholipase C (PLC). PLC cleaves the target membrane lipids to generate two key intracellular second messengers, 1,4,5-inositol trisphosphate (IP_3) and diacylglycerol (DAG).

DAG is responsible for many of the effects of bradykinin. DAG activates the enzyme protein kinase C (PKC), which phosphorylates various cellular proteins, including membrane receptors and ion channels (see Shearman *et al.* 1989). PKC generates an excitatory depolarizing current in nociceptors by opening a type of ion channel that is permeable to monovalent cations (Na^+, K^+, Cs^+) (Burgess *et al.* 1989*a*; McGehee and Oxford 1991). The role of PKC in sensory transduction is supported by experiments with agents that either inhibit or activate this enzyme. Staurosporine, a relatively selective PKC inhibitor, substantially inhibits the response of cultured DRG neurones to bradykinin (Burgess *et al.* 1989*a*) and attenuates afferent fibre stimulation by brady-kinin in the skin (Dray *et al.* 1992). Bradykinin-induced membrane depolarization and the associated calcium entry can be mimicked by phorbol esters that bind to and activate PKC. Furthermore, bradykinin responses in many neurones are reduced or abolished when PKC is inhibited or downregulated by prolonged exposure of the cells to phorbol esters (Burgess *et al.* 1989*a*). Not all the excitatory actions of bradykinin can be ascribed to PKC activation, however, as neither staurosporine nor PKC downregulation by phorbol esters completely abolish the response. In addition, some bradykinin-responsive DRG neurones fail to respond to phorbol esters (Burgess *et al.* 1989*a*). A non-PKC-mediated excitatory mechanism is also suggested by the finding that staurosporine does not inhibit the bradykinin-induced dorsal root depolarization in a rat spinal cord preparation *in vitro* (Dunn and Rang 1990).

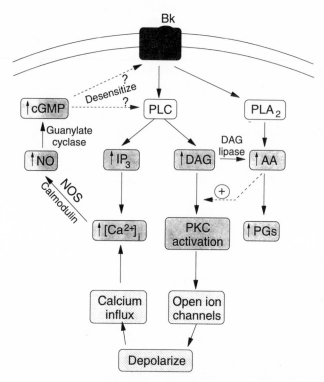

Fig. 12.1 Schematic diagram of the effects of bradykinin (Bk) B_2 receptor (B_2 R) activation. Note that not all reactions may occur in the neurone. Receptor-linked enzymes are shown in open boxes and intracellular mediators in grey boxes. PLC, Phospholipase C; PLA_2, phospholipase A_2; NOS, nitric oxide synthase; DAG, diacylglycerol; AA, arachidonic acid; PG, prostaglandin; I P_3, inositol trisphosphate; PKC, protein kinase C.

Bradykinin evokes a rise in the cytosolic calcium concentration by two separate mechanisms. Depolarization of nociceptors by bradykinin opens voltage-sensitive calcium channels (VSCCs) and allows calcium to enter the cell from the external medium. Increases in intracellular free calcium concentration are also evoked by IP_3 production. IP_3 stimulates the release of calcium from intracellular membrane-bound stores by acting on a specific reactor. The released calcium elevates the concentration of free calcium ions within the cell (Thayer *et al.* 1988). In some other cell types, such as

NG108-15 cells, IP$_3$-mediated elevation of the calcium concentration opens potassium channels (Brown and Higashida 1988), but this has not been observed in DRG neurones in response to bradykinin. The results of one study suggest that IP$_3$ production may have an excitatory role in DRG neurones: internal application of a stable IP$_3$ analogue, inositol 1,4,5-trisphosphothioate (IPS$_3$), mimics and then blocks the ability of brady-kinin to elicit a train of action potentials in response to a depolarizing stimulus. Intracellular application of ryanodine and caffeine, which also mobilize calcium from internal stores, also inhibits the actions of bradykinin, but, unlike IPS$_3$, these agents do not have any initial excitatory effects on their own (McQuirk and Dolphin 1992). The mechanisms that underlie these effects have not been elucidated. The calcium that enters the cell through the VSCCs can stimulate the production of cGMP, although production of the nucleotide is not elicited by the rise in calcium triggered by IP$_3$ (Burgess *et al.* 1989*b*). This difference suggests that the precise location of an intracellular signal is an important factor in determining the overall cellular response.

cGMP appears to be an important regulator of B$_2$ receptor function. Bradykinin-induced IP$_3$ production and activation of sensory neurones are reduced in the presence of cGMP. This effect is downstream of ligand binding to the receptor and could involve desensitization of the receptor, or an inhibitory effect on either the G protein or PLC (Burgess *et al.* 1989*b*; Dray *et al.* 1992; McGehee et al. 1992). The inhibitory effect is initiated by NO production, since inhibitors of the enzyme nitric oxide synthase (NOS) attenuate bradykinin-induced desensitization in cultured sensory neurones (McGehee *et al.* 1992). The likely sequence of events is that the increase in intracellular calcium concentration activates calcium-dependent calmodulin which stimulates NOS to produce NO which, in turn, activates guanylate cyclase to produce cGMP (see Fig. 12.1).

The majority of the available evidence suggests that mammalian sensory nerves produce relatively little or no prostaglandins in response to bradykinin and that the majority of prostanoids (PGE$_2$, PGD$_2$, and PGI$_2$) generated in tissues are produced by non-neuronal cells. Prostanoids do mediate some of the excitatory effects of bradykinin since bradykinin-induced excitation of nociceptors in tissues is reduced, but not abolished, by cyclooxygenase inhibitors (Geppetti *et al.* 1991; Hua and Yaksh 1993; Rueff and Dray 1993). The more pronounced action of the prostaglandins is, however, their well documented ability to sensitize sensory neurones (see below).

Lipoxygenase products of arachidonic acid, such as leukotrienes and hydroxyeico-satetraenoic acids (HETEs), may also play some role in bradykinin-induced excitation as McQuirk and Dolphin (1992) found that the lipoxygenase inhibitor norhydroguaiaretic acid (NDGA) inhibited the ability of bradykinin to elicit trains of action potentials in rat cultured DRG neurones. In contrast, block of the cyclooxygenase enzyme with indomethacin had no effect in their preparation. The release of lipoxygenase products (5-HETE and leukotriene B$_4$) from neutrophils is also stimulated by bradykinin at doses consistent with B$_2$ receptor activation (Nielsen *et al.* 1988), and these may contribute to the overall tissue effects of bradykinin.

Signalling via B$_1$ receptors

The transduction mechanisms associated with bradykinin B$_1$ receptor activation have not been extensively studied. There is no evidence that nociceptors express B$_1$ receptors even under pathopysiological conditions, and it is possible that the effects of B$_1$ agonists on sensory neurones are indirect. For that reason it seems likely that the neuronal effects depend on the production of mediators that can be released from the non-neuronal cells.

B_1 receptor activation stimulates PLC in vascular endothelial-derived cells to generate IP_3 and to elevate intracellular calcium levels. The B_1 receptor transduction mechanisms are generally similar to those for B_2 receptors, although there may be some diversity in the signalling pathways even in a single type of cell (see Smith *et al.* 1995). B_1 receptors can stimulate PLA_2 activity (Hong and Deykin 1982) and eicosanoid (PGI_2, PGE_2) production in a range of cell types including vascular endothelial (D'Orleans-Juste *et al.* 1989), some fibroblast (Cahill *et al.* 1988; but see Goldstein and Wall 1984), dermal (Marceau and Tremblay 1986), and osteoblast-like cells (Ljunggren and Lerner 1990). NO release and production of cGMP have also been reported for endothelial cells (Sung *et al.* 1988; D'Orleans-Juste *et al.* 1989; Wiemer and Wirth 1992). An interaction between bradykinin B_1 receptor activation, prostanoids, and cytokines has been observed in peripheral tissue cells, where B_1 agonists stimulate the release of the cytokines, interleukins, and tumour necrosis factor (TNFα), from vascular cells and macrophages (Toda *et al.* 1987; Cahill *et al.* 1988; D'Orleans-Juste *et al.* 1989; Tiffany and Burch 1989), and B_1, as well as B_2, agonists act synergistically with IL-1 to release PGE_2 from fibroblasts (Lerner and Modeer 1991).

Histamine

Histamine, released from mast cells, acts on sensory neurones to evoke both itch and pain but little is known about the underlying mechanisms. It excites a small population of peripheral sensory nerve fibres (Koppert *et al.* 1993; Mizumura *et al.* 1994) and depolarizes some trigeminal ganglion and visceral (nodose ganglion) neurones, but usually does not evoke action potentials (Hutcheon *et al.* 1993; Undem and Weinreich 1993). The evoked depolarizations are associated with variable changes in membrane conductance, which suggests that histamine can act in several ways. Histamine increases the calcium permeability of sensory neurones (Tani *et al.* 1990), although it is unclear whether this is a 'direct' agonist effect on membrane permeability or is secondary to membrane depolarization. Most of the available evidence indicates that the effects of histamine are mediated by H_1 receptors, which are usually linked to DAG/IP_3 production. H_1 receptors have been described on some sensory neurones (Ninkovic and Hunt 1985), and H_1, but not H_2, antagonists inhibit the histamine-induced rise in calcium levels (Tani *et al.* 1990) as well as the depolarization of some, but not all, trigeminal ganglion neurones (Hutcheon *et al.* 1993).

Adenylate cyclase linked G protein-coupled receptors

5-Hydroxytryptamine (5-HT)

5-HT (serotonin) can be released from platelets and mast cells during tissue damage and acts on sensory neurones either by opening ion channels directly or by operating G-protein-coupled receptors. There is evidence for the presence of members of four groups of 5-HT receptors on sensory neurones (5-HT_{1-4}), but the precise distribution of all of the subtypes is unknown. All but one of the types of 5-HT receptors (5-HT_3) are seven-transmembrane, G-protein-coupled receptors. The 5-HT_1 group of receptors are generally linked negatively to adenylate cyclase to reduce cAMP levels while 5-HT_4

receptor activation increases cAMP. The other major group of receptors, the 5-HT_2 receptors (including the receptor originally described as 5-HT_{1c}), are positively linked to the breakdown of phosphoinositides to produce DAG and IP_3.

5-HT excites sensory neurones, and the application of 5-HT to a blister base in human skin causes a mild and transient pain (Sicuteri *et al.* 1965; Richardson *et al.* 1985). Although most of the noxious effects of 5-HT have been ascribed to an action at 5-HT_3 receptors (see above), stimulation of other 5-HT receptor subtypes that are positively linked to adenylate cyclase can also lead to membrane depolarization. The extent to which increases in adenylate cyclase activity contribute directly to nociception is unclear and the effects may be of more importance for sensitization (see below).

5-HT_4 receptor activation depolarizes vagus nerve preparations (Rhodes *et al.* 1992; Bley *et al.* 1994). The mechanism for this has yet to be fully elucidated, but the observation that application of either the adenylate cyclase activator, forskolin, or 8-bromo-cAMP also depolarizes the preparation (Bley *et al.* 1994) is consistent with the notion that the effect is mediated by an increase in the concentration of cAMP. Elevation of cAMP levels has been reported to produce a modest inhibition of potassium currents in DRG neurones (Akins and McCleskey 1993), and it is possible that the depolarization evoked by 5-HT_4 receptor activation is due to the closure of potassium channels that are open at the resting membrane potential.

Activation of 5-HT_2 receptors depolarizes capsaicin-sensitive DRG neurones by reducing a resting membrane conductance (Todorovic and Anderson 1990), which suggests that this also may be due to closure of potassium channels that are normally open in the resting membrane.

Noradrenaline

Noradrenaline has no obvious excitatory effect on normal nociceptive afferents but does excite some damaged as well as intact neurones after peripheral nerve injury or during inflammation (see, for example, Habler *et al.* 1987; Sato and Perl 1991; Devor *et al.* 1994). This effect is retained in isolated nerve preparations (Koltzenburg *et al.* 1994) and so cannot be simply ascribed to a vascular effect of the agonist. The mechanisms that underlie the excitation are unclear but the pharmacology of the response is typical of an action at α_2 receptors (Levine *et al.* 1986*b*; Sato and Perl 1991), which normally act either by inhibiting adenylate cyclase or by modulating ion channels.

Although the effects of noradrenaline are uncontentious, the location of the receptors is open to question. Levine and colleagues (1986*b*) examined the mechanical hyperalgesia induced by chloroform treatment of rat paws and proposed that noradrenaline, which would normally be released from the sympathetic postganglionic nerves, acts on α_2 receptors on the terminals of these sympathetic nerves. Their hypothesis is that α_2 receptor stimulation elicits the release of prostanoids, which act on the nociceptors. In addition, they have proposed that other agents, such as leukotrienes, are also released and act on polymorphonuclear leucocytes to evoke the release of other lipoxygenase products (8R,15S-di HETE). Other investigators have studied sensory nerve discharges after peripheral nerve constriction (Koltzenburg *et al.* 1994) and adjuvant-induced arthritis (Sato *et al.* 1994) and have shown that noradrenaline-induced excitation is not dependent on the presence of sympathetic nerves. These latter findings suggest that noradrenaline acts directly on nociceptors and would be consistent with the observations that some DRG neurones express mRNA for α_2 receptors (Nicholas *et al.* 1993) and that receptor expression is increased after nerve damage (McMahon 1991).

Nitric oxide and cGMP

Nitric oxide (NO) is a readily diffusible but unstable molecule that is considered to be an important intercellular mediator. NO is formed from L-arginine following the activation of the enzyme nitric oxide synthase (NOS) by calcium and other co-factors, including calmodulin. NO diffuses to its site of action where it modifies cellular processes mainly by the activation of guanylate cyclase and the production of gAMP, although other, non-cGMP-mediated actions of NO, such as activation of cyclooxygenase enzymes and *S*-nitrosylation of proteins, may occur (Bredt and Snyder 1994). Many interactions between NOS, NO, and other intracellular mediators and their synthetic enzymes have been described (see Fig. 12.2) and some of these, at least, probably operate in nociceptive neurones. Studies on the distribution of NOS have shown that NOS activity is found in a wide variety of cells, including many that have some physical association with sensory nerve terminals, and the synthesis of an inducible form of NOS in these cells can be stimulated by products of tissue injury and inflammation, such as cytokines (Moncada 1992).

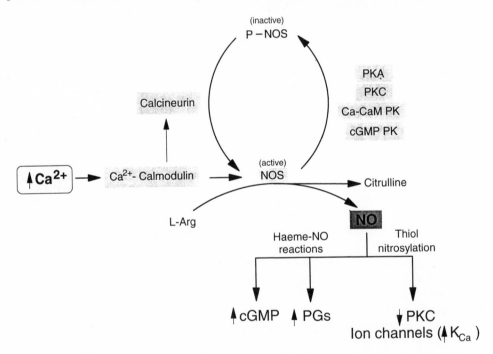

Fig. 12.2 Diagram to illustrate the regulation and activation of nitric oxide synthase (NOS) by calcium ions and some of the possible effects of nitric oxide (NO) production.

Some DRG neurones express NOS under normal conditions, but this appears to depend on the ganglion under study (Steel *et al.* 1994) and suggests some environmental regulation of enzyme expression. The expression of NOS in DRG neurones is upregulated after either nerve section (Verge *et al.* 1992) or partial nerve ligation (Steel *et al.* 1994).

Intradermal injections of NO in human volunteers evoke a concentration-dependent pain sensation with a duration of about 1 minute (Holthusen and Arndt 1994). The involvement of NO in nociception has also been investigated with inhibitors of NOS, such as nitro-L-arginine methyl ester (L-NAME) and compounds that generate NO, such as sodium nitroprusside (SNP). SNP has no obvious direct stimulatory effect on membrane currents in rat cultured DRG neurones, although it enhances bradykinin desensitization in the same cells (see above; McGehee *et al.* 1992) and stimulates the release of calcitonin gene-related peptide (CGRP) and substance P from primary afferent neurones in a spinal cord slice preparation. The peptide release occurs, in part, through an NO-dependent mechanism and can be inhibited by the guanylate cyclase inhibitor, methylene blue (Garry *et al.* 1994). Studies on sectioned nerves, which show spontaneous action potentials, also suggest that NO may regulate neuronal activity. Weisenfeld-Hallin *et al.* (1993) showed that L-NAME inhibited the spontaneous action potentials in damaged nerve but had little or no effect on normal nerve activity. It seems likely that the induced expression of NOS in the damaged nerves contributes to an increased production of NO, although the mechanisms that underlie the postulated excitatory effects of NO have not been elucidated.

One possible effect of NO is a cGMP-mediated regulation of potassium currents, and there is evidence that NO regulates the frequency of action potentials in visceral (nodose) afferents (Cohen *et al.* 1994) where L-NAME almost totally blocked the slow after-hyperpolarization (AHP) without any effect on another calcium-dependent current or on the concentration of free intracellular calcium. This effect can be reversed by co-application of S-nitroso-N-acetylpenicillamine, a nitric oxide releaser, and Cohen *et al.* (1994) suggested that NO regulates ion channel activity by an indirect mechanism that involves a subsequent signal molecule (for example, cGMP). It is difficult to see how the maintenance (or enhancement) of a slow AHP by NO is related to the increased activity of nociceptive neurones, as increased firing is usually associated with inhibition of this potential. It is possible that NO increases nociceptor activity by modulating the activity of other types of ion channels. In addition, NO has been shown to activate cyclooxygenase enzymes to stimulate the production of prostaglandins (Salvemini *et al.* 1993), and this may be an important pathway for NO effects on nociceptive peripheral neurones (see Fig. 12.2).

Intracellular mediators and sensitization

There are at least five basic ways in which one agent can sensitize nociceptive neurones to the actions of a second agent: (1) summation of depolarizing responses, whereby a subthreshold depolarization allows a second depolarizing input to reach a threshold potential and fire a train of action potentials; (2) an increase in membrane resistance produced by a reduction in 'resting' membrane conductance, perhaps by closure of potassium channels, such that an excitatory current evokes a larger depolarization; (3) a subthreshold activation of a stimulatory biochemical pathway that primes the pathway for a second agent; (4) biochemical modification of agonist-operated enzymes and ion channels, such that they show an augmented response when activated; (5) a modification of the ion channels that underlie the action potential either to reduce the threshold for action potential initiation or to increase the number of action potentials evoked by a given stimulus.

A role for arachidonic acid metabolites

The bioactive metabolites of arachidonic acid (eicosanoids) include the products of both the cyclooxygenase and lipoxygenase enzyme pathways, which are produced in increased amounts during inflammation. These lipid-soluble molecules can act as intercellular mediators and, in general, can either excite nociceptors or, more usually, sensitize them to other stimuli. One of the best established mechanisms for sensitization of nociceptive neurones is mediated by prostaglandins. Although the mechanisms are not understood completely, there is persuasive evidence that this process involves, at least in some preparations, an elevation of cAMP concentration and inhibition of potassium currents.

The sensitization of nociceptors by bradykinin involves production of arachidonic acid, which can occur by two major pathways (see Fig. 12.1). In mammalian sensory neurone preparations this involves activation of PLC and metabolism of the resultant DAG which is hydrolysed by the enzyme DAG lipase to generate monoacylglycerol and arachidonic acid (Gammon *et al.* 1989; Allen *et al.* 1992). The activation of DAG lipase may involve calcium entry to the neurone and an opioid peptide, morphiceptin, has been shown to decrease the calcium conductance and block bradykinin-stimulated arachidonic acid release without any inhibition of DAG formation (Gammon *et al.* 1989, 1990). In other cell types, including fibroblasts and endothelial and DRG neurone-derived cells, phospholipase A_2 is responsible for arachidonic acid production (See Burch and Axelrod 1987; Conklin *et al.* 1988; Francel and Dawson 1988). Arachidonic acid is metabolized to a range of biologically active molecules (see below), but most studies on bradykinin have focused on the prostaglandins.

Histamine depolarizes and sensitizes polymodal nociceptors to a second (heat) stimulus (Mizumura *et al.* 1994). It seems unlikely that sensitization is due to summation of the subthreshold histamine-evoked depolarization and the heat-evoked depolarization as sensitization persists after the cessation of histamine-induced action potential discharges (Mizumura *et al.* 1994). Prostanoids are released from some tissues in response to histamine and are obvious candidate mediators of sensitization (Juan and Samtex 1980; Falus and Meretey 1992), although their possible role in histamine-induced sensitization has not been explored (see Mizumura *et al.* 1994). As histamine depolarizes some sensory neurones by acting at an H_1 receptor, it is conceivable that prostanoids generated by H_1 receptor activation are responsible for both the depolarization and the sensitization.

Prostanoids

Prostaglandins (PGs) are produced during inflammatory diseases such as rheumatoid arthritis or after experimental inflammation. There are five naturally occurring prostanoids, PGD_2, PGE_2, PGF2a, PGI_2, and thromboxane A_2, all of which act on seven-transmembrane, G-protein-linked receptors (see Coleman *et al.* 1994). Prostaglandins are generated from arachidonic acid by the action of cyclooxygenase enzymes. A major effect of prostaglandins is to sensitize nociceptors to noxious (chemical, mechanical, and heat) stimuli (see, for example, Mizumura *et al.* 1987; Schaible and Schmidt 1988; Birrell *et al.* 1991), although not all prostaglandins act in this way. While PGE_2 and PGI_2

(prostacyclin) commonly sensitize nociceptors, PGD_2 has been reported to show little or no such activity (Rueff and Dray 1993). The ability of prostaglandins to sensitize nociceptors also depends on the nature of the noxious stimulus. PGE_2 is a potent sensitizer for chemical activation by bradykinin but the same concentrations of PGE_2 do not always sensitize nociceptors to either heat or mechanical stimuli and higher concentrations of PGE_2 (for example, 100-fold) are frequently required to influence the response to temperature and pressure (see Schaible and Schmidt 1988; Grubb *et al.* 1991; Kumazawa *et al.* 1994). This disparity in the concentration of PGE_2 required for sensitization suggests that different receptor subtypes mediate the sensitization process for different noxious stimuli and suggest the presence of multiple sensitization mechanisms.

Prostaglandins do not usually activate cutaneous sensory neurones directly and fail to evoke pain when injected intradermally into human skin (Crunkhorn and Willis 1971) PGE_2 and PGI_2 have, however, been shown to increase the activity of nociceptors in rat articular nerves (Schaible and Schmidt 1988; Birrell *et al.* 1991; Schepelmann *et al.* 1992) and to stimulate the release of substance P from sensory neurones in culture (Nicol *et al.* 1992; Hingtgen and Vasko 1994). Furthermore, PGE_2 has been reported to depolarize cultured DRG neurones (Puttick 1992) as well as sensory neurones in some intact preparations (Yanagisawa *et al.* 1986). These findings suggest that during inflammation prostanoids may contribute directly to the activation of some afferent neurones as well as sensitize them to other stimuli.

Prostanoid receptors have been broadly classified into five categories (EP, DP, FP, IP, and TP) at which one of the naturally occurring prostanoids (PGE_2, PGD_2, etc.) is at least one order of magnitude more potent than any of the other four. There are at least three, probably four, subtypes of EP receptors [EP_{1-4}] (see Coleman *et al.* 1994 for review). The relative occurrence of these receptors, at either the mRNA or protein level, in nociceptive afferents has not been described, but the physiological and pharmacological data point to the existence of at least EP and IP receptors on nociceptors (Birrell and McQueen 1993; Rueff and Dray 1993) with some suggestion that IP receptors may be more widely distributed than EP receptors (Birrell and McQueen 1993). The prostanoid receptors are coupled physiologically to different G proteins (G_s, G_i, and G_q) and activation of each type therefore gives rise to a different cellular response. In general, the evidence from studies on a wide range of cells suggests that stimulation of DP, EP_2, and IP receptors leads to an increase in cAMP levels (via G_s and adenylate cyclase) and activation of FP and TP receptors stimulates IP_3/DAG formation (via G_q and PLC) while EP_3 receptors can couple either to stimulate IP_3/DAG formation (via G_q) or to inhibit cAMP formation (G_i). Activation of EP_1 receptors leads to an increase in intracellular calcium levels, which is consistent with an action via G_q, PLC, and IP_3, although this remains to be substantiated.

cAMP plays a role in sensitization

In some experimental situations, sensitization by prostaglandins involves elevation of cAMP (Ferreira and Nakamura 1979) and agents that elevate cAMP induce hyperalgesia (Taiwo and Levine 1991; Taiwo *et al.* 1992). In contrast, inhibition of PKC with staurosporine has no effect on the PGE_2-induced sensitization (Taiwo and Levine 1991). The experimental evidence is largely consistent with the hypothesis that sensitization to chemical (bradykinin), heat, and mechanical stimuli is due to activation of either EP_3 and/or IP receptors (see, for example, Birrell *et al.* 1991; Schepelmann *et al.* 1992; Kumazawa *et al.* 1994). In contrast, contradictory data from Kumazawa (1994) on testicular polymodal nociceptors indicate that the response to bradykinin is not sensitized by treatments that elevate cAMP levels (Fig. 12.3), whereas EP_3 receptor stimulation, which typically is linked to inhibition of adenylate cyclase and a reduction in cAMP levels, augments the response to bradykinin (Fig. 12.4). A possible explanation for this interaction is that cAMP inhibits PLC activity (Campbell *et al.* 1990) and that the reduced cAMP levels result in greater bradykinin-induced formation of IP_3/DAG. Alternatively, the sensitizing effect may be associated more directly with PLC activation as EP_3 receptors can couple to G_q to activate PLC and thus stimulate the production of IP_3 and DAG.

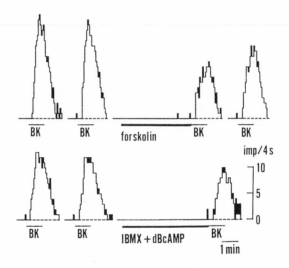

Fig. 12.3 Elevation of cAMP concentration suppresses the bradykinin (BK)-evoked activity of testicular polymodal nociceptive neurones. Data show the number of discharges evoked by 0.1 μM bradykinin. Forskolin (10 μM) or a mixture of membrane-permeable dibutyryl cAMP (dBcAMP, 20 μM) and a phosphodiesterase inhibitor (IBMX, 20 μM) were applied during the period marked by the thick horizontal bar. Reproduced with permission from Kumazawa *et al.* (1994).

5-HT sensitizes nociceptors by lowering their threshold to other stimuli (heat, mechanical, chemical) (Beck and Handwerker 1974; Taiwo and Levine 1992; Rueff and Dray 1992). The available evidence suggests that several mechanisms of 5-HT-evoked sensitization operate, only some of which involve increases in cAMP concentrations. In some preparations, sensitization is independent of $5-HT_3$ receptors and involves either $5-HT_{1a}$ receptors (Taiwo and Levine 1992), which usually decrease cAMP levels but have been reported to elevate cAMP in some cells, or $5-HT_2$ receptors (Rueff and Dray 1992), which stimulate PLC. Sensitization is not blocked by indomethacin, which suggests that cyclooxygenase products are not involved. A role for cAMP is also indicated by the finding that 5-HT-induced mechanical hyperalgesia is blocked by Rp-cAMPS, an inhibitor of cAMP-dependent kinase, and augmented by a phosphodiesterase inhibitor (Taiwo *et al.* 1992) which will elevate the cAMP concentration.

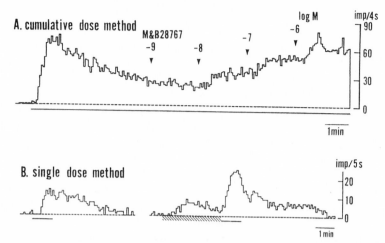

Fig. 12.4 Bradykinin responses of testicular polymodal nociceptive neurones are enhanced by a prostaglandin EP$_3$ receptor agonist (M&B28767). (A) Cumulative dose method. Histogram shows the number of discharges evoked by 1 μM bradykinin applied for the period shown by the lower horizontal line. Increasing concentrations of M&B28767 (1 nM–1 μM) were applied at 2-min intervals as shown by the arrowheads. (B) Single dose method. Responses to 1 mM bradykinin in normal conditions (left) and after a 3-min exposure to 0.1 μM M&B28767 (shown by hatching) (right). Reproduced with permission from Kumazawa *et al.* (1994).

Local application of adenosine has been reported to produce mechanical hyperalgesia in the rat and the pharmacology of the effect is consistent with an action of adenosine at A$_2$ receptors (Taiwo and Levine 1990), which are usually linked positively to adenylate cyclase activation. A role for cAMP is also suggested by the finding that the hyperalgesic effect is prolonged by rolipram, an inhibitor of the enzyme (phosphodiesterase) that breaks down cAMP. In contrast, adenosine A$_1$ receptor activation, which typically inhibits adenylate cyclase, antagonizes the hyperalgesic effects of both A$_1$ receptor agonists and PGE$_2$ (Taiwo and Levine 1990). These findings suggest that adenosine hyperalgesia results from an elevation of cAMP levels and that the hyperalgesia can be antagonized by a reduction in the activity of adenylate cyclase.

Arachidonic acid can be metabolized by the lipoxygenase enzymes to produce the leukotrienes B$_4$–D$_4$ (LTB$_4$–LTD$_4$, products of the 5-lipoxygenase pathway) and other hydroxyeicosatetraenoic acids, such as 8R,15S-diHETE (a product of the 15-lipoxygenase pathway), and there is accumulating evidence that these lipoxygenase products influence the activity of nociceptors. Intradermal injection of either LTB$_4$ or 8R,15S-diHETE deceases the mechanical and thermal thresholds for nociception (Levine *et al.* 1984, 1985, 1986*a*; Bisgaard and Kristensen 1985; Martin *et al.* 1987; Martin 1990) and LTB$_4$ sensitizes dental afferents (Madison *et al.* 1992). The sensitizing actions of LTB$_4$ are slow in onset and this effect is independent of cyclooxygenase activity and requires the presence of polymorphonuclear leucocytes that release sensitizing factors that act on the nerves (Levine *et al.* 1984, 1985). Levine *et al.* (1985, 1986*a*) have postulated that the sensitizing effect of LTB$_4$ is mediated by 8R,15S-diHETE, which has been shown experimentally to produce hyperalgesia by decreasing the mechanical and thermal thresholds of C fibres (Taiwo *et al.* 1989; Taiwo and Levine (1991). The finding that the antagonistic isomer, 8S,15S-diHETE, inhibits the hyperalgesic effect of both 8R,15S-diHETE and LTB$_4$ is consistent with this hypothesis (Levine *et al.* 1986*a*).

The mechanisms by which lipoxygenase products act are not well established and it seems likely that some of the actions involve non-neuronal cells. In general, activation of both LTB$_4$ and LTD$_4$ receptors increases IP$_3$/DAG formation via the enzyme PLC. 8R,15S-diHETE could be formed from arachidonic acid cleaved from DAG by DAG lipase, although the involvement of other metabolic enzymes such as PLA$_2$ cannot be excluded. The sensitization evoked by 8R,15S-diHETE is antagonized by the cAMP antagonist Rp-cAMP (Taiwo and Levine 1991) and augmented by phosphodiesterase inhibitors (Taiwo *et al.* 1989), which argues that this agent acts by elevating cAMP levels.

Potassium channels and sensitization

One known mechanism of sensitization involves inhibition of a potassium current that regulates the frequency of action potentials evoked by a given depolarization of the nerve. This has been well documented for visceral sensory neurones where an increase in excitability is associated with an inhibition of the long-lasting spike afterhyperpolarization (the slow-AHP) generated by a calcium-activated potassium current. The slow-AHP following each action potential limits the number of action potentials that can be evoked by a depolarizing stimulus. Prostaglandins, 5-HT, leukotriene C$_4$, inhibitors of NO synthesis, and bradykinin, through prostanoid formation, inhibit the slow-AHP and allow the cell to fire repetitively in response to a depolarizing stimulus (Weinreich 1986; Weinreich and Wonderlin 1987; Christian *et al.* 1989; Undem and Weinrich 1993; Cohen *et al.* 1994). Thus, the prostanoid sensitization of visceral sensory neurones can be ascribed to the inhibition of a current that regulates action potential frequency (see Fig. 12.5).

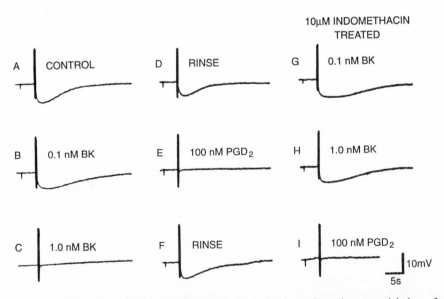

Fig. 12.5 Effects of bradykinin (BK) and prostaglandin D$_2$ (PGD$_2$) on the action potential slow after-hyperpolarization (AHP) in rabbit nodose ganglion neurones. 1 nM bradykinin inhibits the slow-AHP in control conditions (C) but not after treatment with the cyclooxygenase inhibitor indomethacin (H), whereas PGD$_2$ abolishes the AHP in both conditions. Reproduced with permission from Weinreich (1986).

The mechanisms of sensitization in spinal ganglion neurones have yet to be elucidated. Unlike visceral sensory neurones, few spinal ganglion neurones show a pronounced slow-AHP (Gold *et al.* 1994) despite the presence of many calcium-activated potassium channels in their membrane (Naruse *et al.* 1992). One explanation for the relative infrequence of this current is that calcium-activated potassium channels in DRG neurones have a low sensitivity to intracellular calcium and so are not activated by calcium entry during an action potential. A low calcium sensitivity would also explain why DRG neurones, unlike other neuronal-derived cells such as NG108-15 (Brown and Higashida 1988) and F-11 cells (Naruse *et al.* 1992), do not show a bradykinin-stimulated, IP$_3$-mediated potassium current despite a significant rise in intracellular calcium concentration (Naruse *et al.* 1992).

Agents such as prostanoids could also modify the properties of other action potential currents. The properties of many voltage-gated ion channels are regulated by phosphorylation and dephosphorylation, although the extent to which such changes influence action potential characteristics (thresholds and firing frequency) remains to be elucidated.

Other mechanisms of sensitization

Effects on membrane receptors/ion channels

Prostaglandins can also augment receptor-operated responses. PGE$_2$ and PGI$_2$ increase the membrane response to capsaicin (Pitchford and Levine 1991; Hingtgen and Nicol 1994) and this can be mimicked by treatments that elevate the cAMP concentration (Pitchford and Levine 1991). It is possible that this effect may be related to the degree of desensitization of the capsaicin receptor/ion channel, which can be reduced by treatments that inhibit protein phosphatase 2B (calcineurin) activity (Yeats *et al.* 1992). Together the data suggests that phosphorylation increases either the number of available ion channels or the probability that they can be opened by capsaicin. Whether other ligand-gated ion channels are similarly modulated remains to be explored.

Sensitization via ligand-gated ion channels—a calcium-mediated effect

5-HT enhances the pain evoked by bradykinin. This sensitization is blocked by the 5-HT$_3$ antagonist ICS 205.930 (Richardson *et al.* 1985) with a potency that suggests an action at 5-HT$_3$ receptors. At first sight it is difficult to see how the rapid events associated with direct ion channel gating can lead to a long-lasting sensitization. The observation that 5-HT$_3$ receptor activation can lead to cGMP formation in neuronal cells (Reiser and Hamprecht 1989; Reiser 1991) offers a possible explanation. The increase in cGMP is dependent on external calcium ions and can be blocked by NOS inhibitors. These findings suggest that the entry of calcium ions through the activated ion channels triggers NOS activity and cGMP production, which could result in relatively long-lasting biochemical changes. Stimulation of cGMP production is not limited to 5-HT receptors; capsaicin, which also opens a calcium-permeable ion channel, promotes cGMP production in sensory neurones (Wood *et al.* 1989), and this process could be common to all receptors linked to calcium-permeable ion channels.

It is likely that calcium ions stimulate other intracellular processes, some of which may be linked to sensitization. Changes in intracellular calcium levels modify the activity of a wide range of enzymes. Many of these latter effects are mediated by calcium binding to calmodulin and involve a subsequent interaction between the calcium/calmodulin complex and the enzyme. Calmodulin therefore plays a pivotal role in many of the actions of calcium and is responsible for the regulation of proteins including calcium/calmodulin-dependent (CaM) kinase, NOS, calcineurin (protein phosphatase 2B), some membrane receptors, and PLA_2. CaM kinase autophosphorylates upon activation to generate a constitutively active, calcium-independent enzyme. Thus the actions of CaM kinase can outlast the initial calcium signal, which may explain the duration of sensitization. Calcium ions can also stimulate PKC, which will contribute to nociceptor excitation, but this action does not require calmodulin and is mediated by direct calcium binding to the enzyme.

Nerve growth factor and long-term regulation

Recent studies have shown that nociceptors respond, not only to ligands that act via ligand-gated or G protein-coupled receptors, but also to NGF, which acts via a tyrosine kinase receptor. The responses to NGF differ radically from those discussed above and involve regulation of gene transcription by distinct intracellular signalling mechanisms.

NGF is produced in limited amounts in normal tissues by a range of cell types, such as fibroblasts and Schwann cells. It is an essential survival factor for both sensory and sympathetic neurones at early stages of development. In contrast, sensory neurones in adult animals do not require NGF for survival (see Lindsay 1988), but show modified properties in response to alterations in NGF concentration. The full repertoire of phenotypic effects exerted by NGF has yet to be catalogued, but it is already clear that NGF regulates the expression of a number of important proteins, including the sensory neuropeptides, substance P and CGRP (Lindsay and Harmar 1989; Donnerer *et al.* 1992), and the capsaicin receptor/ion channel (Winter *et al.* 1988). The production of NGF increases markedly in experimentally induced inflammation (Donnerer *et al.* 1992; Woolf *et al.* 1994) and elevated NGF levels are found in the synovial fluid from rheumatoid arthritis patients (Aloe *et al.* 1992). The (patho)physiological importance of elevated levels of NGF is illustrated by the observations that application of exogenous NGF and treatments that increase NGF production cause hyperalgesia (Davis *et al.* 1993; Lewin *et al.* 1993; Woolf *et al.* 1994), while administration of a neutralizing antibody to NGF antagonizes the effects of NGF and the hyperalgesia induced by a chronic inflammatory stimulus (Woolf *et al.* 1994).

In general, NGF-induced hyperalgesia develops slowly, which is consistent with an effect on gene transcription. A prolonged mechanical hyperalgesia is first noted several hours after elevation of the systemic NGF concentration. Heat hyperalgesia is also prolonged, but unlike mechanical hyperalgesia develops within an hour. This early phase of hyperalgesia has been attributed to an action of NGF on mast cells that stimulates degranulation (Lewin *et al.* 1993). The early sensitization may therefore be explained by the actions of mast cell products (Histamine, 5-HT) and involve the mechanisms discussed earlier in this chapter.

The mechanisms that mediate the changes in nociceptor phenotype in response to NGF have not been elucidated. NGF produced in the periphery modifies gene transcription in the soma of the neurone by mechanisms that require transport of signals from the periphery to soma as well as from the membrane to the nucleus. The available studies on the effects of NGF on sensory neurones and PC12 cells suggest that the signalling process involves the following general steps (see Heumann 1994). The dimeric NGF molecule binds to a high-affinity transmembrane receptor (tyrosine kinase (trk) or trk A) and cross-links two adjacent trk molecules. Cross-linking of the receptors induces receptor internalization and the receptors are then transported to the soma. Cross-linking also triggers a tyrosine cross-phosphorylation of a cytoplasmic domain on each trk molecule. This stimulates the activity of the small GTP-binding protein p21-Ras (Ras) in DRG neurones (Ng and Shooter 1993) via a pathway that has not been elucidated in sensory neurones.

The likely mechanisms for Ras activation, deduced from PC12 studies, are illustrated in Fig. 12.6 (see Heumann 1994). Tyrosine phosphorylation opens up binding sites for a number of proteins carrying the src-homology motifs (SH2), which are domains of about 100 amino acids with high affinity for phosphorylated tyrosine residues. The SH2 domain proteins are phosphorylated by the receptor kinase, which initiates a signal cascade. Adapter proteins can link one type of phosphorylated SH2 protein to an exchange factor protein that enhances the exchange of GDP for GTP on the Ras protein. Alternatively, the adapter protein can bind to and inhibit the activity of a GTPase-activating protein, and so reduces the breakdown of GTP-bound Ras to GDP-bound Ras. The net result of either reaction is the production of the active GTP-bound form of Ras. The signal is transmitted from Ras through the cytoplasm and to the nucleus by a sequence of phosphorylation events, whereby each protein in the cascade phosphorylates the next number. The final steps in the cascade involve the phosphorylation of transcription factors that bind either directly or indirectly to specific DNA sequences in the promoter sequence of the gene and regulate transcription. The cascade described above is thought to involve a branching network of pathways. NGF activation can therefore stimulate different cellular responses via divergent pathways (D'Arcangelo and Halegoua 1993).

The trk receptor can also activate other proteins via SH2 domains. A subtype of phosphatidylinositol-specific PLC (PLC-γ) and phosphoinositol-3-kinase are SH2 domain proteins that are phosphorylated by direct binding to trk receptors in PC12 cells (Obermeier *et al.* 1993; Stephens *et al.* 1994). Interestingly, phosphoinositol-3 kinase is also phosphorylated by Ras (Rodriguez-Viciana *et al.* 1994), so that trk receptors activate this enzyme by two parallel pathways. Both enzymes are important for inositol phosphate metabolism and activation by trk can lead to IP_3 release (via PLC-γ) in other cell types, although there is no strong evidence, as yet, for this effect in sensory neurones.

A rise in intracellular calcium concentration, evoked by either calcium influx or release from intracellular stores, has been reported to stimulate Ras (Rosen *et al.* 1994) and the $\beta\gamma$ subunits of G proteins can promote protein phosphorylation by a mechanism that depends on Ras (Crespo *et al.* 1994). Although these events remain to be examined in sensory neurones, their occurrence in other cell types raises the possibility of interactions between the 'conventional', rapid signalling pathways and transcriptional control of nociceptor properties.

Another transmembrane receptor, p75, acts as a low-affinity receptor for NGF. This molecule, which is structurally similar to the receptor for tumour necrosis factor-α

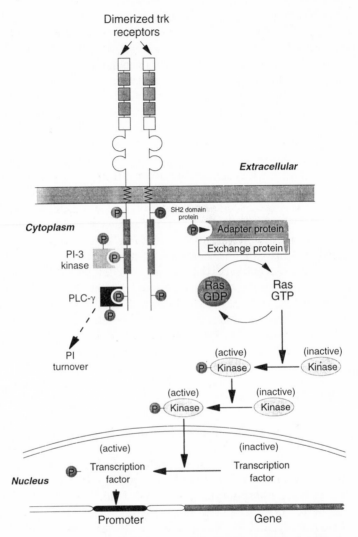

Fig. 12.6 Schematic diagram to show some of the reactions that may underlie signalling by the high-affinity NGF receptor in nociceptors.

(TNF α), was considered to be the NGF receptor before the discovery of the trk family of proteins. The role of p75 in trk signalling is unclear, although there is a body of evidence to suggest that p75 modulates the function of trk in some way. In addition, there are new data to show that NGF acts via p75 to stimulate a sphingomyelin-specific PLC (sphingomyelinase) to break down the membrane lipid sphingomyelin to yield phosphocholine and ceramide (Dobrowsky *et al.* 1994). This breakdown of sphingo-myelin is thought to be an important transduction step for other ligands such as TNFα and IL-1 (Kolesnik and Golde 1994). The functions of ceramide in sensory neurones have yet to be examined but this newly discovered pathway represents a potentially important transduction mechanism for sensory neurones. Studies from other cell types suggest that ceramide stimulates specific (proline-directed, serine/threonine) protein kinases that are distinct from protein kinase C. Ceramide has also been reported to stimulate protein phosphatases (PPs), notably the okadaic acid-sensitive PP2A subtype, and this action may be responsible for many of the biological effects of ceramide (see Liscovitch and Cantley 1994).

Rapid effects of NGF

Although most of the effects of NGF are thought to be mediated by changes in gene transcription, there are several examples of rapid actions that may involve other mechanisms. NGF prolongs the duration of action potentials in sensory neurones *in vitro* via a mechanism that may involve the release of endogenous opioids from DRG neurones (Shen and Crain 1994). The effect occurs within a few minutes and is blocked by antibody to the low-affinity NGF receptor (p75), which suggests that this receptor plays either a direct or a modulatory role in the response. These authors postulated that the released opioids act on κ-opioid receptors to stimulate the G protein, G_s, and so prolong the action potential by augmenting the calcium current. In addition, the amino terminal octapeptide of NGF, which is cleaved from the parent molecule by an endogenous endopeptidase, induces a concentration-dependent, short-lasting (< 2 h) mechanical hyperalgesia in chloroform-treated rat paw (Taiwo *et al.* 1991). The mechanism for this effect is unclear, although the authors suggested an action that is mediated by sympathetic nerves. It is possible that these relatively rapid responses of NGF involve the phosphoinositol/DAG or sphingomyelin pathways noted above.

Concluding remarks

There is still much to be learned about the mechanisms of transduction and sensitization in nociceptive afferent neurones. While we have a reasonable insight into the signalling pathways for a few chemical agents, such as bradykinin, there is little available information for many other agents. Such mechanisms may be inferred from studies on other cell types, but their presence in nociceptors has yet to be investigated. For example, many transduction and sensitization studies have used visceral afferent neurones, but it is far from clear that the mechanisms found in these cells will also operate in nociceptive neurones. Some of the data reviewed here illustrate that a single agent can act in several ways. Indeed, some of the conclusions reached from experiments on different *in vivo* preparations are contradictory, and the reasons for the differences are unclear. Further studies on nociceptors, in isolated preparations and in intact tissues *in vitro* and *in vivo*, are required for us to obtain a broader and more accurate understanding of the inter- and intracellular events in nociceptive signalling.

References

Akins, P.T. and McCleskey, E.W. (1993). Characterization of potassium currents in adult rat sensory neurons and modulation by opioids and cyclic AMP. *Neuroscience* **56**, 759–69.

Allan, A.C., Gammon, C.M., Ousley, A.H., McCarthy, K.D., and Morell, P. (1992). Bradykinin stimulates arachidonic acid release through the sequential actions of an *sn*-1 diacylglycerol lipase and a monoacylglycerol lipase. *J. Neurochem.* **58**, 1130–9.

Aloe, L., Tuveri, M.A., Carcassi, U., and Levi-Montalcini, R. (1992). Nerve growth factor in the synovial fluid of patients with chronic arthritis. *Arthritis Rheumatism* **35**, 351–5.

Bean, B. (1992), Pharmacology and electrophysiology of ATP-activated ion channels. *Trends pharmacol. Sci.* **13**, 87–90.

Beck, P.W. and Handwerker, H.O. (1974). Bradykinin and serotonin effects on various types of cutaneous nerve fibres. *Pflügers Arch.* **347**, 209–22.

Bevan, S. and Docherty, R.J. (1993). Cellular mechanisms of the action of capsaicin. In *Capsaicin in the study of pain* (ed. J.N. Wood), pp. 27–44. Academic Press, London.

Bevan, S. and Geppetti, P. (1994). Protons: small stimulants of capsaicin-sensitive nerves. *Trends Neurosc.* **17**, 509–12.

Bevan, S. and Szolcsányi, J. (1990). Sensory neuron-specific actions of capsaicin: mechanisms and applications. *Trends Pharmacol. Sci.* **11**, 330–3.

Birrell, G.J. and McQueen, D.S. (1993). The effects of capsaicin, bradykinin, PGE$_2$ and cicaprost on the discharge of articular sensory receptors in vitro. *Brain Res.* **611**, 103–7.

Birrell, G.J., McQueen, D.S., Iggo, A., Coleman, R.A., and Grubb, B.D. (1991). PGI$_2$-induced activation and sensitization of articular mechanociceptors. *Neurosci. Lett.* **124**, 5–8.

Bisgaard, H. and Kristensen, J.K. (1985). Leukotriene B$_4$ produces hyperalgesia in humans. *Prostaglandins* **30**, 791–7.

Bleehan, T. and Keele, C.A. (1977). Observations on the algogenic actions of adenosine compounds on the human blister base preparation. *Pain* **3**, 367–77.

Bley, K.R., Eglen, R.M., and Wong, E.H.F. (1994). Characterization of 5-hydroxytryptamine-induced depolarizations in rat isolated vagus nerve. *Eur. J. Pharmacol.* **260**, 139–47.

Bouthillier, J., DeBois, D., and Marceau, F. (1987). Studies on the induction of pharmacological responses to des-Arg^9-bradykinin *in vitro* and *in vivo*. *Br. J. Pharmacol.* **92**, 257–64.

Brake, A.J., Wagenbach, M.J., and Julius, D. (1994). New structural motif for ligand-gated ion channels defined by an ionotropic ATP receptor. *Nature* **371**, 519–23.

Bredt, D.S. and Snyder, S.H. (1994). Nitric oxide: a physiologic messenger molecule. *Ann. Rev. Biochem.* **63**, 175–95.

Brown, D.A. and Higashida, H. (1988). Inositol 1,4,5-triphosphate and diacylglycerol mimic bradykinin effects on mouse neuroblastoma × glioma hybrid cells. *J. Physiol.* **397**, 185–207.

Burch, R.M. and Axelrod, J. (1987). Dissociation of bradykinin-induced prostaglandin formation from phosphoinositol turnover in Swiss 3T3 fibroblasts: evidence for G protein regulation of phospholipase A$_2$. *Proc. natl Acad. Sci., USA* **84**, 6372–8.

Burgess, G.M., Mullaney, J., McNeil, M., Dunn, P., and Rang, H.P. (1989*a*). Second messengers involved in the action of bradykinin on cultured sensory neurons. *J. Neurosci.* **9**, 3314–25.

Burgess, G.M., Mullaney, I., McNeill, M., Coote, P.R., Minhas, A., and Wood, J.N. (1989*b*). Activation of guanylate cyclase by bradykinin in rat sensory neurones is mediated by calcium influx: possible role of the increase in cyclic GMP. *J. Neurochem.* **53**, 1212–18.

Cahill, M., Fishman, J.B., and Polgar, P. (1988). Effect of des-arginine^9-bradykinin and other bradykinin fragments on the synthesis of prostacyclin and the binding of bradykinin by vascular cells in culture. *Agents Actions* **24**, 224–31.

Campbell, M.D., Subramaniam, S., Kotlikoff, M.I., Williamson, J.R., and Fluharty, S.J. (1990). Cyclic AMP inhibits polyphosphate production and calcium mobilization in neuroblastoma × glioma NG108-15 cells. *Mol. Pharmacol.* **38**, 282–8.

Christian, E.P., Taylor, G.E., and Weinreich, D. (1989). Serotonin increases excitability of rabbit C-fibre neurons by two distinct mechanisms. *J. Appl. Physiol.* **67**, 584–91.

Cohen, A.S., Weinreich, D., and Kao, J.P.Y. (1994). Nitric oxide regulates spike frequency accommodation in nodose neurons of the rabbit. *Neurosc. Lett.* **173**, 17–20.

Coleman, R.A., Smith, W.L., and Narumiya, S. (1994). VIII. International Union of Pharmacology classification of prostanoid receptors: properties, distribution, and structure of the receptors and their subtypes. *Pharmacol. Rev.* **46**, 205–229.

Conklin, B.R., Burch, R.M., Steranka, L.R., and Axelrod, J. (1988). Distinct bradykinin receptors mediate stimulation of prostaglandin synthesis by endothelial cells and fibroblasts. *J. Pharmacol. Exp. Therapeut.* **244**, 646–9.

Crespo, P., Xu, N., Simonds, W.F., and Gutkind, J.S. (1994). Ras-dependent activation of MAP-kinase pathway mediated by G protein subunits. *Nature* **369**, 418–20.

Crunkhorn, P. and Willis, A.L. (1971). Cutaneous reaction to intradermal prostaglandins. *Br. J. Pharmacol.* **41**, 49–56.

D'Arcangelo, G. and Halegoua, S. (1993). A branched signalling pathway for nerve growth factor is revealed by Src-, Ras-, and Raf-mediated gene functions. *Mol. Cell Biol.* **13**, 3146–55.

Davis, A.J. and Perkins, M.N. (1994). Induction of B1 receptors *in vivo* in a model of persistent inflammatory mechanical hyperalgesia in the rat. *Neuropharmacology* **33**, 127–33.

Davis, B.M., Lewin, G.R., Mendell, L.M., Jones, M.E., and Albers, K.M. (1993). Altered expression of nerve growth factor in the skin of transgenic mice leads to changes in response to mechanical stimuli. *Neuroscience* **56**, 789–92.

DeBlois, D., Bouthillier, J., and Marceau, F. (1988). Effect of glucocorticoids, monoamines and growth factors on the spontaneously developing responses of the rabbit isolated aorta to des-Arg^9-bradykinin. *Br. J. Pharmacol.* **93**, 969–77.

DeBlois, D., Bouthillier, J., and Marceau, F. (1991). Pulse exposure to protein synthesis inhibitors enhances vascular responses to des-Arg^9-bradykinin: possible role of interleukin-1. *Br. J. Pharmacol.* **103**, 1057–66.

Devor, M., Jänig, W., and Michaelis, M. (1994). Modulation of activity in dorsal root ganglion neurons by sympathetic activation in nerve-injured rats. *J. Neurosci.* **71**, 38–47.

Dobrowsky, R.T., Werner, M.H., Castellino, A.M., and Chao, M.V. (1994). Activation of the sphingomyelin circle through the low affinity neurotrophin receptor. *Science* **265**, 1596–9.

Donnerer, J., Schuligoi, R., and Stein, C. (1992). Increased content and transport of substance P and calcitonin gene-related peptide in sensory nerves innervating inflamed tissue: evidence for a regulatory function of nerve growth factor *in vivo*. *Neuroscience* **49**, 693–8.

D'Orleans-Juste, P., de Nucci, G., and Vane, J.R. (1989). Kinins act on B$_1$ or B$_2$ receptors to release conjointly endothelium-derived relaxing factor and prostacyclin from bovine aortic endothelial cells. *Br. J. Pharmacol.* **96**, 920–6.

Dray, A. and Perkins, M. (1993). Bradykinin and inflammatory pain. *Trends Neurosc.* **16**, 99–104.

Dray, A., Patel, I.A., Perkins, M.N., and Rueff, A. (1992). Bradykinin-induced activation of nociceptors: receptor and mechanistic studies on the neonatal rat spinal cord-tail preparation in vitro. *Br. J. Pharmacol.* **107**, 1129–34.

Dunn, P.M. and Rang, H.P. (1990). Bradykinin-induced depolarisation of primary afferent nerve terminals in the neonatal rat spinal cord *in vitro*. *Br. J. Pharmacol.* **100**, 656–60.

Falus, A. and Meretey, K. (1992). Histamine: an early messenger in inflammatory immune reactions. *Immunol. Today* **13**, 154–6.

Farmer, S.G. and Burch, R.M. (1992). Biochemical and molecular pharmacology of kinin receptors. *Ann. Rev. Pharmacol.* **32**, 511–36.

Ferreira, S.H. and Nakamura, M. (1979). Prostaglandin hyperalgesia: the peripheral analgesic activity of morphine, enkephalin and opioid-antagonists. *Prostaglandins* **18**, 191–200.

Fozard, J.R. (1994). Role of 5-HT$_3$ receptors in nociception. In *5-Hydroxytryptamine-3 receptor antagonists* (ed. F.D. King, B.J. Jones, and G.J. Sanger), pp. 241–53. CRC Press, Boca Raton, Florida.

Francel, P. and Dawson, G. (1988). Bradykinin induces the bi-phasic production of lysophosphatidylinositol and diacylglycerol in a dorsal root × neurotumor hybrid cell line, F11. *Biochem. biophys. Res. Commun.* **152**, 724–31.

Gammon, C.M., Allen, A.C., and Morell, P. (1989). Bradykinin stimulates phosphoinositide hydrolysis and mobilization of arachidonic acid in dorsal root ganglion neurons. *J. Neurochem.* **53**, 95–101.

Gammon, C.M., Lyons, S.A., and Morell, P. (1990). Modulation by neuropeptides of bradykinin-stimulated second messenger release in dorsal root ganglion neurons. *Brain Res.* **518**, 159–65.

Garry, M.G., Richardson, J.D., and Hargreaves, K.M. (1994). Sodium nitroprusside evokes the release of immunoreactive calcitonin gene-related peptide and substance P from dorsal horn slices via nitric oxide-dependent and nitric oxide-independent mechanisms. *J. Neurosc.* **14**, 4329–37.

Geppetti, P., Del Bianco, E., Tramontana, M., Vigano, T., Folco, G.C., Maggi, C.A., Manzini, S., and Fanciullacci, M. (1991). Arachidonic acid and bradykinin share a common pathway to release neuropeptide from capsaicin-sensitive sensory nerve fibers of the guinea pig heart. *J. Pharmacol. exp. Therapeut.* **259**, 759–65.

Gold, M.S., Shuster, M.J., Dastmalchi, S., and Levine, J.D. (1994). Role of a slow Ca^{2+}-dependent afterhyperpolarization in prostaglandin E_2-induced sensitization of cultured rat sensory neurons. *Soc. Neurosc. Abstr.* **20**, 1569.

Goldstein, R.H. and Wall, M. (1984). Activation of protein formation and cell division by bradykinin and des-Arg^9-bradykinin. *J. Biol. Chem.* **259**,9263–8.

Grubb, B.D., Birrell, G.J., McQueen, D.S., and Iggo, A. (1991). The role of PGE_2 in the sensitization of mechanoreceptors in normal and inflamed ankle joints of the rat. *Exp. Brain Res.* **84**, 383–92.

Häbler, H.-J., Jänig, W., and Koltzenburg, M. (1987). Activation of unmyelinated afferents in chronically lesioned nerves by adrenaline and excitation of sympathetic efferents in the cat. *Neurosc. Lett.* **82**, 35–40.

Hall, J.M. (1992). Bradykinin receptor: pharmacological properties and biological roles. *Pharmacol. Therapeut.* **56**, 131–90.

Hess, J.F., Borkowski, J.A., Young, G.S., Strader, C.D., and Ransom, R.W. (1992). Cloning and pharmacological characterization of a human bradykinin (BK-2) receptor. *Biochem. Biophys. Res. Commun. b184*, 260–8.

Heumann, R. (1994). Neurotrophin signalling. *Curr. Opin. Neurobiol.* **4**, 668–79.

Hille, B. (1994). Modulation of ion-channel function by G-protein coupled receptors. *Trends Neurosc.* **17**, 531–6.

Hingtgen, C.M. and Nicol, G.D. (1994). Carba prostacyclin enhances the capsaicin-induced cobalt-loading of rat sensory neurons grown in culture. *Neurosci. Lett.* **1173**, 99–102.

Hingtgen, C.M. and Vasko, M.R. (1994). Prostacyclin enhances the evoked release of substance P and calcitonin gene-related peptide from rat sensory neurons. *Brain Res.* **655**, 51–60.

Holthusen, H. and Arndt, J.O. (1994). Nitric oxide evokes pain in humans on intracutaneous injection. *Neurosci. Lett.* **165**, 71–4.

Hong, S.L. and Deykin, D. (1982). Activation of phospholipase A2 in pig aortic endothelial cells synthesizing prostacyclin. *J. Biol. Chem.* **257**, 7151–4.

Hua, X-Y. and Yaksh, T.L. (1993). Pharmacology of the effects of bradykinin, serotonin and histamine on the release of calcitonin gene-related peptide in the rat trachea. *J. Neurosc.* **13**, 1947–53.

Hutcheon, B., Puil, E., and Spigelman, I. (1993). Histamine actions and comparisons with substance P effects in trigeminal neurons. *Neuroscience* **55**, 521–9.

Juan, H. and Sametz, W. (1980). Histamine-induced release of arachidonic acid and of prostaglandins in the peripheral vascular bed. *Naunyn-Schmiedebergs Arch. Pharmacol.* **314**, 183–90.

Kolesnik, R. and Golde, D.W. (1994). The sphingomyelin pathway in tumor necrosis factor and interleukin-1 signaling. *Cell* **77**, 325–8.

Koltzenburg, M., Kees, S., Budweiser, S., Ochs, G., and Toyka, K.V. (1994). The properties of unmyelinated nociceptive afferents change in a painful chronic constriction neuropathy. In *Proceedings of the 7th World Congress on Pain*, Vol. 2. *Progress in pain management* (ed. G.F. Gebhart, D.L. Hammond, and T.S. Jensen), pp. 511–22. IASP Press, Seattle.

Koppert, W., Reeh, P.W., and Handwerker, H.O. (1993). Conditioning of histamine by bradykinin alters responses of rat nociceptors and human itch sensation. *Neurosc. Lett.* **152**, 117–20.

Kumazawa, T., Mizumura, K., and Koda, H. (1994). Different mechanisms (receptor subtypes and second messenger actions) implicated in PGE_2-induced sensitization of the responses to bradykinin and to heat of polymodal receptors. In *Proceedings of the 7th World Congress on Pain*, Vol. 2. *Progress in pain management* (ed. G.F. Gebhart, D.L. Hammond, and T.S. Jensen), pp. 265–76. IASP Press, Seattle.

Lerner, U.H. and Modeer, T. (1991). Bradykinin B1 and B2 receptor agonists synergistically potentiate interleukin-1-induced prostaglandin biosynthesis in human gingival fibroblasts. *Inflammation* 15, 427–36.

Levine, J.D., Lau, W., Kwiat, G., and Goetzl, E. (1984). Leukotriene produces hyperalgesia that is dependent on polymorphonuclear leukocytes. *Science* 225, 743–5.

Levine, J.D., Gooding, J., Donatoni, P., Borden, L., and Goetzl, E. (1985). The role of the polymorphonuclear leukocyte in hyperalgesia. *J. Neurosc.* 5, 3025–9.

Levine, J.D., Lam, D., Taiwo, Y.O., Donatoni, P., and Goetzl, E.J. (1986a). Hyperalgesic properties of 15-lipoxygenase products of arachidonic acid. *Proc. natl Acad. Sci., USA* 93, 5331–4.

Levine, J.D., Taiwo, Y.O., Collins, S.D., and Tam, J.K. (1986b). Noradrenaline hyperalgesia is mediated through interaction with sympathetic postganglionic neurone terminals rather than activation of primary afferent nociceptors. *Nature* 323, 158–60.

Lewin, G.R., Ritter, A.M., and Mendell, L.M. (1993). Nerve growth factor-induced hyperalgesia in the neonatal and adult rat. *J. Neurosc.* 13, 2136–48.

Lindsay, R.M. (1988). Nerve growth factors (NGF, BDNF) enhance axonal regeneration but are not required for survival of adult sensory neurons. *J. Neurosc.* 8, 2394–405.

Lindsay, R.M. and Harmar, A.J. (1989). Nerve growth factor regulates expression of neuropeptide genes in adult sensory neurons. *Nature* 337, 362–4.

Liscovitch, M. and Cantley, L.C. (1994). Lipid second messengers. *Cell* 77, 329–34.

Ljunggren, O. and Lerner, U.H. (1990). Evidence for BK_1 bradykinin-receptor-mediated prostaglandin formation in osteoblasts and subsequent enhancement of bone resorption. *Br. J. Pharmacol.* 101, 382–6.

McEachern, A.E., Shelton, E.R., Bhakta, S., Obernolte, R., Bach, C., Zuppan, P., Fujisaka, J., Aldrich, R.W., and Jarnagin, K. (1991). Expression cloning of a rat B_2 receptor. *Proc. natl Acad. Sci., USA* 88, 7724–8.

McGehee, D.S. and Oxford, G.S. (1991). Bradykinin modulates the electrophysiology of cultured rat sensory neurons through a pertussis toxin-insensitive G protein. *Mol. Cell. Neurosc.* 2, 21–30.

McGehee, D.S., Goy, M.F., and Oxford, G.S. (1992). Involvement of the nitric oxide–cyclic GMP pathway in the desensitization of bradykinin responses of cultured rat sensory neurons. *Neuron* 9, 315–24.

McIntyre, P., Phillips, E., Skidmore, E., Brown, M., and Webb, M. (1993). Cloned murine bradykinin receptor exhibits a mixed B_1 and B_2 pharmacological selectivity. *Mol. Pharmacol.* 44, 346–55.

McMahon, S.B. (1991). Mechanisms of sympathetic pain. *Br. med. Bull.* 3, 584–600.

McQuirk, S.M. and Dolphin, A.C. (1992). G-protein mediation in nociceptive signal tranduction: an investigation into the excitatory action of bradykinin in a subpopulation of cultured rat sensory neurons. *Neuroscience* 49, 117–28.

Madison, S., Whitsel, E.A., Suarez-Roca, H., and Maixner, W. (1992). Sensitizing effects of leukotriene B_4 on intradental primary afferents. *Pain* 49, 99–104.

Marceau, F. and Regoli, D. (1991). Kinin receptors of the B_1 type and their antagonists. In *Bradykinin antagonists. Basic and clinical research* (ed. R.M. Burch), pp. 33–49. Marcel Dekker, New York.

Marceau, F. and Tremblay, B. (1986). Mitogenic effect of bradykinin and of des-Arg^9-bradykinin on cultured fibroblasts. *Life Sci.* 39, 2351–8.

Martin, H.A. (1990). Leukotriene B_4 induced decrease in mechanical and thermal thresholds of C-fiber mechanociceptors in rat hairy skin. *Brain Res.* 509, 273–9.

Martin, H.A., Basbaum, A.I., Kwiat, G.C., Goetzl, E.J., and Levine, J.D. (1987). Leukotriene and prostaglandin sensitization of cutaneous high threshold C- and A-delta mechanoreceptors in the hairy skin of rat hindlimbs. *Neuroscience* 22, 651–9.

Menke, J.G., Borkowski, J.A., Bierilo, K.K., MacNeil, T., Derrick, A.W., Schneck, K.A., Ransom, R.W., Strader, C.D., Linemeyer, D.L., and Hess, J.F. (1994). Expression cloning of a human B_1 bradykinin receptor. *J. Biol. Chem.* **269**, 21583–6.

Mizumura, K., Sato, J., and Kumazawa, T. (1987). Effects of prostaglandins and other putative chemical intermediaries on the activity of canine testicular polymodal receptors studied in vitro. *Pflügers Arch.* **408**, 565–72.

Mizumura, K., Minagawa, M., Koda, H., and Kumazawa, T. (1994). Histamine-induced sensitization of the heat response of canine visceral polymodal receptors. *Neurosc. Lett.* **168**, 93–6.

Moncada, S. (1992). The L-arginine: nitric oxide pathway. *Acta physiolog. scand.* **145**, 201–27.

Naruse, K., McGehee, D.S., and Oxford, G.S. (1992). Differential response of Ca-activated K channels to bradykinin in sensory neurons and F-11 cells. *Am. J. Physiol.* **262**, C453–C460.

Ng, N.F.L. and Shooter, E.M. (1993). Activation of p21[ras] by nerve growth factor in embryonic sensory neurons and PC12 cells. *J. biol. Chem.* **268**, 25329–33.

Nicholas, A.P., Pieribone, V., and Hökfelt, T. (1993). Distributions of mRNAs for alpha-2 adrenergic receptor subtypes in rat brain: an in situ hybridization study. *J. comp. Neurol.* **328**, 575–94.

Nicol, G.D., Klingberg, D.K., and Vasko, M.R. (1992). Prostaglandin E_2 increases calcium conductance and stimulates release of substance P in avian sensory neurons. *J. Neurosc.* **12**, 1917–27.

Nielsen, O.H., Bukhave, K., Ahnfelt-Ronne, I., and Rask-Madsen, J. (1988). Source of endogenous arachidonate and 5-lipoxygenase products in human neutrophils stimulated by bradykinin and A23187. *Gut* **29**, 319–24.

Ninkovic, M. and Hunt, S.P. (1985). Opiate and histamine H1 receptors are present on some substance P-containing dorsal root ganglion cells. *Neurosc. Lett.* **53**, 133–7.

Obermeier, A., Lammers, R., Wiesmuller, K-H., Jung, G., Schlessinger, J., and Ulrich, A. (1993). Identification of trk binding sites for SHC and phosphatidylinositol 3′-kinase and formation of a multimeric signalling complex. *J. Biol. Chem.* **268**, 22963–6.

Perkins, M.N., Campbell, E., and Dray, A. (1993). Anti-nociceptive activity of the B_1 and B_2 receptor antagonists desArg⁹Leu⁸Bk and HOE 140, in two models of persistent hyperalgesia in the rat. *Pain* **53**, 191–7.

Perkins, M.N. and Kelly, D. (1994). Interleukin-1β induced desArg⁹bradykinin-mediated thermal hyperalgesia in the rat. *Neuropharmacology* **33**, 657–60.

Peters, J.A., Malone, H.M., and Lambert, J.J. (1992). Recent advances in the electrophysiological characterization of 5-HT₃ receptors. *Trends pharmacol. Sc.* **13**, 391–7.

Pitchford, S. and Levine, J.D. (1991). Prostaglandins sensitize nociceptors in cell culture. *Neurosc. Lett.* **132**, 105–8.

Puttick, R.M. (1992). Excitatory action of prostaglandin E_2 on rat neonatal cultured dorsal root ganglion cells. *Br. J. Pharmacol.* **105**, 133P.

Regoli, D., Marceau, F., and Barabe, J. (1978). *De novo* formation of vascular receptors for bradykinin. *Can. J. Physiol. Pharmacol.* **56**, 674–7.

Reiser, G. (1991). Molecular mechanisms of action induced by 5-HT₃ receptors in a neuronal cell line and by 5-HT₂ receptors in a glial cell line. In *Serotonin, molecular biology, receptors and functional effects* (ed. J.R. Fozard and P.R. Saxena), pp. 69–83. Birkhäuser, Basel.

Reiser, G. and Hamprecht, B. (1989). Serotonin raises the cyclic GMP level in a neuronal cell line via 5-HT₃ receptors. *Eur. J. Pharmacol.* **172**, 195–8.

Rhodes, K.F., Coleman, J., and Lattimer, N. (1992). A component of 5-HT-evoked depolarization of the rat isolated vagus nerve is mediated by a putative 5-HT₄ receptor. *Naunyn-Schmiedebergs Arch. Pharmacol.* **346**, 496–503.

Richardson, B.P., Engel, G., Donatsch, P., and Stadler, P.A. (1985). Identification of serotonin M-receptor subtypes and their specific blockade by a new class of drugs. *Nature* **316**, 126–31.

Robertson, B. and Bevan, S. (1991). Properties of 5-hydroxytryptamine₃ receptor-gated currents in adult dorsal root ganglion neurones. *Br. J. Pharmacol.* **102**, 272–6.

Rodriguez-Viciana, P., Warne, P.H., Dhand, R., Vanhaesebroeck, B., Gout, I., Fry, M.J., Waterfield, M.D., and Downward, J. (1994). Phosphatidylinositol-3-OH kinase as a direct target of Ras. *Nature* **370**, 527–32.

Rosen, L.B., Ginty, D.D., and Weber, M.J. (1994). Membrane depolarization and calcium influx stimulate MEK and MAP kinase via activation of Ras. *Neuron* **12**, 1207–21.

Rueff, A. and Dray, A. (1992). 5-Hydroxytryptamine-induced sensitization and activation of peripheral fibres in the neonatal rat are mediated via different 5-hydroxytryptamine-receptors. *Neuroscience* **50**, 899–905.

Rueff, A. and Dray, A. (1993). Sensitization of peripheral afferent fibres in the in vitro neonatal rat spinal cord–tail by bradykinin and prostaglandins. *Neuroscience* **54**, 527–35.

Salvemini, D., Misko, T.P., Masferrer, J.L., Seibert, K., Currie, M.G., and Needleman, P. (1993). Nitric oxide activate cyclooxygenase enzymes. *Proc. natl Acad. Sci., USA* **90**, 7240–4.

Sato, J. and Perl, E. (1991). Adrenergic excitation of cutaneous pain receptors induced by peripheral nerve injury. *Science* **251**, 1608–10.

Sato, J., Suzuki, S., Tamura, R., and Kumazawa, T. (1994). Norepinephrine excitation of cutaneous nociceptors in adjuvant-induced inflamed rats does not depend on sympathetic neurons. *Neurosc. Lett.* **177**, 135–8.

Schaible, H.-G. and Schmidt, R.F. (1988). Excitation and sensitization of fine articular afferents from cat's knee joint by prostaglandin E$_2$. *J. Physiol.* **403**, 91–104.

Schepelmann, K., Messlinger, K., Schaible, H.-G., and Schmidt, R.F. (1992). Inflammatory mediators and nociceptors in the joint: excitation and sensitization of slowly conducting afferent fibers of cat's knee by prostaglandin I$_2$. *Neuroscience* **50**, 237–47.

Shearman, M.S., Sekiguchi, K., and Nishizuka, Y. (1989). Modulation of ion channel activity: a key function of the protein kinase C enzyme family. *Pharmacol. Rev.* **41**, 211–37.

Shen, K.-F. and Crain, S.M. (1994). Nerve growth factor rapidly prolongs the action potential of mature sensory ganglion neurons in culture, and this effect requires the activation of Gs-coupled excitatory k-opioid receptors on these cells. *J. Neurosc.* **14**, 5570–9.

Sicuteri, F., Franciullacci, M., Franchi, G., and Del Bianco, P.L. (1965). Serotonin–bradykinin potentiation on the pain receptors in man. *Life Sci.* **4**, 309–16.

Smith, J.A.M., Webb, C., Holford, J., and Burgess, G.M. (1995). Signal transduction pathways for B$_1$ and B$_2$ bradykinin receptors in bovine pulmonary artery endothelial cells. *Mol. Pharmacol.* **47**, 525–34.

Steel, J.H., Terenghi, G., Chung, J.M., Na, H.S., Carlton, S.M., and Polak, J.M. (1994). Increased nitric oxide synthase immunoreactivity in rat dorsal root ganglia in a neuropathic pain model. *Neurosc. Lett.* **169**, 81–4.

Stephens, R.M., Loeb, D.M., Copeland, T.D., Greene, L.A., and Kaplan, D.R. (1994). trk Receptors use redundant signal transduction pathways involving SHC and PLC-γl to mediate NGF responses. *Neuron* **12**, 691–705.

Sung, C-P., Arleth, A.J., Shikano, K., and Berkowitz, B.A. (1988). Characterization and function of bradykinin receptors in vascular endothelial cells. *J. Pharmacol. exp. Therapeut.* **247**, 8–13.

Taiwo, Y.O., Bjerknes, L.K., Goetzl, E.J., and Levine, J.D. (1989). Mediation of primary afferent peripheral hyperalgesia by the cAMP second messenger system. *Neuroscience* **32**, 577–80.

Taiwo, Y.O. and Levine, J.D. (1990). Direct cutaneous hyperalgesia induced by adenosine. *Neuroscience* **38**, 757–62.

Taiwo, Y.O. and Levine, J.D. (1991). Further confirmation of the role of adenyl cyclase and of cAMP-dependent protein kinase in primary afferent hyperalgesia. *Neuroscience* **44**, 131–5.

Taiwo, Y.O. and Levine, J.D. (1992). Serotonin is a directly-acting hyperalgesic agent in the rat. *Neuroscience* **48**, 485–90.

Taiwo, Y.O., Levine, J.D., Burch, R.M., Woo, J.E., and Mobley, W.C. (1991). Hyperalgesia induced in the rat by the amino-terminal octapeptide of nerve growth factor. *Proc. natl Acad. Sci., USA* **88**, 5144–8.

Taiwo, Y.O., Heller, P.H., and Levine, J.D. (1992). Mediation of serotonin hyperalgesia by the cAMP second messenger system. *Neuroscience* **48**, 479–83.

Tani, E., Shiosaka, S., Sato, M., Ishikawa, T., and Tohyama, M. (1990). Histamine acts directly on calcitonin gene-related peptide- and substance P-containing trigeminal ganglion neurons as assessed by calcium influx and immunocytochemistry. *Neurosc. Lett.* **115**, 171–6.

Thayer, S.A., Perney, T.M., and Miller, R.J. (1988). Regulation of calcium homeostasis in sensory neurons by bradykinin. *J. Neurosci.* **8**, 4089–97.

Tiffany, C.W. and Burch, R.M. (1989). Bradykinin stimulates tumor necrosis factor and interleukin 1 release from macrophages. *FEBS Lett.* **247**, 189–92.

Toda, N., Bian, K., Aikiba, T., and Okamura, T. (1987). Heterogeneity in mechanisms of bradykinin action in canine isolated blood vessels. *Eur. J. Pharmacol.* **135**, 321–9.

Todorovic, S. and Anderson, E.G. (1990). 5-HT2 and 5-HT3 receptors mediate two distinct depolarizing responses in rat dorsal root ganglion neurons. *Brain Res.* **511**, 71–9.

Undem, B.J. and Weinreich, D. (1993). Electrophysiological properties and chemosensitivity of guinea pig ganglion neurons in vitro. *J. autonom. Nerv. Syst.* **44**, 17–33.

Valera, S., Hussy, N., Evans, R.J., Adami, N., North, R.A., Suprenant, A., and Buell, G. (1994). A new class of ligand-gated ion channel defined by P_{2x} receptor for extracellular ATP. *Nature* **371**, 516–19.

Verge, V.M.K., Xu, Z., Xu, X.-J., Wiesenfeld-Hallin, Z., and Hökfelt, T. (1992). Marked increase in nitric oxide synthase mRNA in rat dorsal root ganglia after peripheral axotomy: in situ hybridization and functional studies. *Proc. natl Acad. Sci., USA* **89**, 11617–21.

Weinreich, D. (1986). Bradykinin inhibits a slow spike afterhyperpolarization in visceral sensory nerves. *Eur. J. Pharmacol.* **132**, 61–3.

Weinreich, D. and Wonderlin, W.F. (1987). Inhibition of calcium-dependent spike after-hyperpolarization increases excitability of rabbit visceral sensory neurons. *J. Physiol.* **394**, 415–27.

Wiemer, G. and Wirth, K. (1992). Production of cGMP via activation of B_1 and B_2 kinin receptors in cultured bovine aortic endothelial cells. *J. Pharmacol. exp. Therapeut.* **262**, 729–33.

Wiesenfeld-Hallin, Z., Hao, J.-X., Xu, X.-J., and Hökfelt, T. (1993). Nitric oxide mediates ongoing discharges in dorsal root ganglion cells after peripheral nerve injury. *J. Neurophysiol.* **70**, 2350–535.

Winter, J., Forbes, C.A., Sternberg, J., and Lindsay, R.M. (1988). Nerve growth factor (NGF) regulates adult rat cultured dorsal root ganglion neuron responses to the excitotoxin capsaicin. *Neuron* **1**, 973–81.

Wood, J.N., Coote, P.R., Minhas, A., Mullaney, I., McNeill, M., and Burgess, G.M. (1989). Capsaicin-induced ion influxes increase cGMP but not cAMP levels in rat sensory neurones in culture. *J. Neurochem.* **53**, 1203–11.

Woolf, C.J., Safieh-Garabedian, B., Ma, Q-P., Crilly, P., and Winter, J. (1994). Nerve growth factor contributes to the generation of inflammatory sensory hypersensitivity. *Neuroscience* **62**, 327–31.

Yanagisawa, M.Y., Otsuka, M., and Garcia-Arraras, J.E. (1986). E-type prostaglandins depolarize primary afferent neurons of the neonatal rat. *Neurosci. Lett.* **68**, 351–5.

Yeats, J.C., Boddeke, H.G.M., and Docherty, R.J. (1992). Capsaicin desensitization in rat dorsal root ganglion neurones is due to activation of calcineurin. *Br. J. Pharmacol.* **107**, 238P.

13 Sensitization of polymodal receptors

TAKAO KUMAZAWA

Introduction

The 'coiling reflex' observed in the protochordate is the most primitive vertebrate nervous reflex, exhibited as the body coils away from noxious stimulus (Fig. 13.1). From an evolutionary point of view, all nervous regulatory systems may have been derived from this primitive withdrawal reflex and built on the nociceptive system. Since the very early stages of evolution, before the birth of the nervous system, humoral mechanisms such as primitive immune and inflammatory reactions had played important parts in the bio-warning and defence mechanisms. Various means of signalling, as used by the aboriginal humoral bio-warning systems, would have come into use in the primitive nervous nociceptive systems.

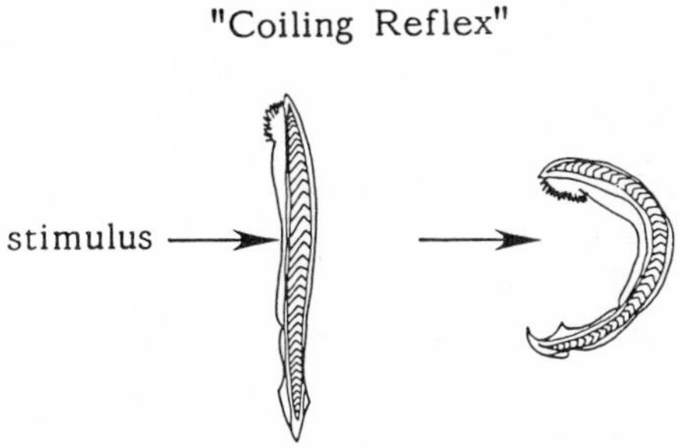

"Coiling Reflex"

Fig. 13.1 'Coiling reflex': a withdrawal reflex, as observed in *Amphioxus*—the most primitive reflex in the vertebrate.

The responsiveness of sensory receptors is often limited to a certain type of stimulus and certain range of intensity. In the skin, which is exposed to various forms of stimuli from the external environment, a number of sensory receptors are differentiated so as to precisely transduce specific types of stimuli including the most minute and subtle changes in the environment (Burgess and Perl 1973). Polymodal receptors (PMRs), however, are characterized by activation from a wide variety of stimuli, including mechanical, chemical, and heat stimuli; thus the term 'polymodal' was coined (Bessou and Perl 1969). These PMRs are widely distributed over the skin as well as in the somatic and visceral deep tissues (Kumazawa and Mizumura 1977*b*, 1980*b*; Kumazawa and Perl 1977; Table 13.1). The unclearly differentiated nature of these PMRs suggests that PMRs are the sensory receptors that conservatively preserve the response characteristics of the most primitive sensory receptors. This chapter reviews the modulations mediated by humoral agents in the activities of the PMRs.

Polymodal receptors (PMRs) (Table 13.1)

Nociceptive function of sensory receptors

Sensory receptors with a high threshold to stimulation, particularly to mechanical stimulation, are generally defined as nociceptors. However, PMRs have a wide dynamic range in the mechanical response. They respond in an intensity-dependent manner not only to distinctly noxious stimuli, but also to non-noxious stimuli (see Cervero, Chapter 9, this volume). The threshold is one means by which to measure and understand the characteristics of sensory receptors; however, the threshold may vary depending on how it is tested. The physical nature of the tissues surrounding the receptive site of the receptor greatly influences the thresholds for mechanical stimulation. Specifically, the mechanical threshold and pattern of evoked discharges will vary depending on where the receptive site is located in the tissue and from which direction the stimulus is applied. More than 80 per cent of the C-fibre afferents recorded in the gastrocnemius muscle of dogs are PMRs, which have been classified according to the responses to mechanical stimulation, to the close-arterial injection of algesic substances, and to noxious heat stimuli in some units (Kumazawa and Mizumura 1977*b*). It was noted in this particular experiment that the thresholds of some units were extremely high when mechanical stimulation was applied on the exposed outer surface of the muscle, but that they dropped to lower levels when tested from the inner surface of the muscle.

Table 13.1 Characteristics and functions of the polymodal receptor

Receptor activity
Wide variety of stimuli (mechanical, chemical, heat)
Wide distribution (skin, muscle, viscera)
Wide dynamic range (from non-noxious to noxious)
Easily modulated (sensitization)
Functions
Nociceptor
Reflex afferent
Local regulatory effector

Experiments on the PMRs of the testis and epididymis, which are located in the natural cavity of the tunica vaginalis, may be another example indicating the importance of methods for testing mechanical responses. Single-unit recordings from canine superior spermatic nerve afferents revealed that about 90 per cent of the units were PMRs responding to mechanical, noxious heat, and algesic chemical stimuli applied to the tunica vaginalis visceralis that was exposed without any injurious handling (Kumazawa and Mizumura 1980*b*). Peterson and Brown (1973) classified three types of testicular afferents on the basis of the pattern of discharges evoked by mechanical stimulation in cats: rapidly adapting mechanoreceptors; nociceptors displaying brief afterdischarges; and nociceptors displaying persistent afterdischarges. Comparison showed that the population of rapidly adapting receptors in the spermatic nerve afferents in cats (Peterson and Brown 1973) was much higher than that in dogs (Kumazawa *et al.* 1987*a*). This may be due to a species difference or, alternatively, it may be explained by reviewing the method of stimulation. In particular, Peterson and Brown (1973) used compression with a rod applied to the testis through the scrotal skin. In our own experiments, however, we noted that slowly adapting responses could often be changed to rapidly adapting ones in the same unit if the stimulus probe was moved slightly from the targeted receptive spot. It should also be noted that slowly adapting responses of single PMR units were followed by afterdischarges when stimulation was strong. The presence of afterdischarges following strong stimulation in a tested unit means that the unit can encode tissue damage that produces changes in the chemical environments where the ending is located (Lim *et al.* 1962; Lim 1970; Peterson and Brown 1973; Kumazawa and Mizumura 1980*b*).

The most important point in defining the nociceptive function is whether the sensory receptor can encode events that are noxious to the tissue surrounding the receptor terminals. Limited types of sensory receptors among a number of different somatic and visceral sensory receptors can encode noxious events. PMRs definitely signal nociceptive information and are especially important in signalling the pathological conditions of tissues. On the other hand, PMRs also respond to stimuli in a non-noxious range and may play important roles as reflex afferents at both non-noxious and noxious levels. For this reason they are referred to as polymodal receptors, instead of polymodal nociceptors.

The skin is exposed to sharp edges and has developed a special class of nociceptors – other than primitive PMRs – that signal precise information on the exact location and timing of the noxious stimulation applied. This is the high-threshold mechanoreceptor, which responds exclusively to intense mechanical stimuli. From a teleological viewpoint, this kind of pure mechanonociceptor may not have a chance to fully develop in deep tissues unexposed to any external environment.

Polymodal receptors in various tissues and in various animal species

The polymodal type of receptors are found in the skin of human beings (Torebjörk and Hallin 1974; Hallin *et al.* 1982), monkeys (Beitel and Dubner 1976; Croze *et al.* 1976; Kumazawa and Perl 1977), cats (Iggo 1959; Bessou and Perl 1969), rabbits (Lynn 1979), and rats (Lynn and Carpenter 1982). These cutaneous PMRs are reportedly conducted by C-fibres in general. The proportion of PMRs to cutaneous C-fibre afferents is almost 100 per cent in humans (Hallin *et al.* 1982), 85–90 per cent in monkeys (Kumazawa and Perl 1977), 35–40 per cent in cats (Bessou and Perl 1969), and about 70 per cent in rabbits (Lynn 1979) and in rats (Lynn and Carpenter 1982). The finding that almost all C-fibre afferents in humans are PMRs may indicate that all other afferents, which are differentiated so as to precisely transduce specific types of stimuli, are myelinated in human beings who are larger in size.

Sensory receptors, the characteristics of which are essentially the same as those of the cutaneous C-fibre PMRs, are also found in the somatic and visceral deep tissues: in the skeletal muscles (Mense 1977, 1981; Kumazawa and Mizumura 1977*b*; Kaufman *et al.* 1982); in the knee joint (Kanaka *et al.* 1985; Schaible and Schmidt 1988); in the cornea (Belmonte *et al.* 1991); in the heart (Nishi *et al.* 1977; Baker *et al.* 1980; Nerdrum *et al.* 1986); and in the testis and epididymis (Kumazawa and Mizumura 1980*a,b*). A substantial number of these receptors in the deep tissues are conducted by Aδ fibres. It should be noted, however, that the latencies measured by stimulation of multiple receptive spots in the single testicular PMR unit were much longer than those measured by stimulation of the nerve trunk at the spermatic cord, indicating that a nerve fibre sends out unmyelinated branches in the receptive region (Kumazawa and Mizumara 1980*b*). A similar phenomenon was reported for vagal and hypogastric afferent fibres (Duclaux *et al.* 1976; Floyd *et al.* 1976).

The characteristics of A- and C-fibre PMRs are essentially similar, although some quantitative differences do exist. For example, units with faster conduction velocities tend to have lower mechanical thresholds (Kumazawa *et al.* 1987*a*). Studies on the receptors in the deep tissues commonly report that bradykinin (BK) evokes discharges that can be augmented by prostaglandins (PGs) or other algesic substances. The effects of phorbol ester on the A- and C-fibre afferents are similar in both the articular (Schepelmann *et al.* 1993) and testicular afferents (Mizumura *et al.* 1994*c*), as described below. The responses to noxious heat and heat-induced sensitization are very important when identifying PMRs in the skin. Although heat stimulation has been tested only to a limited extent in some deep tissues, the results have shown that the effects in the muscle (Kumazawa and Mizumura 1977*b*), testis (Kumazawa and Mizumura 1980*b*), and heart (Nishi *et al.* 1977) are similar to those observed in the skin.

Morphological aspects of PMRs

Electron miscroscope images of the presumptive axonal ending, which was neurophysiologically identified as a receptive spot on a single PMR, often appear as an expansion not surrounded by Schwann cell processes but instead covered by basal lamina (Kruger *et al.* 1988; Kruger and Halata, Chapter 2, this volume). This region generally contains numerous tightly packed, clear spherical vesicles, although several granular vesicles and a few dense-core vesicles may also be present. The absence of any synaptic contact with specialized receptor structures reflects neurophysiological data regarding the response of the receptor to changes in a concentration ratio of Ca and Mg ions in the milieu (Sato *et al.* 1989).

Thin-fibre dorsal root ganglion (DRG) neurones are known to contain several kinds of peptides. Antidromic stimulation of neurophysiologically identified PMR fibres has been shown to produce extravasation (Kenins 1981), indicating that PMRs are implicated in neurogenic inflammation and, consequently, that PMR neurones contain neuropeptides. In testicular DRG neurones labelled by fast blue applied to the superior spermatic nerve, we found substance P (SP)-like and calcitonin-gene related peptide (CGRP)-like immunoreactivities in 66 per cent and 78 per cent of the labelled cells, respectively, and we also found that SP and CGRP were co-localized in 63 per cent of these testicular afferent neurones. More than 80 per cent of the superior spermatic afferents contained at least one of these peptides. Effector functions caused by a release of neuropeptides from the peripheral endings of these neurones are also very important as the local regulatory element of the body.

Sensitization of PMRs by heat stimulation

Sensitization induced by repeated heat stimulations

Heat stimulation above 45°C evokes discharges in PMRs in an intensity-dependent manner (Bessou and Perl 1969; Beck *et al.* 1974; Beitel and Dubner 1976; Croze *et al.* 1976). When the same pattern of ramp- or step-increasing heat stimulations is repeatedly applied at several °C above the threshold, the subsequent responses become enhanced, indicating sensitization of the receptor (Fig. 13.2). Further excessive heat stimuli cause the response to subsequent heating at the same intensity to decrease. These features of the effects of heat stimuli were similarly observed in cutaneous, muscular, and testicular

PMRs (Kumazawa and Mizumura 1977*a,b*, 1980*b*; Kumazawa and Perl 1977). Although heat stimulation in these ranges would probably not occur in the deep tissues in normal life, the response to heat stimulation is one of the most important tests in studying the nature of PMRs, regardless of the location of the receptors.

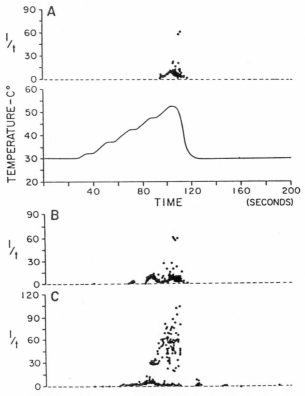

Fig. 13.2 Heat sensitization of a cutaneous PMR. Response (shown by instantaneous frequency of discharges) of a monkey C-fibre PMR to repeated noxious heating (lower graph of (A): thermode temperature near the skin interface). (A) First cycle; (B) third cycle; (C) fifth cycle. From Kumazawa and Perl (1977) with permission.

Sensitization induced by a single stimulation with strong heat

Stimulation at 55°C for 30s (strong heat) induced clear augmentation of the responses to stimulations at 45°C when tested within 10 min (Fig. 13.3). The augmentation of the heat response observed after applying strong heat continued for up to 3 hours. The response to BK was also potentiated after strong heat was applied; both the mean discharge rate and the total number of impulses induced by BK (0.1 μM) significantly increased to approximately double that observed before strong heat was applied (Fig. 13.3). However, the potentiation of the BK response did not last long and was of a lesser magnitude when compared with the potentiation of the heat responses (Fig. 13.3; Kumazawa *et al.* 1988; Mizumura *et al.* 1992). Although one receptive spot in a single unit responded to both heat and BK, the two responses were modulated differently. These differences in the augmentation of the responses to BK and heat suggest that there may be differences in the sensitizing mechanisms, such as in the mediators involved, the sensitizing potencies of a given mediator for these two responses, and/or the intracellular transduction processes involved in these responses.

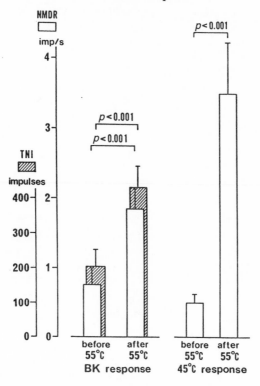

Fig. 13.3 Sensitizing effects of 55°C heating on both the BK response and the response to 45°C in testicular PMR units. Both the responses to BK and to 45°C were tested in the same unit. Net mean discharge rate, NMDR; total number of impulses, TNI; mean ± SEM; *n* = 14. From Mizumura *et al.* (1992), with permission.

Processes involved in the sensitization induced by heat stimulation

Applying strong heat to the tissues causes the release of various chemical mediators (Goodwin *et al.* 1963; Arturson *et al.* 1973; Fazekas *et al.* 1973), which may sensitize PMRs. In the presence of aspirin, the heat responses of PMRs were suppressed depending on the magnitude of the response. Aspirin also reduced the strong heat-induced enhancements of heat and BK responses, although substantial magnitudes of the enhancement were still observed in the presence of aspirin (Mizumura *et al.* 1994*d*). The aspirin dosage used in this particular experiment was sufficiently high to completely suppress cyclooxygenase (Ferreira *et al.* 1971) but was low enough to induce conduction blocking, if present (Riccioppo Neto 1980). These results indicate that PGs also play some role in the heat-induced enhancement of both the heat and BK responses and that other mediators besides the PGs are also implicated in the sensitization process. King *et al.* (1976) reported that suppression of heat sensitization could be obtained only by applying a combination of agents that would inhibit the production of PGs and BK, and would antagonize the effects of serotonin (5–HT) and histamine (HA). Such a report strongly suggests an interaction among various kinds of chemical mediators.

Modulation of PMR activities by inflammatory mediators

The intimate relation between pain and inflammation can be demonstrated by the fact that 'dolor' (pain) has been described as a classical symptom of inflammation. Among the various inflammatory mediators, it is known that BK, PGs, HA, and 5–HT play important roles in inflammatory pain. The activities of PMRs are sensitized by mediators such as PGs (Kumazawa *et al.* 1987*b*; Mizumura *et al.* 1987; Schaible and Schmidt 1988), BK (Lang *et al.* 1990; Kumazawa *et al.* 1991), 5–HT (Kumazawa *et al.* 1987*b*; Mizumura *et al.* 1987; Lang *et al.* 1990), and HA (Mizumura *et al.* 1994*b*).

Effects of BK on the activities of testicular PMRs

The concentration-related effects of BK, PGE_2, 5–HT, and HA on the activities of PMRs were compared using *in vitro* testis–spermatic nerve preparations, and the results are summarized in Fig. 13.4. Among these substances, BK evoked discharges in a concentration-dependent manner, with significance observed at concentrations as low as 10 nM. The other three substances, however, even at concentrations 1000 times greater than that required for BK, did not induce any excitation, although they all enhanced heat responses. This finding may support the concept that BK is the most likely 'endogenous pain-producing substance' (Armstrong *et al.* 1957; Lim 1970). The BK-induced discharges, however, were clearly suppressed by treatments with such cyclooxygenase inhibitors as indomethacin (Kumazawa and Mizumura 1980*a*) and aspirin (Kumazawa *et al.* 1987*b*; Mizumura *et al.* 1987), while, on the other hand, they were enhanced by treatments with PGE_2 and PGI_2 (Mizumura *et al.* 1987, 1991). Such responses indicate that PGs are clearly involved in the BK respose. Bradykinin is known to activate the release of PGs in various tissues (McGiff *et al.* 1972; Ferreira *et al.* 1973), while aspirin-like drugs have been shown to suppress some pseudo-affective reflexes (Hashimoto *et al.* 1964; Lim 1970; Ferreira *et al.* 1973).

Bradykinin-induced discharges were also enhanced by increasing the temperature within the non-noxious range. Compared with responses to the same concentration of BK tested at 30°C, BK responses at 36°C occurred after a shorter latency, with a higher maximum discharge rate and a larger number of impulses evoked during the 1-min stimulation period (Kumazawa *et al.* 1987*c*). These results by focusing on the neuronal impulse activity in the peripheral nociceptors, may explain the hyperalgesic conditions that often develop when the inflammatory tissues are warmed.

Responses to BK were gradually suppressed when tested in a Ca^{2+}-free solution that was made by eliminating Ca^{2+} from the Krebs solution and adding 1 mM EGTA. However, responses to hypertonic saline and KCl were augmented immediately after changing the solution to a Ca^{2+}-free solution. Adding Mg^{2+} to the solution induced a reversal of this augmentation, but Mg^{2+} did not inhibit the Ca^{2+}-free effect on the BK response (Sato *et al.* 1989). It is thus presumed that different mechanisms of action by the Ca ion are involved in these two phenomena. The slower time course reported for the Ca^{2+}-free solution to affect the BK responses may suggest the involvement of the Ca ion in the intracellular signal transduction of the BK response.

Pretreatment with BK significantly enhanced heat responses at concentrations as low as 0.1 nM (Kumazawa *et al.* 1991). The augmenting effects were concentration-dependent and occurred whether BK-induced discharges were present or not. The

BK-induced enhancement of the heat responses, however, did not last long even at a high concentration (10 μM).

The effects of BK on the activities of PMRs are characterized by the facts that: (1) it excites the PMRs at low concentrations; and (2) it also sensitizes the PMRs to enhance the heat response even at much lower concentrations, although this effect is short-lasting.

Modulation of PMR activities by PGE₂, 5–HT, and HA

Prostaglandin E_2 and 5–HT did not evoke significant discharges at concentrations of 0.1–10 μM (Fig. 13.4), but significantly enhanced responses to heat as well as to hypertonic saline and BK whether or not these substances evoked any discharges (Kumazawa *et al.* 1987*b*; Mizumura *et al.* 1987). Prostaglandin E_2 significantly enhanced responses to BK at 10 nM (Mizumura *et al.* 1987) and to heat at 1 μM (Kumazawa *et al.* 1992; Mizumura *et al.* 1993*a*; Fig. 13.5). Prostaglandin I_2 induced similar outcomes on the activities of PMRs to PGE₂, and tended to be effective at a lower concentration than required for PGE₂ (Mizumura *et al.* 1991).

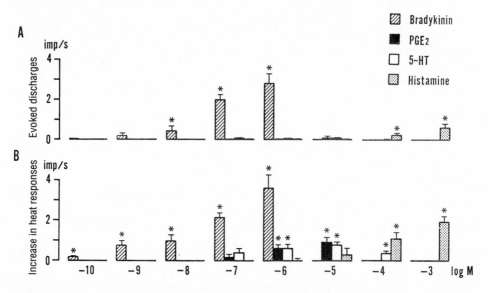

Fig. 13.4 Concentration relationships of evoked discharges and augmenting effects on heat responses induced by various inflammatory mediators. Effects of BK (0.1 nM–1 μM), PGE₂ (100 nM–10 μM), 5-HT (100 nM–10 μM), and HA (1 μM–1 mM) are shown by hatched, black, white, and dotted columns, respectively. (A) Mean discharge rate evoked by each substance; (B) net increase in mean discharge rate evoked by heat stimulation, which was induced by pretreatment with each of these four substances. Abscissa: concentrations in log M. *Significant difference compared to control ($p < 0.05$, paired t-test).

Histamine induced a distinct increase in the discharge rate in some of the units tested (high-responders). An HA-induced discharge pattern is characterized by a slow onset and a slow decline similar to the pattern produced by BK-induced discharges. In contrast, some units failed to induce even a single impulse in response to HA even at concentrations as high as 1 mM (low responders). Conduction velocity in the high-responder group ranged from 0.6 to 5.4 m/s, while in the low-responder group it ranged from 4.0 to 17.5 m/s. Treatment with HA augmented the heat responses, but no significant differences were observed between the high- and low-responder groups (Mizumura *et al.* 1994*b*).

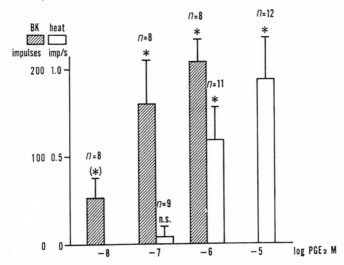

Fig. 13.5 Comparison of the augmenting effects of PGE_2 on the BK and heat responses. Hatched column, net increase in number of impulses evoked by BK (10 nM); white column, net increase in mean discharge rate during heat stimulation. *Significant change ($p < 0.05$). From Kumazawa *et al.* (1992), with permission.

Substance P is known as a mediator of neurogenic inflammation (Lembeck 1983). Substance P neither evoked discharges nor modulated the activity of this receptor to any substantial degree (Kumazawa and Mizumura 1979; Mizumura *et al.* 1987), confirming the results obtained by Lembeck and Gamse (1977) in a study on nociceptive reflexes.

The effects of PGs, 5–HT, and HA on the activities of PMRs are characterized by the facts that: (1) they evoke no discharges of the PMRs even at concentrations much higher than that required for BK; and (2) they sensitize the PMRs even in the absence of any excitatory effect, and these sensitizing effects last longer than any induced by BK.

These observations suggest that various inflammatory mediators affect nociceptor activities, even though the implicated mechanisms may differ among these mediators. To clarify the roles of these mediators in peripheral nociception, the next step would be to investigate the membrane receptors for these substances and to study the intracellular signal transduction mechanisms through these receptors. Findings from our recent experiments investigating these issues are described next.

Receptors and second messengers implicated

Receptors and second messengers implicated in the sensitization of PMRs by BK and HA

Two subtypes of BK receptors, B_1 and B_2, have been proposed (Regoli and Barabe 1980). The B_1 agonist and antagonist neither evoked discharges of testicular PMRs nor suppressed their responses to BK, whereas B_2 antagonists suppressed the BK responses (Mizumura *et al.* 1990). Figure 13.6(A) shows an involvement of the B_2 receptor in the BK-induced excitation and augmentation of heat responses in a testicular PMR unit using a B_2 receptor antagonist, NPC349 (Kumazawa *et al.* 1991). The response to BK was almost completely suppressed when applied along with NPC349 (940 nM) (Fig. 13.6(C)). The application of NPC349 also almost completely eliminated the BK-induced augmentation of the heat response (Fig. 13.6(B)).

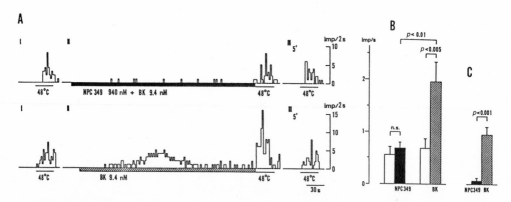

Fig. 13.6 Effects of a B_2 receptor antagonist, NPC349, on the BK-induced discharges and augmentation of heat responses. (A) I, Control responses to 48°C stimulation; II, response to BK (9.4 nM) in the presence or absence of NPC349 (940 nM) and the following heat responses; III, heat responses 5 min after BK application. Black bars, application time for BK plus NPC349; hatched bar, application time for BK alone. (B) Effect of NPC349 on BK-induced augmentation of the heat response. White columns, control heat responses; black columns, responses following BK plus NPC349; hatched columns, responses following BK alone. (C) Effect of NPC349 on the response to BK. Black column, responses to BK plus NPC349; hatched column, BK alone. Concentration of BK, 9.4 nM; concentration of NPC349, 940 nM; $n = 7$. From Kumazawa *et al.* (1991) with permission.

Three subtypes of HA receptors, H_1, H_2, and H_3, have been identified in mammalian tissues (Hill 1990). Our experiments using an H_1 antagonist, D-chlorpheniramine, and an H_2 antagonist, famotidine, revealed that the HA-induced discharges and enhancement of the heat responses were both antagonized by the H_1 but not by the H_2 receptor antagonist.

These results indicate that BK- and HA-induced responses in testicular PMRs are mediated by the B_2 and H_1 receptor subtypes, respectively. Involvement of protein kinase C (PKC) activation is known in both B_2- and H_1-receptor mediated signal transduction (Miller 1987; Hill 1990).

The implication of PKC activation in testicular PMR activities was examined using phorbol esters, phorbol 12, 13-dibutyrate (PDBu) and phorbol 12-myristate 13-acetate (PMA), which are known to readily enter into the cell membrane and activate PKC (Castagna *et al.* 1982; Nishizuka 1984). The application of 10 nM PDBu did not affect the activities of testicular PMRs. At 100 nM it induced excitation in 45 per cent of the units tested, and these PDBu-induced discharges lasted long after rinsing PDBu away (Fig. 13.7(A)). The heat response was clearly augmented by pretreatment with PDBu, and the effect was long-lasting (Fig. 13.7(B)). PMA at 100 nM only occasionally induced a small increase in the discharge rate, while it augmented heat responses weakly but significantly (Mizumura *et al.* 1994*c*). The responses to BK were also significantly augmented when applied along with PDBu (100 nM) but not when applied as a pretreatment. A recent report showed that, in the Aδ and C-fibre knee joint afferents, a PDBu solution at concentrations > 10 μM caused excitation and augmentation of the responses to mechanical stimulation when applied intraarterially close to the knee joint (Schepelmann *et al.* 1993). Involvement of PKC in the effects of the phorbol esters on these afferents is highly probable, but further studies, for example, using PKC inhibitors, will be necessary to verify such a hypothesis.

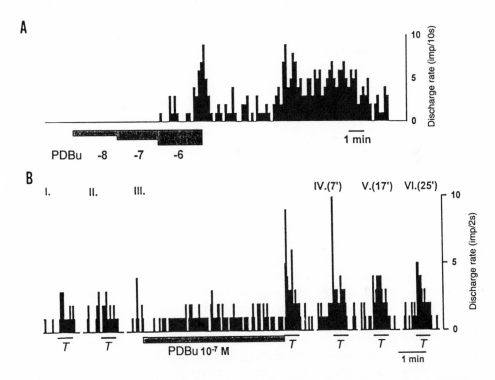

Fig. 13.7 Effects of PDBu, a phorbol ester, on testicular PMRs. (A) Excitatory effects of PDBu at concentrations between 10 nM and 1 μM applied cumulatively. The shaded area indicates the application period of PDBu. (B) Responses to heat (*T*, 46°C) were augmented after an application of PDBu at 100 nM which induced a small excitation. From Mizumura *et al.* (1994*c*), with permission.

The stimulation of phospholipase C (PLC) is one of the main intracellular pathways mediated by the BK receptor, as it produces inositol triphosphate (IP$_3$) and diacylglycerol (DAG) (Yano *et al.* 1984; Higashida *et al.* 1986; Brown and Higashida 1988; Gammon *et al.* 1989). Diacylglycerol is known in turn to activate PKC, which is important in controlling various aspects of neuronal function and in modulating the activity of ion channels (Kaczmarek 1987; Miller 1987). Bradykinin depolarizes neonatal rat DRG neurones, which is mimicked by the activation of PKC (Burgess *et al.* 1989). H$_1$-receptor stimulation is generally associated with inositol phospholipid hydrolysis (Lo and Fan 1987; Hill 1990).

It is noteworthy that in our current study the responses to BK were not augmented either by a pretreatment with HA when the application of His evoked substantial discharges, or by a pretreatment with PDBu. Protein kinase C activation has been shown to desensitize the H_1 receptor-mediated responses in *in vitro* cell lines (Smit *et al.* 1992; Dickenson and Hill 1993). If PKC-activation pathways coupled with B_2 and H_1 receptors can be implicated in the BK- and HA-induced effects on testicular PMRs, some type of cross-tachyphylaxis-like phenomenon may occur in the intracellular signal transduction mechanisms.

Receptors and second messengers implicated in the PGE_2-induced enhancement of BK responses in testicular PMRs

In several experiments we found that PGE_2 enhanced the response of PMRs to heat at concentrations that did not evoke any discharge of the sensory receptor. However, PGE_2 enhanced BK responses at concentrations 100 times lower than those necessary for the heat responses (Mizumura *et al.* 1987, 1991; Kumazawa *et al.* 1992; Fig. 13.5). This marked difference in the concentration of PGE_2 that is effective to induce sensitization of the two responses suggests that different types of PGE receptors are involved in each of these phenomena.

On the basis of pharmacological studies carried out mainly on visceral tissue preparations, PGE receptors have been subdivided into three subtypes: EP_1, EP_2, and EP_3 (Coleman *et al.* 1990). The antagonist and agonists selective for these three subtypes of EP receptors were used to determine which receptor is involved in the PGE_2-induced augmentation of BK responses (Kumazawa *et al.* 1993). AH6809, an EP_1 receptor antagonist, at concentrations between 100 nM and 10 μM, affected neither the resting discharges of PMRs nor the PG-induced enhancement of responses to BK or to heat. The discharges evoked by BK after a 3-min treatment with M&B28767 (100 nM), an EP_3 receptor agonist, were augmented in a fashion similar to that experienced with PGE_2 (100 nM; Fig. 13.8). Treatment with butaprost (1 μM), an EP_2 receptor agonist, however, did not augment the BK response. On average, M&B28767 augmented the BK responses in a concentration-dependent manner, with a significant increase induced by M&B28767 at 10 nM. The effect of butaprost, however, was not substantial even at 10 μM. 17-phen PGE, which is known as a relatively selective agonist for the EP_1 receptor, augmented BK responses at high concentrations, but the enhancement was not affected by AH6809, an EP_1 antagonist. Such outcomes indicate that the EP receptor implicated in the PGE_2-induced enhancement of BK responses is the EP_3 receptor (Kumazawa *et al.* 1993).

Activating the EP_3 receptor subtype causes a reduction in intracellular cyclic adenosine monophosphate (cAMP; Coleman *et al.* 1990). Functional cDNA clones for the EP_3 receptor were recently isolated from a mouse cDNA library, and PGE_2 and M&B28767 were shown to decrease the forskolin-induced cAMP formation in the cells transfected with the cDNA for the EP_3 receptor subtype (Sugimoto *et al.* 1992). If PGE_2-induced enhancements of the BK responses of PMRs are mediated through the EP_3 receptor subtypes, then agents known to elevate intracellular cAMP levels should suppress the BK responses of PMRs. Elevating the cAMP levels by forskolin, an activator of adenylyl cyclase, slightly but significantly suppressed the BK responses (Mizumura *et al.* 1994a).

These data suggest that a process that lowers intracellular cAMP levels enhances BK responses, and further support the above-mentioned implication of the EP_3 receptor subtype in the sensitization of the response of PMRs to BK.

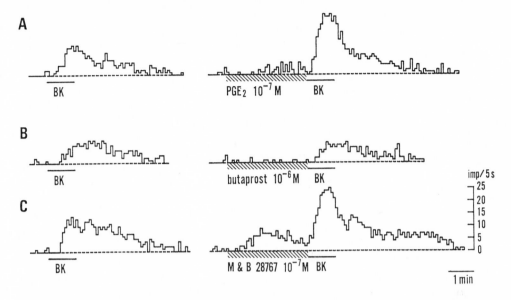

Fig. 13.8 Effects of a pretreatment with PGE_2, EP_2, and EP_3 receptor agonists on BK-evoked discharges in a single PMR unit. Peristimulus time histograms of discharges from a PMR unit with a conduction velocity of 5.9 m/s. The scale (bottom right) applies to all histograms. Bradykinin (1 μM) was applied for 1 min (indicated by a line). PGE analogues were pretreated for 3 min (indicated by hatched area under the right-hand tracings). From Kumazawa *et al.* (1993), with permission.

Receptors and second messengers implicated in the PGE_2–induced enhancement of heat responses in testicular PMRs

We also aimed to identify the EP receptor subtypes implicated in the enhancement of heat responses using the agonist selective for the three receptor subtypes. As shown in Fig. 13.9, a 3-min pretreatment with butaprost, an EP_2 receptor agonist, clearly enhanced the heat responses of a PMR unit in a concentration-dependent manner (Kumazawa *et al.* 1994a). Heat responses after pretreatment with 10 nM of butaprost were increased in all five units tested; the average heat response after butaprost was significantly greater than the control response. It should be noted that butaprost in this concentration range did not affect the BK responses. On the other hand, M&B28767, an EP_3 agonist, which significantly augmented the BK responses at 10 nM, did not significantly augment the heat responses even at 100 nM. The EP_1 agonist, 17-phen PGE, augmented heat responses at higher concentrations, but the enhancement was not antagonized by the EP_1 antagonist, AH6809.

Since stimulation of the EP_2 receptor subtype is known to increase intracellular cAMP (Coleman *et al.* 1990), an elevation in cAMP levels should be expected to augment heat responses. In contrast to the BK responses, a 5-min pretreatment with forskolin as well as a mixture of dibutyryl cAMP (dBcAMP), a membrane-permeable analogue of cAMP, with 3-isobutyl-1-methyl-xanthine (IBMX), an inhibitor of cAMP-degrading enzyme, clearly augmented the heat response as shown in Fig. 13.10. The average heat response after treatment with forskolin (10 μM) was significantly greater than that of the control. In addition, although the augmenting effect induced by a mixture of dBcAMP (100 μM) and IBMX (100 μM) was not as great as that induced by forskolin, it was significant (Mizumura *et al.* 1993b).

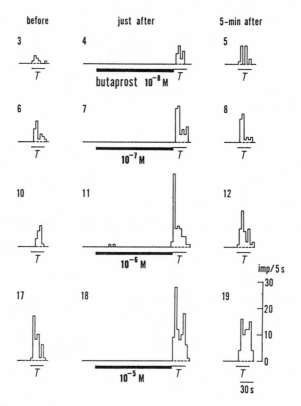

before   just after   5-min after

butaprost 10^{-8} M

10^{-7} M

10^{-6} M

imp/5 s

10^{-5} M

30 s

Fig. 13.9 The EP_2 receptor agonist (butaprost) augmented responses to heat in a concentration-dependent manner. Peristimulus time histograms of heat responses of a single unit, tested repeatedly at intervals > 5 min. (The order of testing is shown by the numeral in the upper left corner of each trace.) Responses to heat (T, 48°C) following 3-min pretreatment with butaprost (10 nM–10 μM, thick lines) are compared with those 5 min before and after the treatment. From Kumazawa *et al.* (1994*b*), with permission.

Sensitization induced under pathological conditions

After setting up partial injuries in the peripheral nerve, sympathetic stimulation and noradrenaline were shown to evoke discharges in a subset of the cutaneous C-fibre PMRs that could be reversed by α_2 adrenergic receptor antagonists (Sato and Perl 1991; see Lisney, Chapter 20, this volume). This indicates that the sensitization of PMRs developed plastically under pathological conditions, since in normal skin sympathomimetic stimulation neither excites nor enhances the activity of PMRs.

In adjuvant-induced chronically inflamed rats, such sympathomimetic stimulations caused excitation in 35–40 per cent of the cutaneous C-fibre PMRs, which could again be reversed by α_2 receptor antagonists (Sato *et al.* 1993; Fig. 13.11). Noradrenaline-induced excitation of PMRs in rats with chronic arthritis was also observed after complete sympathectomy with guanethidine (Sato *et al.* 1994). Hyperalgesia by sympathomimetic stimulation has also been reported in arthritic rats (Levine *et al.* 1986; Gonzales *et al.* 1989, 1991). They showed that PGs released from the sympathetic postganglionic neurone terminals play casual roles. Our own finding, however, indicates that the

A

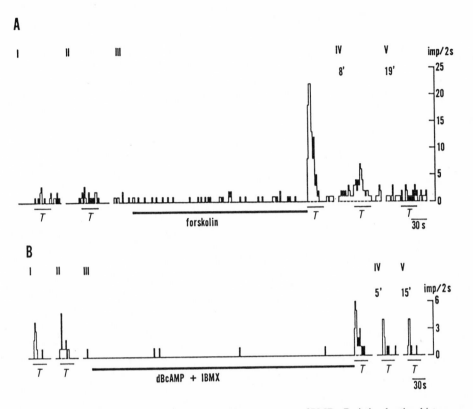

Fig. 13.10 Elevations in intracellular cAMP augmented heat responses of PMRs. Peristimulus time histograms are presented according to the order of testing from I to V. (A) Forskolin (10 μM, thick line) and heat stimulation (*T*, 48°C, thin line) were applied over the periods marked by the lines. (B) A mixture of a membrane-permeable analogue of cAMP (dBcAMP, 100 μM) and an inhibitor of a cAMP-degrading enzyme (IBMX, 100 μM) was applied during the period marked by the thick line. From Mizumura *et al.* (1993*b*), with permission.

appearance of sympathomimetic responsiveness of PMRs in adjuvant rats does not necessarily depend on the sympathetic postganglionic neurone terminals. This notion is further supported by recent reports showing that expression of the α_2 adrenoceptor in the DRG cells can be enhanced during pathological conditions (Nishiyama *et al.* 1993; Perl 1994).

It has been documented in clinical settings as well that stress and other means of activating the sympathetic nervous system can aggravate pain. The above findings suggest that sensitization of the peripheral nociceptors, which is developed plastically under pathological conditions, may also be implicated in sympathetically related pain.

Conclusion

The PMR is characterized by activation from a wide variety of types of stimuli, a wide distribution throughout the body, and a wide dynamic range of stimulus intensity. These three 'wide' factors are what differentiate the PMR from most other types of sensory receptors that have developed to respond to limited types of stimuli. Polymodal-type receptors located in different tissues and with different conduction velocities exhibit essentially the same characteristics, although they may show some quantitative differences. Effector functions developed by releasing peptides from the peripheral endings of PMRs are also markedly different from those of other refined sensory receptors. These particular features of PMRs strongly suggest the primitive nature of this sensory receptor.

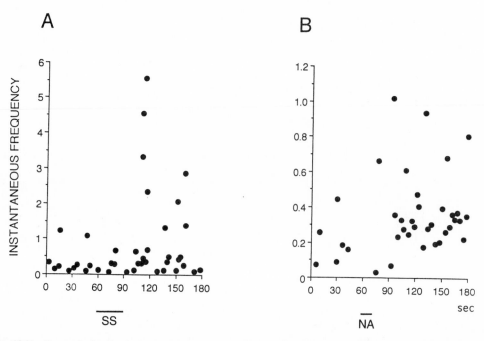

Fig. 13.11 Sympathetic stimulation-induced and noradrenaline-induced abnormal discharges of cutaneous PMRs in chronic arthritis rats. The figure shows the instantaneous frequency of discharges in C-fibre PMRs. (A) Electrical stimulation of lumbar sympathetic chain (SS; 20 Hz, 30 s); (B) close-arterial injection of noradrenaline (NA 400 ng). Rats were given adjuvant either (A) 87 or (B) 68 days before each recording session. From Sato *et al.* (1993), with permission.

Bio-warning and defence mechanisms are the most fundamental functions for the survival of living organisms. The humoral means by which these mechanisms operate at the early stages of development in living organisms would have obvious advantages if put to use in the primitive neural nociceptive mechanisms. The importance of PMRs in the nociceptive function is clear if one studies the sensitization of PMRs induced by chemical substances that are produced in damaged tissues. Investigations of the membrane and intracellular signal transduction mechanisms may provide clues to a better understanding of the transduction mechanisms of PMRs for various physical and chemical stimuli that have not been elucidated to date. This is one aspect that certainly needs to be further investigated in the study of pain.

Acknowledgements

The author is grateful to Ms Yoshiko Yamaguchi for assistance in designing the graphics and preparing this manuscript. This work was supported in part by Grants-in-Aid for Scientific Research from the Ministry of Education, Science, and Culture, Japan.

References

Armstrong, D., Jepson, J.B., Keele, C.A. and Stewart, J.W. (1957). Pain-producing substance in human inflammatory exudates and plasma. *J. Physiol., London* **135**, 350–70.

Arturson, G., Hamberg, M. and Jonsson, C.-E. (1973). Prostaglandins in human burn blister fluid. *Acta physiol. scand.*, **87**, 270–6.

Baker, D.G., Coleridge, H.M., Coleridge, J.C.G. and Nerdrum, T. (1980). Search for a cardiac nociceptor: stimulation by bradykinin of sympathetic afferent nerve endings in the heart of the cat. *J. Physiol., London* **306**, 519–36.

Beck, P.W., Handwerker, H.O. and Zimmermann, M. (1974). Nervous outflow from the cat's foot during noxious radiant heat stimulation. *Brain Res.* **67**, 373–86.

Beitel, R.E. and Dubner, R. (1976). Response of unmyelinated (C) polymodal nociceptors to thermal stimuli applied to monkey's face. *J. Neurophysiol.* **39**, 1160–75.

Belmonte, C., Gallar, J., Pozo, M.A. and Rebollo, I. (1991). Excitation by irritant chemical substances of sensory afferent units in the cat's cornea. *J. Physiol., London* **437**, 709–25.

Bessou, P. and Perl, E.R. (1969). Response of cutaneous sensory units with unmyelinated (C) fibres to noxious stimuli. *J. Neurophysiol.* **32**, 1025–43.

Brown, D.A. and Higashida, H. (1988). Inositol 1,4,5–trisphosphate and diacylglycerol mimic bradykinin effects on mouse neuroblastoma × rat glioma hybrid cells. *J. Physiol., London* **397**, 185–207.

Burgess, G.M., Mullaney, I., McNeill, M., Dunn, P.M. and Rang, H.P. (1989). Second messengers involved in the mechanism of action of bradykinin in sensory neurons in culture. *J. Neurosci.* **9**, 3314–25.

Burgess, P.R. and Perl, E.R. (1973). Cutaneous mechanoreceptors and nociceptors. In *Handbook of sensory physiology*, Vol. 2. *Somatosensory system* (ed. A. Iggo), pp.29–78. Springer, Berlin.

Castagna, M., Takai, Y., Kaibuchi, K., Sano, K., Kikkawa, U. and Nishizuka, Y. (1982). Direct activation of calcium-activated, phospholipid-dependent protein kinase by tumor-promoting phorbol esters. *J. biol. Chem.* **25** 7847–51.

Coleman, R.A., Kennedy, I., Humphrey, P.P.A., Bunce, K. and Lumley, P. (1990). Prostanoids and their receptors. In *Comprehensive medicinal chemistry*, Vol. 3. *Membranes and receptors* (ed. J.C. Emmett), pp.643–714. Pergamon Press, Oxford.

Croze, S., Duclaux, R. and Kenshalo, D.R. (1976). The thermal sensitivity of the polymodal nociceptors in the monkey. *J. Physiol., London* **263**, 539–62.

Dickenson, J.M. and Hill, S.J. (1993). Homologous and heterologous desensitization of histamine H_1- and ATP-receptors in the smooth muscle cell line, DDT_1MF-2: the role of protein kinase C. *Br. J. Pharmacol.* **110**, 1449–56.

Duclaux, R., Mei, N. and Ranieri, F. (1976). Conduction velocity along the afferent vagal dendrites: a new type of fibre. *J. Physiol., London* **260**, 487–95.

Fazekas, I.G., Kosa, F., Viragos-Kis, E. and Basch, A. (1973). Free and total histamine content of the skin in experimental burn injuries. *Z. Rechtsmedizin* **72**, 203–12.

Ferreira, S.H., Moncada, S. and Vane, J.R. (1971). Indomethacin and aspirin abolish prostaglandin release from the spleen. *Nature (New Biology)* **231**, 237–9.

Ferreira, S.H., Moncada, S. and Vane, J.R. (1973). Prostaglandins and the mechanism of analgesia produced by aspirin-like drugs. *Br. J. Pharmacol.* **49**, 86–97.

Floyd, K., Hick, V.E. and Morrison, J.F.B. (1976). Mechanosensitive afferent units in the hypogastric nerve of the cat. *J. Physiol., London* **259**, 457–71.

Gammon, C.M., Allen, A.C. and Morell, P. (1989). Bradykinin stimulates phosphoinositide hydrolysis and mobilization of arachidonic acid in dorsal root ganglion neurons. *J. Neurochem.* **53**, 95–101.

Gonzales, R., Goldyne, M.E., Taiwo, Y.O and Levine, J.D. (1989). Production of hyperalgesic prostaglandin by sympathetiic postganglionic neurons. *J. Neurochem.* **53**, 1595–8.

Gonzales, R., Sherbourne, C.D., Goldyne, M.E. and Levine, J.D. (1991). Noradrenaline-induced prostaglandin production by sympathetic postganglionic neurons is mediated by alpha$_2$-adrenergic receptors. *J. Neurochem.* **57**, 1145–50.

Goodwin, L.G., Jones, C.R., Richards, W.H.G. and Kohn, J. (1963). Pharmacologically active substances in the urine of burned patients. *Br. J. exp. Pathol.* **44**, 551–60.

Hallin, R.G., Torebjörk, H.E. and Wiesenfeld, Z. (1982). Nociceptors and warm receptors innervated by C fibres in human skin. *J. Neurol. Neurosurg. Psychiat.* **45**, 313–19.

Hashimoto, K., Kumakura, S. and Taira, N. (1964). Vascular reflex responses induced by an intraarterial injection of azaazepinophenothiazine, andromedotoxin veratridine, bradykinin and kallikrein and blocking action of sodium salicylate. *Jpn. J. Physiol.* **14**, 299–308.

Higashida, H., Streaty, R.A., Klee, W. and Nirenberg, M. (1986). Bradykinin-activated trans-membrane signals are coupled via N_0 or N_1 to production of inositol 1,4,5-trisphosphate, a second messenger in NG108-15 neuroblastoma-glioma hybrid cells. *Proc. natl. Acad. Sci., USA.* **83**, 942–6.

Hill, S.J. (1990). Distribution, properties, and functional characteristics of three classes of histamine receptor. *Pharmacol. Rev.* **42**, 45–83.

Iggo, A. (1959). Cutaneous heat and cold receptors with slowly conducting C afferent fibres. *Quart. J. exp. Physiol.* **44**, 362–70.

Kaczmarek, L.K. (1987). The role of protein kinase C in the regulation of ion channels and neurotransmitter release. *Trends Neurosci.* **10**, 30–4.

Kanaka, R., Schaible, H.-G. and Schmidt, R.F. (1985). Activation of fine articular afferent units by bradykinin. *Brain Res.* **327**, 81–90.

Kaufman, M.P., Iwamoto, G.A., Longhurst, J.C. and Mitchell, J.H. (1982). Effects of capsaicin and bradykinin on afferent fibres with endings in skeletal muscle. *Circulat. Res.* **50**, 133–9.

Kenins, P. (1981). Identification of the unmyelinated sensory nerves which evoke extravasation in response to antidromic stimulation. *Neurosci. Lett.* **25** 137–41.

King, J.S., Gallant, P., Myerson, V. and Perl, E.R. (1976). The effects of anti-inflammatory agents on the responses and the sensitization of unmyelinated (C) fibre polymodal nociceptors. In *Sensory functions of the skin in primates* (ed. Y. Zotterman), pp.441–54. Pergamon Press, Oxford.

Kruger, L., Kumazawa, T., Mizumura, K., Sato, J. and Yeh, Y. (1988). Observations on electrophysiologically characterized receptive fields on thin testicular afferent axons: a pre-liminary note on the analysis of fine structural specializations of polymodal receptors. *Somatosens. Res.* **5**, 373–80.

Kumazawa, T. and Mizumura, K. (1977*a*). The polymodal receptors in the testis of dog. *Brain Res.* **136**, 553–8.

Kumazawa T. and Mizumura, K. (1977*b*). Thin-fibre receptors responding to mechanical, chemical, and thermal stimulation in the skeletal muscle of the dog. *J. Physiol., London* **273**, 179–94.

Kumazawa, T. and Mizumura, K. (1979). Effects of synthetic substance P on unit-discharges of testicular nociceptors of dogs. *Brain Res.* **170**, 553–7.

Kumazawa, T. and Mizumura, K. (1980*a*). Chemical responses of polymodal receptors of the scrotal contents in dogs. *J. Physiol., London* **299**, 219–31.

Kumazawa, T. and Mizumura, K. (1980*b*). Mechanical and thermal responses of polymodal receptors recorded from the superior spermatic nerve of dogs. *iJ. Physiol., London* **299**, 233–45.

Kumazawa, T. and Perl, E.R. (1977). Primate cutaneous sensory units with unmyelinated (C) afferent fibres. *J. Neurophysiol.* **40**, 1325–38.

Kumazawa, T., Mizumura, K. and Sato, J. (1987*a*). Response properties of polymodal receptors studied using in vitro testis superior spermatic nerve preparations of dogs. *J. Neurophysiol.* **57**, 702–11.

Kumazawa, T., Mizumura, K. and Sato, J. (1987*b*). Modulations of testicular polymodal receptor activity: implication of receptors in inflammatory pain. In *Fine afferent nerve fibres and pain* (ed. R.F. Schmidt, H.-G. Schaible, and C. Vahle-Hinz), pp.147–57. VCH Verlagsgesellschaft, Weinheim.

Kumazawa, T., Mizumura, K. and Sato, J. (1987*c*). Thermally potentiated responses to algesic substances of visceral nociceptors. *Pain* **28**, 255–64.

Kumazawa, T., Mizumura, K. and Sato, J. (1988). Modulation of testicular polymodal receptor activities. In *Progress in brain research*, Vol. 74. *Transduction and cellular mechanisms in sensory receptors* (ed. W. Hamann and A. Iggo), pp.325–30. Elsevier, Amsterdam.

Kumazawa, T., Mizumura, K., Minagawa, M. and Tsujii, Y. (1991). Sensitizing effects of bradykinin on the heat responses of the visceral nocicepter. *J. Neurophysiol.* **66**, 1819–24.

Kumazawa, T., Mizumura, K., Minagawa, M., Koda, H., Tsujii, Y. and Sato, J. (1992). Differences in the response of the polymodal receptor to heat stimulation and to bradykinin. In *Processing and inhibition of nociceptive information* (ed. R. Inoki, Y. Shigenaga, and M. Tohyama), pp.3–8. Elsevier, Amsterdam.

Kumazawa, T., Mizumura, K. and Koda, H. (1993). Involvement of EP_3 subtype of prostaglandin E receptors in PGE_2-induced enhancement of the bradykinin response of nociceptors. *Brain Res.* **632**, 321–4.

Kumazawa, T., Mizumura, K. and Koda, H. (1994*a*). Possible involvement of the EP_2 receptor subtype in PGE_2-induced enhancement of the heat response of nociceptors. *Neurosci. Lett.* **175**, 71–3.

Kumazawa, T., Mizumura, K. and Koda, H. (1994*b*). Different mechanisms (receptor subtypes and second messenger actions) implicated in PGE_2-induced sensitization of the responses to bradykinin and to heat of polymodal receptors. In *Proceedings of the 7th World Congress on Pain. Progress in pain research and management* Vol. 2. (ed. G.F. Gebhart, D.L. Hammond, and T.S. Jensen), pp.265–76. IASP Press, Seattle.

Lang, E., Novak, A., Reeh, P.W. and Handwerker, H.O. (1990). Chemosensitivity of fine afferents from rat skin in vitro. *J. Neurophysiol.* **63**, 887–901.

Lembeck, F., (1983). Sir Thomas Lewis's nocifensor system, histamine and substance-P-containing primary afferent nerves. *Trends Neurosci.,* **6**: 106–8.

Lembeck, F. and Gamse, R. (1977). Lack of algesic effect of substance P on paravascular pain receptors. *Naunyn-Schmiedebergs Arch. Pharmacol.* **299**, 295–303.

Levine, J.D., Taiwo, Y.O., Collins, S.D. and Tam, J.K. (1986). Noradrenaline hyperalgesia is mediated through interaction with sympathetic postganglionic neurone terminals rather than activation of primary afferent nociceptors. *Nature, London* **323**, 158–60.

Lim, R.K.S. (1970). Pain. *Ann. Rev. Physiol.* **32**, 269–88.

Lim, R.K.S., Liu, C.N., Guzman, F. and Braun, C. (1962). Visceral receptors concerned in visceral pain and the pseudaffective response to intra-arterial injection of bradykinin and other algesic agents. *J. Comp. Neurol.* **118** 269–94.

Lo, W.W.Y. and Fan, T.-P.D. (1987). Histamine stimulates inositol phosphate accumulation via the H_1-receptor in cultured human endothelial cells. *Biochem. biophys. Res. Commun.* **148**, 47–53.

Lynn, B. (1979). The heat sensitization of polymodal nociceptors in the rabbit and its independence of the local blood flow. *J. Physiol., London* **287**, 493–507.

Lynn, B. and Carpenter, S.E. (1982). Primary afferent units from the hairy skin of the rat hind limb. *Brain Res.* **238**, 29–43.

McGiff, J.C., Terragno, N.A., Malik, K.U. and Lonigro, A.J. (1972). Release of a prostaglandin E-like substance from canine kidney by bradykinin. *Circulation Res.* **31**, 36–43.

Mense, S. (1977). Nervous outflow from skeletal muscle following chemical noxious stimulation. *J. Physiol., London* **267**, 75–88.

Mense, S. (1981). Sensitization of group IV muscle receptors to bradykinin by 5-hydroxytrypta-mine and prostaglandin E_2. *Brain Res.* **225**, 95–105.

Miller, R.J. (1987). Bradykinin highlights the role of phospholipid metabolism in the control of nerve excitability. *Trends Neurosci.* **10**, 226–8.

Mizumura, K., Sato, J. and Kumazawa, T. (1987). Effects of prostaglandins and other putative chemical intermediaries on the activity of canine testicular polymodal receptors studied in vitro. *Pflügers Arch. – Eur. J. Physiol.* **408**, 565–72.

Mizumura, K., Minagawa, M., Tsujii, Y. and Kumazawa, T. (1990). The effects of bradykinin agonists and antagonists on visceral polymodal receptor activities. *Pain* **40**, 221–7.

Mizumura, K., Sato, J. and Kumazawa, T. (1991). Comparison of the effects of prostaglandins E_2 and I_2 on testicular nociceptor activities studied in vitro. *Naunyn-Schmiedebergs Arch. Pharmacol.* **344**, 368–76.

Mizumura, K., Sato, J., and Kumazawa, T. (1992) Strong heat stimulation sensitizes the heat response as well as the bradykinin response of visceral polymodal receptors. *J. Neurophysiol.* **68**, 1209–15.

Mizumura, K., Minagawa, M., Tsujii, Y. and Kumazawa, T. (1993a). Prostaglandin E_2-induced sensitization of the heat response of canine visceral polymodal receptors in vitro. *Neurosci. Lett.* **161**, 117–19.

Mizumura, K., Koda, H. and Kumazawa, T. (1993b). Augmenting effects of cyclic AMP on the heat response of canine testicular polymodal receptors. *Neurosci. Lett.* **162**, 75–7.

Mizumura, K., Minagawa, M., Koda, H. and Kumazawa, T. (1994a). Forskolin does not augment the bradykinin response of canine visceral polymodal receptors in vitro. *Neurosci. Lett.* **166**, 195–8.

Mizumura, K., Minagawa, M., Koda, H. and Kumazawa, T. (1994b). Histamine-induced sensitization of the heat response of canine visceral polymodal receptors. *Neurosci. Lett.* **168**, 93–6.

Mizumura, K., Koda, H. and Kumazawa, T. (1994c). Phorbol ester-induced excitation and facilitation of the heat response of testicular polymodal receptors in vitro. *Environ. Med.* **38**, 41–4.

Mizumura, K., Sato, J., Minagawa, M. and Kumazawa, T. (1994d). Incomplete suppressive effects of acetylsalicylic acid on the heat sensitization of canine testicular polymodal receptor activities. *J. Neurophysiol.* **72**, 2729–36..

Nerdrum, T., Baker, D.G., Coleridge, H.M. and Coleridge, J.C.G. (1986). Interaction of bradykinin and prostaglandin E_1 on cardiac pressor reflex and sympathetic afferents. *Am. J. Physiol.* **250**, R815–22.

Nishi, K., Sakanashi, M. and Takenaka, F. (1977). Activation of afferent cardiac sympathetic nerve fibres of cats by pain producing substances and by noxious heat. *Pflügers Arch. – Eur. J. Physiol.* **372**, 53–61.

Nishiyama, K., Brighton, B.W., Bossut, D.F. and Perl, E.R. (1993). Peripheral nerve injury enhances alpha$_2$-adrenergic receptor expression by some DRG neurones. *Soc. Neurosci. Abstr.* **19**, 499.

Nishizuka, Y. (1984). The role of protein kinase C in cell surface signal transduction and tumour promotion. *Nature, London* **308**, 693–8.

Perl, E.R. (1994). A reevaluation of mechanisms leading to sympathetically related pain. In *Progress in pain research and management*, Vol. 1. *Pharmacological approaches to the treatment of chronic pain: new concepts and critical issues* (ed. H.L. Fields and J.C. Liebeskind), pp.129–50. IASP Press, Seattle.

Peterson, D.F. and Brown, A.M. (1973). Functional afferent innervation of testis. *J. Neurophysiol.* **36**, 425–33.

Regoli, D. and Barabe, J. (1980). Pharmacology of bradykinin and related kinins. *Pharmacol. Rev.* **32**, 1–46.

Riccioppo Neto, F. (1980). Further studies on the action of salicylates on nerve membranes. *Eur. J. Pharmacol.* **68**, 155–62.

Sato, J. and Perl, E.R. (1991). Adrenergic excitation of cutaneous pain receptors induced by peripheral nerve injury. *Science* **251**, 1608–10.

Sato, J. Mizumura, K. and Kumazawa, T. (1989). Effects of ionic calcium on the responses of canine testicular polymodal receptors to algesic substances. *J. Neurophysiol.* **62**, 119–25.

Sato, J., Suzuki, S., Iseki, T. and Kumazawa, T. (1993). Adrenergic excitation of cutaneous nociceptors in chronically inflamed rats. *Neurosci. Lett.* **164**, 225–8.

Sato, J., Suzuki, S., Tamura, R. and Kumazawa, T. (1994). Norepinephrine excitation of cutaneous nociceptors in adjuvant-induced inflamed rats does not depend on sympathetic neurones. *Neurosci. Lett.* **177**, 135–8.

Schaible, H.–G. and Schmidt, R. F. (1988). Excitation and sensitization of fine articular afferents from cat's knee joint by prostaglandin E_2. *J. Physiol., London* **403**, 91–104.

Schepelmann, K., Messlinger, K. and Schmidt, R.F. (1993). The effects of phorbol ester on slowly conducting afferents of the cat's knee joint. *Exp. Brain Res.* **92**, 391–8.

Smit, M.J., Bloemers, S.M., Leurs, R., Tertoolen, L.G.J., Bast, A., de Laat, S.W. and Timmerman, H. (1992). Short-term desensitization of the histamine H_1 receptor in human HeLa cells: involvement of protein kinase C dependent and independent pathways. *Br. J. Pharmacol.* **107**, 448–55.

Sugimoto, Y., Namba, T., Honda, A., Hayashi, Y., Negishi, M., Ichikawa, A. and Narumiya, S. (1992). Cloning and expression of a cDNA for mouse prostaglandin E receptor EP_3 subtype. *J. biol. Chem.* **267** 6463–6.

Torebjörk, H.E. and Hallin, R.G. (1974). Identification of afferent C units in intact human skin nerves. *Brain Res.* **67**, 387–403.

Yano, K., Higashida, H., Inoue, R. and Nozawa, Y. (1984). Bradykinin-induced rapid breakdown of phosphatidylinositol 4.5-bisphosphate in neuroblastoma × glioma hybrid NG108-15 cells. A possible link to agonist-induced neuronal functions. *J. biol. Chem.* **259**, 10201–7.

PART 4
Functions of nociceptors

14 Functional properties of human cutaneous nociceptors and their role in pain and hyperalgesia

H.E. TOREBJÖRK, M. SCHMELZ, AND
H.O. HANDWERKER

Introduction

The study of peripheral mechanisms of pain was greatly advanced by the technique of microneurography introduced by Hagbarth and Vallbo (1967). This technique not only makes possible experiments on human volunteers instead of on guinea-pigs, but also adds a psychophysical dimension to electrophysiology, since human volunteers are able to describe their stimulus-induced sensations while primary afferent units are recorded. From this additional information one may deduce whether the excitation of a particular type of nerve fibre can possibly contribute to the respective sensory experience. For instance, combined psychophysical and neurophysiological experiments in humans indicate that C-fibre mechanoheat (CMH) nociceptors provide a peripheral neuronal basis for the determination of the heat pain threshold, at least in hairy skin (Van Hees and Gybels 1981; LaMotte et al. 1982). Furthermore, a nearly linear relation found between the mean suprathreshold response functions in a population of CMH nociceptors and the median ratings of pain suggests that these nociceptors provide an essential code for the magnitude of pain sensation in response to heat (Torebjörk et al. 1984a). This is supported by the finding that CMH nociceptors are activated by small increments of 0.1–0.5°C on a base temperature of 48°C, which is matched by the human ability to detect such increments as painful (Robinson et al. 1983).

A typical feature of CMH nociceptors is their sensitization after heat injury to their receptive fields. The lowering of thresholds to heat stimuli and the enhanced responses to suprathreshold stimuli correlate with increased pain ratings, indicating that CMH nociceptors contribute to heat hyperalgesia in hairy skin (LaMotte et al. 1982; Torebjörk et al. 1984a). The situation seems to be different in the glabrous skin of the hand, since neurophysiological studies in monkey have shown that only sensitization of Aδ nociceptors matches the heat hyperalgesia following a burn lesion, while CMH nociceptors are often desensitized (Meyer and Campbell 1981).

The microneurographic recording technique has been supplemented by electrical intraneural microstimulation of single (or small groups of) afferent fibres that were characterized by recording beforehand (Torebjörk and Ochoa 1980; Vallbo 1981). Microstimulation of nociceptor units provided insights into the quality of sensations induced by stimulation of certain types of afferent nerve fibres and into the role of their impulse patterns for sensation. Thus, intraneural microstimulation in C-fibre recording sites evoked dull pain sensations (Ochoa and Torebjörk 1989) that were projected with an accuracy of the order of 1 or 2 cm to the innervation territory of the recorded C nociceptors in the skin of the hand or foot, respectively (Jørum *et al.* 1989; Ochoa and Torebjörk 1989), while intraneural stimulation in Aδ nociceptor recording sites evoked sharp pain projected to the receptive field of the stimulated Aδ nociceptor in the hand (Torebjörk 1985; Torebjörk and Ochoa 1990). Intraneural stimulation of nociceptive fibres with different patterns revealed a close correlation between number of impulses and magnitude of pain and, in addition, showed the importance of temporal summation of nociceptor impulses for the magnitude of pain (Lundberg *et al.* 1992).

However, criticism has also been raised against microneurography and microstimulation. In one review it was conjectured that single-unit recordings in human nerves may only be possible while the metal microelectrode functionally blocks the conduction in the majority of the neighbouring axons (Wall and McMahon 1985). In experimental studies conducted on the much smaller nerves of rats these conjectures were subsequently tested (Calancie and Stein 1988; Rice *et al.* 1993). As discussed in several reviews, the claim of a blocking of most fibres is probably exaggerated (Torebjörk *et al.* 1987), although individual nerve fibres may indeed be functionally blocked by the tip of the microelectrode (Vallbo 1976).

For the purpose of this chapter it is of minor interest if a single unit from which recordings were obtained actually conducted beyond the point of recording since most sensations certainly are mediated by the excitation of large populations of afferent nerve fibres. However, microneurography and microstimulation studies help to answer questions such as: is it likely that a particular type of primary afferent unit contributes to a particular sensation? Which aspects of a stimulus-induced pain report can be explained by the discharge patterns of individual nociceptors?

This chapter will discuss the insights into the peripheral neural mechanisms of pain and hyperalgesia recently gained by microneurography. The most abundant and probably the most important class of nociceptor units in the skin are unmyelinated (C) fibres, and hence most of this review will be dedicated to this fibre class. The myelinated fibres contributing to withdrawal reflexes and pain, which are generally slowly conducting Aδ fibres, will also be considered. Mechanisms of hyperalgesia involving low-threshold mechanoreceptor units and central nervous plasticity will be briefly discussed.

Properties of nociceptor units in human skin

The problem of bias in single-unit recording

The standard procedure used in microneurography experiments has been described elsewhere in detail (Vallbo and Hagbarth 1968). Briefly, for single-unit recordings a metal microelectrode isolated with a coating of lacquer or Teflon except at the very tip is inserted transcutaneously into a nerve. Most recordings of cutaneous nociceptor activity were performed in the peroneal and radial nerves innervating the lower leg and the dorsum of the hand, respectively, but recordings from other regions including the glabrous skin of the hand and the facial area were also obtained (for reviews see Vallbo *et al.* 1979; Hagbarth *et al.* 1993).

One salient problem of all types of electrophysiological single-unit analysis is the possible recording bias in favour of certain nervous elements. In microneurography mechanical stimuli, for example, stiff von Frey bristles, were usually used for searching (for a review see Handwerker and Kobal 1993). Obviously, only mechanically responsive units were thus encountered. Most of these units did also respond to heat and were classified as C polymodal nociceptors (Bessou and Perl 1969) or C mechanoheat (CMH) nociceptors (LaMotte *et al.* 1982). However, it has long been recognized that there exist in the monkey skin several types of C nociceptors that respond differentially to mechanical, mechanothermal, or thermal stimuli (Georgopoulos 1976). Improved experimental techniques with electrical search stimuli (Meyer and Campbell 1988) have led to the discovery of very-high-threshold or insensitive cutaneous nociceptors that are primarily activated by inflammation processes. They are frequent in the hairy skin of monkey (Meyer *et al.* 1991; Davis *et al.* 1993) and rat (Handwerker *et al.* 1991*b*; Kress *et al.* 1992) and also in non-cutaneous tissues such as the knee joint (Schaible and Schmidt 1985, 1988; Grigg *et al.* 1986) and the urinary bladder of cat (Häbler *et al.* 1988, 1990). Some of these unresponsive units were activated and/or sensitized to subsequent mechanical and thermal stimulation by chemical irritant substances (Neugebauer *et al.* 1989; Handwerker *et al.* 1991*b*; Kress *et al.* 1992; Davis *et al.* 1993). Moreover, the study of different forms of hyperalgesias in man has led to the theoretical assumption that there would be specific chemosensitive nociceptors in human skin (LaMotte 1988, 1992).

In order to study the full spectrum of C nociceptors of various classes in human skin we recently changed the experimental protocol from the traditional mechanical search stimuli to a search procedure employing electrical stimuli to recruit units independently of their sensitivity to natural stimulation (Schmidt *et al.* 1995). In addition, a computerized version of a method utilizing interactions between naturally and electrically evoked discharges (Hallin and Torebjörk 1974; Torebjörk 1974; Torebjörk and Hallin 1976) allowed reliable testing of the responsiveness of individual C units in multiunit recordings frequently encountered in microneurography (Forster and Handwerker 1990; Schmidt *et al.* 1995). This method utilizes the slowing of conduction velocity due to the slow recovery of Na^+ channels during the relative refractory period after activation, which lasts a particularly long time in C fibres.

In our experiments electrical stimuli delivered from a surface electrode were used to locate individual C units. Once the innervation territory of a C unit was found, the respective skin site was encircled with a pen and a pair of uninsulated steel needles were inserted intracutaneously with one needle inside the innervation territory and the other one placed transversely at a distance of 5–10 mm. We then used the needle electrodes for continuously stimulating this and other adjacent C units at intervals of 3–4 s at a moderately painful intensity (10–30 V, 0.2 ms).

Figure 14.1 shows an example of a recording in which two C units with action potentials of similar shape and amplitude were recorded from the foot dorsum. The conduction delays to the recording site at the ankle level were 150 and 205 ms, respectively. The conduction velocities were 0.93 and 0.68 m/s. The lower panel of the figure shows only the action potentials elicited by the repetitive intracutaneous electrical stimuli, written from top to bottom. Additional excitation of a unit induced an increased conduction delay due to slowing during the relative refractory period and this 'marking' was used as an indication of a response to the respective stimulus. Whereas the unit labelled 'b' in Fig. 14.1 was insensitive to mechanical stimuli (and also to heat stimulation, not shown), unit 'a' was activated from the same skin site. This unit showed graded responses to suprathreshold stimuli in the noxious intensity range, as seen by the greater conduction delays following stimulation with stronger von Frey filaments.

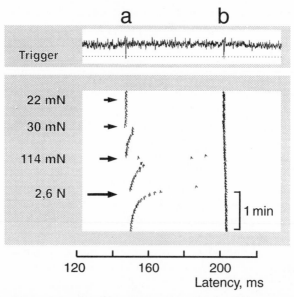

Fig. 14.1   Illustration of the marking technique. Upper panel, A suitable time segment of the C-fibre response to electrical intradermal stimulation is shown. Two C units, labelled 'a' and 'b', exceed the lower trigger level. Lower panel, Successive recordings from top to bottom of the same units during electrical stimulation at 4-s intervals. As seen from the transient increases in latency, unit 'a' responded in a graded fashion to von Frey filaments of increasing strength (indicated to the left). Unit 'b' did not respond, as seen by the constant latency.

Employing the marking method we were able to identify in human skin not only the classical CMH units but also other types of afferent C fibres that lack mechanical sensitivity. Sympathetic efferent units were identified by their responsiveness to stimuli provoking sympathetic reflexes.

Obviously, the validity of these results depends on the sensitivity of the marking technique. Slowing of an individual C fibre clearly indicates the activation of the respective unit. However, the proof of unresponsiveness to a particular stimulus depends on the sensitivity of the method to detect the slowing induced by a few, or even by one single additional spike.

The sensitivity of the marking technique

To investigate the sensitivity of the marking technique we used conditioning electrical stimuli. By variation of the number and temporal position of suprathreshold electrical pulses interpolated between regularly delivered stimuli we studied the effect of number and position of additional spike responses on the latency shifts of C units in the peroneal nerves of humans. The conduction velocity and the distance between stimulating and recording electrodes were also taken into account as potential additional factors (Schmelz *et al.* 1995).

The left panel of Fig. 14.2 shows an example of such an analysis, performed on a C unit with its receptive field on the dorsum of the foot and recorded in the peroneal nerve at knee level. Repetitive electrical stimulation in the innervation territory at 4-s intervals evoked a spike response at a latency of 522 ms in this particular case (conduction velocity 0.84 m/s). Additional electrical pulses delivered within the 4-s interstimulus interval (dark symbols and arrows in the insets in left panel of Fig. 14.2) caused reliable latency shifts with a subsequent slow recovery back to the previous latency. Since the units studied did not show spontaneous activity and since each stimulus induced just one spike, the number of additional stimuli and the number of spikes were identical. It is obvious from the specimen record shown in the left panel of Fig. 14.2 that an increasing number of additional pulses leads to increasing latency shifts.

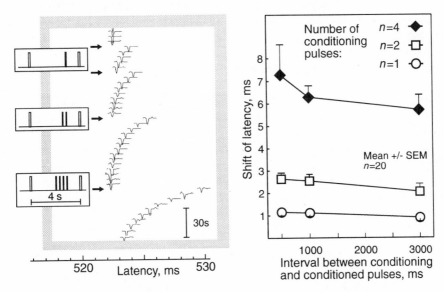

Fig. 14.2 Sensitivity of the marking technique. Left panel, Latency shifts in the responses of a C unit to one, two, or four extra impulses (dark symbols in the insets) delivered between the regular stimuli every 4 s (open symbols in the insets). One extra impulse was given twice and 2 and 4 impulses were given once (arrows). It is seen that a single extra impulse was sufficient to produce a noticeable latency shift and that this effect was increased by additional impulses. Right panel, Mean±SEM of latency shifts in 20 C units recorded in the peroneal nerve at knee level in response to intracutaneous stimulation in the lower leg or foot. The conduction distance was more than 20 cm. One, two, or four stimuli were given 500, 1000, or 3000 ms before the next regular pulse. In all instances one extra impulse caused a latency shift of the order of 1 ms, and additional impulses led to increased changes in latency.

Latency shifts were assessed in 20 C units after one, two, and four additional conditioning stimuli delivered at three different intervals from the last interposed to the next ordinary pulse (500, 1000, 3000 ms). This stimulus protocol with nine permutations was repeated at least twice in each unit. The results of this analysis are shown in the right panel of Fig. 14.2. We always found a clear effect of the number of additional stimuli on the latency shifts. While one additional stimulus pulse caused a latency shift of 1.2 ± 0.2 ms (mean $\pm$ SEM), the latency increase was approximately doubled after two additional pulses to 2.3 ± 0.3 ms, and four pulses induced a fivefold delay (5.9 ± 0.7 ms; right panel of Fig. 14.2), that is, the delays were almost linearly correlated to the number of additional spikes.

The closer the interposed pulses were given to the regular pulse, the more pronounced was the effect on latency shifts. In comparison to number of pulses this effect was smaller, but still significant ($t = -2.3$; partial correlation coefficient -0.17; $p = 0.02$).

However, latency shifts caused by additional pulses given 500 and 3000 ms before the regular pulse differed by only 17 per cent on average.

Even though the magnitude of the delay was dependent to some degree on the distance between the recording and stimulating electrodes, the number of additional spikes was by far the most important factor. We thus conclude that the marking technique is indeed sensitive enough to even detect responses consisting of single spikes. Due to the other intervening variables (for example, conduction velocity, temperature, and latency between intervening spike and next stimulus), the marking method cannot easily be used for quantitative evaluation of the number of spike discharges induced by a particular stimulus. However, our finding that conduction delay and number of intervening spikes are almost linearly related may render the conduction delay a useful measure for semiquantitative estimations, for example, of the proportion of discharges induced by different stimuli.

An example is shown in Fig. 14.3. In this experiment a C unit was tested with short mechanical impact stimuli (Kohllöffel *et al.* 1991; Koltzenburg and Handwerker 1994). A weaker impact induced six spikes in this particular unit, a stronger impact 13 spikes (Fig. 14.3, left). The latency shifts were approximately proportional to the magnitude of the response (Fig. 14.3, right). With the marking method it is possible to prove that a particular C unit responds to a particular stimulus and, if the recording is good enough for waveform recognition, additional analysis of ongoing discharges allows the quantification of the response.

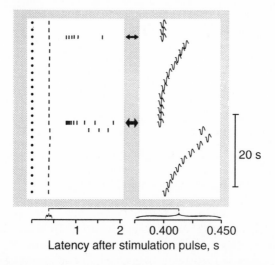

Fig. 14.3 Semiquantitative estimation of the proportion of a C-fibre response to stimuli of different intensity. Left panel, Electrical shock artefacts are shown as round dots and the C-unit response as vertical bars. A weak mechanical impact induced six spikes in this particular unit; a stronger impact 13 spikes (arrows). Right panel, The latency delays were approximately proportional to the magnitude of the response. Notice the different time base in the left and right panels.

The marking technique has opened up the possibility of collecting large C-unit samples in human skin nerves. Since C fibres tend to aggregate and remain as neighbours for considerable distances in the human peroneal nerve (Jørum *et al.* 1989), several C-fibre responses to electrical skin stimulation are often encountered in one recording site. Due to the long distance between the innervation territory in the foot or lower leg and the recording site in the peroneal nerve at knee level, units with slightly different conduction velocities are dispersed and can be identified individually, even if they have similar spike forms. Computer processing using dedicated software greatly facilitates on-line and off-line analysis of their response characteristics (Forster and Handwerker 1990).

Classes of afferent C units in human skin

Employing the marking technique, a sample of 220 C units was analysed in recent experiments and most of this sample has been published (Schmidt *et al.* 1995). Electrical search stimuli were largely used to avoid the bias induced by searching with mechanical stimuli. However, searching with electrical stimuli delivered from a pointed probe that is systematically moved on the skin is not entirely without bias either. This strategy will clearly favour detection of fibres with many widespread terminal branches in the skin, whereas fibres with just one or a few closely apposed endings are easily missed. This may be one explanation as to why we have encountered only one specific C warm unit in our present material, since these units typically have small spot-like receptive fields in human skin (Hensel 1976; Hallin *et al.* 1982). As is true for efferent fibres, afferent axons with deep endings are not likely to be recruited by this superficial search strategy.

Another shortcoming of the marking method is that it cannot easily be used to study the effects of cooling stimuli since cooling induces a slowing of conduction velocity similar to marking. Therefore, for the evaluation of responses to cooling we still depend on conventional methods.

Thus, the proportions of different unit classes discussed here are only tentative, and we realize that these proportions may vary depending on different experimental approaches.

CMH units

About 45 per cent of the 220 C fibres encountered were classified as CMH, that is, the conventional polymodal nociceptor type. Their mechanical thresholds shall be discussed in the next paragraph. However, they were in the same range as in other studies using conventional estimations (Torebjörk 1974; Van Hees and Gybels 1981; Adriaensen *et al.* 1983) suggesting that the electrical stimulation *per se* did not influence thresholds to any considerable degree.

CM units

Another 20 per cent of the C units responded to mechanical but not to heat stimuli up to the tolerance level of the subjects (usually 50–52°C). The mechanical thresholds of these CM units were not significantly different from the thresholds of CMH units. Furthermore, most of the CM and CMH units responded in a graded fashion to suprathreshold stimuli in the noxious intensity range, supporting the conclusion that many of them could be regarded as nociceptors. In the past, little if any attention has been paid to this class of human nociceptors. Yet, we cannot exclude that some CM units were actually low-threshold C mechanoreceptors of the type commonly encountered in hairy skin in the cat (Iggo 1960) and less commonly found in proximal parts of the extremities in the monkey (Kumazawa and Perl 1977) and in the human forehead (Nordin 1990). A typical feature of these low-threshold C mechanoreceptors is their responsiveness to cooling. As judged from the acoustically monitored discharges, no low-threshold cold responsive units were encountered in the present sample.

CH units

Eight units in the entire material (4 per cent) responded to heating with thresholds ranging from 45°C to 48°C but were not activated by mechanical stimulation even with a rather stiff von Frey filament (1.2–1.6 N). An example is shown in Fig. 14.4. There were no latency shifts in response to sympathetic provocation for any of these units, thus excluding the hypothesis that the heat responses might have been due to sympathetic reflexes. This type of CH unit has been reported before in animals albeit rarely (Georgopoulos 1976; Welk *et al.* 1984; Baumann *et al.* 1991), but it was not known previously that CH nociceptors also exist in human skin. One unit was mechano-insensitive but had a low threshold (34°C) to warming stimuli, and hence was classified as a *warm-specific C unit*.

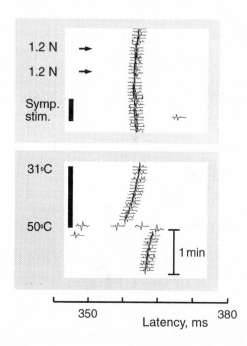

Fig. 14.4 Heat-specific C unit. Upper panel, This unit type was unresponsive to stiff von Frey filaments (arrows) and to sympathetic reflex provocation (Symp. stim.). Lower panel, During skin warming from 31 to 50°C the latency of the unit responses became shorter in the beginning due to a temperature-dependent increase of conduction velocity. The unit was activated at 48°C and, as a consequence, the latency was increased.

Sympathetic units

Twenty-four sympathetic units were identified. They constituted 11 per cent of all units tested. None of them responded to mechanical or heat stimuli. In contrast to afferent C units, most of them were spontaneously active, as seen by latency increases in the absence of any intentional manoeuvre. These units showed marked increases in latency during sympathetic reflex provocation. Sympathetic units may be underrepresented in our sample, since probably not all units participated in the sympathetic reflex provocation that we used (shouting, deep breathing, quick mental arithmetic). Furthermore, many of them may terminate at deeper structures in the skin making them less accessible to electrical surface stimuli.

Mechano- and heat-insensitive units

Seventeen per cent of the units were insensitive to mechanical and heating stimuli (mechanical stimulation up to 1.6 N von Frey bristle, and heating up to 50°C). If only the units encountered with a strict electrical search technique are regarded, this proportion was even higher (above 20 per cent in the study of Schmidt *et al.* 1995). These units were labelled CM_iH_i as suggested in a recent review (Handwerker and Kobal 1993). Even though there are differences in search techniques and classification criteria this proportion is in a range similar to that of the 30 per cent insensitive C units that have been found in the hairy skin in monkey (Meyer *et al.* 1991) and the 26 per cent recorded *in vivo* and the 15 per cent found *in vitro* in the hairy skin in rat (Kress *et al.* 1992).

These units may have been either efferent or afferent. However, silent and unresponsive postganglionic sympathetic units probably constitute at best a minor part of the CM_iH_i population, since the proportion of efferent C fibres is generally much lower than that of afferent ones in nerves supplying hairy skin in mammals (Baron *et al.* 1988).

The most striking argument in favour of the afferent nature of most CM_iH_i units is provided by the fairly high percentage of them that were activated or sensitized by irritant substances (see below). Figure 14.5 shows the different C-fibre classes in cutaneous fascicles of the human peroneal nerve and their relative frequency.

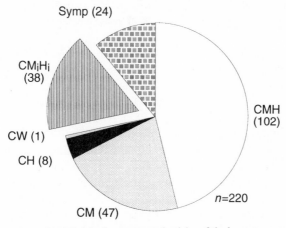

Fig. 14.5 Relative proportions of 220 C units in cutaneous fascicles of the human peroneal nerve. Number of units within brackets.

Mechanical and thermal thresholds of nociceptive and other slowly conducting afferents

Aδ fibres were less frequently studied than C fibres in human skin nerves. In the hairy skin of the extremities they seem to be less crucial than C fibres for pain and hyperalgesia as suggested by unchanged heat and pressure pain thresholds and unchanged hyper-algesia to heating and pressure during differential block of the myelinated nerve fibres (for a review see Handwerker and Kobal 1993).

In one study on 66 mechanoreceptive Aδ fibres recorded in the superficial radial nerve with conventional microneurography methods (Adriaensen *et al.* 1983), a low-threshold group (von Frey hair thresholds <9 mN) was found that had some characteristics in common with the 'down hair' receptors found in animal experiments (Brown *et al.* 1967). The other units had thresholds to von Frey hair stimulation comparable to those of CMH units (see Fig. 14.6). Twenty per cent of these Aδ fibres were also activated by noxious heat (Adriaensen *et al.* 1983) and, generally, heat-sensitive Aδ fibres also responded to chemical irritants (Adriaensen *et al.* 1980).

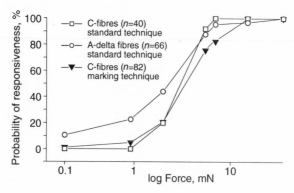

Fig. 14.6   Cumulative mechanical thresholds of one population of mechanoresponsive C nociceptors (*n* = 40) and one population of mechanoresponsive Aδ units (*n* = 66) recorded with the conventional technique (data from Adriaensen *et al.* 1983). In addition, C unit data obtained with our marking technique are shown (*n* = 82). Whereas in the Aδ group a subpopulation of units with very low mechanical thresholds was encountered, the two populations of C fibres are not different.

Mechanoheat-sensitive Aδ units (AMH) have also been described in other primates. According to their thresholds to heating they have been subdivided into two classes, AMH I and II (Meyer *et al.* 1985*a*). AMH I units have very high thermal thresholds that are considerably lowered in inflamed skin. They may play a role in heat hyperalgesia in the glabrous skin (Meyer and Campbell 1981). AMH II units seem to be more frequent in the hairy than in the glabrous skin of the monkey. They have thermal and mechanical thresholds similar to those of the CMHs. Most AMH units described in human hairy skin are similar to the AMH II type of unit, but there are findings that indicate that AMH I units occur in the glabrous skin of the human hand (Torebjörk 1985; Torebjörk and Ochoa 1990).

Aδ fibres are less frequent than C fibres in skin nerves, and the results from micro-neurography experiments indicate that, in addition, in human hairy skin the proportion of heat-sensitive elements is smaller in the Aδ than in the C-fibre group. Heat thresholds of the human AMH type II were 37–47°C, and hence in the same range as those of CMH units, 36–49°C.

Generally, heat thresholds of human nociceptors are often lower by some degree than pain thresholds and this indicates that some central summation is required for activation of central nervous structures involved in pain processing. Graded responses to supra-threshold noxious stimulation seem to be a more suitable indication of the nociceptive function of a particular primary afferent unit than mere consideration of thresholds (Handwerker and Kobal 1993). The discrepancy between pain threshold and the activation threshold of cutaneous C and Aδ units is greater when the mechanical thresholds to stimulation with von Frey hairs are regarded (Van Hees and Gybels 1981). This discrepancy may be due to less spatial summation, that is, activation of fewer C nociceptors with a punctate stimulus as opposed to the more widespread heat stimulus from a light bulb, or it may be the consequence of central gating of nociceptive input by simultaneous activation of low-threshold mechanoreceptor input caused by the von Frey stimulus.

Figure 14.6 shows the cumulative thresholds of two populations of mechanorespon-sive C nociceptors recorded with the conventional and the marking technique, respec-tively, and of one population of mechanoresponsive Aδ units. Whereas in the Aδ group a subpopulation of units with very low mechanical thresholds was encountered, the two populations of C fibres are not different. This can be regarded as another proof of the sensitivity of the marking method. It should be pointed out, however, that mechano-insensitive units are missed with the conventional technique, and those recorded with the marking technique are not included in Fig. 14.6.

Chemical excitation and sensitization of nociceptors

Excitability by chemical irritants was tested with mustard oil (allyl-iso-thiocyanate) and capsaicin (8-methyl-*N*-vanillyl-6-noneamide). Both agents are known to excite nocicep-tors and to induce inflammation (Jancsó 1960; Jancsó *et al.* 1967; Carpenter and Lynn 1981; Reeh *et al.* 1986; Handwerker *et al.* 1991*a*). For stimulation, pieces of filter paper soaked with a 100 per cent solution of mustard oil were applied for 3 to 5 min under the cover of a plastic film to prevent evaporation. After the treatment the skin site was reddened. Some units were subsequently also tested with capsaicin (1 per cent solution dissolved in ethanol and applied for 30 min).

Altogether, about 40 per cent of the afferent C units were activated by mustard oil. Among CMH units the proportion of activated units was almost 60 per cent, and in the class of CM units the respective proportion was still 36 per cent (Schmidt *et al.* 1995). Some of the units that were not excited by mustard oil were activated by subsequent capsaicin treatment of their receptive fields. Figure 14.7 demonstrates a CMH unit activated by capsaicin application. Among the CM$_i$H$_i$ units about one-third were activated by mustard oil and/or capsaicin and these units can be regarded as chemo-nociceptors.

The inflammation induced by mustard oil and capsaicin is known to result in hyperalgesia to heating, pressure, and stroking the skin. Hyperalgesia to heating and pressure is probably due to sensitization of nociceptors (see below). In the context of hyperalgesia it is significant that part of the C units had changed their responsiveness when tested with physical skin stimuli after application of mustard oil and/or capsaicin. For example, almost half of the CM units tested became heat-responsive after induction of an inflammation. An example is shown in Fig. 14.8. Similarly, two of three CH units were excited by mustard oil and one became sensitized to mechanical stimuli afterwards.

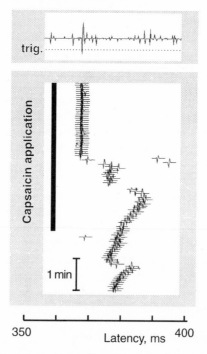

Fig. 14.7   Excitation of a CMH unit by topical application of capsaicin in the receptive field. This unit was not excited by previous treatment with mustard oil.

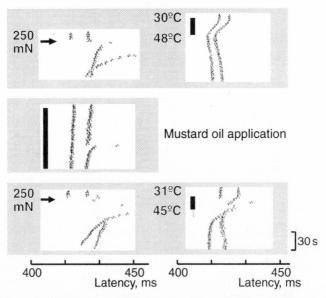

Fig. 14.8   Sensitization of CM units after topical application of mustard oil. Upper panel, Two C units responded to mechanical stimulation with 250 mN von Frey filament but not to heating up to 48°C before treatment. Middle panel, The second unit was weakly excited during mustard oil application. Lower panel, Afterwards, both units were activated by mechanical stimuli, and the first and probably also the second unit responded to heat as a sign of sensitization to a new stimulus modality.

In the class of the CM_iH_i units, two of 18 units tested with mustard oil became responsive to heating but not to mechanical stimuli, a further unit was sensitized to mechanical stimulation but not to heat, and one unit was sensitized to both. Some CM_iH_i units (5 of 12) that were neither excited nor sensitized by mustard oil became sensitized to heat or mechanical stimulation or both by the subsequent capsaicin treatment. Thus, about 40 per cent of CM_iH_i units became sensitized after chemical irritation. Figure 14.9 shows a specimen record. This CM_iH_i unit was not excited by mustard oil and capsaicin; however, after capsaicin treatment it became responsive to mechanical stimulation and to heating. It is important to note that the sensitizations to mechanical and heat stimuli occurred independently of each other and of a previous excitation by the irritant substance. In conclusion, more than 50 per cent of CM_iH_i units were either excited or sensitized by chemical inflammation and were thus proven to be afferent.

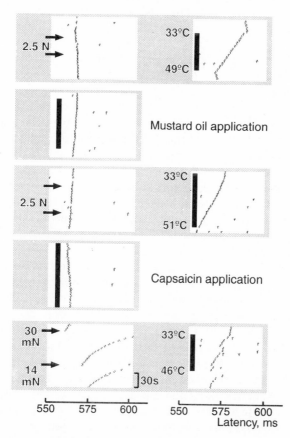

Fig. 14.9 Sensitization of a CM_iH_i unit. Top panel, This unit was insensitive to mechanical stimuli with von Frey filament 2.5 N and heating up to 49°C. Middle panels, Mustard oil did not excite the unit, and it remained insensitive to mechanical and heat stimuli afterwards. Topical capsaicin was also an ineffective stimulus. Bottom panel, However, after the capsaicin treatment this unit was greatly sensitized to mechanical stimuli and responded to 30 and 14 mN von Frey hairs. In addition, the unit had acquired a new sensitivity to heat.

Sensitization of 'silent' C-fibre branches

The expansion of receptive fields for mechanical stimulation during inflammation has been demonstrated in animal experiments, for example, in monkey hairy skin for high-threshold (HTM) Aδ and CMH nociceptors after a heat injury (Thalhammer and LaMotte 1982) and in Aδ but not C units after noxious mechanical stimulation in the rat tail (Reeh *et al.* 1987). These reports are compatible with the idea that there exist different terminal branches in nociceptive units some of which are insensitive to mechanical stimuli but which become responsive following sensitization by inflammatory mediators.

To test this hypothesis in human skin on the lower leg we conducted experiments in which the marking technique was used to electrically map the extension of the terminal cutaneous branches of individual C units (electrical receptive fields: eRFs). These electrically mapped terminals were compared with the receptive fields to mechanical stimulation (mRFs) with a von Frey hair of suprathreshold strength (Schmelz *et al.* 1994).

For this purpose a pair of needles, 0.2 mm in diameter, were inserted intracutaneously 5–10 mm apart at a site from which the C-fibre responses were elicited. We then used these needle electrodes to continuously stimulate the respective C unit at regular intervals of 4 s at a moderately painful intensity (0.3-ms pulses of 4–20 V). As described above, the latency shifts of the evoked C-fibre responses to these intracutaneous stimuli were used for assessment of the excitation of the respective C fibre. For mapping the eRFs, the tip of a pointed steel electrode (area 1.5 mm) was moistened with electrode gel and gently appositioned on the skin for unipolar electrical stimulation with the indifferent electrode (steel plate, 3 × 5 cm) attached to the dorsomedial aspect of the lower thigh. Trains of three pulses were delivered from a constant-current stimulator at a moderately painful intensity (2–3 mA; duration 0.2 ms; interval, 200 ms). A skin area with a radius of at least 2.5 cm around the intracutaneous stimulation needles was searched for mapping the maximal extension of the eRF.

Points from which mechanical or transcutaneous electrical stimuli activated the C unit, as indicated by slowing of its conduction velocity, were carefully marked on the skin. Stimulation points within and at the borders of RFs were spaced by about 2–3 mm.

Forty-seven CMH units were tested. The borders of the mRFs and those of the eRFs were largely identical apart from 15 cases in which mechano-insensitive fields were found. Figure 14.10 shows an example of such an analysis. In this case the eRF had a distal extension that was not susceptible to noxious mechanical stimulation. Mustard oil was exclusively applied to this distal extension for 5 min. After that, this part of the eRF was sensitized to mechanical stimulation and the borders of the eRF and mRF were coincident. It has to be mentioned that the thresholds for heating and mechanical stimulation of the untreated part of the eRF were unchanged.

One has to concede that our data on receptive fields with complex forms and properties also allow an alternative interpretation to the branching of C fibres, namely, stable ephaptic coupling of different C fibres. If, for example, a CMH unit and a 'silent' unit are coupled, the latter could appear as the 'silent branch' of the former. Indeed, using the nerve split technique, Meyer *et al.* (1985*b*) demonstrated coupling of afferent C fibres in monkey, but no data on the incidence of couplings were provided. In another study on cat hairy skin, coupling was fund to be rare in normal nerves (Blumberg and Jänig 1982). In a recent study on C fibres in the human peroneal nerve we found 20 per cent 'silent' units, the majority of which were probably afferent, and which were apparently not ephaptically coupled to other types of C fibres (Schmidt *et al.* 1995).

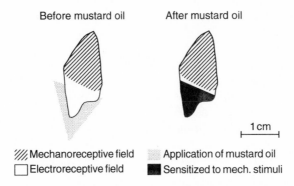

Before mustard oil   After mustard oil

1 cm

⧄ Mechanoreceptive field   ░ Application of mustard oil
□ Electroreceptive field   ■ Sensitized to mech. stimuli

Fig. 14.10 Sensitization of silent branches of a CMH unit. Left panel, The electroreceptive field of this unit overlapped with the mechanoreceptive field (hatched area), but, in addition, had a distal extension outside the mechanoreceptive border (unfilled area). Right panel, After mustard oil application to this distal extension, this part of the electroreceptive field was sensitized to mechanical stimulation (black area) and the borders of the electroreceptive and mechanoreceptive fields were coincident.

Thus, even though it cannot be excluded that some of the 'silent branches' were in reality silent units ephaptically coupled to 'conventional' C nociceptors, there is no evidence that coupling occurs often enough as to explain the expansion of mRFs in about one-third of the units tested. Furthermore, it has to be pointed out that coupled axons and dichotomized axons would lead to the same physiological effect. Regardless of whether inflammation induces recruitment of silent branches or silent units, the net effect will be an increased population of C fibres driven by a particular stimulus, and hence spatial summation at central synapses. This may be of importance for hyperalgesia in addition to the increased firing of sensitized 'conventional' nociceptors.

Nociceptor sensitization, central modulation, and different forms of hyperalgesia

From the above it is evident that human cutaneous nociceptors are heterogeneous and that their receptive properties may change considerably following tissue injury and inflammation. The lowering of thresholds, the enhanced responses to supraliminal stimuli, and the acquisition of responsiveness to new stimulus modalities as demonstrated here probably will contribute to hyperalgesia to heat and to mechanical stimulation as seen in the area of inflammation following topical application of mustard oil or capsaicin (see Meyer *et al.*, Chapter 15, this volume).

There has been a long-standing debate about the relative importance of peripheral and central nervous mechanisms in generating hyperalgesia by inflammatory processes. Initially, the excitability increase of either peripheral (Lewis 1935, 1942) or central

(Hardy *et al.* 1952*a, b*) neural pathways was favoured. Recently, it has been suggested that peripheral and central mechanisms may contribute differentially depending on the type of tissue injury and sensory modality being tested (Kilo *et al.* 1994).

The known plasticity changes of human nociceptors following mild inflammation may be important for several kinds of hyperalgesia phenomena, in particular, in the case of primary hyperalgesias restricted to the area of tissue injury or inflammation. The following forms of hyperalgesia have been explored to some extent.

Hyperalgesia to heating

It has been demonstrated in several studies on human and monkey skin that topical capsaicin treatment is able to lower the heat thresholds of CMH units by about 5°C or more (Baumann *et al.* 1991; LaMotte *et al.* 1992). Similar changes were seen after burning lesions (LaMotte *et al.* 1983; Torebjörk *et al.* 1984*a, b*). Such sensitization of nociceptors may well explain primary hyperalgesia to heating. Probably CM and CM_iH_i units by becoming sensitized to heating (Schmidt *et al.* 1995) contribute to spatial summation at central synapses during subliminal stimulation and hence to hyperalgesia.

Hyperalgesia to tonic blunt pressure

Like heat hyperalgesia, hyperalgesia to tonic blunt pressure was found only in the area of capsaicin application and not in the surroundings (primary hyperalgesia) (Koltzenburg *et al.* 1992; Kilo *et al.* 1994). It is known to persist when the A fibres are differentially blocked and it is diminished by cooling the skin which reduces the activity in sensitized C fibres (Culp *et al.* 1989; Koltzenburg *et al.* 1992). However, some studies have demonstrated that the discharges of CMH units upon blunt pressure stimulation are not increased after topical capsaicin (LaMotte *et al.* 1992) or mustard oil (Handwerker *et al.* 1991*a*). Therefore, the recruitment of sensitized CH and 'silent' CM_iH_i units (Schmidt *et al.* 1995) and the recruitment of silent branches (Schmelz *et al.* 1994) may be more important for this type of hyperalgesia.

Hyperalgesia to mechanical impact

However, using mechanical stimulation, it can easily be demonstrated that changing the stimulus parameters or the type of inflammation might change the tendency to hyperalgesia. For example, after topical capsaicin no *hyperalgesia to phasic impact stimuli* was found though it was clearly demonstrated in a skin area traumatized by freezing (Kilo *et al.* 1994). These differential effects deserve further investigation.

Hyperalgesia to gentle stroking

Tenderness in the surroundings of a focal inflammation, that is, secondary hyperalgesia, has been clearly demonstrated for different forms of mechanical stimulation (see LaMotte, Chapter 16, this volume). LaMotte *et al.* (1991) found secondary hyperalgesia to gentle stroking in a wide area around a capsaicin injection site. Recordings from nociceptors around that area in monkeys (Baumann *et al.* 1991) and humans (LaMotte *et al.* 1992) have not shown any evidence of peripheral sensitization to tactile stimuli. Instead, experiments with selective nerve blocks revealed that the tactile hyperalgesia was only detectable in the presence of intact conduction in large myelinated fibres, and could be mimicked by intraneural electrical microstimulation of low-threshold mechanoreceptive afferents that normally signal non-painful touch (Torebjörk *et al.* 1992). Indeed, neurones in the spinal cord of monkey getting nociceptor input displayed increased excitability to A-fibre input following capsaicin injections (Simone *et al.* 1991).

It appears that this type of hyperalgesia (*touch-evoked hyperalgesia* or allodynia) is related to a sensitization of central neurones that is critically dependent on ongoing activity in nociceptive afferents, and the hyperalgesia quickly disappears when that input is stopped. Thus, the magnitude of touch-evoked hyperalgesia after a topical application of mustard oil or capsaicin was linearly dependent on the degree of background pain, and hence probably on the amount of nociceptor barrage (Koltzenburg *et al.* 1992). The hyperalgesia disappeared when the ongoing activity in the sensitized nociceptors was stopped by cooling the skin, as directly observed in microneurographic recordings (LaMotte *et al.* 1992). The linear relationship between background pain and touch-evked hyperalgesia has been observed also in patients with various forms of neuralgia, regardless of whether the pain condition was sympathetically maintained or not (Koltzenburg *et al.* 1994). Thus, it appears that this particular form of touch-evoked secondary hyperalgesia represents a physiological response of the central nervous system and is a consequence of an ongoing nociceptor barrage, regardless of its underlying pathophysiological cause (Torebjörk 1992). This nociceptive input does not need to be very strong, since the phenomenon of transient touch-evoked hyperalgesia could be demonstrated after slowly heating the skin without causing detectable pain (Cervero *et al.* 1993).

Pinprick hyperalgesia

However, another form of secondary hyperalgesia to punctuate stimuli with pins or von Frey bristles has a much longer time course and covers a larger skin area after capsaicin injection (LaMotte *et al.* 1991). It probably also represents an example of central sensitization since no clear signs of nociceptor sensitization to this form of stimulation were found in microneurography experiments (LaMotte *et al.* 1992). Pinprick hyper-algesia may be initiated by changes in responsiveness of central projecting units due to the initial nociceptor barrage but can be maintained for some time in the absence of such input (Kilo *et al.* 1994).

Putative mechanisms for hyperalgesia

In summary, there is evidence that of the five forms of hyperalgesia studied, namely, in response to: (1) heating; (2) blunt pressure; (3) mechanical impacts; (4) gentle stroking; and (5) pointed pressure, the first three occur in the primary area after capsaicin application and to some extent these may be directly due to excitability changes of nociceptors. The two remaining forms of mechanical hyperalgesia occur in the primary and secondary zone after capsaicin and these forms—at least in the secondary zone—seem to be largely due to plasticity changes in central neurones initiated and/or maintained by nociceptor input. In their attempt to explain the mechanisms for secondary hyperalgesia, LaMotte *et al.* (1991) postulated the existence in humans of chemonociceptors, which were thought to be particularly powerful in their actions to produce central sensitization. Our finding that there are insensitive C units in human skin that are activated and sensitized by chemical irritants is of considerable interest in this context.

Conclusions

Novel classes of human nociceptors are described, including C units that are insensitive even to very strong mechanical and heat stimuli in normal skin but are excited by chemical agents and become sensitive to mechanical and/or heat stimuli after chemical irritation. The receptive fields of mechanoresponsive C nociceptors are complex with insensitive branches that can be sensitized by chemical irritation and then acquire sensitivity to mechanical stimuli. Thus, human nociceptors are heterogeneous and complex and their receptive properties may change considerably following tissue injury and inflammation. Such peripheral sensitization of nociceptors probably contributes to primary hyperalgesia to heat and to pressure following tissue injury or inflammation. In addition, the temporal and spatial summation of nociceptor impulses after such injury will affect the signal processing in the central nervous system and lead to various forms of secondary hyperalgesia.

References

Adriaensen, H., Gybels, J., Handwerker, H.O., and Van Hees, J. (1980). Latencies of chemically evoked discharges in human cutaneous nociceptors and of the concurrent subjective sensations. *Neurosci. Lett.* **20**, 55–9.

Adriaensen, H., Gybels, J., Handwerker, H.O., and Van Hees, J. (1983). Response properties of thin myelinated (A-delta) fibers in human skin nerves. *J. Neurophysiol.* **49**, 111–22.

Baron, R., Jänig, W., and Kollmann, W. (1988). Sympathetic and afferent somata projecting in hindlimb nerves and the anatomical organization of the lumbar sympathetic nervous system of the rat. *J. comp. Neurol.* **275**, 460–8.

Baumann, T.K., Simone, D.A., Shain, C.N., and LaMotte, R.H. (1991). Neurogenic hyperalgesia: the search for the primary cutaneous afferent fibers that contribute to capsaicin-induced pain and hyperalgesia. *J. Neurophysiol.* **66**, 212–27.

Bessou, P. and Perl, E.R. (1969). Responses of cutaneous sensory units with unmyelinated fibers to noxious stimuli. *J. Neurophysiol.* **32**, 1025–43.

Blumberg, H. and Jänig, W. (1982). Changes in unmyelinated fibers including sympathetic postganglionic fibers of a skin nerve after peripheral neuroma formation. *J. auton. nerv. Syst.* **6**, 173–83.

Brown, A.G., Iggo, A., and Miller, S. (1967). Myelinated afferent nerve fibers from the skin of the rabbit ear. *Exp. Neurol.* **18**, 338–49.

Calancie, B. and Stein, R.B. (1988). Microneurography for the recording and selective stimulation of afferents: an assessment. *Muscle Nerve* **11**, 638–45.

Carpenter, S.E. and Lynn, B. (1981). Vascular and sensory responses of human skin to mild injury after topical treatment with capsaicin. *Br. J. Pharmacol.* **73** 755–8.

Cervero, F., Gilbert, R., Hammond, R.G.E., and Tanner, J. (1993). Development of secondary hyperalgesia following nonpainful thermal stimulation of the skin—a psychophysical study in man. *Pain* **54** 181–9.

Culp, W.J., Ochoa, J.L., Cline, M., and Dotson, R. (1989). Heat and mechanical hyperalgesia induced by capsaicin. Cross modality threshold modulation in human C nociceptors. *Brain* **112**, 1317–31.

Davis, K.D., Meyer, R.A., and Campbell, J.N. (1993). Chemosensitivity and sensitization of nociceptive afferents that innervate the hairy skin of monkey. *J. Neurophysiol* **69**, 1071–81.

Forster, C. and Handwerker, H.O. (1990). Automatic classification and analysis of microneurographic spike data using a PC/AT. *J. Neurosci. Meth.* **31**, 109–18.

Georgopoulos, A.P. (1976). Functional properties of primary afferent units probably related to pain mechanisms of primate glabrous skin. *J. Neurophysiol.* **39**, 71–84.

Grigg, P., Schaible, H-G., and Schmidt, R.F. (1986). Mechanical sensitivity of group III and IV afferents from posterior articular nerve in normal and inflamed cat knee. *J. Neurphysiol.* **55**, 635–43.

Häbler, H.J., Jänig, W., and Koltzenburg, M. (1988). A novel type of unmyelinated chemosensitive nociceptor in the acutely inflamed urinary bladder. *Agents Actions* **25**, 219–21.

Häbler, H.J., Jänig, W., and Koltzenburg, M. (1990). Activation of unmyelinated afferent fibres by mechanical stimuli and inflammation of the urinary bladder in the cat. *J. Physiol., London*, **425**, 545–62.

Hagbarth, K.E., and Vallbo, A.B. (1967). Mechanoreceptor activity recorded percutaneously with semimicroelectrodes in human peripheral nerves. *Acta physiol. scand.* **69**, 121–2.

Hagbarth, K.E., Torebjörk, H.E., and Wallin, B.G. (1993). Microelectrode explorations of human peripheral nerves. In *Peripheral neuropathy*, (ed. P.J. Dyck, P.K. Thomas, J.W. Griffin, P.A. Low, and J.F. Poduslo), pp. 658–71. W.B. Saunders Co, Philadelphia.

Hallin, R.G. and Torebjörk, H.E. (1974). Methods to differentiate electrically induced afferent and sympathetic C unit responses in human cutaneous nerves. *Acta physiol. scand.* **92**, 318–31.

Hallin, R.G., Torebjörk, H.E., and Wiesenfeld, Z. (1982). Nociceptors and warm receptors innervated by C fibres in human skin. *J. Neurol. Neurosurg. Psychiat.* **45**, 313–19.

Handwerker, H.O., and Kobal, G. (1993). Psychophysiology of experimentally induced pain. *Physiol. Rev.* **73**, 639–71.

Handwerker, H.O., Forster, C., and Kirchhoff, C. (1991*a*). Discharge patterns of human C fibers induced by itching and burning stimuli. *J. Neurophysiol.* **66**, 307–15.

Handwerker, H.O., Kilo, S., and Reeh, P.W. (1991*b*). Unresponsive afferent nerve fibers in the sural nerve of the rat. *J. Physiol.* **435**, 229–42.

Hardy, J.D., Wolff, H.G., and Goodell, H. (1952*a*). *Pain sensations and reactions*. Williams & Wilkins, Baltimore.

Hardy, J.D., Wolff, H.G., and Goodell, H. (1952*b*). Experimental evidence on the nature of cutaneous hyperalgesia. *J. clin. Invest.* **29**, 115–40.

Hensel, H. (1976). Correlations of neural activity and thermal sensation in man. In *Sensory functions of the skin in primates* (ed. Y. Zotterman), pp. 331–52. Pergamon Press, Oxford.

Iggo, A. (1960). Cutaneous mechanoreceptors with afferent C fibres. *J. Physiol., London*, **152**, 337–53.

Jancsó, N. (1960). Role of the nerve terminals in the mechanism of inflammatory reactions. *Bull. Millard Fillmore Hosp., Buffalo, NY* **7**, 53–77.

Jancsó, N., Jancsó Gabor, A., and Szolcsányi, J. (1967). Direct evidence for neurogenic inflammation and its prevention by denervation and by pretreatment with capsaicin. *Br. J. Pharmacol.* **31**, 138–51.

Jørum, E., Lundberg, L.E., and Torebjörk, H.E. (1989). Peripheral projections of nociceptive unmyelinated axons in the human peroneal nerve. *J. Physiol., London*, **416**, 291–301.

Kilo, S., Schmelz, M., Koltzenburg, M., and Handwerker, H.O. (1994). Different patterns of hyperalgesia induced by experimental inflammations in human skin. *Brain* **117**, 385–96.

Kohllöffel, L.U.E., Koltzenburg, M., and Handwerker, H.O. (1991). A novel technique for the evaluation of mechanical pain and hyperalgesia. *Pain* **46**, 81–7.

Koltzenburg, M. and Handwerker, H.O. (1994). Differential ability of human cutaneous nociceptors to signal mechanical pain and to produce vasodilatation. *J. Neurosci.* **14**, 1756–65.

Koltzenburg, M., Lundberg, L.E.R., and Torebjörk, H.E. (1992). Dynamic and static components of mechanical hyperalgesia in human hairy skin. *Pain* **51**, 207–19.

Koltzenburg, M., Torebjörk, H.E., and Wahren, L.K. (1994). Nociceptor modulated central sensitisation causes mechanical hyperalgesia in acute chemogenic and chronic neuropathic pain. *Brain* **117**, 579–91.

Kress, M., Koltzenburg, M., Reeh, P.W., and Handwerker, H.O. (1992). Responsiveness and functional attributes of electrically localized terminals of cutaneous C-fibers in vivo and in vitro. *J. Neurophysiol.* **68**, 581–95.

Kumazawa, T. and Perl, E.R. (1977). Primate cutaneous sensory units with unmyelinated (C) afferent fibres. *J. Neurophysiol.* **40**, 1325–39.

LaMotte, R.H. (1988). Psychophysical and neurophysiological studies of chemically induced cutaneous pain and itch. The case of the missing nociceptor. *Prog. Brain Res.* **74**, 331–5.

LaMotte, R.H. (1992). Subpopulations of 'nocifensor neurons' contributing to pain and allodynia, itch and alloknesis. *Am. Pain. Soc. J.* **1**, 115–26.

LaMotte, R.H., Thalhammer, J.G., Torebjörk, H.E., and Robinson, C.J. (1982). Peripheral neural mechanisms of cutaneous hyperalgesia following mild injury by heat. *J. Neurosci.* **2**, 765–81.

LaMotte, R.H., Thalhammer, J.G., and Robinson, C.J. (1983). Peripheral neural correlates of magnitude of cutaneous pain and hyperalgesia: a comparison of neural events in monkey with sensory judgments in human. *J. Neurophysiol.* **50**, 1–26.

LaMotte, R.H., Shain, C.N., Simone, D.A., and Tsai, E.F. (1991). Neurogenic hyperalgesia: psychophysical studies of underlying mechanisms. *J. Neurophysiol.* **66**, 190–211.

LaMotte, R.H., Lundberg, L.E.R., and Torebjörk, H.E. (1992). Pain, hyperalgesia and activity in nociceptive C units in humans after intradermal injection of capsaicin. *J. Physiol.* **448**, 749–64.

Lewis, T. (1935). Experiments relating to cutaneous hyperalgesia and its spread through somatic nerves. *Clin. Sci.* **2**, 373–423.

Lewis, T. (1942). *Pain*. Macmillan, New York.

Lundberg, L.E.R., Jørum, E., Holm, E., and Torebjörk, H.E. (1992). Intraneural electrical stimulation of cutaneous nociceptive fibres in humans: effects of different pulse patterns on magnitude of pain. *Acta physiol. scand.* **146**, 41–8.

Meyer, R.A. and Campbell, J.N. (1981). Myelinated nociceptive afferents account for the hyperalgesia that follows a burn to the hand. *Science* **213**, 1527–9.

Meyer, R.A. and Campbell, J.N. (1988). A novel electrophysiological technique for locating cutaneous nociceptive and chemospecific receptors. *Brain Res.* **441**, 81–6.

Meyer, R.A., Campbell, J.N., and Raja, S.N. (1985a). Peripheral neural mechanisms of cutaneous hyperalgesia. In *Advances in pain research and therapy*, Vol. 9 (ed. H.L. Fields, R. Dubner, and F. Cervero), pp. 53–71. Raven Press, New York.

Meyer, R.A., Raja, S.N., and Campbell, J.N. (1985b). Coupling of action potential activity between unmyelinated fibers in the peripheral nerve of monkey. *Science* **227**, 184–7.

Meyer, R.A., Davis, K.D., Cohen, R.H., Treede, R.D., and Campbell, J.N. (1991). Mechanically insensitive afferents (mias) in cutaneous nerves of monkey. *Brain Res.* **561**, 252–61.

Neugebauer, V., Schaible, H-G., and Schmidt, R.F. (1989). Sensitization of articular afferents to mechanical stimuli by bradykinin. *Pflügers Arch.* **415**, 330–5.

Nordin, M. (1990). Low-threshold mechanoreceptive and nociceptive units with unmyelinated (C) fibres in the human supraorbital nerve. *J. Physiol. London*, **426**, 229–40.

Ochoa, J.L. and Torebjörk, H.E. (1989). Sensations evoked by intraneural microstimulation of C nociceptor fibres in human skin nerves. *J. Physiol. London*, **415**, 583–99.

Reeh, P.W., Kocher, L., and Jung, S. (1986). Does neurogenic inflammation alter the sensitivity of unmyelinated nociceptors in the rat? *Brain Res.* **384**, 42–50.

Reeh, P.W., Bayer, J., Kocher, L., and Handwerker, H.O. (1987). Sensitization of nociceptive cutaneous nerve fibers from the rat's tail by noxious mechanical stimulation. *Exp. Brain Res.* **65**, 505–12.

Rice, A.S.C., McMahon, S.B., and Wall, P.D. (1993). The electrophysiological consequences of electrode impalement of peripheral nerves in the rat. *Brain Res.* **631**, 221–6.

Robinson, C.J., Torebjörk, H.E., and LaMotte, R.H. (1983). Psychophysical detection and pain ratings of incremental thermal stimuli: a comparison with nociceptor responses in humans. *Brain Res.* **274**, 87–106.

Schaible, H-G. and Schmidt, R.F. (1985). Effects of an experimental arthritis on the sensory properties of fine articular afferent units. *J. Neurophysiol.* **54**, 1109–22.

Schaible, H-G. and Schmidt, R.F. (1988). Time course of mechanosensitivity changes in articular afferents during a developing experimental arthritis. *J. Neurophysiol.* **60**, 2180–95.

Schmelz, M., Schmidt, R., Ringkamp, M. Handwerker, H.O., and Torebjörk, H.E. (1994). Sensitization of insensitive branches of C nociceptors in human skin. *J. Physiol.* **480**, 389–94.

Schmelz, M., Forster, C., Schmidt, R., Ringkamp, M., Handwerker, H.O., and Torebjörk, H.E. (1995). Delayed responses to electrical stimuli reflect C-fiber responsiveness in human microneurography. *Exp. Brain Res.* **104**, 331–6.

Schmidt, R., Schmelz, M., Forster, C., Ringkamp, M., Torebjörk, H.E., and Handwerker, H.O. (1995). Novel classes of responsive and unresponsive C nociceptors in human skin. *J. Neurosci.* **15**, 333–41.

Simone, D.A., Sorkin, L.S., Oh, U., Chung, J.M., Owens, C., LaMotte, R.H., and Willis, W.D. (1991). Neurogenic hyperalgesia: central neural correlates in responses of spinothalamic tract neurons. *J. Neurophysiol,* **66**, 228–46.

Thalhammer, J.G. and LaMotte, R.H. (1982). Spatial properties of nociceptor sensitization following heat injury of the skin. *Brain Res.* **231**, 257–65.

Torebjörk, H.E. (1974). Afferent C units responding to mechanical, thermal and chemical stimuli in human non-glabrous skin. *Acta physiol. scand.* **92**, 374–90.

Torebjörk, H.E. (1985). Nociceptor activation and pain. *Phil. Trans. R. Soc., London,* **308**, 227–34.

Torebjörk, H.E. (1992). Nociceptive and non-nociceptive afferents contributing to pain and hyperalgesia in humans. In *Hyperalgesia and allodynia,* (ed. W.D. Willis), pp. 135–9. Raven Press, New York.

Torebjörk, H.E. and Hallin, R.G. (1976). A new method for classification of C-unit activity in intact human skin nerves. In *Advances in pain research and therapy,* Vol. 1 (ed. J.J. Bonica and D. Albe-Fessard), pp. 29–34. Raven Press, New York.

Torebjörk, H.E. and Ochoa, J.L. (1980). Specific sensations evoked by activity in single identified sensory units in man. *Acta physiol. scand.* **110**, 445–7.

Torebjörk, H.E. and Ochoa, J.L. (1990). New method to identify nociceptor units innervating glabrous skin of the human hand. *Exp. Brain Res.* **81**, 509–14.

Torebjörk, H.E., LaMotte, R.H., and Robinson, C.J. (1984*a*). Peripheral neural correlates of magnitude of cutaneous pain and hyperalgesia: simultaneous recordings in humans of sensory judgments of pain and evoked responses in nociceptors with C-fibers. *J. Neurophysiol.* **51**, 325–39.

Torebjörk, H.E., Schady, W., and Ochoa, J.L. (1984*b*). Sensory correlates of somatic afferent fibre activation. *Hum. Neurobiol.* **3**, 15–20.

Torebjörk, H.E., Vallbo, Å.B., and Ochoa J.L. (1987). Intraneural microstimulation in man. Its relation to specificity of tactile sensations. *Brain* **110**, 1509–29.

Torebjörk, H.E., Lundberg, L.E.R., and LaMotte, R.H. (1992). Central changes in processing of mechanoreceptive input in capsaicin-induced secondary hyperalgesia in humans. *J. Physiol.* **448**, 765–80.

Vallbo, Å.B. (1976). Prediction of propagation block on the basis of impulse shape in single unit recordings from human nerves. *Acta physiol. scand.* **97**, 66–74.

Vallbo, Å.B. (1981). Sensations evoked from the glabrous skin of the human hand by electrical stimulation of unitary mechanosensitive afferents. *Brain Res.* **215**, 359–63.

Vallbo, Å.B. and Hagbarth, K.E. (1968). Activity from skin mechanoreceptors recorded percutaneously in awake human subjects. *Exp. Neurol.* **21**, 270–89.

Vallbo, Å.B., Hagbarth, K.E., Torebjörk, H.E., and Wallin, B.G. (1979). Somatosensory, proprioceptive and sympathetic activity in human peripheral nerves. *Physiol. Rev.* **59**, 919–57.

Van Hees, J. and Gybels, J. (1981). C nociceptor activity in human nerve during painful and non painful skin stimulation. *J. Neurol. Neurosurg. Psychiat.* **44**, 600–7.

Wall, P.D. and McMahon, S.B. (1985). Microneuronography and its relation to perceived sensation. A critical review. *Pain* **21**, 209–29.

Welk, E., Fleischer, E., Petsche, U., and Handwerker, H.O. (1984). Afferent C-fibres in rats after neonatal capsaicin treatment. *Pflügers Arch.* **400**, 66–71.

15 Neural mechanisms of primary hyperalgesia

RICHARD A. MEYER, SRINIVASA N. RAJA,
AND JAMES N. CAMPBELL

Hyperalgesia is a consistent characteristic of tissue injury and inflammation. For example, pain in response to gentle warming and light touch is common after a sun burn. Pharyngitis is associated with hyperalgesia in the pharyngeal tissues, such that merely swallowing induces pain. In inflammatory arthritis, slight movement of the joint leads to pain. Micturition in the presence of a urinary tract infection is painful, again reflecting the presence of hyperalgesia. In this chapter, we will focus our attention on the hyperalgesia that develops in cutaneous tissue. We will discuss how hyperalgesia depends on: (1) the stimulus modality being tested (for example, heat, cold, mechanical, or chemical stimuli); (2) the type of injury; (3) the type of cutaneous tissue (for example, hairy versus glabrous skin); and (4) neurogenic factors (for example, axonal reflex, sympathetic efferents).

Hyperalgesia occurs not only at the site of injury but also in the surrounding uninjured area. Hyperalgesia at the site of injury is termed *primary hyperalgesia*, while hyperalgesia in the uninjured skin surrounding the injury is termed *secondary hyperalgesia* (Lewis 1942). In this chapter, we will discuss the evidence that primary hyperalgesia is due, in large part, to the sensitization of primary afferent receptors. As will be discussed in detail later (LaMotte, Chapter 16, this volume), secondary hyperalgesia appears to be due to sensitization in the central nervous system.

Taxonomy: hyperalgesia versus allodynia

One of the first issues to address is nomenclature. The IASP Subcommittee on Taxonomy has recommended that hyperalgesia be defined as an increased response to a stimulus that is normally painful and that hyperalgesia should not be associated with a lowering of threshold (Merskey and Bogduk 1994, pp. 210–12). It is suggested that 'allodynia' refer to pain due to a stimulus that does not normally produce pain.

The term 'allodynia' stems from the Greek term *allos*, which means 'other' or 'another' and is a common prefix for medical conditions that are different from the expected. The term allodynia appears to be appropriate when pain arises from channels of perceptual information not ordinarily concerned with pain. For example, a patient may be said to have allodynia if pain arises from activity in low-threshold mechanoreceptors.

The distinction between hyperalgesia and allodynia suggested by Merskey and Bogduk (1994) poses many difficulties. The term hyperalgesia has been in the literature for decades and was used by Lewis (1942) and Hardy and co-workers (1952) to refer to a lowering of the pain threshold as well as increased pain in response to suprathreshold stimuli. If secondary hyperalgesia develops because low-threshold receptors attain the capacity to evoke pain, should the term secondary hyperalgesia be discarded and replaced by the term secondary allodynia?

When nociceptors are subjected to an injury to their receptive field, they often develop a lowered threshold and an increased response to suprathreshold stimuli (see, for example, Fig. 15.1(B)). Should pain provoked by a normally non-painful stimulus that is due to activity in sensitized nociceptors be termed allodynia? Do we have to know the neural mechanism involved in order to decide how to describe a given individual's altered pain state?

Hypo-algesia is associated with an increased pain threshold and decreased pain in response to suprathreshold stimuli. If 'hyper' is the opposite of 'hypo', a lowered threshold seems implicitly to be an attribute of hyperalgesia. If a lowered threshold is implicit in the term hyperalgesia, pain due to a normally non-painful stimulus should be an aspect of hyperalgesia.

In discussing the psychophysics of pain we need a vocabulary that allows an individual's condition to be described without using terms that presuppose a mechanism. We believe that the term hyperalgesia should be used as the umbrella term to refer to enhanced pain in general (LaMotte 1992; Meyer *et al.* 1992*b*). Thus, hyperalgesia refers to any lowering of pain threshold (even to non-noxious stimuli) and/or increase in response to suprathreshold stimuli. Allodynia is reserved as a term to describe the special situation where pain arises from activation of sensory channels not ordinarily involved in pain (for example, low-threshold mechanoreceptors).

Hyperalgesia in response to different stimulus modalities

Hyperalgesia to heat stimuli

A distinguishing characteristic of primary hyperalgesia is the observation of hyperalgesia to heat stimuli. In the zone of secondary hyperalgesia, hyperalgesia to heat is not observed (see, for example, Raja *et al.* 1984; Ali *et al.* 1994; Kilo *et al.* 1994). Substantial evidence favours the concept that the primary hyperalgesia to heat stimuli is mediated by sensitization of nociceptors (Meyer and Campbell 1981*a*; LaMotte *et al.* 1982). Sensitization is defined as a leftward shift of the stimulus–response function that relates the magnitude of the neural response to stimulus intensity. Sensitization is characterized by a decrease in threshold, an augmented response to suprathreshold stimuli, and ongoing spontaneous activity (Bessou and Perl 1969; Beck *et al.* 1974; Beitel and Dubner 1976). These properties correspond to the properties of hyperalgesia.

In one study of the neural mechanisms of heat hyperalgesia, a burn was applied to the glabrous skin of the hand, and heat pain ratings were determined before and after this heat injury (Meyer and Campbell 1981*a*). As illustrated in Fig. 15.1(A), a marked hyperalgesia to heat developed. There was a leftward shift in the stimulus–response function relating the magnitude of pain sensation to the temperature of the heat stimulus. The threshold for pain decreased, and the pain to suprathreshold stimuli increased. This heat hyperalgesia was reduced during a selective A-fibre block (Meyer and Campbell 1981*a*).

A corresponding sensitization to heat stimuli was observed for A-fibre nociceptors that innervate the glabrous skin of the anaesthetized monkey (Fig. 15.1(B)). In contrast, the response of the C-fibre nociceptors was suppressed following the burn (Fig. 15.1(C)). Thus, in normal skin, heat pain near threshold appears to be signalled by activity in C-fibre nociceptors (Meyer and Campbell 1981*b*; see also Chapter 5, this volume). However, after injury, the hyperalgesia to heat that develops on glabrous skin appears to be due to the sensitization to heat of primary afferent A-fibre nociceptors.

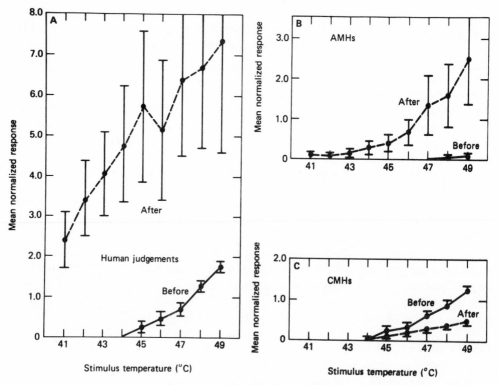

Fig. 15.1 Hyperalgesia and nociceptor sensitization after a cutaneous burn injury. Responses to heat stimuli were obtained 5 min before and 10 min after a 53°C, 30-s burn to the glabrous skin of the hand. The burn resulted in increases in the magnitude of pain (hyperalgesia) in human subjects that were matched by enhanced responses (sensitization) in A-fibre nociceptors (AMHs) in the monkey. In contrast, C-fibre nociceptors (CMHs) exhibited decreased sensitivity after the burn. (A) Human judgements of pain ($n = 8$). (B) Responses of AMHs in monkeys ($n = 14$). (C) Responses of CMHs in monkeys ($n = 15$). The first stimulus of the heat sequence was always 45°C. The remaining nine stimuli ranged from 41° to 49°C in 1°C increments and were presented in random order. Human judgements of pain were measured with a magnitude-estimation technique. Subjects assigned an arbitrary number (the modulus) to the magnitude of pain evoked by the first 45°C stimulus and judged the painfulness of all subsequent stimuli as a ratio of this modulus. The response to a given stimulus was normalized by dividing by the modulus for each human subject or by the average response to the first 45°C stimulus for the CMHs. Because the AMHs did not respond to the 45°C stimulus before the burn, the AMH data were normalized by dividing by the response to the first 45°C after the burn. Reproduced with permission from Meyer and Campbell (1981*a*).

Hyperalgesia to cold stimuli

Primary hyperalgesia to cold is not apparent following a cutaneous injury. If anything, applying cold to the injury site leads to a decrease in the ongoing pain and a decrease in the size of the zone of secondary hyperalgesia (LaMotte *et al.* 1991; Koltzenburg *et al.* 1992*b*). In contrast, hyperalgesia to cold has been reported to occur in the zone of secondary hyperalgesia (Gracely *et al.* 1993) and is often observed in neuropathic pain states (Frost *et al.* 1988; Wahren *et al.* 1991).

Hyperalgesia to mechanical stimuli

In contrast to heat hyperalgesia, mechanical hyperalgesia develops in both the primary and secondary hyperalgesia zones. Different forms of mechanical hyperalgesia have been identified based on the nature of the stimulus. 'Punctate' hyperalgesia is characterized by enhanced pain in response to punctate mechanical stimuli (for example, needle pricks, von Frey probes), 'stroking' hyperalgesia is characterized by enhanced pain in response to gentle stroking of the skin (for example, with a soft brush or a cotton swab), and 'pressure' hyperalgesia is characterized by enhanced pain in response to blunt pressure (Culp *et al.* 1989; LaMotte *et al.* 1991; Koltzenburg *et al.* 1992*b*; Kilo *et al.* 1994). Punctate and stroking hyperalgesia are observed in both the primary and secondary hyperalgesia zones, whereas pressure hyperalgesia is observed only in the primary zone (Koltzenburg *et al.* 1992*b*). Stroking (or dynamic) hyperalgesia and pressure (or static) hyperalgesia are also observed in neuropathic pain patients (Ochoa and Yarnitsky 1989).

The pressure hyperalgesia that develops only at the site of tissue injury is probably due to an enhanced response of primary afferent nociceptors. Nociceptor sensitization can be manifest as a lowering of threshold for activation, an enlargement of the receptive field size, and/or an enhanced response to suprathreshold stimuli. The form of sensitization appears to be dependent on the injury type. For example, a heat injury does not lead to a decrease in threshold of either mechanoheat-sensitive C fibres (CMHs) or mechanoheat-sensitive A fibres (AMHs), as measured with punctate von Frey hairs (Campbell *et al.* 1979, 1988; Thalhammer and LaMotte 1982), but the receptive fields of AMH fibres as well as those of some CMH fibres expand into the area of an adjacent heat (Thalhammer and LaMotte 1982) or mechanical (Reeh *et al.* 1987) injury. As a result of this expansion, heat or mechanical stimuli delivered after the injury will activate a greater number of fibres. This spatial summation would be expected to induce more pain.

Inflammation may lead to pronounced sensitization of nociceptors to mechanical stimuli. This has perhaps been shown most clearly following experimentally induced inflammation of the knee joint where joint afferents that were previously insensitive to mechanical stimuli become responsive to normally innocuous movements of the knee joint (Schaible and Schmidt 1988). Similarly, intradermal injection of mediators thought to be responsible for inflammatory pain may cause cutaneous nociceptors to become sensitized to mechanical as well as heat stimuli (Martin *et al.* 1987; K.D. Davis *et al.* 1993). Mechanically insensitive afferents (MIAs) have also been identified in skin (see Campbell and Meyer, Chapter 5, this volume). Cutaneous MIAs can become mechanically responsive after administration of algesic chemicals (K.D. Davis *et al.* 1993). Figure 15.2 shows the response of a cutaneous MIA to mechanical stimuli before and after exposure to a mixture of algesic inflammatory mediators (bradykinin, histamine, serotonin, and prostaglandin E_1). The von Frey threshold of this Aδ-fibre nociceptor decreased from 10 to 4 bar, and the receptive field size increased from 9 to 88 mm^2. Mechanically insensitive branches of C-fibre nociceptors in human skin also become mechanically responsive after application of mustard oil or capsaicin (Schmelz *et al.* 1994).

There is some evidence that the acidic pH of inflamed skin is the primary factor responsible for nociceptor sensitization to mechanical stimuli (K.H. Steen *et al.* 1992). Another possibility is that the apparent mechanical sensitization is just chemical stimulation in disguise: the pressure may cause a redistribution of inflammatory mediators that activate the nociceptor.

An enhanced response of primary afferent nociceptors may also be due to a change in transmission of the stimulus to the receptor. Thus, changes in tissue biomechanics may play a role in the apparent nociceptor sensitization. For example, simple wetting of the skin can increase the response of nociceptors to punctate stimuli (Kenins 1988) and to wool fabrics (Garnsworthy *et al.* 1988). In addition, the oedema associated with inflammation alters the biomechanical properties of the tissue and may lead to changes in the response properties (Cooper 1993).

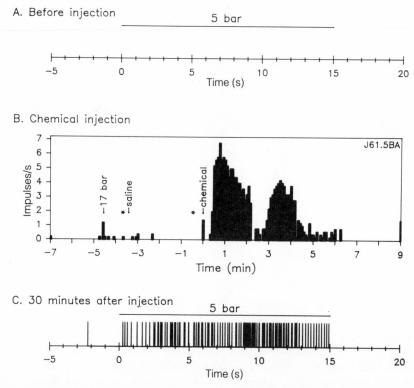

Fig. 15.2 Example of sensitization to mechanical stimuli following a chemical injection for an Aδ-fibre nociceptor. (A) The fibre did not respond to application of a 5-bar stimulus for 15 s to the most sensitive area within its receptive field. The initial mechanical threshold for this fibre was 10 bar and therefore it was a mechanically insensitive afferent (MIA). (B) This fibre had a strong response following injection into its receptive field of a mixture of inflammatory mediators including bradykinin, serotonin, histamine, and prostaglandin E_1. (Each asterisk indicates time of needle insertion; bin size, 5 s.) (C) Sensitization to mechanical stimuli was demonstrated in this fibre 30 min after the chemical injection. The fibre now responded to application of the 5-bar stimulus. Each vertical line corresponds to time of occurrence of an action potential. The von Frey threshold decreased (from 10 to 4 bar) and the receptive field area increased (from 9 to 88 mm^2). No response to heat was observed either before or after the injection. Reproduced with permission from K.D. Davis *et al.* (1993).

Punctate and stroking hyperalgesia of a similar magnitude are observed in the zone of primary and secondary hyperalgesia. For example, the pain threshold to punctate von Frey probes decreased from 12 to 5 bar at the site of a burn injury as well as in the adjacent zone of secondary hyperalgesia (Raja *et al.* 1984). Thus, the neural mechanisms for punctate and stroking hyperalgesia in the primary zone may be the same as that in the secondary zone. As will be discussed in detail by LaMotte in Chapter 16, this volume, stroking hyperalgesia appears to be due to a central sensitization to input from low-threshold mechanoreceptors. Several lines of evidence indicate that punctate hyper-algesia has a different neural mechanism and is due to central sensitization to input from nociceptors.

1. In the zone of secondary hyperalgesia, the area of punctate hyperalgesia is consistently larger than that of stroking hyperalgesia (LaMotte *et al.* 1991; Kilo *et al.* 1994).
2. Stroking hyperalgesia after capsaicin injection lasts 1 to 2 hours, whereas punctate hyperalgesia lasts 13 to 24 hours (LaMotte *et al.* 1991).
3. Punctate hyperalgesia, not stroking hyperalgesia, developed after intradermal capsaicin injection into the arm of a patient with a severe large-fibre neuropathy (Treede and Cole 1993). This suggests that punctate hyperalgesia is mediated by small-diameter (presumably nociceptive) fibres.
4. Punctate hyperalgesia persists after an A-fibre block, whereas stroking hyperalgesia disappears (LaMotte *et al.* 1991; Kilo *et al.* 1994).
5. The pain produced by touching the skin with different wool fabrics was greatly increased in the region of secondary hyperalgesia (Cervero *et al.* 1994). The pain was proportional to the prickliness of the fabrics. Since nociceptors, and not low-threshold mechanoreceptors, exhibit a differential response to different wool fabrics (Garnsworthy *et al.* 1988), activity in nociceptors probably contributes to this form of secondary hyperalgesia to wool fabrics.

Other observations support the concept that punctate hyperalgesia is due to central sensitization to input from nociceptive fibres. The development of punctate and stroking hyperalgesia is abolished or markedly reduced when capsaicin is injected into an area rendered temporarily anaesthetized by a proximal nerve block (LaMotte *et al.* 1991). Thus, the initial nociceptive input is important in the induction of stroking and punctate hyperalgesia. When the area of primary hyperalgesia is anaesthetized, however, punctate hyperalgesia persists, whereas stroking hyperalgesia is eliminated. Therefore, stroking hyperalgesia has an ongoing dependence on inputs from the sensitized area, whereas punctate hyperalgesia is more enduring and less dependent on ongoing discharge from the sensitized area.

Since hyperalgesia to heat does not occur in the zone of secondary hyperalgesia, punctate hyperalgesia cannot be due to generalized central sensitization to polymodal nociceptive inputs. This suggests that the central sensitization applies to the inputs from nociceptors sensitive only to mechanical stimuli and not to inputs from nociceptors sensitive to heat stimuli.

Hyperalgesia to chemical stimuli

Whether hyperalgesia to chemical stimuli develops in the zone of primary or secondary hyperalgesia has not been determined. However, when the forearm skin of human subjects was experimentally made acidotic to mimic the conditions observed during inflammation (Steen and Reeh 1993), the pain in response to intradermal injection of a combination of inflammatory mediators (bradykinin, serotonin, histamine, and prostaglandin E_2 was enhanced (A.E. Steen *et al.* 1993). In addition, enhanced pain in response to bradykinin is observed after administration of serotonin (Sicuteri *et al.* 1965; Richardson and Engel 1986). An enhanced response of nociceptors to chemical stimuli following injury has also been observed, which would predict that primary hyperalgesia to chemical stimuli should be present. For example, an enhanced response of nociceptors to bradykinin is observed following a heat (Lang *et al.* 1990) or ultraviolet radiation (Szolcsányi 1987) injury or following inflammation induced by carrageenan (Kirchhoff *et al.* 1990). This sensitization to bradykinin may be due to the release of prostaglandins by the injury since prostaglandins have been shown to sensitize nociceptors to bradykinin (Lang *et al.* 1990; Mizumura *et al.* 1991; Rueff and Dray 1993; Nicol and Cui 1994).

Dependence of hyperalgesia on the type of injury

Different injury models have been used to explore the mechanisms of primary hyperalgesia. These include natural injuries of tissue (for example, by heating, freezing, ultraviolet radiation, and mechanical trauma) as well as exposure of the tissue to endogenous mediators of inflammation or exogenous algesic substances (for example, capsaicin, mustard oil, carrageenan).

Most natural injuries to the skin result in primary hyperalgesia. Although many injuries such as a burn or mechanical trauma are painful, hyperalgesia can develop even if the injury itself does not produce pain. For example, freezing the skin or exposing the skin to ultraviolet radiation does not necessarily induce pain at the time of injury, but during the subsequent period of inflammation hyperalgesia develops. Thus, nociceptor sensitization does not require an initial activation of the nociceptor. A change in the milieu surrounding the nociceptor due to the release of substances by surrounding damaged cells or inflammatory cells can lead to sensitization. For example, exposure to ultraviolet radiation did not lead to direct activation of the nociceptors (Szolcsányi 1987), but after 30 minutes spontaneous activity developed and the response of the nociceptors to heat and chemical stimuli was enhanced (Szolcsányi 1987; Andreev *et al.* 1994). Similarly, A-fibre nociceptors can develop a heat response following an injury that does not activate the receptors (Campbell *et al.* 1979). In addition, some mechanically insensitive afferents in humans became responsive to mechanical and/or heat stimuli after the administration of mustard oil and/or capsaicin which in itself did not elicit a response (Schmidt *et al.* 1995).

One strategy for understanding the mechanisms of primary hyperalgesia has been to determine how various substances released during inflammation alter the response properties of nociceptors. The list of substances found at elevated concentrations in the inflammatory soup includes bradykinin, prostaglandins, leukotrienes, serotonin, substance P, histamine, excitatory amino acids, thromboxanes platelet-activating factor, protons, nerve growth factor, adenosine, interleukins, nitric oxide, and free radicals. Some of these chemicals activate nociceptors and therefore are directly involved in producing pain, while others lead to a sensitization of the nociceptor response to natural stimuli and therefore play a role in primary hyperalgesia.

Bradykinin

Perhaps one of the most frequently investigated substances is bradykinin. Bradykinin is released upon tissue injury and is present in inflammatory exudates (Rocha e Silva and Rosenthal 1961; Melmon *et al.* 1967; DiRosa *et al.* 1971). Bradykinin has been shown to produce pain in man when given intradermally, intraarterially, or intraperitoneally (Cormia and Dougherty 1960; Guzman *et al.* 1962; Coffman 1966; Lim *et al.* 1967; Ferreira 1983; Manning *et al.* 1991). A pronounced tachyphylaxis of the evoked pain is observed following repeated presentations of bradykinin to the same location (Manning *et al.* 1991). As illustrated in Fig. 15.3(A), intradermal injection of bradykinin in humans produces hyperalgesia to heat but not to mechanical stimuli (Manning *et al.* 1991). This suggests that the neural mechanisms of primary hyperalgesia to heat and mechanical stimuli differ. In contrast, behavioural evidence for mechanical hyperalgesia is observed following the injection of bradykinin into the rat paw (Levine *et al.* 1986). This suggests a species difference in the neural mechanisms of bradykinin-induced hyperalgesia.

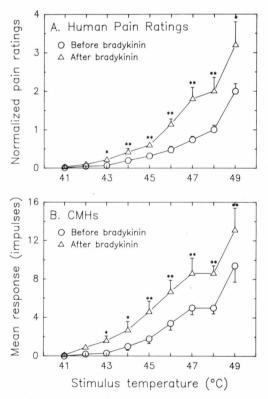

Fig. 15.3 Intradermal injection of bradykinin leads to hyperalgesia to heat in human subjects and sensitization to heat in CMH receptors of the monkey. Heat testing was done before and after intradermal injection of bradykinin (10 nmol in 10 μl). The heat sequence described in Fig. 15.1 was used. (A) Bradykinin produces hyperalgesia to heat stimuli in human subjects. Pain ratings to heat stimuli presented to the volar forearm were obtained before and after injections of bradykinin ($n=22$). Adapted with permission from Manning *et al.* (1991). (B) Bradykinin produces sensitization to heat of CMHs in the monkey ($n=10$). Adapted with permission from Khan *et al.* (1992). ($* = p \leqslant 0.05$; $** = p \leqslant 0.01$)

Administration of bradykinin in the region of the receptive field of unmyelinated and myelinated nociceptors results in an evoked response in the fibres (Beck *et al.* 1974; Lang *et al.* 1990; Mizumura *et al.* 1990; Khan *et al.* 1992). A pronounced tachyphylaxis of the evoked response is observed following the initial presentation of bradykinin. As illustrated in Fig. 15.3(B), intradermal injection of bradykinin leads to a transient sensitization of the response of nociceptors to heat but not to mechanical stimuli (Kirchhoff *et al.* 1990; Kumazawa *et al.* 1991; Khan *et al.* 1992; Koltzenburg *et al.* 1992*a*). This correlates with the transient hyperalgesia to heat but not mechanical stimuli observed in humans (Fig. 15.3(A)).

The acute activation of nociceptors by bradykinin in normal animals appears to be mediated by the bradykinin B_2 receptor (Haley *et al.* 1989; Steranka *et al.* 1989; Dray and Perkins 1993). Similarly, the acute pain induced by bradykinin in humans appears to be mediated by the B_2 receptor (Whalley *et al.* 1987). However, recent evidence indicates that the bradykinin B_1 receptor may be expressed in certain persistent inflammatory conditions (Perkins *et al.* 1993; A.J. Davis and Perkins 1994).

Several observations suggest that bradykinin *by itself* is not the sole mediator of nociceptor sensitization after tissue injury.

1. Bradykinin injected into the skin induces hyperalgesia in response to heat but not to mechanical stimuli (Manning *et al.* 1991). Tissue injury induces both heat and mechanical hyperalgesia.
2. Tachyphylaxis to the algesic effects of bradykinin is prominent. It is therefore unlikely that bradykinin by itself could account for the pain that lasts many minutes.
3. Bradykinin is believed to be derived from serum. Yet, in the *in vitro* preparations where presumably there is no source of bradykinin, nociceptors sensitize in a fashion similar to that of nociceptors in the *in vivo* preparation (Kress *et al.* 1992).
4. In a patient with a documented kininogen deficiency, normal hyperalgesia developed after a cutaneous injury (Raja *et al.* 1992).

Nitric oxide

Nitric oxide (NO) is a novel neuronal messenger that is not stored in synaptic vesicles but is produced on demand (Bredt and Snyder 1990; Moncada *et al.* 1991; Snyder 1992). It can act as an intercellular and possibly intracellular messenger in the nervous system, including the nociceptive pathways. Although NO does not appear to play a role in normal nociception, it may play a role in facilitating nociceptive processing during states of enhanced neuronal excitability (Haley *et al.* 1992; Kitto *et al.* 1992; Meller *et al.* 1992; Malmberg and Yaksh 1993; for review see Meller and Gebhart 1993).

Nitric oxide appears to be involved at both the peripheral and central sites of nociceptive processing. Inflammatory mediators such as substance P and bradykinin can induce the release of NO from endothelial cells. Ferreira and co-workers (1991) suggest a role for NO in the peripheral *anti*nociceptive actions of morphine and acetylcholine in a rat model of prostaglandin-induced hyperalgesia. They observed that substances that release NO, such as nitroglycerine, cause peripheral analgesia, and that NO synthesis inhibitors antagonized peripheral morphine analgesia (Ferreira *et al.* 1992). In contrast to the behavioural studies, Haley and co-workers (1992) observed that the administration of nitro-L-arginine methyl ester (L-NAME), an NO synthesis inhibitor, into the receptive field of dorsal horn neurones decreased the responses of these neurones to formalin injection. NO can also increase vascular permeability and oedema formation following carrageenan-induced inflammation (Ialenti *et al.* 1992) and contribute to the sensitization of high-threshold mechanoreceptors (Cooper 1993). The summed effects of these potentially opposing peripheral actions of NO on hyperalgesia are unclear.

Nerve growth factor

There is increasing evidence that nerve growth factor (NGF) plays a role in the hyperalgesia associated with inflammation (Lewin and Mendell 1993; also see Chapter 19, this volume). An increase in the tissue levels of NGF occurs within hours of the initiation of inflammation (Weskamp and Otten 1987; Aloe *et al.* 1992). The production of NGF can be upregulated by inflammatory mediators such as cytokines and growth factors (Lindholm *et al.* 1987; Yoshida and Gage 1992). Adult rats develop a prolonged thermal and mechanical hyperalgesia following a single systemic dose of NGF (Lewin *et al.* 1993). Although the heat hyperalgesia is evident within 15 min after the injection, the mechanical hyperalgesia is observed only after several hours. Lewin and co-workers postulate that the NGF-induced mechanical and heat hyperalgesia may involve two different mechanisms. The mechanical hyperalgesia may involve central changes, while the heat hyperalgesia is likely to result, in part, from sensitization of nociceptors (Lewin *et al.* 1993). Recent studies indicate that NGF-induced thermal hyperalgesia in adult rats may involve the activation of B_1 bradykinin receptors (Rueff and Mendell 1994). In addition, the mechanisms of NGF-induced mechanical hyperalgesia differ in neonatal and adult rats. In the case of neonatal rats, mechanical hyperalgesia could be explained by sensitization of Aδ nociceptors to mechanical stimuli, while in adult rats no sensitization was observed. B.M. Davis and co-workers (1993) showed that an increase or decrease in basal levels of NGF expression in the skin of transgenic mice resulted in profound hyperalgesia or hypo-algesia, respectively. In addition to the direct actions of NGF on sensory neurones, NGF may induce hyperalgesia by indirect mechanisms. NGF causes mast cell degranulation that leads to the release of substances such as 5-hydroxytryptamine and histamine that could, in turn, sensitize nociceptors. NGF also increases the synthesis, the axoplasmic transport, and the neuronal content of peptides such as substance P and calcitone gene-related peptide (CGRP). Thus, greater amounts of these peptides will be available for release from central and peripheral terminals of sensory neurones. In summary, the role of NGF in nociception appears to be diverse and is dependent on the developmental stage of the animal (Lewin and Mendell 1993; Lewin *et al.* 1994).

pH

Inflamed tissues have an acidic pH. Steen and co-workers have hypothesized that local acidosis may contribute to the pain and hyperalgesia associated with inflammation. Continuous administration of acid buffer solutions into human skin causes pain and hyperalgesia to mechanical stimuli (K.H. Steen and Reeh 1993). This correlates with the observation that low pH induces excitation and sensitization of nociceptors to mechanical stimuli (K.H. Steen *et al.* 1992). Topical acetylsalicyclic acid and salicylic acid block the pain and hyperalgesia and suppress the excitation of nociceptors induced by low pH (K.H. Steen *et al.* 1994; Stefanidis *et al.* 1994).

Serotonin

Serotonin causes pain when applied to a human blister base (Richardson and Engel 1986) and can also potentiate the pain induced by bradykinin (Sicuteri *et al.* 1965; Richardson and Engel 1986). Serotonin can activate nociceptors (Fock and Mense 1976; Lang *et al.* 1990) and enhance the response of nociceptors to bradykinin (Fjallbrant and Iggo 1961; Hiss and Mense 1976; Nakano and Taira 1976; Mense 1981; Lang *et al.* 1990).

Eicosanoids

The eicosanoids are a large family of arachidonic acid metabolites that includes the prostaglandins, thromboxanes, and leukotrienes. The eicosanoids are generally considered not to directly activate nociceptors, but rather to sensitize them to natural stimuli and other endogenous chemicals. This sensitizing effect of eicosanoids may play an important role in hyperalgesia associated with inflammation (for recent reviews see Levine and Taiwo 1994; Dray and Bevan 1993).

Excitatory amino acids

The role of excitatory amino acids and *N*-methyl-D-aspartate (NMDA) receptors in central sensitization is well established. However, recent reports indicate that the NMDA receptor is also present in the dorsal root ganglion and is transported down the peripheral nerve (Liu *et al.* 1994). These observation raise the possibility that excitatory amino acids acting via NMDA receptors may play a role in the peripheral modulation of nociceptive processing. A recent behavioural study demonstrated that the peripheral administration of L-glutamate, not D-glutamate, resulted in hyperalgesia to heat stimuli in rats (Jackson *et al.* 1994). In contrast, the peripheral administration of aspartate resulted in antinociception. These behavioural studies are consistent with neurophysiological observations in a rat spinal cord–tail preparation that peripherally administered glutamate activates certain primary afferent neurones (Ault and Hildebrand 1993). These preliminary studies suggest that excitatory amino acids may modulate pain behaviour via a peripheral action on nociceptor responsiveness.

Platelet-activating factors

Platelets store and, when stimulated, can release substances such as serotonin, histamine, and precursors of bradykinin that are capable of exciting and/or sensitizing nociceptors (Ringkamp *et al.* 1994*a,b*). Neurophysiological studies in an *in vitro* preparation indicate that cutaneous nociceptors can be excited and sensitized by activated platelets. Preliminary studies reveal that the nociceptor excitation by activated platelets is not blocked by serotonin antagonists or by cyclooxygenase inhibitors, suggesting that this excitation does not depend on serotonin or prostanoids (Ringkamp *et al.* 1994*a*).

Dependence of hyperalgesia on the type of tissue

There is some evidence that the neural mechanisms of hyperalgesia depend on tissue type (Campbell and Meyer 1983). As shown in Fig. 15.4(A), the hyperalgesia to heat that develops after a burn to the hairy skin is quite different from the hyperalgesia to heat that develops after a burn to the glabrous skin (Fig. 15.1(A)). Although a decrease in pain threshold and an increase in pain ratings are seen at low temperature for both skin types, pain ratings at the high temperatures were not enhanced on the hairy skin. In addition, C-fibre nociceptors on hairy skin can become sensitized following a thermal injury (Fig. 15.4(B)), whereas they are not sensitized on glabrous skin (Fig. 15.1(C)). Thus, both A-fibre and C-fibre nociceptors may play an important role in the hyperalgesia to heat that develops on hairy skin.

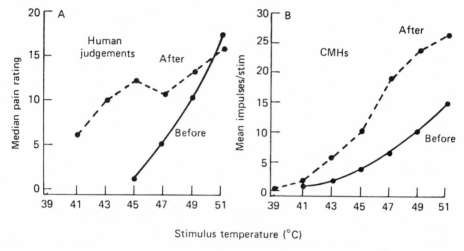

Fig. 15.4 Responses to heat stimuli immediately before and 10 min after a 50°C, 100-s burn to the hairy skin of the forearm. The burn resulted in a decrease in the pain threshold and an increase in the painfulness in response to mild heat stimuli (for example, 43°C), but a decrease in painfulness in response to intense heat stimuli (for example, 51°C). In contrast, the burn resulted in enhanced responses of the CMHs at all temperatures. The heat test consisted of an ascending sequence of seven stimuli ranging from 39°C to 51°C in 2°C increments. The stimuli were 5 s in duration and were presented every 30 s. (A) Median maximum pain rating for 13 human subjects. (B) Mean total number of impulses per stimulus in 12 CMHs recorded from anaesthetized monkey. Adapted with permission from LaMotte *et al.* (1983).

Role of neurogenic factors in primary hyperalgesia

Axon reflex and spreading sensitization of nociceptors

Activation of nociceptors leads to a flare response. This response is neurogenic in the sense that it depends on intact innervation of the skin by nociceptors. The flare response occurs within, but also extends well outside, the area of initial injury. One explanation of the flare response is that it involves a spreading activation of nociceptors. Activation of one nociceptor leads to a release of chemicals that activate neighbouring nociceptors, leading to a further release of chemicals and activation of additional nociceptors. Lewis (1942) believed that a similar mechanism, which he termed spreading sensitization, accounted for secondary hyperalgesia (and also contributed to primary hyperalgesia). Activation and sensitization of one nociceptor leads to spread of this sensitization to another nociceptor, due possibly to the effects of a sensitizing substance released from the nociceptor initially activated.

A number of lines of evidence suggest that spreading sensitization does not occur. Antidromic stimulation of nociceptive fibres in the monkey (Meyer *et al.* 1988) and the rat (Reeh *et al.* 1986) does not cause sensitization to heat stimuli. Heat injury to one-half of the receptive field of nociceptors does not alter the sensitivity of the other half to heat stimuli (Thalhammer and LaMotte 1982). Similarly, mustard oil applied to one-half of a nociceptor in human sensitized that half but not the other half to heat stimuli (Handwerker *et al.* 1994). An injury adjacent to the receptive field of nociceptors also fails to alter the responses of CMHs in monkey (Campbell *et al.* 1988) and rat (Reeh *et al.* 1986). The psychophysical observation that hyperalgesia to heat is not observed in the zone of secondary hyperalgesia (Raja *et al.* 1984; Ali *et al.* 1994) despite the presence of axon reflexive flare in this region provides strong evidence that spreading sensitization to heat does not occur.

These data suggest that neurogenic factors that occur at a distance from the injury site and that therefore require propagation of neural activity are not important in primary and secondary hyperalgesia. This does not rule out the possibility that non-propagating neurogenic factors are important (see below).

Sympathetic nervous system

Traditionally, the sympathetic nervous system (SNS) has been characterized as an effector organ. However, the SNS may also influence the presence and severity of pain. Although experimental and clinical observations suggest that the SNS may play a role in neuropathic pain states (Loh and Nathan 1978; Devor and Jänig 1981; Raja *et al.* 1991; Sato and Perl 1991), the part played by the SNS in acute pain states such as post-operative pain is unclear (Forrest 1992). Some studies indicate that the sympathetic nervous system may contribute to inflammatory pain (Levine and Taiwo 1994).

In healthy tissue, the SNS does not appear to be involved in the production of pain (Jänig 1989). Studies in normal cutaneous tissues have failed to demonstrate an excitation of either thinly myelinated or unmyelinated nociceptive afferent fibres by sympathetic stimulation (Roberts and Elardo 1985; Shea and Perl 1985; Barasi and Lynn 1986). These neurophysiological observations are consistent with psychophysical observations in humans that intradermal injections of adrenergic agonists in normal skin are not associated with pain (Wallin *et al.* 1976; K.D. Davis *et al.* 1991). Moreover, sympathectomy is not associated with alterations in pain perception or the development of hyperalgesia (Meyer *et al.* 1992*a*). A psychophysical study in normal subjects, however, provides pharmacological evidence that sympathetic nerve fibres may exert an inhibitory effect on C-fibre responses in normal skin via an α-adrenoceptor mechanism (Le Vasseur *et al.* 1993). These investigators observed that capsaicin caused more pain and increased flare when administered to skin pretreated with phentolamine than when administered to skin pretreated with a saline control.

In a series of behavioural studies in rat, Levine and associates (Levine *et al.* 1986; Taiwo and Levine 1988; Gonzales *et al.* 1989) present evidence for a role of the sympathetic efferents in the production of hyperalgesia. Topical application of chloroform to the hindpaw resulted in hyperalgesia to mechanical stimuli that was enhanced by local administration of noradrenaline (NA). The hyperalgesia was abolished by yohimbine but not by prazosin, suggesting that NA acts in inflamed tissues via an α_2-adrenoceptor mechanism. Sympathectomy prevented the chloroform-induced hyperalgesia and the effect of NA. The authors postulate that adrenergic agents released from the sympathetic postganglionic terminals activate autoreceptors in the same terminals, resulting in the release of prostaglandins, which may be the final mediators of the hyperalgesia (Taiwo and Levine 1988; Gonzales *et al.* 1989; Levine *et al.* 1993). Donnerer and co-workers (1991), however, failed to demonstrate a significant contribution of the sympathetic postganglionic nerves to the sensory function or to neurogenic or non-neurogenic inflammation in rat skin. A peripheral sympathetic component, possibly mediated by a D_1 dopamine receptor, has been suggested in carrageenan-induced hyperalgesia (Nakamura and Ferreira 1987). A role of the SNS in primary hyperalgesia in humans has recently been suggested (Drummond 1995; Meyer and Raja 1996).

On the basis of the effects of chemical sympathectomy, Levine and co-workers (1986) postulated that the mechanical hyperalgesia induced by bradykinin depends on the production of prostaglandins by the sympathetic postganglionic terminals. However, the hyperalgesia to heat that develops after bradykinin injection in humans was not altered in a patient following a surgical sympathectomy (Meyer *et al.* 1992*a*). Also, the sensitization to heat of CMHs in rat skin was not altered following a sympathectomy (Koltzenburg *et al.* 1992*a*). Thus, it is not clear whether sympathetic terminals play an important role in bradykinin-induced hyperalgesia.

Whereas sympathetic efferents do not have marked effects on nociceptor function in healthy tissues, type I AMHs can be activated by sympathetic stimulation following sensitization by a heat injury (Roberts and Elardo 1985). This activation was blocked by phentolamine, suggesting an α-adrenoceptor-mediated mechanism. Sanjue and Jun (1989) reported that cutaneous polymodal nociceptors in rats that had been sensitized by the injection of a mixture of inflammatory mediators into the receptive field responded to sympathetic stimulation and local arterial injection of NA. Sato and co-workers (1993) also observed that sympathetic nerve stimulation or intraarterial NA administration excited a proportion of cutaneous C-fibre afferents in adjuvant-induced inflammation. The sympathetic activation of C-fibres was blocked or attenuated by the α_2-adrenergic antagonist yohimbine, but less so by the α_1-adrenergic antagonist prazosin.

In summary, behavioural and neurophysiological studies in experimental animals indicate a role of the sympathetics in hyperalgesia or sensitization following injury. Recent psychophysical studies suggest that such a mechanism may play a role in humans as well.

Acknowledgements

We appreciate the editorial assistance of Jennifer L. Turnquist. This research was supported by NIH grants NS-14447, NS-26363, and NS-32386 and by an unrestricted gift from the Bristol–Myers Squibb Corporation.

References

Ali, Z., Meyer, R.A., Meleka, S.M., and Campbell, J.N. (1994). Capsaicin produces secondary hyperalgesia to mechanical but not heat stimuli. *Soc. Neurosci. Abstr.* **20**, 1570.

Aloe, L., Tuveri, M.A., and Levi-Montalcini, R. (1992). Studies on carrageenan-induced arthritis in adult rats: presence of nerve growth factor and role of sympathetic innervation. *Rheumatol. Int.* **12**, 213–16.

Andreev, N., Urban, L., and Dray, A. (1994). Opioids suppress spontaneous activity of polymodal nociceptors in rat paw skin induced by ultraviolet irradiation. *Neuroscience* **58**, 793–8.

Ault, B. and Hildebrand, L.M. (1993). L-glutamate activates peripheral nociceptors. *Agents Actions* **39**, C142–4.

Barasi, S. and Lynn, B. (1986). Effects of sympathetic stimulation on mechanoreceptive and nociceptive afferent units from the rabbit pinna. *Brain Res.* **378**, 21–7.

Beck, P.W., Handwerker, H.O., and Zimmermann, M. (1974). Nervous outflow from the cat's foot during noxious radiant heat stimulation. *Brain Res.* **67**, 373–86.

Beitel, R.E. and Dubner, R. (1976). Response of unmyelinated (C) polymodal nociceptors to thermal stimuli applied to monkey's face. *J. Neurophysiol.* **39**, 1160–75.

Bessou, P. and Perl, E.R. (1969). Response of cutaneous sensory units with unmyelinated fibers to noxious stimuli. *J. Neurophysiol.* **32**, 1025–43.

Bredt, D.S. and Snyder, S.H. (1990). Isolation of nitric oxide synthase. A calmodulin-requiring enzyme. *Proc. natl. Acad. Sci., USA* **87**, 682–5.

Campbell, J.N. and Meyer, R.A. (1983). Sensitization of unmyelinated nociceptive afferents in the monkey varies with skin type. *J. Neurophysiol.* **49**, 98–110.

Campbell, J.N., Meyer, R.A., and LaMotte, R.H. (1979). Sensitization of myelinated nociceptive afferents that innervate monkey hand. *J. Neurophysiol.* **42**, 1669–79.

Campbell, J.N., Khan, A.A., Meyer, R.A., and Raja, S.N. (1988). Responses to heat of C-fiber nociceptors in monkey are altered by injury in the receptive field but not by adjacent injury. *Pain* **32**, 327–32.

Cervero, F., Meyer, R.A., and Campbell, J.N. (1994). A psychophysical study of secondary hyperalgesia: evidence for increased pain to input from nociceptors. *Pain* **58**, 21–8.

Coffman, J.D. (1966). The effect of aspirin on pain and hand flow responses to intra-arterial injection of bradykinin in man. *Clin. Pharmacol. Ther.* **7**, 26–37.

Cooper, B. (1993). Contribution of edema to the sensitization of high-threshold mechanoreceptors of the goat palatal mucosa. *J. Neurophysiol.* **70**(2), 512–21.

Cormia, F.E. and Dougherty, J.W. (1960). Proteolytic activity in development of pain and itching: cutaneous reactions to bradykinin and kallikrein. *J. Invest. Dermatol.* **35**, 21–6.

Culp, W.J., Ochoa, J., Cline, M., and Dotson, R. (1989). Heat and mechanical hyperalgesia induced by capsaicin. Cross modality threshold modulation in human C nociceptors. *Brain* **112**, 1317–31.

Davis, A.J. and Perkins, M.N. (1994). Induction of B1 receptors in vivo in a mode of persistent inflammatory mechanical hyperalgesia in rat. *Neuropharmacology* **33**, 127–33.

Davis, B.M., Lewin, G.R., Mendell, L.M., Jones, M.E, and Albers, K.M. (1993). Altered expression of nerve growth factor in the sin of transgenic mice leads to changes in response to mechanical stimuli. *Neuroscience* **56**, 788–92.

Davis, K.D., Treede, R.-D., Raja, S.N., Meyer, R.A., and Campbell, J.N. (1991). Topical application of clonidine relieves hyperalgesia in patients with sympathetically-maintained pain. *Pain* **47**, 309–17.

Davis, K.D., Meyer, R.A., and Campbell, J.N. (1993). Chemosensitivity and sensitization of nociceptive afferents that innervate the hairy skin of monkey. *J. Neurophysiol.* **69**, 1071–81.

Devor, M. and Jänig, W. (1981). Activation of myelinated afferents ending in a neuroma by stimulation of the sympathetic supply in the rat. *Neurosci. Lett.* **24**, 43–7.

DiRosa, M., Giroud, J.P., and Willoughby, D.A. (1971). Studies of the mediators of the acute inflammatory response induced in rats in different sites by carrageenan and turpentine. *J. Pathol.* **104**, 15–29.

Donnerer, J., Amann, R., and Lembeck, F. (1991). Neurogenic and non-neurogenic inflammation in the rat paw following chemical sympathectomy. *Neuroscience* **45**, 761–5.

Dray, A. and Bevan, S. (1993). Inflammation and hyperalgesia: highlighting the team effort. *Trends Pharmacol. Sci.* **14**, 287–90.

Dray, A. and Perkins, M. (1993). Bradykinin and inflammatory pain. *Trends Neurosci,* **16**, 99–104.

Drummond, P.D. (1995). Noradrenaline increases hyperalgesia to heat in skin sensitized by capsaicin. *Pain* **60**, 311–15.

Ferreira, S.H. (1983). Peripheral and central analgesia. In *Advances in Pain Research and Therapy*, Vol. 5 (ed. J.J. Bonica, U. Lindblom, and A. Iggo), pp. 627–34. Raven Press, New York.

Ferreira, S.H., Duarte, I.D.G., and Lorenzetti, B.B. (1991). Molecular actions of acetyl choline and morphine analgesia. *Agents Actions* **32**, 101–6.

Ferreira, S.H., Lorenzetti, B.B., and Faccioli, L.H. (1992). Blockade of hyperalgesia and neurogenic edema by topical application of nitroglycerin. *Eur. J. Pharmacol.* **217**, 207–9.

Fjallbrant, N. and Iggo, A. (1961). The effect of histamine, 5-hydroxytryptamin and acetylcholine on cutaneous afferent fibres. *J. Physiol.* **156**, 578–90.

Fock, S. and Mense, S. (1976). Excitatory effects of 5-hydroxytryptamine, histamine and potassium ions on muscular group IV afferent units: a comparison with bradykinin. *Brain Res.* **105**, 459–69.

Forrest, J.B. (1992). Sympathetic mechanisms in postoperative pain. *Can. J. Anaesthesiol.* **39**, 523–7.

Frost, S.A., Raja, S.N., Campbell, J.N., Meyer, R.A., and Khan, A.A. (1988). Does hyperalgesia to cooling stimuli characterize patients with sympathetically maintained pain (reflex sympathetic dystrophy)? In *Proceedings of the 5th World Congress on Pain* (ed. R. Dubner, G.F. Gebhart, and M.R. Bond), pp. 151–6, Elsevier, New York.

Garnsworthy, R.K., Gully, R.L., Kenins, P., Mayfield, R.J., and Westerman, R.A. (1988). Identification of the physical stimulus and the neural basis of fabric-evoked prickle. *J. Neurophysiol.* **59**, 1083–97.

Gonzales, R., Goldyne, M.E., Taiwo, Y.O., and Levine, J.D. (1989). Production of hyperalgesic prostaglandins by sympathetic postganglionic neurons. *J. Neurochem.* **53**, 1595–8.

Gracely, R.H., Lynch, S., and Bennett, G.J. (1993). Evidence for A-beta low-threshold mechanoreceptor-mediated allodynia and cold hyperalgesia following intradermal capsaicin injection in the foot dorsum. 7th World Congress on Pain (abstract), p. 31.

Guzman, F., Braun, C., and Lim, R.K.S. (1962). Visceral pain and the pseudaffective response to intra-arterial injection of bradykinin and other algesic agents. *Arch. Int. Pharmacodyn.* **136**, 353–84.

Haley, J.E., Dickenson, A.H., and Schachter, M. (1989). Electrophysiological evidence for a role of bradykinin in chemical nociception in the rat. *Neurosci. Lett.* **97**, 198–202.

Haley, J.E., Dickenson, A.H., and Schachter, M. (1992). Electrophysiological evidence for a role of nitric oxide in prolonged chemical nociception in the rat. *Neuropharmacology* **31**, 251–8.

Handwerker, H.O., Schmelz, M., Schmidt, R., Ringkamp, M., and Torebjörk, H.E. (1994). Heat sensitization of parts of receptive fields in human skin C nociceptors. *Soc. Neurosci. Abstr.* **20**, 763.

Hardy, J.D., Wolff, H.G., and Goodell, H. (1952). *Pain sensations and reactions.* Williams & Wilkins, Baltimore.

Hiss, E. and Mense, S. (1976). Evidence for the existence of different receptor sites for algesic agents at the endings of muscular group IV afferent units. *Pflügers Arch.* **362**, 141–6.

Ialenti, A., Ianora, A., Moncada, S., and DiRosa, M. (1992). Modulation of acute inflammation by endogenous nitric oxide. *Eur. J. Pharmacol.* **211**, 177–82.

Jackson, D.L., Richardson, J.D., and Hargreaves, K.M. (1994). Peripheral administration of excitatory amino acids modulate nociceptive behavior in rats. *Soc. Neurosci. Abstr.* **20**, 1390.

Jänig, W. (1989). The sympathetic nervous system in pain: physiology and pathophysiology. In *Pain and the sympathetic nervous system* (ed. M. Stanton-Hicks), pp. 17–89. Kluwer, London.

Kenins, P. (1988). The functional anatomy of the receptive fields of rabbit C polymodal nociceptors. *J. Neurophysiol.* **59**, 1098–115.

Khan, A.A., Raja, S.N., Manning, D.C., Campbell, J.N., and Meyer, R.A. (1992). The effects of bradykinin and sequence-related analogs on the response properties of cutaneous nociceptors in monkeys. *Somatosens. Motor Res.* **9**, 97–106.

Kilo, S., Schmelz, M., Koltzenburg, M., and Handwerker, H.O. (1994). Different patterns of hyperalgesia induced by experimental inflammation in human skin. *Brain* **117**, 385–96.

Kirchhoff, C., Jung, S., Reeh, P.W., and Handwerker, H.O. (1990) Carrageenan inflammation increases bradykinin sensitivity of rat cutaneous nociceptors. *Neurosci. Lett.* **111**, 206–10.

Kitto, K.F., Haley, J.E., and Wilcox, G.L. (1992). Involvement of nitric oxide in spinally mediated hyperalgesia in the mouse. *Neurosci. Lett.* **148**, 1–5.

Koltzenburg, M., Kress, M, and Reeh, P.W. (1992a). The nociceptor sensitization by bradykinin does not depend on sympathetic neurons. *Neuroscience* **46**, 465–73.

Koltzenburg, M., Lundberg, L.E.R., and Torebjörk, H.E. (1992b). Dynamic and static components of mechanical hyperalgesia in human hairy skin. *Pain* **51**, 207–19.

Kress, M., Koltzenburg, M., Reeh, P.W., and Handwerker, H.O. (1992). Responsiveness and functional attributes of electrically localized terminals of cutaneous C-fibers in vivo and in vitro. *J. Neurophysiol.* **68**, 581–95.

Kumazawa, T., Mizumura, K., Minagawa, M., and Tsujii, Y. (1991). Sensitizing effects of bradykinin on the heat responses of the visceral nociceptor. *J. Neurophysiol.* **66**, 1819–24.

LaMotte, R.H. (1992). Subpopulations of 'nocifensor neurons' contributing to pain and allodynia, itch and alloknesis. *Am. Pain Soc. J.* **2**, 115–26.

LaMotte, R.H., Thalhammer, J.G., Torebjörk, H.E., and Robinson, C.J. (1982). Peripheral neural mechanisms of cutaneous hyperalgesia following mild injury by heat. *J. Neurosci.* **2**, 765–81.

LaMotte, R.H., Thalhammer, J.G., and Robinson, C.J. (1983). Peripheral neural correlates of magnitude of pain and hyperalgesia: a comparison of neural events in monkey with sensory judgements in human. *J. Neurophysiol.* **50**, 1–26.

LaMotte, R.H., Shain, C.N., Simone, D.A., and Tsai, E.-F.P. (1991). Neurogeic hyperalgesia: psychophysical studies of underlying mechanisms. *J. Neurophysiol.* **66**, 190–211.

Lang, E., Novak, A., Reeh, P.W., and Handwerker, H.O. (1990). Chemosensitivity of fine afferents from rat skin in vitro. *J. Neurophysiol.* **63**, 887–901.

LeVasseur, S.A., Khalil, Z., and Helme, R.D. (1993). Measurement of alpha-adrenoceptor modulation of nociceptive sensory nerve function in normal human skin. 7th World Congress on Pain (abstract).

Levine, J.D. and Taiwo, Y. (1994). Inflammatory pain. In *Textbook of pain* (ed. P.D. Wall and R. Melzack), pp. 45–56. Churchill Livingstone, Edinburgh.

Levine, J.D., Taiwo, Y.O., Collins, S.D., and Tam, J.K. (1986). Noradrenaline hyperalgesia is mediated through interaction with sympathetic postganglionic neurone terminals rather than activation of primary afferent nociceptors. *Nature* **323**, 158–60.

Levine, J.D., Fields, H.L., and Basbaum, A. (1993). Peptides and the primary afferent nociceptor. *J. Neurosci.* **13**, 2273–86.

Lewin, G.R. and Mendell, L.M. (1993). Nerve growth factor and nociception. *Trends Neurosci.* **16**, 353–9.

Lewin, G.R., Ritter, A.M., and Mendell, L.M. (1993). Nerve growth factor-induced hyperalgesia in the neonatal and adult rat. *J. Neurosci.* **13**, 2136–48.

Lewin, G.R., Koltzenburg, M., Toyka, K.V, and Barde, Y.-A. (1994). Involvement of neurotrophins in the phenotypic specifications of chick cutaneous afferents. *Soc. Neurosci. Abstr.* **20**, 1094.

Lewis, T. (1942). *Pain*. Macmillan, New York.

Lim, R.K.S., Miller, D.G., Guzman, F., Rodgers, D.W., Wang, R.W., Chao, S.K., and Shih, T.Y. (1967). Pain and analgesia evaluated by intraperitoneal bradykinin-evoked pain method in man. *Clin. Pharmacol. Ther.* **8**, 521–42.

Lindholm, D., Heumann, R., Meyer, M., and Thoenen, H. (1987). Interleukin-1 regulates synthesis of nerve growth factor in non-neural ells of rat sciatic nerve. *Nature* **330**, 658–9.

Liu, H., Wang, H., Sheng, M., Jan, L.Y., Jan, Y.N., and Basbaum, A.I. (1994). Evidence for presynaptic NMDA autoreceptors in the spinal dorsal horn. *Soc. Neurosci. Abstr.* **20**, 482.

Loh, L. and Nathan, P.W. (1978). Painful peripheral states and sympathetic blocks. *J. Neurol. Neurosurg. Psychiat.* **41**, 664–71.

Malmberg, A.B. and Yaksh, T.L. (1993). Spinal nitric oxide synthesis inhibition blocks NMDA-induced thermal hyperalgesia and produces antinociception in the formalin test in rats. *Pain* **54**, 291–300.

Manning, D.C., Raja, S.N., Meyer, R.A., and Campbell, J.N. (1991). Pain and hyperalgesia after intradermal injection of bradykinin in humans. *Clin. Pharmacol. Ther.* **50**, 721–9.

Martin, H.A., Basbaum, A.I., Kwiat, G.C., Goetzl, E.J., and Levine, J.D. (1987). Leukotriene and prostaglandin sensitization of cutaneous high-threshold C- and A-delta mechanoreceptors in the hairy skin of rat hindlimbs. *Neuroscience* **22**, 651–9.

Meller, S.T. and Gebhart, G.F. (1993). Nitric oxide (NO) and nociceptive processing in the spinal cord. *Pain* **52**, 127–36.

Meller, S.T., Pechman, P.S., Gebhart, G.F., and Maves, T.J. (1992). Nitric oxide mediates the thermal hyperalgesia produced in a model of neuropathic pain in the rat. *Neuroscience* **50**, 7–10.

Melmon, K.L., Webster, M.E., Goldfinger, S.E., and Seegmiller, J.E. (1967). The presence of a kinin in inflammatory synovial effusion from arthritides of varying etiologies. *Arthritis Rheumatism* **10**, 13–20.

Mense, S. (1981). Sensitization of group IV muscle receptors to bradykinin by 5-hydroxytryptamine and prostaglandin E2. *Brain Res.* **225**, 95–105.

Merskey, H. and Bogduk, N. (ed.) (1994). *Classification of chronic pain: descriptions of chronic pain syndromes and definition of pain terms,* (2nd ed). IASP Press, Seattle.

Meyer, R.A. and Campbell, J.N. (1981*a*). Myelinated nociceptive afferents account for the hyperalgesia that follows a burn to the hand. *Science* **213**, 1527–29.

Meyer, R.A. and Campbell, J.N. (1981*b*). Peripheral neural coding of pain sensation. *Johns Hopkins Appl. Phys. Lab. Tech. Dig.* **2**, 164–71.

Meyer, R.A. and Raja, S.N. (1996). Intradermal norepinephrine produces a dose-dependent hyperalgesia to heat in humans, *VIIIth World Congress on Pain*, Vancouver, Canada (abstract).

Meyer, R.A., Campbell, J.N., and Raja, S.N. (1988). Antidromic nerve stimulation in monkey does not sensitize unmyelinated nociceptors to heat. *Brain Res.* **441**, 168–72.

Meyer, R.A., Davis, K.D., Raja, S.N., and Campbell, J.N. (1992*a*). Sympathectomy does not abolish bradykinin induced cutaneous hyperalgesia in man. *Pain* **51**, 323–7.

Meyer, R.A., Treede, R.-D., Raja, S.N., and Campbell, J.N. (1992*b*). Peripheral versus central mechanisms for secondary hyperalgesia: is the controversy resolved? *Am. Pain Soc. J.* **1**, 127–31.

Mizumura, K., Minagawa, M., Tsujii, Y., and Kumazawa, T. (1990). The effects of bradykinin agonists and antagonists on visceral polymodal receptor activities. *Pain* **40**, 221–7.

Mizumura, K., Sato, J., and Kumazawa, T. (1991). Comparison of the effects of prostaglandins E2 and I2 on testicular nociceptor activities studied in vitro. *Naunyn-Schmiedebergs Arch. Pharmacol.* **344**, 368–76.

Moncada, S., Palmer, R.M.J., and Higgs, E.A. (1991). Nitric oxide: Physiology, pathophysiology, and pharmacology. *Pharmacol. Rev.* **43**, 109–42.

Nakamura, M. and Ferreira, S.H. (1987). A peripheral sympathetic component in inflammatory hyperalgesia. *Eur. J. Pharmacol.* **135**, 145–53.

Nakano, T. and Taira, N. (1976). 5-Hydroxytryptamine as a sensitizer of somatic nociceptors for pain-producing substances. *Eur. J. Pharmacol.* **38**, 23–9.

Nicol, G.D. and Cui, M. (1994). Enhancement by prostaglandin E2 of bradykinin activation of embryonic rat sensory neurons. *J. Physiol., London* **480**, 485–92.

Ochoa, J.L. and Yarnitsky, D. (1989). Mechanical hyperalgesia in neuropathic pain patients: dynamic and static types. *Ann. Neurol.* **33**, 465–72.

Perkins, M.N., Campbell, E., and Dray, A. (1993). Antinociceptive activity of the bradykinin B1 and B2 receptor antagonists, des-Arg^9, [Leu^8]-BK and HOE 140, in two models of persistent hyperalgesia in the rat. *Pain* **53**, 191–7.

Raja, S.N., Campbell, J.N., and Meyer, R.A. (1984). Evidence for different mechanisms of primary and secondary hyperalgesia following heat injury to the glabrous skin. *Brain* **107**, 1179–88.

Raja, S.N., Treede, R.-D., Davis, K.D., and Campbell, J.N. (1991). Systemic alpha-adrenergic blockade with phentolamine: a diagnostic test for sympathetically maintained pain. *Anesthesiology* **74**, 691–8.

Raja, S.N., Campbell, J.N., Meyer, R.A., and Colman, R.W. (1992). Role of kinins in pain and hyperalgesia: psychophysical studies in a patient with kininogen deficiency. *Clin. Sci.* **83**, 337–41.

Reeh, P.W., Kocher, L., and Jung, S. (1986). Does neurogenic inflammation alter the sensitivity of unmyelinated nociceptors in the rat? *Brain Res.* **384**, 42–50.

Reeh, P.W., Bayer, J., Kocher, L., and Handwerker, H.O. (1987). Sensitization of nociceptive cutaneous nerve fibers from the rat tail by noxious mechanical stimulation. *Exp. Brain Res.* **65**, 505–12.

Richardson, B.P. and Engel, G. (1986). The pharmacology and function of 5-HT3 receptors. *Trends Neurosci.* **9**, 424–7.

Ringkamp, M., Schmelz, M., Allwang, M., Ogilvie, A., and Reeh, P.W. (1994*a*). Nociceptor excitation by platelets is not due to 5-HT or prostanoids released. *Soc. Neurosci. Abstr.* **20**, 1569.

Ringkamp, M., Schmelz, M., Kress, M., Allwang, M., Ogilvie, A., and Reeh, P.W. (1994*b*). Activated human platelets in plasma excite nociceptors in rat skin, in vitro. *Neurosci. Lett.* **170**, 103–6.

Roberts, W.J. and Elardo, S.M. (1985). Sympathetic activation of A-delta nociceptors. *Somatosens. Res.* **3**, 33–44.

Rocha e Silva, M. and Rosenthal, S.R. (1961). Release of pharmacologically active substances from the rat skin in vivo following thermal injury. *J. Pharmacol. exp. Ther.* **132**, 110–16.

Rueff, A. and Dray, A. (1993). Sensitization of peripheral afferent fibers in the in vitro neonatal rat spinal cord–tail preparation by bradykinin and prostaglandins. *Neuroscience.* **54**, 527–35.

Rueff, A. and Mendell, L.M. (1994). NGF-induced thermal hyperalgesia in adult rats involves the activation of bradykinin B_1-receptors. *Soc. Neurosci. Abstr.* **20**, 671.

Sanjue, H. and Jun, Z. (1989). Sympathetic facilitation of sustained discharges of polymodal nociceptors. *Pain* **38**, 85–90.

Sato, J. and Perl, E.R. (1991). Adrenergic excitation of cutaneous pain receptors induced by peripheral nerve injury. *Science* **251**, 1608–10.

Sato, J., Suzuki, S., Iseki, T., and Kumazawa, T. (1993). Adrenergic excitation of cutaneous nociceptors in chronically inflamed rats. *Neurosci. Lett.* **164**, 225–8.

Schaible, H.-G. and Schmidt, R.F. (1988). Time course of mechanosensitivity changes in articular afferents during a developing experimental arthritis. *J. Neurophysiol.* **60**, 2180–95.

Schmelz, M., Scmidt, R., Ringkamp, M., Handwerker, H.O., and Torebjörk, H.E. (1994). Sensitization of insensitive branches of C nociceptors in human skin. *J. Physiol., London* **480**, 389–94.

Schmidt, R., Schmelz, M., Forster, C., Ringkamp M., Torebjörk, H.E., and Handwerker, H.O. (1995). Novel classes of responsive and unresponsive C nociceptors in human skin. *J. Neurosci.* **15**, 333–41.

Shea, V.K. and Perl, E.R. (1985). Failure of sympathetic stimulation to affect responsiveness of rabbit polymodal nociceptors. *J. Neurophysiol.* **54**, 513–19.

Sicuteri, F., Fanciullacci, M., Franchi, G., and Del Bianco, P.L. (1965). Serotonin–bradykinin potentiation on the pain receptors in man. *Life Sci.* **4**, 309–16.

Snyder, S.H. (1992). Nitric oxide: first in a new class of neurotransmitters. *Science* **257**, 494–6.

Steen, A.E., Reeh, P.W., Kreysel, H.W., and Steen, K.H. (1993). Experimental tissue acidosis potentiates pain induced by inflammatory mediators. 7th World Congress on Pain (abstract), pp. 39–40.

Steen, K.H. and Reeh, P.W. (1993). Sustained graded pain and hyperalgesia from harmless experimental tissues acidosis in human skin. *Neurosci. Lett.* **154**, 113–16.

Steen, K.H., Reeh, P.W., Anton, F., and Handwerker, H.O. (1992). Protons selectively induce lasting excitation and sensitization to mechanical stimulation of nociceptors in rat skin. *J. Neurosci.* **12**, 86–95.

Steen, K.H., Reeh, P.W., and Kreysel, H.W. (1994). Dose-dependent competitive block by topical acetylsalicylic and salicylic acid of pH-induced cutaneous pain. *Soc. Neurosci. Abstr.* **20**, 763.

Stefanidis, D., Reeh, P.W., Kreysel, H.W., and Steen, K.H. (1994). Acetylsalicylic and salicylic acid suppress pH induced excitation of rat nociceptors. *Soc. Neurosci. Abstr.* **20**, 15.

Steranka, L.R., Farmer, S.G., and Burch, R.M. (1989). Antagonists of B_2 bradykinin receptors. *FASEB J.* **3**, 2019–25.

Szolcsányi, J. (1987). Selective responsiveness of polymodel nociceptors of the rabbit ear to capsaicin, bradykinin, and ultraviolet irradiation. *J. Physiol.* **388**, 9–23.

Taiwo, Y.O. and Levine, J.D. (1988). Characterization of the arachidonic acid metabolites mediating bradykinin and noradrenaline hyperalgesia. *Brain Res.* **458**, 402–6.

Taiwo, Y.O., Levine, J.D., Burch, R.M., Woo, J.E., and Mobley, W.C. (1991). Hyperalgesia induced in the rat by the amino-terminal octapeptide of nerve growth factor. *Proc. natl Acad. Sci., USA* **88**, 5144–8.

Thalhammer, J.G. and LaMotte, R.H. (1982). Spatial properties of nociceptor sensitization following heat injury of the skin. *Brain Res.* **231**, 257–65.

Treede, R.-D. and Cole, J.D. (1993). Dissociated secondary hyperalgesia in a subject with large fibre sensory neuropathy. *Pain* **53**, 169–74.

Wahren, L.K., Torebjörk, E., and Nystrom, B. (1991). Quantitative sensory testing before and after regional guanethidine block in patients with neuralgia in the hand. *Pain* **46**, 23–30.

Wallin, B.G., Torebjörk, E, and Hallin, R.G. (1976). Preliminary observations on the pathophysiology of hyperalgesia in the causalgic pain syndrome. In *Sensory functions of the skin of primates with special reference to man* (ed. Y. Zotterman), pp. 489–99. Pergamon, Oxford.

Weskamp, G. and Otten, U. (1987). An enzyme-linked immunoassay for nerve growth factor (NGF): a tool for studying regulatory mechanisms involved in NGF production in brain and peripheral tissues. *J. Neurochem.* **48**, 1779–86.

Whalley, E.T., Clegg, S., Stewart, J.M., and Vavrek, R.J. (1987). The effects of kinin agonists and antagonists on the pain response of the human blister base. *Arch. Pharmacol.* **336**, 652–5.

Yoshida, K. and Gage, F.H. (1992). Cooperative regulation of nerve growth factor synthesis and secretion in fibroblasts and astrocytes by fibroblast growth factor and other cytokines. *Brain Res.* **569**, 14–25.

16 Secondary cutaneous dysaesthesiae

ROBERT H. LAMOTTE

A localized irritation of the skin, if sufficiently potent, produces a remarkable change in the quality of mechanically evoked sensations in a large area surrounding the injury. In the case of a particularly noxious stimulus—a burn, a cut, or crush—the skin becomes hyperalgesic: normally painful stimuli such as a pinprick elicit abnormally intense and prolonged sensations of pain (punctate hyperalgesia), and the threshold for pain may be lowered so that normally innocuous stimuli such as a light touch are painful ('allodynia') (Lewis 1936; Hardy *et al.* 1950; LaMotte *et al.* 1991; Koltzenburg *et al.* 1992; Meyer *et al.* 1993).

In the case of an itch-producing irritation such as a mosquito bite, the quality of mechanically evoked sensations in the skin surrounding the region of wheal and local redness is also changed. But instead of hyperalgesia, a state of hyperknesis is produced ('knesis' from the ancient Greek word for itching). A stimulus that can evoke itch in uninjured skin (such as a prickly hair) now elicits an abnormally intense itch (punctate hyperknesis) (unpublished observations) and gently stroking the skin with an innocuous cotton swab evokes itch and/or exacerbates an ongoing itch ('alloknesis') (Bickford 1938; Graham *et al.* 1951; Simone *et al.* 1987, 1991*a*; LaMotte 1992).

The unpleasant, abnormal sensory states (dysaesthesiae) of hyperalgesia and hyperknesis are qualitatively very different as illustrated by the different sensations and reactions in response to the same stimuli. In hyperalgesic skin, a prickly hair elicits pain as does light stroking with a cotton swab. These unpleasant sensations are accompanied by behavioural reactions of protecting the skin from further mechanical contact. In contrast, when the same stimuli are applied to hyperknesic skin, they evoke sensations of itch and reactions of scratching the stimulated area. The dysaesthesiae of hyperalgesia or hyperknesis when elicited within the area of cutaneous irritation are called 'primary'. Those evoked by stimuli delivered outside this primary area are termed 'secondary' (Hardy *et al.* 1950, 1951). In the following, I will discuss the contributions of primary cutaneous peripheral nerve fibres to the cutaneous dysaesthesiae of secondary hyperalgesia and secondary hyperknesis.

Sensory descriptions of experimentally produced cutaneous secondary dysaesthesiae

Secondary hyperalgesia

Cutaneous secondary hyperalgesia can easily be produced in the laboratory by a variety of localized injuries of the skin including those resulting from electrical, thermal, mechanical, and chemical stimuli (Lewis 1936; Hardy *et al.* 1950). It can also be induced by the electrical stimulation of a cutaneous nerve (Lewis 1936), although it is then uncertain to what extent the hyperalgesia arises from resulting injury of tissues in and surrounding the nerve as opposed to the peripheral release of neurochemicals by electrically evoked activity in afferent nerve fibres (Hardy *et al.* 1950, 1952).

In the case where the external stimulus is physical, it is possible that the real stimuli are the inflammatory chemical mediators that are produced in response to the injury rather than an injury of afferent nerve terminals *per se*.

Exogenous chemical irritants can produce secondary hyperalgesia. An intradermal injection of capsaicin, the algesic chemical in hot peppers, produces an area of secondary hyperalgesia not unlike that produced by a localized physical injury of the skin. The area of hyperalgesia depends on the concentration of capsaicin in a constant volume of 10 μl injected into the skin (Simone *et al.* 1989). The chemical produces no long-lasting signs of injury, and its effectiveness and, therefore, the duration of the 'injurious stimulus' is short-lived (about an hour) (LaMotte *et al.* 1991).

The area and time course of hyperalgesia after an injection of 100 μg of capsaicin was determined for a group of human subjects after a single injection of capsaicin into the volar forearm (LaMotte *et al.* 1991). The injection produces an intense sensation of burning pain, which reaches a peak magnitude within 15 s, gradually subsides, and disappears within 10–30 min. The 4-mm diameter bleb produced by the injection is analgesic to pinprick. This area is surrounded by a ring (radius 1 to 2 cm) of cutaneous hyperalgesia to heat. Within and surrounding this region is an area of mechanical hyperalgesia to innocuous stroking with a cotton swab (allodynia) and to punctate stimulation with a von Frey-type filament (Fig. 16.1). The results of experiments in which capsaicin is injected adjacent to the receptive fields of cutaneous nociceptors suggest that the capsaicin typically remains within the bleb and that the surrounding hyperalgesias are of the secondary and not the primary type (Baumann *et al.* 1991). The absence of hyperalgesia to heat within the area of secondary hyperalgesia to mechanical stimuli confirms the results of a study of hyperalgesia after a burn injury (Raja *et al.* 1984).

A flare reaction is also present and its area is determined from the outline of a visible reddening of the skin. The areas of flare and hyperalgesia are fully developed within 10–30 min and then gradually decrease in size. The hyperalgesia disappears after 1–3 h for heat and stroking stimuli but shrinks more gradually for punctate stimuli—disappearing after 13–24 h. The flare is no longer visible after an hour or two. Thus, the area of hyperalgesia to punctate stimuli is larger and lasts longer than the area of flare and the areas of hyperalgesia to stroking and heat.

With minor exceptions, the general features of secondary hyperalgesia after capsaicin injection are similar to those obtained after a thermal, mechanical, or electrical injury (Hardy *et al.* 1950, 1951; Lewis 1936; Raja *et al.* 1984).

Secondary hyperknesis

Itchy skin can be experimentally produced by stimuli that induce itching including mild intensities of the same stimuli that produce secondary hyperalgesia (see, for example, Bickford 1938). Histamine is particularly effective. Puncturing the skin through droplets of histamine, rubbing the skin with cowhage spicules, or intradermally injecting histamine each produces itch, flare, and a surrounding area of alloknesis to stroking the skin (Bickford 1938; Graham *et al.* 1951; Shelley and Arthur 1955; Tuckett 1982; Simone *et al.* 1991*a*).

Capsaicin   Histamine

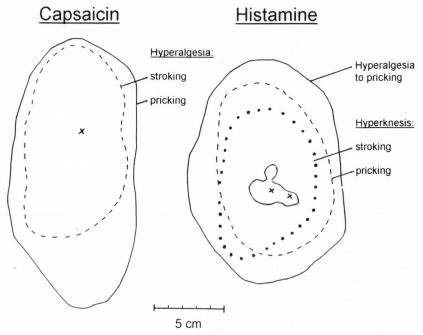

5 cm

Fig. 16.1   Two kinds of experimentally produced cutaneous dysaesthesiae to pricking and stroking the skin: hyperalgesia and hyperknesis. (Left side) An intradermal injection of 100 μg of capsaicin into the volar forearm (x) resulted in an enhanced pain response to pricking the skin with a fine, stiff probe (50 μm diameter) and pain in response to gently stroking the skin with a cotton swab (within the areas enclosed by solid and dashed lines, respectively). Outside the dysaesthetic areas, stroking evoked sensations of touch, not pain, and pricking evoked a weak sensation of pain followed, on occasion, by a second sensation described as itch. 30 min after the injection, after the pain in response to capsaicin had disappeared, an intradermal injection of 20 μg of histamine dihydrochloride was given within the dashed area 5 cm proximal (below) the capsaicin injection. Neither itch nor hyperknesis developed, suggesting that this state was suppressed by the presence of hyperalgesia. (Right side) On another day, the same subject was given two intradermal injections of 10 μg of histamine dihydrochloride into the volar forearm (xs). This produced both hyperalgesia and hyperknesis. Within the outer, solid line, pricking with the fine probe produced a greater than normal sensation of pricking pain followed, on occasion, by a normal sensation of itch. Within the dashed line, pricking evoked an enhanced sensation of pricking pain followed in every case by a greater than normal sensation of itch. Within the dotted line, stroking the skin with a cotton swab evoked an itch or sometimes increased the magnitude of any background itching.

An effective way of grading the magnitude and duration of itch is to vary the amount of histamine injected in a constant volume of 10 μl of vehicle injected intradermally (Simone *et al.* 1987). An intradermal injection of 10 μg of histamine hydrochloride in saline into the volar forearm in humans typically elicits a sensation of itch with little or no pain that begins about 10 s after injection, reaches a maximal magnitude within 1 to 2 min, and disappears in a mean of 13 min. A wheal forms at the injection site and is surrounded by a flare. An area of alloknesis to stroking the skin surrounding the wheal begins almost immediately with the onset of itch and reaches a maximum within 10 min. It then decreases in size during the next 25 to 40 min (Simone *et al.* 1991*a*). A mean maximum area of 44 cm was found for seven subjects given an injection of 10 μg on the volar forearm. This is comparable to areas described by Graham *et al.* (1951) after application of cowhage spicules and Bickford (1938) after pricking histamine into the forearm.

Recently, it was discovered that the area of alloknesis to stroking is surrounded by a slightly larger area of punctate hyperknesis (unpublished observations) and hyperalgesia (Fig. 16.1). This area is revealed by indenting the skin with a stiff, small-diameter probe (50 μm diameter) mounted at the end of a nylon filament that produces a bending force of 2 g-wt. Before the injection of histamine, this stimulus elicits a faint sensation of pricking pain (a 'prickle') followed in about 0.5–1 s by a second sensation described as itch. The prickle is evoked on most applications, whereas the itch is more easily elicited on the volar wrist and is fainter and more intermittent on the middle volar forearm. Within minutes after an injection of 10 μg of histamine, an area of enhanced sensations of pain and itch surrounds the area of alloknesis to stroking, reaches a maximum area within about 10 min, and disappears only after 1–4 h. The enhanced second sensation of itch is best elicited by the 50-μm diameter probe and is weak or absent in response to probes of much larger diameter.

The 50-μm probe evokes pain but no itch within the area of secondary hyperalgesia produced by an injection of capsaicin. The magnitude and duration of the pain is greater after capsaicin than it is after an injection of histamine (unpublished observations).

The importance of these findings is that two different chemicals, capsaicin and histamine, elicit two qualitatively different kinds of sensations each accompanied by different secondary cutaneous dysaesthesiae that are each evoked in response to the same mechanical stimuli. Capsaicin evokes pain and not itch, whereas the reverse is true for histamine. Gently stroking the skin elicits pain and not itch after capsaicin and itch but not pain after histamine. Poking the skin with a probe that is stiff and of sufficiently small diameter evokes a first sensation of enhanced pricking pain for both capsaicin and histamine; but a second sensation of itch occurs in the case of histamine but not capsaicin. It is hypothesized below that the central nervous system alters the sensory quality and behavioural reactions to the information conveyed by two sets of mechanosensitive primary afferent nerve fibres depending on which of two classes of chemosensitive nociceptive nerve fibres has been activated.

Another piece of evidence in support of the important role of central neural mechanisms in processing information about itch and itchy skin is that sensations of itch and the state of hyperknesis are suppressed both by painful stimulation (unpublished observations and Bickford 1938) and, in the absence of ongoing pain, by the presence of cutaneous hyperalgesia (Graham *et al.* 1951). Bickford (1938) proposed that painful cutaneous stimulation sets up an 'antipruritic state' in the central nervous system that blocks the itch and itchy skin that normally result from puncturing the skin with histamine. However, our recent observations (unpublished) suggest that hyperalgesia and hyperknesis can coexist if the hyperalgesia is mild, as it is after an injection of histamine, but not if it is strong, as it is after an injection of capsaicin.

Peripheral neurones contributing to secondary cutaneous dysaesthesiae

The following discussion will be based primarily on the mechanically evoked dysaesthesiae evoked by an intradermal injection of capsaicin or histamine and will pertain to four kinds of primary afferent neurones: neurones contributing to the sensation of pain (or itch) produced by the injection; neurones contributing to the initiation of the secondary dysaesthesia and its spread in the skin away from the injection site; neurones that become sensitized (develop enhanced responses) to cutaneous stimuli in the area of secondary dysaesthesia; and, lastly, neurones that respond to the pricking and stroking stimuli used to evoke the dysaesthesia. For some topics, data are incomplete or lacking— particularly on the mechanisms of hyperknesis. In these instances, suggestions and hypotheses for future research are proposed.

Neurones contributing to the chemically evoked sensations of pain and itch

A selective block of conduction in small- or large-diameter primary afferent nerve fibres in humans reveals that capsaicin-evoked pain and histamine-evoked itch are mediated by small-diameter peripheral nerve fibres (Bickford 1938; Graham *et al.* 1951; LaMotte *et al.* 1991; Torebjörk *et al.* 1992). These are probably unmyelinated (C) fibres although a contribution from slowly conducting, thinly myelinated (Aδ) fibres has not been entirely ruled out.

Capsaicin excites only heat-sensitive and/or chemosensitive receptors with unmyelinated or thinly myelinated fibres (see, for example, Baumann *et al.* 1991). These include C fibres with either heat nociceptors (CHs), polymodal nociceptors (for example, mechanoheat nociceptors or CMHs), chemonociceptors (Cchems), low-threshold warm receptors, and type II A fibres with mechanoheat nociceptors. Of these, CHs are the best candidates, so far, as major contributors to the magnitude and duration of pain but the responses of chemonociceptors have not yet been adequately evaluated.

The discharge rates of evoked responses in high-threshold (HT) and wide-dynamic-range (WDR) spinothalamic tract cells in the monkey correlate with estimates of magnitude of pain in humans after an intradermal injection of capsaicin (Simone *et al.* 1991*b*). Thus, chemically evoked pain in response to capsaicin is mediated by the responses of a subpopulation of small-diameter nociceptive afferents in the periphery and certain spinothalamic tract neurones in the dorsal horn of the spinal cord.

The available evidence suggests that the sensation of itch is mediated in the periphery by subpopulations of CMH and chemospecific (mechanically insensitive) nociceptors (Torebjörk 1974; Tuckett and Wei 1987; Lang *et al.* 1990; Handwerker *et al.* 1991*a*; Meyer *et al* 1991). In the rat, a subpopulation of CMH fibres responds to bradykinin and also to histamine (see, for example, Lang *et al.* 1990). In the monkey, a subpopulation of mechanically and thermally insensitive afferents with C or Aδ fibres responds to intracutaneous injections of histamine (Meyer *et al.* 1991). Iontophoresis of histamine into the skin activates a subpopulation of nociceptors with C or A fibres in humans (Handwerker *et al.* 1991*a*). CMHs in human respond to bradykinin and to histamine but, for some fibres, the response to histamine is more vigorous. Intraneural electrical stimulation of CMH fibres in humans typically evokes the sensation of pain but occasionally elicits itch instead. In these cases, variations in the frequency of stimulation, while keeping intensity constant, altered the magnitude of itch but not the quality of sensation (Torebjörk and Ochoa 1981; Schmidt *et al.* 1993).

The responses of identified spinothalamic tract cells in the primate to histamine need to be studied. Preliminary recordings from WDR cells in the dorsal horn of the spinal cord in the cat revealed a subpopulation that responded both to histamine and to capsaicin (Hirata *et al.* 1990). Other WDRs responded to capsaicin but not to histamine, while a third group responded to neither chemical. Thus, unless histamine-specific peripheral and/or central nociceptive neurones can be found that respond selectively to histamine, a plausible hypothesis is that the sensation of itch is mediated by the activity of histamine-sensitive nociceptive neurones in the absence of significant activity in histamine-insensitive nociceptive cells (see, for example, Handwerker 1992; LaMotte 1992). The 'antipruritic state' described by Bickford (1938) could occur as a result of the central inhibition of histamine-responsive cells in the dorsal horn by activity in histamine-unresponsive nociceptive neurones.

Neurones responsible for the initiation of secondary cutaneous dysaesthesiae

Primary afferent neurones that elicit pain may not be the same as those that initiate secondary hyperalgesia. This hypothesis is supported by experiments that demonstrate a non-correspondence between the magnitude of pain and the magnitude of hyperalgesia produced by a given stimulus. For example, an intradermal injection of histamine can produce secondary hyperalgesia with minimal or no pain (Fig. 16.1 and unpublished observations). Secondary hyperalgesia can also occur after the skin is painlessly frozen (Lewis 1936) or given long-duration, non-painful heat (Hardy *et al.* 1950; Cervero *et al.* 1993). Conversely, equally painful stimuli may not result in equal magnitudes of secondary hyperalgesia. When the temperature of a noxious heat stimulus delivered to one arm was adjusted so that the magnitude and time course of pain was matched with the pain evoked by 10 μg of capsaicin injected at the same time into the other arm, the area of secondary hyperalgesia was greater on the capsaicin-injected arm (LaMotte *et al.* 1991). One interpretation of these results is that there exist chemosensitive neurones that are effective in eliciting secondary dysaesthesia and that are not the same ones that contribute to pain. These chemosensitive afferents may be more readily excited by capsaicin than by the algesic inflammatory chemicals released by the heat stimulus used in this experiment. Also, the heat-sensitive nociceptive afferents may play less of a role than the hypothesized chemosensitive afferents in releasing neurochemicals that initiate central sensitization and secondary hyperalgesia.

Neurones responsible for the spread of secondary cutaneous dysaesthesiae

When the centre of a small area of locally anaesthetized skin is physically injured (Lewis 1936), punctured, injected with histamine (Bickford 1938), or injected with capsaicin (LaMotte *et al.* 1991), cutaneous dysaesthesia does not develop in the surrounding skin at least until after recovery from the anaesthetic. Thus, the dysaesthesiae in the large area of skin surrounding a localized physical injury or an intradermal injection of histamine or capsaicin are of the secondary type and do not result from the transport or diffusion of chemical substances away from the injury site. Instead, the spread of the dysaesthesia is 'neurogenic', that is, it occurs as a result of neuronal activity.

What is the pathway by which injury- or chemically induced activity in nerve fibres innervating one region of skin influences the activity of sensory neurones responsive to mechanical stimulation of the skin (stroking, pricking) in remote cutaneous areas? Lewis (1936) demonstrated that the spread of secondary hyperalgesia resulting from a localized cutaneous injury could be blocked by small barriers of local anaesthetic injected into the skin. Subsequently, Bickford (1938) obtained a similar result for a histamine puncture. A long, thin mediolateral strip of anaesthetized skin prevented alloknesis on one side of the strip from spreading to the other side.

Hardy and his colleagues (1950, 1952), hypothesized that central and not peripheral neuronal mechanisms were responsible for the development of secondary hyperalgesia and alloknesis. But they did not publish any comments on the anaesthetic-barrier experiments carried out by previous investigators. Recently, experiments in which a mediolateral strip of anaesthetized skin was produced close to an injection of capsaicin (LaMotte *et al.* 1991) or histamine (Simone *et al.* 1991*a*) replicated the results of Lewis and Bickford. The cutaneous dysaesthesia developed normally on the side of the injected irritant but was absent or reduced on the opposite side (Fig. 16.2). The dysaesthesiae tested were hyperalgesia (to stroking and poking the skin) and alloknesis to stroking. Experiments are needed to test whether an anaesthetic barrier will block the spread of punctate hyperknesis.

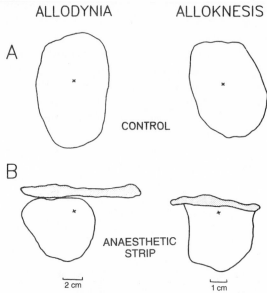

ALLODYNIA   ALLOKNESIS

A

CONTROL

B

ANAESTHETIC
STRIP

2 cm   1 cm

Fig. 16.2 A narrow strip of cutaneous anaesthesia blocked the spread of a secondary dysaesthesia to stroking the skin. (A) Fully developed areas of allodynia (left) and alloknesis (right) after injections (x) of capsaicin and histamine, respectively, into the volar forearms of two human subjects (see main text). (B) Capsaicin (left) and histamine (right) were then given into the opposite forearm immediately after anaesthetizing a mediolateral strip of skin (stippled area). Hyperalgesia to gentle stroking developed normally on the capsaicin side of the anaesthetic strip but was absent on the opposite side. Similarly, alloknesis to stroking developed only on the side of the histamine injection (punctate stimuli were not used in these experiments).

The results of the anaesthetic-barrier experiments strongly support, although they do not prove, the hypothesis that neuronal activity evoked by chemical injection or a physical injury 'spreads' radially away from the injury set in peripheral nerve fibres within or beneath but in close proximity to the skin to surrounding cutaneous regions as originally hypothesized by Lewis (1936). The anaesthetic-strip experiment provides strong evidence for a peripheral mechanism contributing to the radial spread of secondary hyperalgesia. Alternatively, one must hypothesize a more complex mechanism such as a central facilitation of the 'spread' of neural activity from capsaicin- or histamine-activated spinal neurones to spinal neurones that are activated by and become sensitized to cutaneous stimulation of skin remote to the injury. What set of primary afferents might bring about such a facilitation? One must suppose that they are normally spontaneously active because only then could their activity be eliminated by the anaesthetic strip. The low-threshold slowly adapting type II mechanoreceptors and thermoreceptors, but not nociceptors, exhibit ongoing activity. But a selective block of activity in large-diameter peripheral nerve fibres mediating the sense of touch does not necessarily eliminate secondary mechanical hyperalgesia, nor does a cold or warm strip of metal laid mediolaterally across the skin (which would suppress ongoing activity in warm and cold fibres, respectively) affect the lateral spread of hyperalgesia (LaMotte *et al.* 1991). Thus, there is no compelling evidence supporting the hypothesis of central facilitation.

Which set of peripheral nerve fibres might convey neuronal activity within the skin over large distances? While there is presently no direct evidence for such fibres, there are a few hypotheses and a small amount of indirect evidence. One hypothesis (LaMotte 1988) is that there are chemosensitive primary afferent nerve fibres that branch widely within the skin. These receptive fields would have to be larger than those of the common CMH nociceptors (Torebjörk 1974; but see Schmelz *et al.* 1994) recorded in human subjects. One set would be maximally responsive to itch-producing stimuli such as histamine, the other to algesic chemicals such as capsaicin or to certain inflammatory mediators. Neither would respond well to thermal or mechanical stimuli—but could respond to the endogenous chemicals released as a consequence of such stimulation. Each set of fibres would have a particularly powerful effect on the response properties of second-order neurones in the dorsal horn of the spinal cord—resulting in an increased excitability (lowered threshold and enhanced suprathreshold responses) when sufficiently excited. The evidence for the sensitization of central neurones is discussed subsequently. A third set of widely branching fibres would have to be postulated as contributing to the neurogenic flare, since the flare and secondary hyperalgesia can be dissociated under certain conditions (see, for example, LaMotte *et al.* 1991).

There is some support for the existence of primary afferent fibres that branch widely in the periphery. Certain fibres with receptive fields in the tooth pulp of the cat were shown to have proximal branches at distances of 1–5 cm (Lisney and Matthews 1978). A small proportion of cutaneous nociceptors in the monkey were found to have multiple receptive fields separated by unresponsive zones extending over a distance of 4 cm (Meyer *et al.* 1991). One or more of the zones was relatively insensitive to mechanical or thermal stimuli. A similar kind of fibre was recently recorded in human (Schmelz *et al.* 1994). These fibres may belong to a class of nociceptors in animals and humans that are normally insensitive to mechanical or thermal stimuli but that respond to chemical irritants or to inflammatory chemical mediators, which, in some studies, have included histamine (Schaible and Schmidt 1985; Grigg *et al.* 1986; Häbler *et al.* 1990; Handwerker *et al.* 1991*b*; Kress *et al.* 1992; Davis *et al.* 1993; Schmidt *et al.* 1994). Therefore, there is at least preliminary evidence for the existence of widely branching chemosensitive peripheral nerve fibres. However, more studies are needed in which the search stimuli are chemical and electrocutaneous (see, for example, Meyer and Campbell 1988;

Handwerker *et al.* 1991*b*; Meyer *et al.* 1991) as opposed to the mechanical stimulation that is typically used.

A second hypothesis is that the putative chemoreceptors are not widely branching but instead have ordinary sized receptive fields that are somehow functionally coupled so that activity in one fibre elicits responses in its neighbours. A functional coupling was demonstrated in the monkey for about 3 per cent of the unmyelinated nerve fibres sampled (Meyer *et al.* 1985, 1988). It is possible that nerve impulses traveling anti-dromically along the stimulated nerve activate the peripheral endings of another sensory nerve either ephaptically or by means of the release of neurochemicals. Sensations can sometimes be evoked in human patients when the distal portion of a severed nerve is electrically stimulated (Foerster 1927). It is possible that nerve impulses traveling antidromically along the stimulated nerve, distal to the transection, activate the peripheral endings of another sensory nerve, for example, by the release of excitatory neurochemicals.

Perhaps certain nociceptive fibres have both afferent and efferent peripheral terminals (Szolcsányi 1988). The cutaneous vasodilatation that occurs after antidromic stimulation of dorsal roots and the flare that develops around a local cutaneous injury may involve similar effector mechanisms, for example, the release of vasodilating peptides such as substance P and calcitonin gene-related peptide (CGRP) (see, for example, Holzer 1988; Lisney and Bharali 1989). The flare has an underlying neurogenic mechanism since it persists after peripheral nerve section until the nerve degenerates (see review by Chapman *et al.* 1961). Since capsaicin can have a toxic effect on small-diameter neurones containing substance P, and repeated topical applications of capsaicin can block the flare and antidromic vasodilatation (Bernstein *et al.* 1981; Carpenter and Lynn 1981; Fitzgerald 1983), the flare is probably mediated by activity in certain C and possibly Aδ fibres (Holzer 1988; Jänig and Lisney 1989; Lisney and Bharali 1989).

One mechanism by which activity in one peripheral chemosensitive fibre could induce activity in its neighbour would be by the release of a neuromodulator that would produce a depolarization of an adjacent terminal (Lynn 1988). Another mechanism might involve a cascade of events that involve blood-borne substances and mast cells coupled with the neurogenic release of a neuromodulator (Lembeck and Gamse 1982).

The sensitized neurones contributing to secondary cutaneous dysaesthesiae

The neurogenic activation of one fibre's peripheral terminal by another does not necessarily imply that the activated fibre becomes sensitized, that is, that it develops an enhanced responsiveness to physical or chemical stimulation. Indeed, there is little evidence for the remote sensitization of cutaneous receptors. First, antidromic electrical stimulation of C fibres does not result in the sensitization of these fibres—at least of CMH nociceptive C fibres in the rat and monkey (Reeh *et al.* 1986; Meyer *et al.* 1988). Second, a mechanical or heat injury of one-half of the receptive fields of cutaneous nociceptors with A or C fibres does not change the responsiveness of the fibre to stimuli delivered to the other half (Thalhammer and LaMotte 1982; Campbell *et al.* 1988*a*,*b*; Schmelz *et al.* 1994). However, there is one study demonstrating that cutaneous nociceptors with A fibres (but not those with C fibres) in the rat can become sensitized to mechanical stimuli after a noxious mechanical conditioning stimulus delivered adjacent to the receptive field (Reeh *et al.* 1987).

An intradermal injection of capsaicin or of histamine outside, adjacent to, or within the cutaneous receptive fields of nociceptive and low-threshold afferent fibres in the monkey failed to sensitize, that is, lower the response thresholds or enhance suprathreshold responses of, any class of fibres to heat or mechanical stimuli. The same finding was obtained, using capsaicin, in a study of CMH nociceptors in humans (LaMotte *et al.* 1992). (The effects of remote injections of histamine have not been tested in human subjects.) Thus, the sensitization of peripheral cutaneous receptors is probably not responsible for the development of secondary cutaneous dysaesthesiae.

The results of four additional kinds of experiments support the conclusion that central and not peripheral neuronal sensitization contributes to the secondary hyperalgesia produced by an injection of capsaicin. Comparable experiments have not yet been carried out to determine the role of central sensitization in secondary hyperknesis from histamine. In the first experiment, capsaicin was injected into a cutaneous area that was rendered anaesthetic by the infiltration of a proximal part of a cutaneous nerve with a local anaesthetic (Fig. 16.3). Upon complete recovery from the anaesthetic, 0.5 to 3 h later, the usual areas of hyperalgesia to stroking and punctate mechanical stimuli were either absent or greatly reduced in comparison to those obtained in the absence of a nerve block (LaMotte *et al.* 1991). The implication is that the proximal nerve block prevented neuronal activity from reaching and then sensitizing neurones in the spinal cord.

In the second experiment (Torebjörk *et al.* 1992), non-painful tactile sensations, evoked in humans by intraneural electrical stimulation of myelinated peripheral nerve fibres, were referred to a 'projection field' on the skin (Fig. 16.4). When a remote injection of capsaicin produced an area of allodynia that enveloped the projection field, the electrically evoked tactile sensation was then accompanied by pain. This condition persisted until the hyperalgesia receded away from the field, whereupon the original painless tactile sensation was obtained. This finding is consistent with the hypothesis that a change in the central processing of the tactile input had occurred after capsaicin injection when nociceptive spinal neurones became sensitized to input from low-threshold mechanoreceptive peripheral neurones.

In the third experiment, which supported the role of central sensitization, it was found that both wide-dynamic-range and high-threshold nociceptive spinothalamic tract cells in the anaesthetized monkey became sensitized to both punctate and stroking mechanical stimulation after an injection of capsaicin into their cutaneous receptive fields (Simone *et al.* 1991*b*).

In a fourth experiment, it was shown that the electrical stimulation of large-diameter myelinated fibres in the proximal end of a cut dorsal rootlet evoked a greater response in those spinothalamic tract cells that had received an intracutaneous injection of capsaicin (sensitizing them to cutaneous mechanical stimulation) than in cells that had not (Simone *et al.* 1991*b*). The conclusion is that capsaicin-evoked activity in certain peripheral neurones had made the spinothalamic tract neurones more excitable to input from low-threshold mechanoreceptors.

Additional evidence for central sensitization has been provided by animal models of hyperalgesia produced by thermal, mechanical, or chemical injury of the skin in the rat (see, for example, Woolf 1983; McMahon and Wall 1984; Coderre and Melzack 1987; Laird and Cervero 1989; Dubner 1991; Guilbaud *et al.* 1992) and by articular inflammation in the cat (Schaible *et al.* 1987).

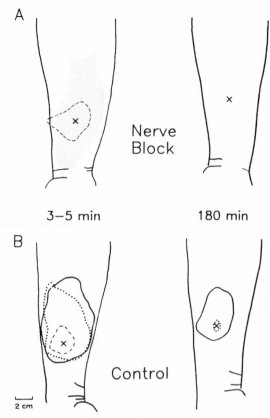

Fig. 16.3 The effects of an anaesthetic nerve block on the development of secondary hyperalgesia. Capsaicin was injected into a cutaneous area made anaesthetic by a proximal nerve block. Secondary hyperalgesia did not develop and was absent after the block wore off. (A) A flare (- - - -) but no hyperalgesia developed within or outside the anaesthetic area (stippled) 3–5 min after the capsaicin injection. Hyperalgesia was still absent 180 min after the capsaicin injection even though the effects of the anaesthetic had worn off. (B) Areas of secondary hyperalgesia to stroking (. . . .) and to punctate (————) stimuli and flare (- - - -) on the control arm 3–5 min after capsaicin and again at 180 min. Reproduced with permission from LaMotte *et al.* (11991).

Maintenance of secondary cutaneous dysaesthesiae by activity in peripheral neurones

It is hypothesized that the primary afferent neurones responsible for the initiation and spread of secondary cutaneous dysaesthesiae have certain functional properties (LaMotte 1992). First, their peripheral terminals have chemoreceptors. Probably there are two classes of chemoreceptive fibres. One is maximally responsive to histamine (possibly other chemicals as well) and functionally linked in the spinal cord to neurones mediating secondary hyperknesis. The other class is responsive to algesic substances and linked to central neurones that contribute to secondary hyperalgesia while also inhibiting neighbouring neurones mediating itch and hyperknesis. Second, these peripheral neurones have normally sized receptive fields that are chemically or electrically coupled or, alternatively, their peripheral endings branch widely (in order to account for the effects of anaesthetic barriers). Third, their major role is more that of effectors ('noceffectors'; Kruger 1988; Kruger *et al.* 1989; Kruger and Halata, Chapter 2, this volume) rather than of sensory organs. Evidence has been presented for a lack of correspondence at times between pain and secondary hyperalgesia (see, for example, Cervero *et al.* 1993). Further evidence of the same kind is provided by the fact that the secondary cutaneous dysaesthesiae outlast the primary sensations of pain or itch and yet are maintained in part by continued activity in certain peripheral afferent neurones.

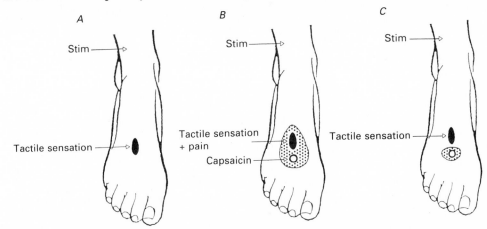

Fig. 16.4 The development of secondary hyperalgesia reversibly altered the quality of sensation evoked by intraneural microstimulation. (A) Electrical microstimulation within the superficial peroneal nerve evoked a non-painful tactile sensation that was referred to a local area of skin (the 'projection field') on the dorsum of the foot (black, filled area). (B) Once secondary hyperalgesia (allodynia to stroking with a cotton swab) induced by a capsaicin injection (open circle) enveloped the projection field, the same intensity of electrical stimulation was perceived as pain in addition to touch. (C) When the area of allodynia receded from the projection field, 39 min after the capsaicin injection, the same electrical stimulus again evoked the tactile sensation without pain. The results suggest that a change occurred in the central processing of mechanoreceptive input from myelinated fibres that normally evoke tactile and not pain sensations. Reproduced with permission from Torebjörk *et al.* (1992).

Support for the partial maintenance of secondary dysaesthesiae by peripheral neuronal activity comes from experiments in which the site of injection of capsaicin or histamine was anaesthetized by xylocaine or by cooling after the dysaesthesia had developed (LaMotte *et al.* 1991; Simone *et al.* 1991a). Cooling the histamine injection site to 1–4°C, rendered the skin beneath the thermode (1 cm diameter) anaesthetized to pinpricks and significantly reduced the area of alloknesis to stroking of the skin. Rewarming to 38°C increased the area of alloknesis back to its original size (hyperknesis to prickling was not tested). Similar results were obtained in experiments with capsaicin. That is, cooling the capsaicin injection site (or infiltrating the site with a xylocaine) significantly reduced the area of allodynia to stroking, while, in the case of cooling, rewarming for 2–5 min enlarged it to its previous state. In contrast, the area of hyperalgesia to punctate stimuli was typically unaffected by anaesthetizing the injection site. However, the magnitude of enhanced pain in response to pricking the skin was reduced. The major conclusion to be drawn from these experiments is that the hypothesized noceffector neurones responsible for initiating secondary dysaesthesiae continue to be active and to contribute at least in part to the maintenance of the dysaesthesia long after the primary sensation of itch or pain evoked by the injection has disappeared.

The return of allodynia within 5 min of rewarming is faster than the 15 min or so required for the maximal area to be reached after the initial injection of capsaicin. This suggests that the change in central processing responsible for secondary dysaesthesia, while slow to develop initially, continues to exist in an inactivated state when sustaining nociceptive peripheral input is reduced and then reactivates quickly when this input is restored (Gracely *et al.* 1992).

Mechanosensitive peripheral neurones contributing to mechanically evoked secondary dysaesthesiae

Several lines of evidence support a role for low-threshold mechanoreceptors with myelinated fibres in evoking dysaesthetic sensations in response to innocuous mechanical stimulation of the skin in the zone of secondary hyperalgesia. In neurophysiological experiments, it was found that spinothalamic tract neurones that became sensitized to innocuous mechanical stimulation of the skin after an intradermal injection of capsaicin also became sensitized to the near-threshold electrical stimulation of the proximal end of a cut-dorsal-rootlet stimulation that activated only Aβ fibres (Simone *et al.* 1991*b*). Similarly, the non-painful tactile sensation evoked by intraneural electrical stimulation of large-diameter peripheral nerve fibres in humans became painful once the skin supplied by the nerve became hyperalgesic after a remote injection of capsaicin (Torebjörk *et al.* 1992).

There is also evidence that low-threshold mechanoreceptors with unmyelinated fibres (Nordin 1990; Vallbo *et al.* 1993) contribute to mechano-allodynia. In sensory tests of the hyperalgesic skin surroundings a capsaicin injection, pain could often be evoked by the gentle movement of hairs—a stimulus that elicits activity in low-threshold mechanoreceptors with myelinated axons. Little or no pain was elicited by static pressure applied with a blunt object such as a cotton swab. However, when the swab was stroked across the skin, the initial sense of tactile contact was accompanied by pain. Each stroke evoked an immediate sense of pain or soreness followed 3–10 s later by a second pain described as burning (LaMotte *et al.* 1991). A pressure of ischaemic block of conduction in myelinated nerve fibres eliminated the first sensation of pain but, for some subjects, left the second sensation intact (LaMotte *et al.* 1991). When measurements were made prior to the block of conduction in thinly myelinated fibres (as evidenced by an intact but delayed sense of cool), some subjects still felt the dual sensation of pain in response to each stroke, that is, a short-latency first pain followed several seconds later by a second pain, while others felt only the second pain—all occurring in the absence of tactile sensations. In a study of brushing-evoked 'first' pain in secondary hyperalgesic skin surrounding a topical application of mustard oil, it was concluded that large myelinated afferents were responsible because the hyperalgesia disappeared with the loss of tactile sensation after an ischaemic nerve block (Koltzenburg *et al.* 1992). However, the second pain in response to stroking was not measured. Since the sense of cool was said to be intact but of lesser magnitude on the nerve-blocked skin, it is possible that certain thinly myelinated fibres with low-threshold mechanoreceptors (Merzenich and Harrington 1969; Adriaensen *et al.* 1983) were impaired.

Taken together, the results of these studies suggest that both thickly and thinly myelinated fibres contribute to the first pain from stroking secondary hyperalgesic skin and that unmyelinated fibres contribute to the second pain. Innocuous stroking does not evoke sensations under ischaemic block of conduction in large-diameter peripheral nerve fibres when the skin is uninjured. Also, a patient with a rare sensory neuropathy that eliminated function in Aβ fibres but left normal function in Aδ and C fibres had no sense of touch or vibratory sensitivity (Treede and Cole 1993). Thus, the activity of low-threshold mechanoreceptors with thinly myelinated (see, for example, Adriaensen *et al.* 1983) or unmylinated (Nordin 1990; Vallbo *et al.* 1993) fibres may normally be masked in the central nervous system only to be unmasked by the onset of secondary hyperalgesia.

What are the small-diameter nerve fibres activated by innocuous stroking? In the hairy skin of humans, these are low-threshold mechanoreceptors with Aβ, Aδ, or C fibres. In addition, a small proportion of nociceptive fibres with high thresholds for noxious thermal stimuli exhibit a weak response to innocuous stroking of the skin (unpublished observations and Meyer *et al.* 1991). The amount of activity and the number of active nerve fibres with nociceptors as opposed to low-threshold mechanoreceptors would depend on how innocuous or noxious the stroking stimulus was—for example, fabrics made of smooth cotton versus those made of prickly wool (Cervero *et al.* 1994). The abrasiveness of an object and thus the degree of nociceptor activation and the amount of pain evoked when the object is stroked across the skin depend upon such variables as the sizes, spacing, and shapes of the raised elements on its surface (see, for example, LaMotte 1995).

There is relatively little research on cutaneous punctate mechanical pressure. Normally painful punctate stimuli are perceived as more painful in an area of secondary hyperalgesia (Lewis 1936; Hardy *et al.* 1950; LaMotte *et al.* 1991; Cervero *et al.* 1994) suggesting a contribution from mechanically sensitive nociceptors. In order to obtain a maximal area of secondary hyperalgesia the probe must not only be sufficiently stiff but small in diameter (LaMotte 1994). A von Frey-type filament (220 mN) that evoked pricking pain in human hairy skin excited the majority of mechanosensitive nociceptors with A and C fibres tested in the monkey before and after an intradermal injection of capsaicin outside the receptive field (Baumann *et al.* 1991). The same filament failed to evoke any sensation in the skin surrounding a capsaicin injection in two human subjects tested during a proximal nerve block of conduction in A fibres that had eliminated the sensations of touch and cool (LaMotte *et al.* 1991). Thus, it is hypothesized that activity in (unsensitized) Aδ nociceptors contributes to the enhanced sense of pricking pain in the skin surrounding an injection of capsaicin.

It is therefore hypothesized that the allodynia to innocuous stroking is served by three sets of nerve fibres with low-threshold mechanoreceptors (C, Aδ, and Aβ). Hyperalgesia to abrasive stroking or to punctate stimulation with a sharp object is hypothesized as being mediated by nociceptors with Aδ fibres and possibly nociceptors with C fibres.

The central neural mechanisms mediating the secondary hyperalgesias to innocuous stroking and noxious punctate stimulation after capsaicin are believed to differ. The allodynia to stroking occupies a smaller area on the skin than that for punctate hyperalgesia, has a shorter time course (typically just a few hours), and is greatly reduced in size by anaesthetizing the injection site. An area of punctate hyperalgesia, while gradually decreasing in size, persisted for a much longer time (a median of 13 h) and is typically changed very little after local cutaneous anaesthesia. There is also clinical evidence for differing mechanisms serving these two types of hyperalgesia. A patient who suffered a loss of function in large-diameter (Aβ) fibres developed a normal area of punctate secondary hyperalgesia after an injection of capsaicin but no mechano-allodynia to lightly stroking the skin (Treede and Cole 1993). The punctate hyperalgesia was interpreted as resulting from the sensitization of central pain-signalling neurones to input from nociceptive primary afferent fibres.

In the spinal dorsal horn, *N*-methyl-D-aspartic acid (NMDA) and non-NMDA receptors participate in somatosensory neurotransmission with NMDA receptors being selectively recruited by activity in nociceptive primary afferents (for a review, see Wilcox 1993). Recordings have been made of the responses of spinothalamic tract (STT) cells to the co-application of neurokinin peptides (for example, substance P) and NMDA and non-NMDA agonists (see, for example, Dougherty *et al.* 1993). The discharge frequency of both nociceptive-specific and wide-dynamic-range STT cells in laminae I–VI of the dorsal horn increases in response to NMDA. This increase was enhanced and prolonged by a single co-application of substance P (SP) and accompanied by an increased response to innocuous and noxious mechanical stimulation of the skin (Dougherty and Willis 1991). Responses of nociceptive cells in the dorsal horn to the non-NMDA agaonists, DL-alpha-amino-3-hydroxy-5-methyl-isoxamole proprinate (AMPA) and quisqualic acid (QUIS), are also enhanced by a co-application with substance P (Budhai *et al.* 1992; Rusin *et al.* 1992; Dougherty *et al.* 1993). In contrast to the long-lasting response evoked by QUIS with SP, the enhancement of the response to AMPA by SP was short-lasting and ceased as soon as the peptide was removed. Based on these results, and the effects of antagonists for these agents, it was recently hypothesized that the long-lasting secondary hyperalgesia to punctate mechanical stimuli is mediated by the SP-enhanced responses of STT cells to excitatory amino acids acting on NMDA receptors (Dougherty *et al.* 1993, 1994). It was also hypothesized that the shorter-lasting secondary allodynia to stroking was mediated by SP-enhanced responses of STT cells to excitatory amino acids acting at AMPA receptors. This might help to explain why the anaesthetization of the injury site had a greater effect in reducing the allodynia to stroking than in reducing the hyperalgesia to punctate stimulation.

Selective nerve blocks in humans and recordings from primary afferent as well as STT neurones in experimental animals must be carried out in order to investigate the role of mechanosensitive peripheral nerve fibres in mediating hyperknesis to pricking and stroking stimuli. Does itch from pricking or from stroking remain after a block of Aδ and/or Aβ fibres? Which nociceptors respond best to the stiff, small-diameter probes required to evoke itch in normal and itchy skin? Why is itch (along with pain) evoked when the probe diameter is small but only pain and not itch when it is slightly larger? In the latter case, perhaps the itch is masked centrally, for example, due to a recruitment of additional fibre populations when the diameter is increased. Alternatively, there might be a previously undescribed subpopulation of mechanonociceptors that respond selectively to stiff, small-diameter probes.

There are further unanswered questions. Are there histamine-responsive neurones in the dorsal horn that become sensitized to input from low-threshold, myelinated and high-threshold, unmyelinated mechanoreceptive primary afferent fibres after an injection of histamine? What neurotransmittors and neuropeptides contribute to hyperknesis and to the inhibition of itch and itchy skin by pain and hyperalgesia? Further research will help to clarify which classes of peripheral neurones and what kinds of central neural mechanisms contribute to mechanically evoked itch in itchy skin.

Secondary cutaneous dysaesthesiae from peripheral nerve injury

An injury that transects, demyelinates, or by some other means chronically excites peripheral axons can induce a hyperexcitability, manifested by spontaneous impulse discharges and abnormal sensitivity to mechanical, thermal, and chemical stimuli at the injury site and more proximal locations along the neurone particularly at the soma (for a review see Devor 1994). There is ample evidence that pain and painful cutaneous dysaesthesiae can result from such injuries presumably as a direct result of activity in nociceptive primary afferent fibres as well as any resulting central sensitization of nociceptive neurones in the spinal dorsal horn (for reviews see Treede *et al.* 1992; Devor 1994; Walters 1994). In contrast, it is uncommon for chronic hyperknesis and/or itch to result from a peripheral nerve injury (Bernhard 1994), possibly because hyperalgesia and/or pain predominate and activate an 'antipruritic state' that suppresses activity in central neurones mediating itch and hyperknesis.

Behavioural evidence for pain and/or hyperalgesia has been obtained in rats after denervation by complete transection of the sciatic nerve (see, for example, Wall *et al.* 1979; Wiesenfeld and Lindblom 1980) or after a partial denervation due to a loose litation of the sciatic that produces in-continuity neuromas (Bennett and Xie 1988), a tight ligation of a portion of the sciatic (Seltzer *et al.* 1990), or a tight ligation of one or two of the lumbar spinal nerves (Kim and Chung 1992). Neuroma endbulbs, sprouts in A and C fibres, and local regions of demyelination in A fibres can become hyperexcitable and loci of ectopic impulse generation can be accompanied in some instances by abnormal responses to thermal stimuli and/or increased responsiveness to mechanical stimulation or to a variety of endogenous metabolic and chemical agents (see, for example, Wall and Gutnick 1974*b*; Govrin-Lippmann and Devor 1978; Blumberg and Jänig 1984; Burchiel 1984; Matzner and Devor 1987; Zimmermann *et al.* 1987; Welk *et al.* 1990; Devor *et al.* 1992). For example, certain neurones with injured peripheral axons develop an abnormal responsiveness to noradrenaline and to electrical stimulation of postganglionic sympathetic efferents (Wall and Gutnick 1974*a,b*; Devor and Jänig 1981; Korenman and Devor 1981; Häbler *et al.* 1987; Sato and Perl 1991; McLachlan *et al.* 1993; Devor *et al.* 1994; Xie *et al.* 1995) possibly as a result of an upregulation of α adrenoceptors (see, for example, Nishiyama *et al.* 1993). The increased responsiveness of nociceptive neurones to noradrenaline is thought to contribute to pain and hyperalgesia in patients with the sympathetically maintained pain of reflex sympathetic dystrophy (RSD) (see, for example, Nathan 1947; Wall and Gutnick 1974*a,b*; McMahon 1991; Campbell *et al.* 1992).

Sites of spontaneous activity and abnormal sensitivities to stimuli can develop at the injury and/or at loci along the nerve and in the dorsal root ganglion (see, for example, Wall and Devor 1983; Burchiel 1984; Kajander *et al.* 1992). Ephaptic coupling between different neurones can sometimes develop at one or more of these sites (see, for example, Seltzer and Devor 1979; Rasminsky 1980; Lisney and Pover 1983), which could conceivably provide a substrate for activation of nociceptive afferent neurones by activity in low-threshold receptors. There can also be 'crossed afterdischarge' in Aδ fibres—but typically not in C fibres—by activity in Aβ afferents (Lisney and Devor 1987; Amir and Devor 1992) that can occur normally in the dorsal root ganglion or pathologically between nerve endings in a neuroma (Devor and Wall 1990). Crossed afterdischarge is believed to result in the release of K^+ and neurotransmitters from repetitively activated neurones resulting in a delayed activation of neighbouring cells (Devor and Wall 1990; Utzschneider *et al.* 1992). The coupling could amplify the effects of abnormal activity in injured neurones and thus contribute to the pain, aftersensations, and hyperalgesia in neuropathic pain syndromes.

Ectopic impulse electrogenesis could occur as a result of an increased concentration of functional voltage-sensitive sodium channels in cellular membranes at various sites from soma to peripheral endings (for reviews, see Titmus and Faber 1990; Devor 1994). Alterations in calcium and/or potassium and other conductances could occur as well. Subunit proteins for sodium channels, stretch-activated channels, α adrenoceptor channels, channels activated by inflammatory mediators, and so on are presumably synthesized in the cell body and then transported preferentially into and down the axon (by fast axoplasmic transport) possibly while they are being assembled into completed channels (see, for example, Lombet *et al.* 1985; for reviews see Titmus and Faber 1990; Devor 1994). Damage to the axon could disturb the axonofugal transport mechanism, alter the rate of turnover or synthesis of the channels, and/or cause channels to accrue at the soma by a 'damming effect' (see, for example, Roederer and Cohen 1983; Titmus and Faber 1986). An accumulation of extra sodium channels alone at any site could produce a region of hyperexcitability such that current generated through ion channels activated by stretch or various chemicals such as noradrenaline would be sufficient to depolarize the cell and produce action potentials (see, for example, Matzner and Devor 1992; Devor 1994).

A tonic excitation of nociceptive primary afferent neurones would be expected to cause pain. Furthermore, if some of these afferents are the kind that induce central sensitization, for example, by the same mechanisms evoked by capsaicin injection, then an enhanced excitability of nociceptive neurones in the spinal dorsal horn would result in widespread mechanical hyperalgesia. Discharges evoked by innocuous cutaneous mechanical stimulation in low-threshold Aβ mechanoreceptive afferents as well as spontaneous activity in injured Aβ fibres might then be expected to evoke pain. Indeed, there is considerable evidence that mechano-allodynia in certain patients with neuropathic pain of peripheral origin is mediated by input from large-diameter, rapidly conducting, low-threshold Aβ mechanoreceptive primary afferents (see, for example, Lindblom and Verrillo 1979; Ochoa 1982; Meyer *et al.* 1985; Campbell *et al.* 1988*a*; Price *et al.* 1989; Treede *et al.* 1991; Gracely *et al.* 1992; but see Cline *et al.* 1989).

Evidence that mechano-allodynia can be maintained by ongoing activity in nociceptive afferents comes from patients in whom the cutaneous dysaesthesia is spatially remote from a cutaneous region that, when anaesthetized, eliminates it and normalizes sensations from the hyperalgesic skin (Gracely *et al.* 1992; Fig. 16.5). In another study, a positive correlation was found between the magnitude of a patient's neuropathic pain, which was modulated by changing local skin temperature, and the intensity of mechanically evoked pain in an area of cutaneous hyperalgesia (Koltzenburg *et al.* 1992).

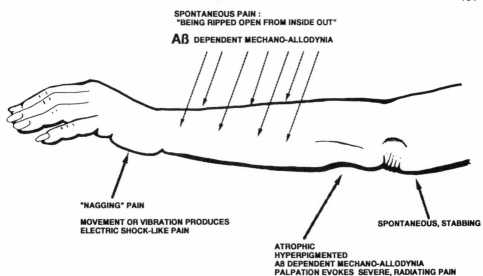

SPONTANEOUS PAIN :
"BEING RIPPED OPEN FROM INSIDE OUT"

Aβ DEPENDENT MECHANO-ALLODYNIA

"NAGGING" PAIN

MOVEMENT OR VIBRATION PRODUCES
ELECTRIC SHOCK-LIKE PAIN

SPONTANEOUS, STABBING

ATROPHIC
HYPERPIGMENTED
Aβ DEPENDENT MECHANO-ALLODYNIA
PALPATION EVOKES SEVERE, RADIATING PAIN

Fig. 16.5 Pain symptoms that developed in a patient after ulnar nerve transposition surgery. The patient suffered from spontaneous pain on the forearm and around the elbow—the latter including a hyperpigmented area. In addition, there was mechano-allodynia in the elbow, forearm, and hand such that a light touch or brushing evoked sharp, shooting pain and a localized burning pain. Selective nerve blocks and electrical stimulation at low intensities demonstrated that the innocuous mechanically evoked pain was mediated by activity in large-diameter, myelinated (Aβ) peripheral nerve fibres. Finger movement evoked electrical shock-like pain that radiated from fingers to forearm. A local anaesthetic block of the hyperpigmented cutaneous area eliminated the spontaneous pains and the mechano-allodynia thereby returning cutaneous sensation to normal until some time after the block wore off. Reprinted with permission from Gracely *et al.* (1992).

While pruritus is rarely described as an important element of most neuropathic syndromes, there are cases of peripheral neuropathies resulting from injury or disease in which localized itching is the predominant symptom (Bernhard 1994). For example, 'notalgia paraesthetica' is the term that characterizes the itching in the scapular or midscapular region of the back resulting apparently from damage or entrapment of spinal nerves T2 through T6 (Astwazaturow 1934; Massay and Pleet 1981; see Bernhard 1994 for review). The itching can be relieved by the topical application of creams containing capsaicin (Wallengren 1991), after which a remission of several months ensues. This suggests the possibility that chemosensitive nerve fibres mediating itch, and possibly capable of inducing hyperknesis, had become hyperexcitable after the nerve injury but then could be temporarily desensitized by capsaicin.

Peripheral nerve injury might bring about structural changes in the central nervous system that could contribute to long-term central sensitization. A loose ligation of the sciatic nerve, resulting in cutaneous hyperalgesia and mechano-allodynia, produced, under certain conditions, a transsynaptic degeneration of small, putative inhibitory, interneurones in the spinal dorsal horn (Sugimoto *et al.* 1990). A subsequent discovery suggesting that the loose-ligation injury resulted in a decrease in primary afferent depolarization and presynaptic inhibition (Laird and Bennett, 1992) supports the hypothesis that spontaneously active nociceptive afferents produce chronic depolarization, excitotoxicity and resulting death of small inhibitory interneurones (Sugimoto *et al.* 1988). Another structural change was found to occur in the central terminals of myelinated Aβ peripheral axons in a sciatic nerve that had been ligated and sectioned. These central terminals of neurones that had presumably been low-threshold mechanoreceptors penetrated into lamina II on to neurones that normally receive monosynaptic contact from nociceptive C fibres and not A fibres (Woolf *et al.* 1992). It was hypothesized that novel contacts between these low-threshold A fibres and nociceptive interneurones in lamina II could contribute to allodynia after peripheral nerve injuries.

Nocifensors

Two classes of primary sensory neurones are hypothesized in this review as contributing to cutaneous secondary dysaesthesiae. The first class comprises neurones with small-diameter axons and peripheral chemoreceptors that differ according to whether they

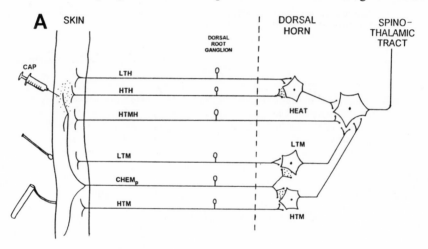

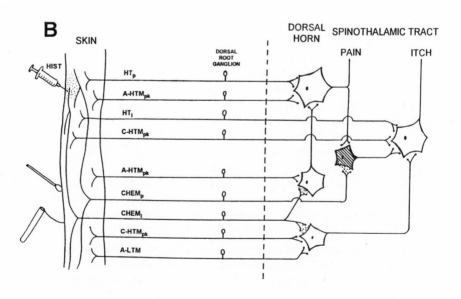

respond to pruritic and/or algesic chemicals and that have a powerful capacity to sensitize certain neurones in the dorsal horn of the spinal cord. These spinal neurones, which differ according to their roles in mediating hyperalgesia and hyperknesis, receive a convergent input from mechanosensitive primary afferent neurones in the second class. Neurones of the second class have peripheral nociceptors with thinly myelinated axons or low-threshold mechanoreceptors with either thinly or thickly myelinated axons. It is hypothesized that there are other primary nociceptive afferent neurones that subserve pain, itch, and the corresponding reflexes to algesic or pruritic peripheral stimulation but that do not elicit central sensitization. Similarly, there are primary afferents that do not contribute to one type of dysaesthesia but do to another. A neuronal model of each type of secondary cutaneous dysaesthesia is presented in Fig. 16.6.

The observations of a lack of correlation between the development of secondary hyperalgesia and the magnitude of pain experienced (see, for example, Hardy *et al.* 1952; LaMotte *et al.* 1991; Cervero *et al.* 1993) are consistent with the hypothesis that the major

---

Fig. 16.6 Models of two kinds of secondary cutaneous dysaesthesia. (A) A model of secondary hyperalgesia. Interneurones in the dorsal horn are sensitized by the release of neuromodulator from chemosensitive, noceffective peripheral nerve fibres (CHEM), which branch widely within the skin and which are activated by algesic chemicals produced at the site of an injury (or, in this case, the algesic chemical, capsaicin). One type of interneurone (HT MECH) receives a convergent input from high-threshold mechanonociceptive fibres while the other type (LT MECH) receives input from low-threshold mechanoreceptive fibres. These fibres supply a large area of skin surrounding the injection site. A third type of interneurone receives a convergent input from low- and high-threshold peripheral nerve fibres responsive to heat stimulations in the immediate vicinity of the injection site. These three types of interneurones increase the excitability of spinothalamic tract (STT) neurones to heat stimulations at (but not remote to) the injection site and to innocuous and nociceptive mechanical stimuli delivered within a large, surrounding area. The widely branching chemosensitive fibres are postulated in order to account for the finding that the spread of mechanical hyperalgesia away from the injection site is blocked by an intracutaneous barrier of anaesthetic. Reproduced with permission from LaMotte *et al.* (1991). (B) A model of secondary hyperknesis and the inhibition of itch and hyperknesis by pain and secondary hyperalgesia. It is postulated that pain and itch are served by different populations of spinothalamic tract neurones, STT_p and STT_i and that the former population, if sufficiently activated, inhibits the latter via inhibitory interneurones (cross-hatched cell). Of those high-threshold peripheral nerve fibres selectively responsive to noxious cutaneous stimuli (for example, those with polymodal nociceptors), there is a subpopulation (HI_i that projects to STT_i cells and that responds readily to itch-producing stimuli such as histamine and another (HT_p), projecting to STT_p cells that does not. A population of high-threshold peripheral nerve fibres is hypothesized to be particularly responsive to stiff, small-diameter mechanical stimuli that evoke prickle. Some of those with A fibres (A-$HTM)_{pk}$ project to STT_p neurones and mediate the sense of pricking pain while others, with C fibres (C-HTM), project to STT_i cells and serve the sense of pricking itch. Two sets of chemosensitive noceffective peripheral nerve fibres are hypothesized to branch widely within the skin—one responding best to pruritic and the other to algesic chemicals ($CHEM_i$ and $CHEM_p$ respectively). $CHEM_i$ neurones are capable of releasing a neuromodulator that sensitizes two kinds of interneurones in the spinal dorsal horn: (1) HTM_i, which receives a convergent input from low-threshold (A-LTM) and high-threshold (C-HTM_{pk}) mechanoreceptive nerve fibres and (2) HTP_p, which receives input from A-HTM_{pk} fibres. These interneurones receive input from fibres with receptive fields at various locations in a large cutaneous area surrounding the injection site. The HTM_i interneurones, when sensitized, increase the excitability of STT_i cells thereby accounting for the secondary hyperkinesis to pricking and alloknesis to stroking the skin after a histamine injection. The HTM_p interneurones slightly increase the excitability of STT_p cells thereby accounting for the mild secondary hyperalgesia to pricking (but this increase is not sufficient to inhibit STT_i cells via inhibitory neurones). The $CHEM_p$ peripheral neurones release a neuronmodulator that sensitizes the interneurones that inhibit STT_i cells thereby accounting for the finding that a histamine injection evokes little or no itch or hyperknesis in an area of strong secondary hyperalgesia produced by a prior injection of capsaicin.

role of certain primary afferent neurones is trophic and not sensory, that is, they act as 'noceffectors' (Kruger 1988; Kruger *et al.* 1989; Kruger and Halata, Chapter 2, this volume). This means that they produce central sensitization or aid in peripheral inflammation (see, for example, Szolcsányi 1988; Lam and Ferrell 1991) and wound healing and do not act as 'nociceptors' in contributing to pain and reflexes. Possible noceffectors include those primary afferent neurones termed 'silent afferents', 'sleeping nociceptors', or 'mechanically insensitive afferents' (Schaible and Schmidt 1985; Grigg *et al.* 1986; Häbler *et al.* 1990; Handwerker *et al.* 1991*b*; Kress *et al.* 1992; Davis *et al.* 1993; Schmidt *et al.* 1994), that typically do not respond to short-lasting thermal or mechanical stimuli but that become active after tissue becomes chemically irritated or inflamed.

A term broader than the conventional word, 'nociceptive', is required to include functions not necessarily correlated with pain and injury such as: (1) the trophic or effector responses of certain primary afferent neurones containing neuropeptides— responses that may not lead directly to pain sensations or nociceptive reflexes; (2) the responses of certain primary sensory neurones to non-injurious algesic chemicals; and (3) responses of certain neurones to pruritic chemicals and other pruritic stimuli. For this purpose, the term 'nocifensive', coined by Lewis (1936), is proposed to label all those somatic and visceral primary afferent neurones that act to protect the body against injury (LaMotte 1992).

One class of nocifensive neurones serves the function of eliciting sensations of pain or itch along with the associated protective reflexes. A second type is capable of becoming sensitized to peripheral stimuli. That is, their response thresholds are lowered and their suprathreshold responses enhanced. These neurones contribute to primary dyaesthesiae within an area of injury or irritation and serve the protective functions of enhancing avoidance and escape behaviour to stimuli restricted to this area. The third type of nocifensive neurone releases chemicals (for example, neuropeptides) in the periphery resulting, for example, in increased vascular permeability, vasodilatation, degranulation of mast cells, and tissue growth (see, for example, Levine *et al.* 1985; Nilsson *et al.* 1985; Ferrel and Russell 1986; Lynn 1988). This serves the protective functions of promoting the health of normal cells and facilitating their repair and recovery after injury. The fourth class of nocifensive neurones releases neurochemicals such as neuropeptides in the dorsal horn thereby enhancing the excitability of STT cells and other nociceptive neurones in the somatovisceral afferent pathways. This extends the dysaesthesia beyond the area of injury and primary dysaesthesia and thus protects, by eliciting avoidance and escape behaviour, a larger portion of the body against further injury.

These four classes are not mutually exclusive and there may be primary afferent neurones that possess the functional properties of more than one or perhaps even all four classes. What is certain is that nocifensive neurones are an extremely heterogeneous population differing widely in their sensitivities to physical and chemical stimuli, in their central projections, and in the kinds of chemicals they release in the periphery and in the chemicals released in the central nervous system.

References

Adriaensen, H., Gybels, J. Handwerker, J.O., and Van Hees, J. (1983) Response properties of thin myelinated (A-delta) fibers in human skin nerves. *J. Neurophysiol.* **49**, 111–22.

Amir, R. and Devor, M. (1992). Axonal cross-excitation in nerve-end neuromas: comparison of A- and C-fibers. *J. Neurophysiol.* **68**, 1160–6.

Astwazaturow, M. (1934). Uber paresthetische Neuralgien und eine besondere Form derselben—Notalgia paresthetica. *Deut. Arch. Nervenheilkd.* **133**, 188.

Baumann, T.K., Simone, D.A., Shain, C.N., and LaMotte, R.H. (1991). Neurogenic hyperalgesia: The search for the primary cutaneous afferent fibers that contribute to capsaicin-induced pain and hyperalgesia. *J. Neurophysiol.* **66**, 212–27.

Bennett, G.J. Neuropathic pain. In *Textbook of pain* (3rd edn) (eds. P. Wall and R. Melzack), pp. 79–100. Churchill Livingstone, New York.

Bennett, G.J. and Xie, Y.-K. (1988). A peripheral mononeuropathy in rat that produces disorders of pain sensation like those seen in man. *Pain* **33**, 87–107.

Bernhard, J.D. (1994). *Itch: mechanisms and management of pruritus.* McGraw-Hill Inc, New York.

Bernstein, J.E., Swift, R.M., Soltani, K., and Lorincz, A.L. (1981). Inhibition of axon reflex casodilatation by topically applied capsaicin. *J. invest. Dermatol.* **76**, 394–5.

Bickford, R.G. (1938). Experiments relating to the itch sensation, its peripheral mechanism, and central pathways. *Clin. Sci.* **3**, 377–86.

Blumberg, H. and Jänig, W. (1984). Discharge pattern of afferent fibres from a neuroma. *Pain* **20**, 335–53.

Budai, D., Wilcox, G.L., and Larson, A.A. (1992). Modulation of N-methyl-D-aspartate and (R,S)-alpha-amino-3-hydroxy-5-methyl-isoxazole-4-proprionate (AMPA) responses of spinal nociceptive neurons by a N-terminal fragment of substance P. *Eur. J. Pharmacol.* **216**, 441–4.

Burchiel, K.J. (1984). Spontaneous impulse generation in normal and denervated dorsal root ganglia: sensitivity to alpha-adrenergic stimulation and hypoxia. *Exp. Neurol.* **85**, 257–72.

Campbell, J.N., Raja, S.N., Meyer, R.A., and Mackinnon, S.E. (1988*a*). Myelinated afferents signal the hyperalgesia associated with nerve injury. *pain* **32**, 89–94.

Campbell, J.N., Khan, A.A., Meyer, R.A., and Raja, S.N. (1988*b*). Responses to heat of C-fiber nociceptors in monkey are altered by injury in the receptive field but not by adjacent injury. *Pain* **32**, 327–32.

Campbell, J.N., Meyer, R.A., and Raja, S.N. (1992). Is nociceptor activation by alpha-1 adrenorecptors the culprit in sympathetically maintained pain? *Am. Pain Soc. J.* **1**, 3–11.

Carpenter, S.E. and Lynn, B. (1981(. Vascular and sensory responses of human skin to mild injury after topical treatment with capsaicin. *Br. J. Pharmacol.* **73**, 755–8.

Cervero, F., Gilbert, R., Hammond, R.G.E., and Tanner, J. (1993), Development of secondary hyperalgesia following non-painful thermal stimulation of the skin: a psychophysical study in man. *Pain* **54**, 181–9.

Cervero, F., Meyer, R.A., and Campbell, J.N. (1994). A psychophysical study of secondary hyperalgesia: evidence for increased pain to input from nociceptors. *Pain* **58**, 21–8.

Chapman, L.F., Ramos, A.O., Goodell, H., and Wolff, H.G. (1961). Neurohumoral features of afferent fibres in man. *Am. Med. Assoc. Arch. Neurol.* **4**, 617–50.

Cline, M.A., Ochoa, J., and Torebjörk, H.E. (1989). Chronic hyperalgesia and skin warming caused by sensitized C nociceptors. *Brain* **112**, 621–47.

Coderre, T.J. and Melzack, R. (1987). Cutaneous hyperalgesia: contributions of the peripheral and central nervous systems to the increase in pain sensitivity after injury. *Brain Res.* **404**, 95–106.

Davis, K.D., Meyer, R.A., and Campbell, J.N. (1993). Chemosensitivity and sensitization of nociceptive afferents that innervate the hairy skin of monkey. *J. Neurophysiol.* **69**, 1071–81.

Devor, M. (1994). The pathophysiology of damaged peripheral nerves. In *Textbook of pain* (3rd edn) (ed. P. Wall and R. Melzack), pp. 79–100. Churchill Livingstone, New York.

Devor, M. and Jänig, W. (1981). Activation of myelinated afferent ending in a neuroma by stimulation of sympathetic supply in the rat. *Neurosci. Lett.* **24**, 43–7.

Devor, M. and Wall, P.D. (1990). Cross-excitation in dorsal root ganglia of nerve-injured and intact rats. *J. Neurophysiol.* **64**, 1733–46.

Devor, M., White, D.M., Goetzl, E.J., and Levine, J.D. (1992). Eicosanoids, but not tachykinins, excite C-fibre endings in rat sciatic nerve-end neuromas. *Neuro Report* **3**, 21–4.

Devor, M., Govrin-Lippmann, R., and Angelides, K. (1993). Na$^+$ channel immunolocalization in peripheral mammalian axons and changes following nerve injury and neuroma formation. *J. Neurosci.* **13**(5), 1976–92.

Devor, M., Jänig, W., and Michaelis, M. (1994). Modulation of activity in dorsal root ganglion neurons by sympathetic activation in nerve-injured rats. *J. Neurophysiol.* **71**(1), 38–47.

Dougherty, P.M. and Willis, W.D. (1991). Enhancement of spinothalamic neuron responses to chemical and mechanical stimuli following combined micro-iontophoretic application of N-methyl-D-aspartic acid and substance P. *Pain* **47**, 85–93.

Dougherty, P.M., Palecek, J., and Willis, W.D. (1993). Does sensitization of responses to excitatory amino acids underlie the psychophysical reports of two modalities of increased sensitivity in zones of secondary hyperalgesia? *Am. Pain Soc. J.* **2**, 276–9.

Dougherty, P.M., Mittman, S. and Sorkin, L.S. (1994). Hyperalgesia and amino acids: receptor selectivity based on stimulus intensity and a role for peptides. *Am. Pain Soc. J.* **3**, 240–8.

Dubner, R. (1991). Neuronal plasticity and pain following peripheral tissue inflammation or nerve injury. In *Proceedings of the 6th World Congress on Pain* (ed. M.R. Bond, J.E. Charlton, and C.J. Woolf), pp. 263–76. Elsevier, Amsterdam.

Ferrell, W.R. and Russell, J.W. (1986). Extravasation in the knee induced by antidromic stimulation of articular C fibre afferents of the anaesthetized cat. *J. Physiol.* **379**, 407–16.

Fitzgerald, M. (1983). Capsaicin and sensory neurones—a review. *Pain* **15**, 109–30.

Foerster, O. (1927). *Die Leituungsbahnen des Schmerzgefuhls und die chirurgische Behandlung der Schmerzzustande*. Urban and Schwarzenber, Berlin.

Govrin-Lippmann, R. and Devor, M. (1978). Ongoing activity in severed nerves: source and variation with time. *Brain Res.* **159**, 406–10.

Gracely, R.H., Lynch, S.A., and Bennett, G.J. (1992). Painful neuropathy: altered central processing maintained dynamically by peripheral input. *Pain* **51**, 175–94.

Graham, D.T., Goodell, H., and Wolff, H.G. (1951). Neural mechanisms involved in itch, 'itchy skin', and tickle sensations. *J. clin. Invest.* **30**, 37–49.

Grigg, P., Schaible, H.-G., and Schmidt, R.F. (1986). Mechanical sensitivity of group II and IV afferents from the posterior articular nerve in normal and inflamed cat knee. *J. Neurophysiol.* **55**, 635–43.

Guilbaud, G., Kayser, V., Attal, N., and Benoist, J-M. (1992). Evidence for a central contribution to secondary hyperalgesia. In *Hyperalgesia and allodynia* (ed. W.D. Willis), pp. 187–201. Raven Press, New York.

Häbler, H-J., Jänig, W., and Koltzenburg, M. (1987). Activation of unmyelinated afferents in chronically lesioned nerves by adrenaline and excitation of sympathetic efferents in the cat. *Neurosci. Lett.* **82**, 35–40.

Häbler, H.-J., Jänig, W., and Koltzenburg, M. (1990). Activation of unmyelinated afferents by mechanical stimuli and inflammation of the urinary bladder. *J. Physiol., London* **425**, 545–63.

Handwerker, H.O. (1992). Pain and allodynia, itch and alloknesis: an alternative hypothesis. *Am. Pain Soc. J.* **1**, 135–8.

Handwerker, H.O., Kilo, S., and Reeh, P.W. (1989). Afferent C-fibres from rat hairy skin not driven by natural stimulation. *Soc. Neurosci. Abst.* **15**, 1265.

Handwerker, H.O., Forster, C., and Kirchhoff, C. (1991a). Discharge properties of human C-fibres induced by itching and burning stimuli. *J. Neurophysiol.* **66**, 307–15.

Handwerker, H.O., Kilo, S., and Reeh, P.W. (1991b). Unresponsive afferent nerve fibres in the sural nerve of the rat. *J. Physiol;., London* **435**, 229–42.

Hardy, J.D., Wolff, H.G., and Goodell, H. (1950). Experimental evidence on the nature of cutaneous hyperalgesia. *J. clin. Invest.* **29**, 115–40.

Hardy, J.D., Wolff, H.G., and Goodell, H. (1952). *Pain sensations and reactions*. Williams & Wilkins, Baltimore.

Hirata, H., Uchida, H., Kishikawa, K., Collins, J.G., and LaMotte, R.H. (1990). Responses of dorsal horn neurons in cats to intracutaneous injections of histamine and capsaicin. *Soc Neurosci. Abstr.* **16**, 231.

Holzer, P. (1988). Local effector functions of capsaicin-sensitive sensory nerve endings: involvement of tachykinins, calcitonin gene-related peptide and other neuropeptides. *Neuroscience* **24** 739–68.

Jänig, W. and Lisney, S.J.W. (1989). Small diameter myelinated afferents produce vasodilatation but not plasma extravasation in rat skin. *J. Physiol.* **415**, 477–86.

Kajander, K.C., Wakisaka, S., and Bennett, G.J. (1992). Spontaneous discharge originates in the dorsal root ganglion at the onset of a painful peripheral neuropathy in rat. *Neurosci. Lett.* **138**, 225–8.

Kim, S.H. and Chung, J.M. (1991). Sympathectomy alleiates mechanical allodynia in an experimental animal model for neuropathy in the rat. *Neurosci. Lett.* **134**, 131–4.

Kim, S.H. and Chung, J.M. (1992). An experimental model for peripheral neuropathy produced by segmental spinal nerve ligation in the rat. *Pain* **50**, 355–63.

Koltzenburg, M. and McMahon, S.B. (1989). Plasma extravasation in the rat urinary bladder following mechanical, electrical and chemical stimuli: evidence for a new population of chemosensitive primary sensory neurones. *Neurosci. Lett.* **7**, 352–6.

Koltzenburg, M., Lundberg, L.E.R., and Torebjörk, H.E. (1992). Dynamic and static components of mechanical hyperalgesia in human hairy skin. *Pain* **51**, 207–19.

Korenman, E.M.D. and Devor, M. (1981). Ectopic adrenergic sensitivity in damaged peripheral nerve axons in the rat. *Exp. Neurol.* **72**, 63–81.

Koschorke, G.M., Meyer, R.A., Tillman, D.B., and Campbell, J.N. (1991). Ectopic excitability of injured nerves in monkey: entrained responses to vibratory stimuli. *J. Neurophysiol.* **65**, 693–701.

Kress, M., Koltzenburg, M., Reeh, P.W., and Handwerker, H.O. (1992). Responsiveness and functional attributes of electrically localized terminals of cutaneous C-fibres in vivo and in vitro. *J. Neurophysiol.* **68**, 581–95.

Kruger, L. (1988). Morphological features of thin sensory afferent fibres: a new interpretation of 'nociceptor' function. In *Progress in brain research*, Vol. 74 (ed. W. Hamann and A. Iggo), pp. 253–7.

Kruger, L., Silverman, J.D., Mantyh, P.W., Sternini, C., and Brecha, N.C. (1989). Peripheral patterns of calcitonin-gene-related peptide general somatic sensory innervation: cutaneous and deep terminations. *J. comp. Neurol.* **280**, 291–302.

Laird, J.M.A. and Bennett, G.J. (1992). Dorsal root potentials and afferent input to the spinal cord in rats with an experimental peripheral neuropathy. *Brain Res.* **584**, 181–90.

Laird, J.M. and Cervero, F. (1989). A comparative study of the changes in receptive-field properties of multireceptive and nociceptive rat dorsal horn neurons following noxious mechanical stimulation. *J. Neurophysiol.* **62**, 854–63.

Lam, F.Y. and Ferrell, W.R. (1991). Neurogenic component of different models of acute inflammation in the rat knee joint. *Ann. rheum. Dis.* **50**, 747–51.

LaMotte, R.H. (1988). Psychophysical and neurophysiological studies of chemically induced cutaneous pain and itch. The case of the missing nociceptor. In *Progress in brain research*, Vol. 74 (ed. W. Hamann and A. Iggo), pp. 331–5.

LaMotte, R.H. (1992). Subpopulations of 'nocifensor neurons' contributing to pain and allodynia, itch and alloknesis. *Am. Pain Soc. J.* **1**, 115–26.

LaMotte, R.H. (1994). Mechanically evoked secondary hyperalgesia in the primate. In *Peripheral neurons in nociception: physio-pharmacological aspects* (ed. J.M. Besson, G. Gilbaud, and H. Ollat). John Libey..

LaMotte, R.H., Simone, D.A., Baumann, T.K., Shain, C.N., and Alreja, M. (1988). Hypothesis for novel classes of chemoreceptors mediating chemogenic pain and itch. In *Proceedings of the 5th World Congress on Pain* (ed. R. Dubner, G.F. Gebhart, and M.R. Bond), pp. 529–35.

LaMotte, R.H., Shain, C.N., Simone, D.A., and Tsai, E. (1991). Neurogenic hyperalgesia: psychophysical studies of underlying mechanisms. *J. Neurophysiol.* **66**, 190–211.

LaMotte, R.H., Lundbert, L.E.R., and Torebjörk, H.E. (1992). Pain, hyperalgesia and activity in nociceptive C units in humans after intradermal injection of capsaicin. *J. Physiol.* **448**, 749–64.

Lang, E., Novak, A., Reeh, P.W., and Handwerker, H.O. (1990). Chemosensitivity of fine afferents from rat skin in vitro. *J. Neurophysiol.* **63**, 887–901.

Lembeck, F. and Gamse, R. (1982). Substance P in peripheral nervous processes. In *Substance P in the nervous system*, Ciba Foundation Symposium no. 91 (ed. R. Porter and M. O'Connor), pp. 35–49.

Levine, J.D., Moskowitz, M.A., and Basbaum, A.I. (1985). The contribution of neurogenic inflammation in experimental arthritis. *J. Immunol.* **135**, 843s–847s.

Lewis, T. (1936). Experiments relating to cutaneous hyperalgesia and its spread through somatic nerves. *Clin. Sci.* **2**, 373–423.

Lindblom, U. and Verrillo, R.T. (1979). Sensory functions in chronic neuralgia. *J. Neurol. Neurosurg. Psychiat.* **42**, 422–35.

Lisney, S.J.W. and Bharali, L.A.M. (1989), The axon reflex: an outdated idea or a valid hypothesis? *News physiol. Sci.* **4**, 45–48.

Lisney, S.J.W. and Devor, M. (1987). Afterdischarge and interactions among fibers in damaged peripheral nerve in the rat. *Brain Res.* **415**, 122–36.

Lisney, S.J.W. and Matthews, B. (1978). Branched afferent nerves supplying tooth-pulp in the cat. *J. Physiol.* **279**, 509–17.

Lisney, S.J.W. and Pover, C.M. (1983). Coupling between fibers involved in sensory nerve neuromata in cats. *J. neurol. Sci* **59**, 255–64.

Lombet, A., Laduron, P., Mourre, C., Jacomet, Y., and Lazdunski, M. (1985). Axonal transport of the voltage-dependent Na^+ channel protein identified by its tetrodotoxin binding site in rat sciatic nerves. *Brain Res.* **345**, 153–8.

Lynn, B. (1988). Neurogenic inflammation. *Skin Pharmacol.* **1**, 217–24.

McLachlan, E.M., Jänig, W., Devor, M., and Michaelis, M. (1993). Peripheral nerve injury triggers noradrenergic sprouting within dorsal root ganglia. *Nature* **363**, 543–5.

MacMahon, S.B. (1991). Mechanisms of sympathetic pain. *Br. med. Bull.* **47**, 584–600.

MacMahon, S.B. and Wall, P.D. (1984). Receptive fields of rat lamina 1 projection cells move to incorporate a nearby region of injury. *Pain* **19**, 2355–47.

Massey, E.W. and Pleet, A.B. (1981). Electromyographic evaluation of notalgia paresthetica. *Neurology* **31**, 642.

Matzner, O. and Devor, M. (1987). Contrasting thermal sensitivity of spontaneously active A- and C-fibers in experimental nerve-end neuromas. *Pain* **30**, 373–84.

Matzner, O. and Devor, M. (1992). Na^+ conductance and the threshold for repetitive neuronal firing. *Brain Res.* **597**, 92–8.

Merzenich, M.M. and Harrington, T. (1969). The sense of flutter-vibration evoked by stimulation of the hairy skin of primates: comparison of human sensory capacity with the responses of merchanoreceptive afferents innervating the hairy skin of monkeys. *Exp. Brain Res.* **9**, 236–60.

Meyer, R.A. and Campbell, J.N. (1988). A novel electrophysiological technique for locating cutaneous nociceptive and chemospecific receptors. *Brain Res.* **441**, 81–6.

Meyer, R.A., Raja, S.N., and Campbell, J.N. (1985). Coupling of action potential activity between unmyelinated fibers in the peripheral nerve of monkey. *Science* **227**, 184–7.

Meyer, R.A., Campbell, J.N., and Raja, S.N. (1988). Antidromic nerve stimulation in monkey does not sensitize unmyelinated nociceptors in heat. *Brain Res.* **441**, 168–72.

Meyer, R.A., Davis, K.D., Cohen, R.H., Treede R-D., and Campbell, J.N. (1991). Mechanically insensitive afferents (MIAs) in cutaneous nerves of monkey. *Brain Res.* **561**, 252–61.

Meyer, R.A., Campbell, J. N., and Raja, S.N. (1993). Peripheral neural mechanisms of nociception. In *Textbook of pain* (3rd edn) (ed. P. Wall and R. Melzack), pp. 79–100. Churchill Livingstone, New York.

Nathan, P.V. (1947). On the pathogenesis of causalgia in peripheral injuries. *Brain* **70**, 145–70.

Nilsson, J., von Euler, A.M., and Dalsgard, C.J. (1985). Stimulation of connective tissue cell growth by substance P and substance K. *Nature* **315**, 61–3.

Nishiyama, K., Brighton, B.W., Bossut, D.F., and Perl, E.R. (1993). Peripheral nerve injury enhances α_2-adrenergic receptor expression by some DRG neurons. *Soc. Neurosci. Abstr.* **19**, 207.

Nordin, M. (1990). Low-threshold mechanoreceptive and nociceptive units with unmyelinated (C) fibres in the human supraorbital nerve. *J. Physiol.* **426**, 229–40.

Ochoa, J. (1982). Pain in local nerve lesions. In *Abnormal nerves and muscles as impulse generators* (ed. W.J. Culp and J. Ochoa), pp. 568–87.

Price, D.D., Bennett, G.J., and Rafii, A. (1989). Psychophysical observations on patients with neuropathic pain relieved by a sympathetic block. *Pain*, **36**, 237–88.

Raja, S.N., Campbell, J.N., and Meyer, R.A. (1984). Evidence for different mechanisms of primary and secondary hyperalgesia following heat injury to the glabrous skin. *Brain* **107**, 1179–88.

Rasminsky, M. (1980). Ephaptic transmission between single nerve fibers in the spinal nerve roots of dystrophic mice. *J. Physiol., London* **305**, 151–69.

Reeh, P.W., Kocher, L., and Jung, S. (1986). Does neurogenic inflammation alter the sensitivity of unmyelinated nociceptors in the rat? *Brain Res.* **384**, 42–50.

Reeh, P.W., Bayer, J., Kocher, L., and Handwerker, H.O. (1987). Sensitization of nociceptive cutaneous nerve fibers from the rat tail by noxious mechanical stimulation. *Exp. Brain Res.* **65**, 505–12.

Roederer, E. and Cohen, M.J. (1983). Regeneration of an identified central neuron in the cricket. II. Electrical and morphological responses of the soma. *J. Neurosci.* **3**, 1848–59,

Rusin, K.L., Ryu, P.D., and Randic, M. (1992). Modulation of excitatory amino acid responses in rat dorsal horn neurons by tachykinins. *J. Neurophysiol.* **68**, 265–86.

Sato, J. and Perl, E.R. (1991). Adrenergic excitation of cutaneous pain receptors induced by peripheral nerve injury. *Science* **251**, 1608–10.

Scadding, J.W. (1981). The development of ongoing activity, mechanosensitivity and adrenaline sensitivity in severed peripheral nerve axons. *Exp. Neurol.* **73**, 345–64.

Schaible, H-G. and Schmidt, R.F. (1985). Effects of an experimental arthritis on the sensory properties of fine articular afferent units. *J. Neurophysiol.* **54**, 1109–22.

Schaible, H-G., Schmidt, R.F., and Willis, W.D. (1987). Enhancement of the responses of ascending tract cells in the cat spinal cord by acute inflammation of the knee joint. *Exp. Brain Res.* **66**, 489–99.

Schmelz, M., Schmidt, R., Ringkamp, M., Handwerker, H., and Torebjörk, H.E. (1994). Sensitization of insensitive branches of C nociceptors in human skin. *J. Physiol.* **480**, 389–94.

Schmidt, R., Torebjörk, E., and Jørum, E. (1993). Pain and itch from intraneural microstimulation. 7th World Congress on Pain (abstract), p. 143.

Schmidt, R., Schmelz, M., Forster, C., RIngkamp, M., Torebjörk, E., and Handwerker, H. (1994). Novel classes of responsive and unresponsive C nociceptors in human skin. *J. Neurosci.* **15**, 333–41.

Seltzer, Z. and Devor, M. (1979). Ephaptic transmission in chronically damaged peripheral nerves. *Neurology* **29**, 1061–4.

Seltzer, Z., Dubner, R., and Shir, Y. (1990). A novel behavioral model of neuropathic pain disorders produced in rats by partial sciatic nerve injury. *Pain* **43**, 205–18.

Shelley, W.B. and Arthur, R.P. (1955). Studies on cowhage (Mucuna pruriens) and its pruritogenic proteinase, Mucunain. *Arch. Dermatol.* **72**, 399–406.

Simone, D.A., Ngeow, J.Y.F., Whitehouse, J., Becerra-Cabal, L., Putterman, G.J., and LaMotte, R.H. (1987). The magnitude and duration of itch produced by intracutaneous injections of histamine. *Somatosens. Res.* **5**, 81–92.

Simone, D.A., Baumann, T.K., and LaMotte, R.H. (1989). Dose-dependent pain and mechanical hyperalgesia in humans after intradermal injection of capsaicin. *Pain* **38**, 99–107.

Simone, D.A., Alreja, M., and LaMotte, R.H. (1991a). Psychophysical studies of the itch sensation and itchy skin ('alloknesis') produced by intracutaneous injection of histamine. *Somatosens. Motor Res.* **8**, 271–9.

Simone, D.A., Sorkin, L.S., Oh, U., Chung, J.M., Owens, C., LaMotte, R.H., and Willis, W.D. (1991b). Neurogenic hyperalgesia: central neurol correlates in responses of spinothalamic tract neurons. *J. Neurophysiol.* **66**, 228–46.

Sugimoto, T., Bennett, G.J., and Kajander, K.C. (1990). Transsynaptic degeneration in the superficial dorsal horn after sciatic nerve injury: effects of a chronic constriction injury, transection and strychnine. *Pain* **42**, 205–13.

Szolcsányi, J. (1988). Antidromic vasodilation and neurogenic inflammation. *Agents Actions* **23**, 4–11.

Thalhammer, J.G. and LaMotte, R.H. (1982). Spatial properties of nociceptor sensitization following heat injury of the skin. *Brain Res.* **231**, 257–65.

Titmus, M.J. and Faber, D.S. (1986). Altered excitability of goldfish Mauthner cell following axotomy. II. Localization and ionic basis. *J. Neurophysiol.* **55**, 1440–4.

Titmus, M.J. and Faber, D.S. (1990). Axotomy-induced alterations in the electrophysiological characteristics of neurons. *Prog. Neurobiol.* **35**, 1–51.

Torebjörk, H.E. (1974). Afferent C units responding to mechanical, thermal and chemical stimuli in human non-glabrous skin. *Acta physiol. scand.* **92**, 374–90.

Torebjörk, H.E. and Ochoa, J.L. (1981). Pain and itch from C-fiber stimulation. *Soc. Neurosci. Abstr.* **7**, 228.

Torebjörk, H.E., Lundberg, L.E.R., and LaMotte, R.H. (1992). Central changes in processing of mechanoreceptive input in capsaicin-induced secondary hyperalgesia in humans. *J. Physiol.* **448**, 763–80.

Treede, R.-D. and Cole, J.D. (1993). Dissociated secondary hyperalgesia in a subject with a large-fibre sensory neuropathy. *Pain* **53**, 169–74.

Treede, R.-D., Raja, S.N., Davis, K.D., Meyer, R.A., and Campbell, J.N. (1991). Evidence that peripheral α-adrenergic receptors mediate sympathetically maintained pain. In *Proceedings of the 6th World Congress on Pain*, Vol. 4. *Pain research and clinical management* (ed. M.R. Bond, J.E. Charlton, and C.J. Woolf), pp. 377–82. Elsevier, Amsterdam.

Treede, R-D., Meyer, R.A., Srinivasa, N.R., and Campbell, J.N. (1992). Peripheral and central mechanisms of cutaneous hyperespondsalgesia. *Prof. Neurobiol.* **38**, 397–421.

Tuckett, R.P. (1982). Itch evoked by electrical stimulation of the skin. *J. invest. Dermatol.* **79**, 368–73.

Tuckett, R.P. and Wei, J.Y. (1987). Response to an itch-producing substance in cat, II. Cutaneous receptor populations with unmyelinated axons. *Brain Res.* **413**, 995–103.

Utzschneider, D., Kocsis, J., and Devor, M. (1992). Mutual excitation among dorsal root ganglion neurons in the rat. *Neurosci. Lett.* **146**, 53–6.

Vallbo, A., Olausson, H., Wessberg, J., and Norrsell, U. (1993). A system of unmyelinated afferents for innocuous mechanoreception in the human skin. *Brain Res.* **628**, 301–4.

Wall, P.D. and Devor, M. (1983). Sensory afferent impulses originate from dorsal root ganglia as well as from the periphery in normal and nerve injury rats. *Pain* **17**, 321–39.

Wall, P.D. and Gutnick, M. (1974a). Properties of afferent nerve impulses originating from a neuroma. *Nature* **284**, 740–3.

Wall, P.D. and Gutnick, M. (1974b). Ongoing activity in peripheral nerve: the physiology and pharmacology of impulses originating from a neuroma. *Exp. Neurol.* **43**, 580–93.

Wall, P.D., Devor, M., Inbal, R., Scadding, W., Schonfeld, D., Seltzer, Z., and Tomkiewicz, M.M. (1979). Autotomy following peripheral nerve lesions: experimental anaesthesia dolorosa. *Pain* **7**, 103–13.

Wallengren, J. (1991). Treatment of notalgia paresthetica with topical capsaicin. *J. Am. Acad. Dermatol.* **24**, 286–8.

Walters, E.T. (1994). Injury-related behavior and neuronal plasticity: An evolutionary perspective on sensitization, hyperalgesia, and analgesia. *Int. Rev. Neurobiol.* **36**, 325–427.

Welk, E., Leah, J.D., and Zimmermann, M. (1990). Characteristics of A- and C-fibers ending in a sensory nerve neuroma in the rat. *J. Neurophysiol.* **63** (4), 759–66.

Wiesenfeld, Z. and Lindblom, U. (1980). Behavioural and electrophysiological effects of various types of peripheral nerve lesions in the rat: a comparison of possible models for chronic pain. *Pain* **8**, 285–98.

Wilcox, G.L. (1993). Spinal mediators of nociceptive neurotransmission and hyperalgesia: relationships among synaptic plasticity, analgesic tolerance and blood flow. *Am. Pain Soc. J.* **2**, 265–75.

Woolf, C.J. (1983). Evidence for a central component of post-injury pain hypersensitivity. *Nature* **306**, 686–8.

Woolf, C.J., Shortland, P., and Coggeshall, R.E. (1992). Peripheral nerve injury triggers central sprouting of myelinated afferents. *Nature* **335**, 75–8.

Xie, Y.-K., Zhang, J.-M., Petersen, M., and LaMotte, R.H. (1995). Functional changes in dorsal root ganglion cells after chronic nerve constriction in the rat. *J. Neurophysiol.* **73**, 1811–20..

Zimmermann, M., Koschorke, G-M., and Sanders, K. (1987). Response characteristics of fibers in regenerating and regenerated cutaneous nerves in cat and rat. In *Effects of injury on trigeminal and spinal somatosensory systems* (ed. S.M. Pubols and B.J. Sessle), pp. 93–106.

17 Efferent function of nociceptors

BRUCE LYNN

Introduction

Nociceptors are defined as afferent fibres signalling strong, injury-threatening stimuli or the presence of chemical irritants, including many inflammatory mediators. Yet, uniquely amongst afferent neurones, many nociceptors also have efferent actions in the tissue that they innervate. When excited, they release vasoactive peptides with potent actions on local blood vessels and on cells of the immune system. This phenomenon is termed neurogenic inflammation. Additionally, in some tissues substances released from nociceptive terminals may cause smooth muscle contraction, and in the airways may trigger the secretion of mucus. In this chapter several aspects of these efferent actions of nociceptors will be examined. First, a brief historical review will introduce the main features of neurogenic inflammation. Next, the question of which nociceptors are involved in different efferent actions will be addressed. The way these neurones can be selectively excited and often functionally blocked by capsaicin will be examined. Then, the nature of the released substances and their actions be considered. Finally, the evidence for a significant role for nociceptors (1) in triggering inflammation and (2) in the pathophysiology of some diseases (for example, arthritis, asthma) will be reviewed.

Historical background

That some somatosensory neurones had vasodilator actions was known before there was any clear definition of afferent classes such as nociceptors. Vasodilatation in response to stimulation of the dorsal (sensory) roots was first reported by Stricker in 1876 and was studied in detail by Bayliss (1901, 1902) who described clearly the main features (Fig. 17.1). This phenomenon of antidromic vasodilatation was shown to involve fibres with cell bodies in the posterior roots, to occur with relatively low-frequency stimulation, and to be slow in onset and recovery. Interest at this time centred on how this observation contradicted the Bell–Magendie law of separation of function (that is, dorsal roots sensory; ventral roots motor) and on the possible role of such fibres in reflex control of blood flow. Bayliss in fact presents indirect evidence for a role in reflex vasodilatation following stimulation of aortic baroreceptors (Bayliss 1902). Direct evidence for central activation of dorsal root afferents has, however, not been forthcoming. A clear description of how such fibres might be activated was provided by Bruce (1913) (Fig. 17.2). Bruce was studying the local inflammatory reaction following application of the chemical irritant mustard oil and found that this was reduced or abolished by chronic sensory denervation or by application of local anaesthetics. He therefore proposed that some afferent fibres might have, in addition to their afferent terminals, a second type of terminal that was motor to blood vessels (Fig. 17.2). The terminals on blood vessels would be activated following stimulation of the sensory terminals via an axon reflex, and would, of course, also be activated on antidromic stimulation of sensory nerves. Bruce also showed that this system of nerves could cause not only vasodilatation, but also—at least in the conjunctiva—marked oedema. Thus afferent neurones could produce two of the cardinal signs of inflammation, being able to increase vascular permeability as well as to dilate vessels.

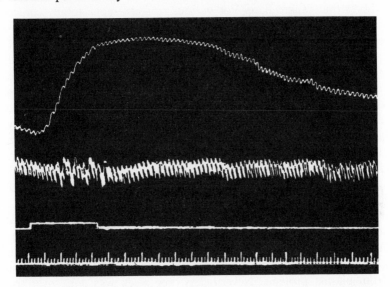

Fig. 17.1 Effect of electrical stimulation of the L7 dorsal root on blood flow in the paw of an anaesthetized dog. Upper trace, limb volume recorded by plethysmography. Second trace from top, blood pressure. Third trace, stimulus marker. Stimulus was at 40 Hz. Bottom trace, time marker, seconds and 5 seconds. Note the latent period of several seconds and the slow time course. From Bayliss (1901).

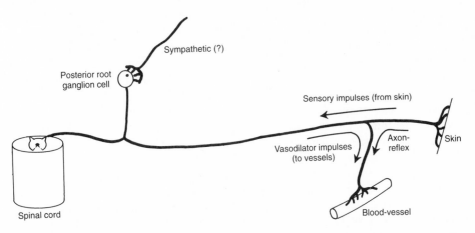

Fig. 17.2 Original diagram explaining how afferent neurones might generate inflammation by axon reflexes and on antidromic stimulation. From Bruce (1913).

The idea that local injury or irritation could trigger vascular changes by an axon reflex was taken up by Lewis (Lewis and Grant 1924; Lewis 1927). Lewis was investigating the 'triple response' of human skin to injury. He noted that the flare surrounding injuries was lost following chronic, but not acute, denervation. It therefore seemed likely to be due to the sort of axon reflex described by Bruce. Lewis was interested in the nature of the nerve fibres that caused flare. For various reasons—none totally convincing—he argued that true afferents were not involved. Instead he proposed a special system of non-sensory 'nocifensor' fibres arising from the dorsal root ganglia (DRG) whose function was to activate defensive changes at tissue level. As well as vasodilatation, Lewis proposed that nocifensor nerves could sensitize the true nociceptors and so cause hyperalgesia (Lewis 1937a,b). He believed that these fibres played a key role in secondary hyperalgesia, the increase in pain sensitivity in the flare zone around skin injuries. The idea of a non-sensory nocifensor system has never received much support. There is, after all, no great difficulty in assigning the efferent actions on blood vessels to fibres that also have an afferent function. Current ideas on the generation of secondary hyperalgesia are addressed by LaMotte, Chapter 16, this volume, and it is of interest to note that some recent studies have led to renewed suggestions that a special set of modulatory fibres without a direct sensory role may be involved (LaMotte 1992).

Between the 1930s and 1970s rather little attention was given to neural influences on inflammation. The axon reflex remained in texts of general pathology, but the emphasis had swung completely towards the control of inflammation by chemical mediators derived from non-neural cells (mast cells, polymorphonuclear leucocytes, macrophages, etc.) or from plasma proteins. Nevertheless, key work was done over this period. Antidromic vasodilatation was linked to C-fibre activation (Hinsey and Gasser 1930), and neurogenic vasodilator responses were shown to need noxious levels of stimulation and thus to involve nociceptors (Celander and Folkow 1953). But the most important studies were being carried out by N. Jancsó in Hungary. Jancsó was investigating the pharmacology of capsaicin, the active ingredient in hot peppers. Capsaicin could cause strong vasodilatation in innervated skin, but not in chronically denervated or locally anaesthetized skin. The inflammatory response to agents like capsaicin and mustard oil was termed neurogenic inflammation (N. Jancsó et al. 1967). As in the earlier work described above, Jancsó explained the actions of capsaicin in terms of the activation of nociceptor terminals. The important new finding of Jancsó was that capsaicin not only initially excited neurogenic inflammation, but could also, with sufficiently strong or repeated treatment, block neurogenic inflammation for variable, often long, periods. Capsaicin pretreatment thus provided a probe for investigating the nature of the fibres involved in neurogenic inflammation, and also a way of assessing, for any particular inflammatory model, whether there was a significant neurogenic contribution.

The discovery that re-stimulated widespread interest in neurogenic inflammation in the 1970s was that substance P, a peptide with known vascular actions, was preferentially located in small DRG neurones (Hökfelt et al. 1975) and their terminals. The subsequent characterization of calcitonin gene-related peptide (CGRP) and the demonstration that this also was present in many DRG neurones and afferent terminals (Rosenfeld et al. 1983) gave a further boost to interest in this area. The role of these potent vasoactive peptides following their release from afferent neurones clearly had to be taken seriously and there has been an explosion of interest in this area in the last two decades. The rest of this review will attempt to summarize this work.

Which nociceptors have what sorts of efferent actions?

In skin, marked vasodilatation follows C-fibre stimulation (Hinsey and Gasser 1930), and, at least in rats, increases in microvascular permeability leading to plasma extravasation also occur (N. Jancsó *et al.* 1967, 1968). A weaker dilatation can, however, be detected in rat and rabbit following Aδ-fibre stimulation (Lynn and Shakhanbeh 1988*a*; Jänig and Lisney 1989; Kolston and Lisney 1993). A-fibre stimulation does not produce plasma extravasation, however, unlike stimulation of C fibres (Jänig and Lisney 1989). The types of stimuli that evoke flare-like dilatations in skin are in the noxious range, so it appears that the non-nociceptive afferent C fibres (mechanoreceptors and thermoreceptors) are not involved. Most C-fibre nociceptors in skin are polymodal, responding to strong pressure, heat, and irritant chemicals, whilst a few appear to be mechanical nociceptors, responding only to strong pressure (see Campbell and Meyer, Chapter 5, this volume). The level of mechanical stimulation needed to evoke local vasodilatation in rat skin is well towards the upper end of the response range of C polymodal nociceptors (Lynn and Cotsell 1992). This result appears to indicate that the fibres involved must be among the least sensitive to pressure. However, direct stimulation of fine nerve filaments indicates that the majority of C polymodal units can evoke plasma extravasation (Kenins 1981; Bharali and Lisney 1992). At first sight these two results appear inconsistent. A possible reason may be that two distinct subpopulations of C nociceptors are involved. Certainly, the sites of action within the microvasculature are different since the vasodilation involves an action on arterioles, while the increases in microvascular permeability are restricted to postcapillary venules (Kenins 1984; Kowalski *et al.* 1990). If two subpopulations exist, then the C nociceptors involved in vasodilatation would have to be less mechanically sensitive than those that produce plasma extravasation. Or it may be that mechanical stimulation of terminals is not as effective in activating peptide release as is antidromic invasion of the terminals. Further work is needed to clarify the role of different C nociceptors in neurogenic inflammation in the skin. Recent work in the pig has revealed another type of cutaneous nociceptor with strong vasodilator actions (Pierau *et al.* 1995). These are heat nociceptors, C-fibre afferents that respond well to noxious heating and irritant chemicals, but weakly or not at all to pressure. On stimulating filaments containing such afferents, small zones of vasodilatation restricted to their afferent receptive fields were consistently found. This population of afferents comprises about 20 per cent of C fibres in the pig and similar units have been reported to comprise around 7 per cent of C fibres from monkey skin (Baumann *et al.* 1991). Note that heat units are not found in cutaneous nerves in the rat (Lynn and Carpenter 1982).

In other tissues the evidence is again that nociceptive C fibres cause neurogenic inflammation. In the knee joint of the cat, antidromic stimulation of C fibres, but not of Aδ fibres, causes increased vascular permeability (Ferrell and Russell 1986). In the gastrointestinal (GI) tract, antidromic afferent fibre stimulation causes increased blood flow in the stomach and the same fibre system appears to be activated by noxious chemical stimuli (high acidity, ethanol) (see review by Holzer 1993).

The GI tract is one of several tissues where stimuli likely to preferentially stimulate nociceptor terminals cause smooth muscle contractions that are lost after capsaicin pretreatment. These effects in the GI tract have been reviewed by Holzer (1993). Smooth muscle contractions associated with local activation of afferent, probably nociceptive, terminals are also seen in the bladder (Maggi and Meli 1986), iris (Mandahl and Bill 1981, 1984), and in the airways (see Lundberg 1993).

The airways are of particular interest since, in addition to constrictions, vasodilatation, and increased vascular permeability, two other effect of afferent nerves have been demonstrated. These are stimulation of mucus secretion (Tokuyama *et al.* 1990; Ramnarine and Rogers 1994; Ramnarine *et al.* 1994) and leucocyte adhesion (McDonald 1988). The afferents involved in all these actions appear to be the irritant receptors with C-fibre axons (Coleridge and Coleridge 1984), sensory units with a clearly nociceptor response profile. It appears that the unique vulnerability of the airways to air-borne particles and pathogens may have led to the development of particularly wide-ranging local defence mechanisms. In particular, fast reactions triggered by axon reflexes appear to be particularly important in the airways and operate alongside 'proper' reflexes, triggered in part by the same C nociceptors, such as coughing and sneezing.

Capsaicin

As well as eliciting a characteristic hot, painful sensation, capsaicin causes marked vasodilatation. This dilatation is absent in tissues with chronic sensory denervation and presumably arises due to the action of vasoactive mediators released from sensory nerve endings. Capsaicin is highly selective in its excitatory actions. In rat and rabbit, only C polymodal nociceptors are excited, and A-fibre nociceptors and A and C thermoreceptors and mechanoreceptors are not fired (Szolcsányi 1987; Szolcsányi *et al.* 1988). In primate skin, both polymodal and heat nociceptors are excited (Baumann *et al.* 1991).

Exposure to capsaicin at anything other than low doses leads to desensitization, and further applications of capsaicin are ineffective in causing vasodilatation or afferent excitation. The duration of desensitization depends on the dose, the route of administration, and the number of treatments (see Holzer 1991). In addition, there are species differences and the effects are different in neonatal and adult animals. Desensitization following topical application is usually temporary. For example, in man, repeated applications over 24 h reduce flare responses for 10–14 days (Carpenter and Lynn 1982). Direct application of capsaicin to nerve trunks in the rat almost completely abolishes neurogenic inflammation and the effects last at least 1 month (G. Jancsó *et al.* 1980*a*). A single injection in rats in the neonatal period (up to 2 days postnatal) is enough to permanently reduce neurogenic inflammation (G. Jancsó *et al.* 1980*b*). Single injections or a small number of repeat injections are less effective in adult rats and reduce neurogenic inflammation only transiently (G. Jancsó *et al.* 1980*b*). However, in the adult guinea-pig a single injection of capsaicin can permanently reduce neurogenic inflammation (N. Jancsó 1960, 1968). Some species are much less sensitive than rats or guinea-pigs. For example, application of capsaicin to a cutaneous nerve in the rabbit causes only a partial reduction in the neurogenic plasma extravasation due to mustard oil application (Lynn and Shakhanbeh 1988*b*). Birds appear to be completely insensitive to capsaicin (Szolcsańyi *et al.* 1986).

What is the mechanism of capsaicin desensitization? Initial studies focused on the fall in neuropeptide levels following capsaicin treatment, both in the nervous system and in non-nervous tissues (Jessell *et al.* 1978; Gamse *et al.* 1980; Nagy *et al.* 1980; Skofitsch and Jacobowitz 1985). For example, a single topical treatment of rat skin leads to halving of substance P levels for 1–4 days (Lynn *et al.* 1992). With nerve application or systemic treatment there are also large falls in tissue substance P levels. In these situations, however, there is an associated reduction in C-fibre numbers (G. Jancsó *et al.* 1985; Pini *et al.* 1990). In rats treated neonatally, the reduction in C-fibre numbers may be very large, falls of up to 94 per cent being reported (Nagy *et al.* 1983). Clearly, in the rat capsaicin acts as a C-fibre neurotoxin, and the changes in peptide levels are a consequence of C-fibre degeneration. With adult treatment in rats, loss of C fibres is highly selective with just a proportion of C polymodal nociceptors being lost and no effect on other classes of C fibre or on A-fibre afferents (Pini *et al.* 1990; Pini and Lynn 1991; Fig. 17.3). Neonatal treatment, in contrast, leads to loss of all types of C afferent approximately equally (Lynn 1984; Welk *et al.* 1984) and even loss of some A fibres at high doses (Nagy *et al.* 1983).

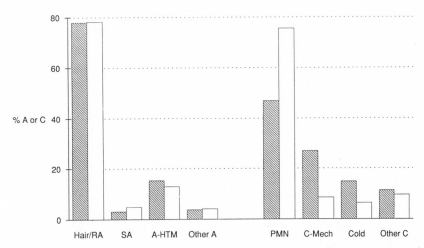

Fig. 17.3 Selective loss of polymodal nociceptors following capsaicin treatment. The proportions of different classes of afferent unit isolated from the rat saphenous nerve 1–46 days after application of 1 per cent capsaicin (hatched bars) or vehicle (open bars) to the nerve. Data for A fibres (*n* = 248, vehicle; *n* = 459, capsaicin) in the left half, for C-fibres (*n* = 94, vehicle; *n* = 115, capsaicin) in the right half. Hair/RA, sensitive, rapidly adapting mechanoreceptors usually associated with hair follicles; SA, slowly adapting mechanoreceptors, mostly type I; A-HTM, mechanical nociceptor units; PMN, polymodal nociceptor units; C-Mech, sensitive slowly adapting mechanoreceptors; Cold, cold-sensitive thermoreceptor units. Note that A-fibre proportions are unchanged in the capsaicin group, but the PMN group shows a large fall, while other C-fibre groups show a relative rise. Since absolute C-fibre numbers fall following the treatment, the actual numbers of non-PMN C afferents do not change significantly.

Most examples given above are for neurogenic inflammation in the skin. However, capsaicin also acts in many other tissues to reduce neurogenic inflammation in parallel with reductions in numbers of nerve fibres and terminals and in neuropeptide content. Detailed information is available for the airways (see review by Lundberg 1993), the bladder (see Maggi and Meli 1988), and the GI tract (see Holzer 1993). In some tissues capsaicin also abolishes elements of normal physiological responses, for example, changes in motility in the stomach (Laird *et al.* 1991) and inotropic actions on heart muscle in the guinea-pig (Miyauchi *et al.* 1987; Maggi *et al.* 1988). There must be some question as to whether the neurons involved in these effects are nociceptors. It may be that, in some visceral areas, capsaicin is affecting non-nociceptive as well as nociceptive neurones. An alternative possibility is that the neurones in question belong to the 'wide dynamic range' or 'intensity encoding' type described in some visceral nerves (see Cervero and Jänig 1992; Cervero, Chapter 9, this volume).

With its rather selective action on the afferent neurones that have efferent actions, capsaicin has proved a useful tool in investigating whether these efferent actions make a significant contribution to physiological or pathological processes. Before moving on to this topic, however, the question of how the efferent actions of nociceptors are brought about will be addressed.

How nociceptors cause their effects

As described by Lawson (Chapter 3, this volume), a feature of many somatovisceral neurones is that they contain one or more peptides of the 'neuropeptide' group, including substance P, neurokinin A (NKA), CGRP, and vasoactive intestinal peptide (VIP). In particular, large numbers of the smaller DRG neurones, with small myelinated (Aδ) or unmyelinated (C) axons contain either substance P or CGRP or both. Since a high proportion of these small neurones are nociceptors, it follows that many nociceptors will contain neuropeptides. In the rat, application of capsaicin to a cutaneous nerve leads to: (1) an 85 per cent fall in skin substance P levels; and (2) a selective loss of nociceptive fibres of the polymodal type (Pini and Lynn 1991; Fig. 17.3). It therefore appears that, in rat skin, substance P is largely present only in polymodal nociceptors. The evidence that nociceptors exert their pro-inflammatory actions by releasing neuropeptides into the tissues that they innervate is now strong and three aspects will be considered here: (1) the release of neuropeptides following nociceptor stimulation; (2) the actions of exogenously administered neuropeptides compared with the effects of nociceptor stimulation; and (3) the block of nociceptor-induced affects by selective neuropeptide antagonists.

Release of neuropeptides following nociceptor stimulation

Direct evidence for neuropeptide release following nerve stimulation was first found in the feline tooth pulp where, following afferent nerve stimulation, substance p-like immunoreactivity was detected in superfusates and the tissue content fell (Olgart *et al.* 1977; Brodin *et al.* 1981). Subsequently, nerve stimulation has been shown to release substance P in the rabbit eye (Bill *et al.* 1979) and the rat skin (White and Helme 1985) and lungs (Saria *et al.* 1988). Clearly, stimulation-evoked substance P release is widespread across a range of tissues and species. Other studies have shown release of NKA (for example Saria *et al.* 1988) and CGRP (for example, Wahlesdedt *et al.* 1986). Noxious stimuli can also provoke neuropeptide release in normally innervated tissues, but not after denervation or capsaicin pretreatment. Thus intermittent skin heating to 50°C evoked substance P release in normally innervated rat skin, but not after chronic denervation (Helme *et al.* 1986). Capsaicin itself can evoke immediate release of neuropeptides, for example release of substance P, NKA, and an eledoisin-like peptide from lungs or ureter in the rat (Saria *et al.* 1985; Hua *et al.* 1986). Finally, bradykinin and low pH, two other effective stimuli for C-fibre nociceptors, can release CGRP from various tissues. Bradykinin caused release from guinea-pig atrial strips (Geppetti *et al.* 1990*b*) and acid solutions evoked release from guinea-pig bladder (Geppetti *et al.* 1990*a*), and heart (Franco-Cereceda *et al.* 1993) and from gastric tissue in the rat (Geppetti *et al.* 1991).

Release of neuropeptides from nerve terminals appears to be from vesicles by a conventional calcium-dependent mechanism (Maggi 1993). Neuropeptides are present in nerve terminals in many tissues and appear to be localized in large dense-cored vesicles (for example CGRP and substance P, Gulbenkian *et al.* 1986; VIP, Lee *et al.* 1984). Release of neuropeptides following electrical stimulation is calcium-dependent and is blocked by the calcium channel blocker omega conotoxin in several tissues (Maggi 1991; Lou *et al.* 1992; Lundberg *et al.* 1992).

Actions of neuropeptides

All the neuropeptides mentioned above, the neurokinins (substance P, neurokinin A), CGRP, and VIP, are vasodilators in a range of tissues. CGRP is the most potent and has the longest duration of action. Thus the concentration for half maximal effect (EC$_{50}$ for arteriolar dilatation in the superfused hamster cheek pouch is approximately 2.10^{-11} M (Hall and Brain 1992), while when injected into human or rabbit skin, doses of 25 fmol in 0.1 ml cause significant vasodilatation (Brain *et al.* 1985). CGRP also causes dilatation in many other tissues and species including skeletal muscle (rabbit, Ohlen *et al.* 1987), coronary vessels (human, Franco-Cereceda and Rudehill 1989; rat, Holman *et al.* 1986), mesentery (rat, Marshall *et al.* 1986; human, Tornebrandt *et al.* 1987) and other parts of the splanchnic circulation (see Holzer 1993), cerebral arteries (McCulloch *et al.* 1986; Uddman *et al.* 1986), and the knee joint (rat, Lam and Ferrell 1993). Substance P is less potent than CGRP, but still causes marked vasodilatation at quite low concentrations in some tissues. For example, 3 nM substance P superfused over the hamster cheek pouch can cause significant arteriolar dilatation (Hall *et al.* 1994) and 10 nM will cause a 100 per cent increase in diameter in vessels in skeletal muscle in rabbits (Ohlen *et al.* 1987). Substance P also dilates vessels in rat skeletal muscle (Baptist and Marshall 1993) and in tooth pulp (cat, Gazelius *et al.* 1981; Rosell *et al.* 1981), pial arteries (cat, Edvinsson *et al.* 1981), and knee joint (rat, Lam and Ferrell 1993). In contrast, in rabbit skin substance P has almost no vasodilatory effect (Brain *et al.* 1985). NKA has been shown to dilate hamster cheek pouch arterioles (Hall *et al.* 1994) and skeletal muscle vessels (Ohlen *et al.* 1987), but with 10 times less potency than substance P. VIP is a very effective dilator in rabbit skin, with an EC$_{50}$ of approximately 100 nM for intradermal injection (Williams 1982). VIP also dilates cerebral arteries (Lee *et al.* 1984; Edvinsson *et al.* 1985) and mesenteric vessels (Tornebrandt *et al.* 1987).

Substance P can cause increased microvascular permeability in skin (Hagermark *et al.* 1978; Chahl 1979; Foreman *et al.* 1983). As with nerve stimulation, the effect is limited to venules (Kenins *et al.* 1984). Plasma extravasation is also seen in response to substance P in bladder (Koltzenburg and McMahon 1986; Lundberg *et al.* 1984), airways (Saria *et al.* 1983), and in parts of the splanchnic circulation (Lundberg *et al.* 1984; Szolcsányi 1988). The closely related neurokinin NKA has much lower potency than substance P whether tested in skin (Andrews *et al.* 1989) or the airways (Saria *et al.* 1983). CGRP (Gamse and

Saria 1985) and VIP (Chahl 1979; Gamse *et al.* 1980; Williams 1982) have no effect on microvascular permeability.

The contraction of smooth muscle in the guinea-pig ileum was for many years a standard bioassay for substance P. Substance P can also contract smooth muscle of the airways (see Lundberg 1993), the ureters (Hua and Lundberg 1986; Maggi *et al.* 1986*b*), bladder (Maggi and Meli 1986), and the iris (Hall *et al.* 1993*b*). Neurokinin A also contracts many smooth muscle preparations and is particularly effective on airway smooth muscle, where it is much more potent than substance P (see Lundberg 1993). CGRP, on the other hand, is a smooth muscle relaxant, for example, in the rat duodenum (Maggi *et al.* 1986*a*) and the ureter (Hua *et al.* 1986; Maggi *et al.* 1986*b*).

Stimulation of mucus secretion from the airways is another action of nociceptors that is mimicked by substance P. For example, nasal secretion is stimulated in the rat (Malm and Peterson 1985) and mucus secretion is stimulated from ferret trachea (Ramnarine *et al.* 1994) and human bronchi (Rogers *et al.* 1989). NKA is less potent than substance P (Ramnarine *et al.* 1994) and CGRP has only weak actions (Webber *et al.* 1991).

The final area where there is evidence for efferent actions of nociceptors is that of leucocyte adhesion. Here there is again strong evidence for parallel actions of neuropeptides. For example, in human skin, substance P, CGRP, and VIP all promote neutrophil influx into the dermis following intradermal injection (Smith *et al.* 1993). This influx is accompanied in endothelial cells by translocation of P-selectin to the luminal surface and the upregulation of E-selectin. Expression of the cell adhesion molecules, VCAM-1 and ECAM-1, was unchanged over the 8-h study period. Substance P, but not CGRP or VIP, induced eosinophils, as well as neutrophils, to enter the human dermis (Smith *et al.* 1993). Leucocyte aggregation has also been seen in the microcirculation of rabbit skeletal muscle following topical application of substance P, but not with CGRP (Ohlen *et al.* 1987). In addition to neuropeptide actions on leucocyte adhesion, a large number of other stimulatory actions on cells of the immune system have been reported, mostly from *in vitro* studies (see Stein, Chapter 18, this volume). Most of these actions, such as leucocyte chemotaxis or activation of macrophages, have not so far been studied following selective nociceptor activation.

Block of nociceptor-induced affects by selective neuropeptide antagonists

Recently, the first effective competitive antagonist for CGRP has become available ($CGRP_{8-37}$) (Han *et al.* 1990; Hughes and Brain 1991) and the first selective, high-affinity antagonists for individual neurokinin receptor subtypes NK_1, NK_2, and NK_3 (preferred endogenous ligands substance P, neurokinin A, and neurokinin B, respectively; For example, see reviews by Hall *et al.* 1993*a*; Maggi *et al.* 1993). Note that some of the early neurokinin antagonists turned out to have substantial side-effects; for example, the local anaesthetic-like action of [D-Pro^2,D-Trp^{7,9}] substance P, an early substance P antagonist (Post *et al.* 1985) and calcium channel blocking by CP-96,345, the first non-peptide neurokinin antagonist (Schmidt *et al.* 1992; see also Maggi *et al.* 1993). It is thus necessary to be careful in interpreting results with these compounds purely in terms of neuropeptide actions.

Neurogenic vasodilatation following topical capsaicin is completely inhibited by $CGRP_{8-37}$ in rat and rabbit skin and vasodilatation in response to nerve stimulation is inhibited by 76 per cent (Escott and Brain 1993; Hughes and Brain 1994). This antagonist also significantly blocks acid- and capsaicin-induced vasodilatation in gastric mucosa and dilatation from electrical field stimulation in mesenteric arteries (Han *et al.* 1990; Kawasaki *et al.* 1991; Li *et al.* 1992). The antagonist data fits well with the powerful vasodilatory action of CGRP and shows that vasodilatation due to nociceptor activation is largely due to CGRP release.

The plasma extravasation that follows nerve stimulation is also reduced by $CGRP_{8-37}$ (Escott and Brain 1993). However, since CGRP itself does not increase vascular permeability, this effect is likely to be secondary to the increased blood flow, a change that will enhance any extravasation due to permeability increases induced by other mediators (Brain and Williams 1986, 1989). Plasma extravasation following nerve stimulation in the rat skin is totally inhibited by NK_1-selective antagonists (Garret *et al.* 1991; Lembeck *et al.* 1992) and by other neurokinin antagonists (Xu *et al.* 1991). Plasma extravasation in the airways following vagal stimulation is also greatly reduced or abolished by NK_1 antagonists (Lembeck *et al.* 1992; Ball *et al.* 1993; see review by Lundberg 1993). Of the endogenous neurokinins, substance P has the highest affinity for the NK_1 receptor. Therefore, these results, together with the efficacy of substance P in causing plasma extravasation and its release following nerve stimulation, provide strong evidence for a major role for substance P in nociceptor-induced increases in vascular permeability. Mucus secretion from the ferret trachea following electrical stimulation in the presence of autonomic blocking drugs is also significantly inhibited (by 73 per cent) by selective NK_1 antagonists, but not by NK_2 antagonists (Ramnarine *et al.* 1994). Airway mucus secretion therefore appears to be another nociceptor efferent action that depends on substance P release.

Smooth muscle contraction due to electrical stimulation of nerve terminals in the iris is completely inhibited by NK_1 antagonists (Hall *et al.* 1993c). In the airways, bronchoconstriction due to nerve stimulation or capsaicin is greatly reduced in the guinea-pig by NK_2 antagonists, while NK_1 blockers have less effect (see Lundberg 1993). This fits with the greater potency of NKA in causing airway constriction in the guinea-pig (and other species). Airway constriction is at present the only action of nociceptors that has been clearly shown to involve NKA.

Overview of neuropeptide involvement in nociceptor-mediated efferent actions

The evidence that neuropeptides are the main mediators of the efferent actions of nociceptors is now extensive, covering the different actions of nociceptors in a range of tissues and species. Vasodilatation appears to be largely due to CGRP release. Increased microvascular permeability, on the other hand, seems to be largely a substance P-mediated effect. A role for NKA has only been clearly established for smooth muscle contraction in the airways. The main nociceptor-mediated effects and the mediators involved are shown in Fig. 17.4 for the skin (A) and the airways (B). Co-release of substance P and NKA has been demonstrated in the lung (Saria *et al.* 1988), and presumably this is the usual pattern since they are synthesized from the same precursor protein (Nawa *et al.* 1983; Carter and Krause 1990; see Maggi *et al.* 1993). Many neurones also have both substance P and CGRP present and they are co-released. Functionally, co-release of a dilator (CGRP) and a mediator that increases vascular permeability (substance P) will lead to enhanced plasma extravasation and oedema. The ability of nociceptor stimulation to trigger leucocyte infiltration may also be a neuropeptide effect, but no data using specific receptor antagonists is available. The ability of substance P to attract and activate cells of the immune system has, however, been repeatedly demonstrated. Whether such effects occur *in vivo* following nociceptor activation merits investigation.

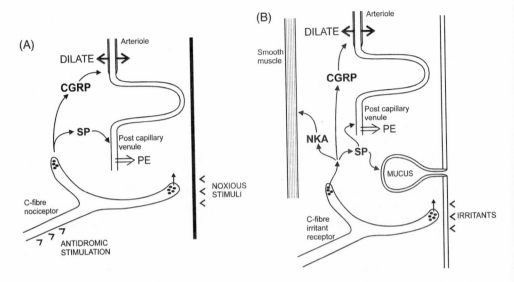

Fig. 17.4 The main efferent actions of nociceptors and the mediators involved in (A) skin and (B) airways. The attraction of leucocytes is not shown, but is a known effect of neuropeptides in skin, and of nerve stimulation in the airways. SP, Substance P; NKA, neurokinin A; CGRP, calcitonin gene-related peptide; PE, plasma extravasation.

How important is neuropeptide release from nociceptive endings in inflammation, other tissue reactions, and in diseases?

The demonstration that neuropeptides released from nociceptors can have major actions, for example, on the microvasculature or on smooth muscle, leads to consideration of whether such actions play an important role in pathophysiology. For example, in real inflammatory diseases do the nociceptor endings contribute to the pathological processes? Three types of experiments have been done to investigate such questions. First, the effects of chronic denervation have been examined, although interpretation can be tricky since cutting nerves can lead to changes in use of a body part, possibly leading to secondary changes in function not directly related to the innervation itself. Also, section of a peripheral nerve often removes at least part of the autonomic innervation, again complicating the interpretation of any changes in function. A second approach is to use capsaicin pretreatment. This is always more selective than total denervation, although with large neonatal dosage the effect may not be restricted to nociceptors. Adult systemic or local treatment in the rat does seem to target just C-fibre nociceptors and, particularly, the ones that cause efferent actions. Capsaicin treatment has therefore proved extremely useful in establishing whether a neurogenic, nociceptor-derived element is present in many conditions. The third approach is to use neuropeptide antagonists. The newer, high-affinity neurokinin antagonists are proving particularly useful. However, it is important to remember that in the GI tract there are neurokinin-containing neurones within the intrinsic, enteric, nervous elements.

Acute inflammatory models

Clearly, inflammatory responses such as flare are completely blocked by any treatment that interferes with the afferent innervation of the skin. So are vasodilatation and plasma extravasation caused by 'neurogenic' irritants such as capsaicin and mustard oil. But is there a nociceptor-related component in more general inflammatory models that are not normally thought of as neurogenic? The inflammation that follows injection of carrageenan into the rat paw is a commonly used model system for investigating inflammatory mediators, and several studies have looked for a neurogenic component, with variable results. One study found no significant reduction in paw oedema either with chronic denervation, capsaicin pretreatment, or injection of spantide, an early substance P antagonist (Ohkubo *et al.* 1990). Similarly, no significant effect of capsaicin treatment could be detected by Newbold and Brain (1993). On the other hand, Jamieson *et al.* (1986) did find a 30 per cent reduction in oedema after nerve treatment with capsaicin. Finally, treatment with neurokinin antagonists have been found to cause quite large reductions in paw oedema by two groups (Birch *et al.* 1992; Yamamoto *et al.* 1993), although the effect of one of the antagonists (CP-96,345) was not stereospecific (Yamamoto *et al.* 1993). On balance, it looks as though release of neuropeptides by nociceptors may be part of the response to carrageenan, but is certainly not all of it.

A similar pattern of mostly modest reductions in acute inflammation has been seen in a range of experimental systems, either due to capsaicin pretreatment or neurokinin antagonists, for example, skin oedema from noxious heating (Saria 1984; Haegerstrand *et al.* 1987), passive cutaneous anaphylaxis (Brain and Wolstencroft 1993), and adjuvant-induced arthritis in the rat (Colpaert *et al.* 1983; Jamieson *et al.* 1986; Levine *et al.* 1986). Rather larger effects have been reported on the increase in lung solute clearance that follows antigen challenge (Sestina *et al.* 1989). Not much attention has been paid to CGRP, but there is evidence from studies using the antagonist $CGRP_{8-37}$ that a significant part of the long-lasting cutaneous hyperaemia that follows exposure to ultraviolet light is due to CGRP (Gillardon *et al.* 1993).

The role of neurogenic factors in disease

There has been much discussion of possible neurogenic components in disease (see, for example, Lynn 1988; Maggi *et al.* 1993). Clearly, disorders where inflammation is a prime feature are possible candidates and several groups have proposed an involvement of nociceptors in rheumatoid arthritis (Colpaert *et al.* 1983; Levine *et al.* 1985; Kidd *et al.* 1990). The airways, with the extensive neurogenic responses found there, are another promising area and Barnes (1986, 1989, 1990) has proposed a possible role in asthma. Moving away from strictly inflammatory disorders, it has been proposed that neurogenic mechanisms, probably involving CGRP release from nociceptors, are responsible for protecting the gastrointestinal mucosa and that defects in this system may lead to formation of gastric or duodenal ulcers (see Holzer 1993 for a review). Another potentially important pathological action of nociceptors is in the causation of headache. Trigeminal fibres innervating the pial vessels can cause marked dilatation, and it has been proposed that this system is involved in headache (Moskowitz *et al.* 1983;

Moskowitz and Buzzi 1991). An extensive list of further conditions where a neurogenic component is suspected, such as chronic inflammation of the GI tract and ocular inflammatory disease, is given by Maggi *et al.* (1993).

Conclusions

A major function of nociceptors is to signal to the central nervous system (CNS) about inflammation, injury, and the threat of injury, and most of this book is concerned with this topic. However, it is clear that a subset of nociceptors with C-fibre axons can also directly trigger rapid local defensive responses. That is, they play a nocifensor role, combining nociception with a direct local defence role. These efferent actions involve release of CGRP and neurokinins. The importance of the local changes triggered by nociceptors, compared with the parallel effects triggered directly by the blood vessels or by cells of the immune system, remains to be established. However, there is evidence for a significant role in many tissues and the availability of high-affinity NK antagonists is leading to further discoveries in this area.

These reactions of the tissue to injury are summarized in Fig. 17.5. This figure also makes the further point that not only can nociceptors release pro-inflammatory agents, but also that many of the classical mediators of inflammation can excite or sensitize

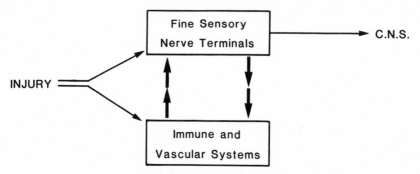

Fig. 17.5   Diagram summarizing the effects of injury on nociceptors and the immune and vascular systems. Note that the reciprocal links between nociceptors and the immune and vascular systems, representing neurogenic inflammation and nociceptor sensitization respectively, form a potential positive-feedback loop.

nociceptor endings (see Kress and Reeh, Chapter 11 and Meyer *et al.*, Chapter 15, this volume). Further, the existence of ongoing inflammation can actually lead to increases in neuropeptide-containing nerve terminals, for example, as seen in inflamed joint tissues in arthritis models in the rat (Levine *et al.* 1985) and cat (Hanesch *et al.* 1994). These two-way interactions between the cellular and vascular components of inflammation and the nociceptor terminals form a potential positive-feedback loop. This system could run out of control and possibly does in some disease states. Obviously, there need to be controls to ensure that normally this cannot happen. In fact, the ways in which the efferent function of nociceptors are controlled have not been extensively examined. Several compounds are known to reduce neurogenic inflammation including opioids, cortico-trophin-releasing factor (CRF), and galanin (another neuropeptide in afferent neurones) (see Maggi 1991 for further examples). There is also evidence for autoreceptors for neuropeptides on nociceptor terminals, for example, CGRP (Nuki *et al.* 1994). To understand the role of these inhibitory systems is one of several challenges that face us in the continuing investigation of this unique efferent role of somatovisceral 'afferent' neurones.

References

Andrews, P.V., Helme, R.D., and Thomas, K.L. (1989). NK-1 receptor mediation of neurogenic plasma extravasation in rat skin. *Br. J. Pharmacol.* **97**, 1232–8.

Ball, D.I., Pendry, Y.D., and Sheldrick, R.L.G. (193). Characterization of tachykinin receptors mediating vagally-induced bronchoconstriction and plasma-protein extravasation in the guinea-pig. *Neuropeptides* **24**, 191.

Baptist, G. and Marshall, J.M. (1993). Vasodilatation mediated by the sensory nerve fibres in the arterioles of skeletal muscle of the anaesthetized rat. *J. Physiol.* **467**, 35P.

Barnes, P.J. (1986). Asthma as an axon reflex. *Lancet* **i**, 242–4.

Barnes, P.J. (1989). Airway neuropeptides: roles in fine tuning and in disease? *News physiol. Sci.* **4**, 116–20.

Barnes, P.J. (1990). Neurogenic inflammation in airways and its modulation. *Arch. int. Pharmacodyn,* **303**, 67–82.

Baumann, T.K., Simone, D.A., Shain, C.H., and LaMotte, R.H. (1991). Neurogenic hyperalgesia: the search for the primary cutaneous afferent fibers that contribute to capsaicin-induced pain and hyperalgesia. *J. Neurophysiol.* **66**, 212–27.

Bayliss, W.M. (1901). On the origin from the spinal cord of the vaso-dilator fibres of the hind-limb, and on the nature of these fibres. *J. Physiol.* **26**, 173–209.

Bayliss, W.M. (1902). Further researches on antidromic nerve-impulses. *J. Physiol.* **28**, 276–99.

Bharali, L.A. and Lisney, S.J.W. (1992). The relationship between unmyelinated afferent type and neurogenic plasma extravasation in normal and reinnervated rat skin. *Neuroscience* **47**, 703–12.

Bill, A., Stjernschantz, J., Mandahl, A., Brodin, E., and Nilsson, G. (1979). Substance P: release on trigeminal nerve stimulation, effects in the eye. *Acta physiol. scand.* **106**, 371–3.

Birch, P.J., Harrison, S.M., Hayes, A.G., Rogers, H., and Tyers M.B. (1992). The nonpeptide NK_1 receptor antagonist, (+/−)-CP-96,345, produces antinociceptive and anti-edema effects in the rat. *Br. J. Pharmacol.* **105**, 508–10.

Brain, S.D. and Williams, T.J. (1986). Inflammatory oedema induced by synergism between calcitonin gene-related peptide (CGRP) and mediators of increased vascular permeability. *Br. J. Pharmacol.* **86**, 855–60.

Brain, S.D. and Williams, T.J. (1989). Interactions between tachykinins and calcitonin gene-related peptide lead to the modulation of oedema formation and blood flow in rat skin. *Br. J. Pharmacol.* **97**, 77–82.

Brain, S.D. and Wolstencroft, P. (193). The inhibition of substance P, neurokinin A and allergic oedema formation in guinea-pig skin by RP67580. *Neuropeptides* **24**, 196.

Brain, S.D., Williams, T.J., Tippins, J.R., Morris, H.R., and McIntyre, I. (1985). Calcitonin gene-related peptide is a potent vasodilator. *Nature* **313**, 54–6.

Brodin, E., Gazelius, B., Olgart, L., and Nilsson G. (1981). Tissue concentration and release of substance P-like immunoreactivity in the dental pulp. *Acta physiol. scand.* **111**, 141–9.

Bruce, A.N. (1913). Vaso-dilator axon-reflexes. *Quart. J. exp. Physiol.* **6**, 339–54.

Carpenter, S.E. and Lynn, B. (1982). Vascular and sensory responses of human skin to mild heat injury after topical treatment with capsaicin. *Br. J. Pharmacol.* **73**, 453–9.

Carter, M.S. and Krause, J.E. (1990). Structure expression and some regulatory mechanisms of the rat preprotachykinin gene ecoding substance P, neurokinin A, neuropeptide K and neuropeptide . *J. Neurosci.* **10**, 2203.

Calender, O. and Folkow, B. (1953). The nature and the distribution of afferent fibres provided with the axon reflex arrangement. *Acta physiol. scand.* **29**, 359–70.

Cervero, F. and Jänig, W. (1992). Visceral nociceptors: a new world order? *Trends Neurosci.* **15**, 374–8.

Chahl, L.A. (1979). The effect of putative peptide neurotransmitters on cutaneous vascular permeability in the rat. *Nannyn-Schmiedebergs Arch. Pharmacol.* **309**, 159–163.

Coleridge, J.C.G. and Coleridge, H.M. (1984). Afferent vagal C-fibre innervation of the lungs and airways and its functional significance. *Rev. Physiol. Biochem. Pharmacol.* **99**, 1–110.

Colpaert, F.J., Donnerer, J., and Lembeck, F. (1983). Effects of capsaicin on inflammation and on the substance P content of nervous tissues in rats with adjuvant arthritis. *Life Sci.* **32**, 1827–34.

Edvinsson, L., McCulloch, J., and Uddman, R. (1981). Substance P: immunohistochemical localization and effect upon cat pial arteries in vitro and in situ. *J. Physiol.* **318**, 251–8.

Edvinsson, L., Fredholm, B.B., Hamel, E., Jansen, I., and Verrecchia, C. (1985). Perivascular peptides relax cerebral arteries concomitant with stimulation of cyclic adenosine monophosphate accumulation or release of an endothelium-derived relaxing factor in the cat. *Neurosci. Lett.* **58**, 213–17.

Escott, K.J. and Brain, S.D. (1993). Effect of a calcitonin gene-related peptide antagonist (CGRP8-37) on skin vasodilatation and oedema induced by stimulation of the rat saphenous nerve. *Br. J. Pharmacol.* **110**, 772–6.

Ferrell, W.R. and Russell, N.J.W. (1986). Extravasation in the knee induced by antidromic stimulation of articular C-fibre afferents of the anaesthetised cat. *J. Physiol.* **379**, 407–16.

Foreman, J.C., Jordan, C.C., Oehme, P., and Renner, H. (1983). Structure–function relationships for some substance P-related peptides that cause wheal and flare reactions in human skin. *J. Physiol.* **335**, 449–65.

Franco-Cereceda, A. and Rudehill, A. (1989). Capsaicin-induced vasodilatation of human coronary arteries in vitro is mediated by calcitonin gene-related peptide rather than substance P or neurokinin A. *Acta physiol. scand.* **136**, 575–80.

Franco-Cereceda, A., Kallner, G., and Lundberg, J.M. (1993). Capsazepine-sensitive release of calcitonin gene-related peptide from C-fibre afferents in the guinea-pig heart by low pH and lactic acid. *Eur. J. Pharmacol.* **238**, 311–16.

Gamse, R. and Saria, A. (1985). Potentiation of tachykinin-induced plasma protein extravasation by calcitonin gene-related peptide. *Eur. J. Pharmacol.* **114**, 61–6.

Gamse, R., Holzer, P. and Lembeck, F. (1980). Decrease of substance P in primary afferent neurones and impairment of neurogenic plasma extravasation by capsaicin. *Br. J. Pharmacol.* **68**, 207–13.

Garret, C., Carruette, A., and Fardin, V., Moussaoui, S., Peyronel, J.F., Blanchard, J.C., and Laduron P.M. (1991). Pharmacological properties of a potent and selective nonpeptide substance P antagonist. *Proc. natl Acad. Sci. USA* **88**, 10208–12.

Gazelius, B., Brodin, E., Olgart, L., and Panopoulos, P. (1981). Evidence that substance P is a mediator of antidromic vasodilatation using somatostatin as a release inhibitor. *Acta physiol. scand.* **113**, 155–9.

Geppetti, P., Tramontana, M., Patacchini, R., Del-Bianco, E., Santicioli, P., and Maggi, C.A. (1990*a*). Neurochemical evidence for the activation of the 'efferent' function of capsaicin-sensitive nerves by lowering of the pH in the guinea-pig urinary bladder. *Neurosci. Lett.* **114**, 101–6.

Geppetti, P., Tramontana, M., Santicioli, P., Del-Bianco, E., Giuliani, S., and Maggi, C.A. (1990*b*). Bradykinin-induced release of calcitonin gene-related peptide from capsaicin-sensitive nerves in guinea-pig atria: mechanism of action and calcium requirements. *Neuroscience* **38**, 687–92.

Geppetti, P., Tramontana, M., Evangelista, S., Renzi, D., Maggi, C.A., Fusco, B.M., and Del-Bianco, E. (1991). Differential effect on neuropeptide release of different concentrations of hydrogen ions on afferent and intrinsic neurons of the rat stomach. *Gastroenterology* **101**, 1505–11.

Gillardon, F., Eschenfelder, C., Benrath, J., and Zimmermann, M. (1993). The sunburn reaction in rat skin: evidence for a neurogenic component in cutaneous inflammation following ultraviolet irradiation. *Neuropeptides* **24**, 195.

Gulbenkian, S., Merighi, A., Wharton, J., Varndell, I.M., and Polak, J.M. (1986). Ultrastructural evidence for the coexistence of calcitonin gene-related peptide and substance P in secretory vesicles of peripheral nerves in the guinea pig. *J. Neurocytol.* **15**, 535–42.

Haegerstrand, A., Dalsgaard, C-J., and Jonsson, C-E. (1987). Effects of capsaicin pretreatment on the inflammatory response to scalding injury in the rat. *Acta physiol. scand.* **130**, 345–8.

Hagermark, O., Hökfelt, T., and Pernow, B. (1978). Flare and itch induced by substance P in human skin. *J. invest. Dermatol.* **71**, 233–5.

Hall, J.M. and Brain S.D. (1992). Quantification of the vasodilator effects of CGRP, Amylin and [Cys(ACM)2–7]-hCGRPalpha on the microvasculature of the hamster cheek pouch in vivo. *Neuropeptides* **24**, 207.

Hall, J.M., Caulfield, M.P., Watson, S.P., and Guard, S. (1993a). Receptor subtypes or species homologues: relevance to drug discovery. *Trends pharmacol. Sci.* **14**, 376–83.

Hall, J.M., Mitchell, D., and Morton, I.K. (1993b). Does substance P release mediate NANC nerve-mediated responses to field stimulation and ligands, in the rabbit isolated sphincter pupillae? *Regulat. Peptides* **46**, 278–81.

Hall, J.M., Mitchell, D., and Morton, I.K. (1993c). Tachykinin receptors mediating responses to sensory nerve stimulation and exogenous tachykinins and analogues in the rabbit isolated iris sphincter. *Br. J. Pharmacol.* **109**, 1008–13.

Hall, J.M., Butt, S., and Brain, S.D. (1994). SR140333 inhibits NK$_1$-receptor mediated vasodilatation in hamster cheek pouch microvasculature. *Neuropeptides* **26** (April suppl. 1), 39.

Han, S.P., Naes, L., and Westfall, T.C. (1990). Inhibition of periarterial nerve stimulation-induced vasodilation of the mesenteric arterial bed by CGRP (8–37) and CGRP receptor desensitization. *Biochem. Biophys. Res. Commun.* **168**, 786–91.

Hanesch, U., Heppelmann, B., and Schmidt, R.F. (1994). Acute monoarthritis of the cat's knee joint alters the proportion of CGRP-immunoreactive articular fibres. *Neuropeptides* **26**, 57.

Helme, R.D., Koschorke, G.M., and Zimmermann, M. (1986). Immunoreactive substance P release from skin nerves in the rat by noxious thermal stimulation. *Neurosci. Lett.* **63**, 295–9.

Hinsey, J.C. and Gasser, H.S. (1930). The component of the dorsal root mediating vasodilatation and the Sherrington contracture. *Am. J. Physiol.* **92**, 679–89.

Hökfelt, T., Kellerth, J.O., Nilsson, G., and Pernow, B. (1975). Substance P: localization in the central nervous system and in some primary sensory neurons. *Science* **190**, 889–90.

Holman, J.J., Craig, R.K., and Marshall, I. (1986). Human alpha- and beta-CGRP and rat alpha-CGRP are coronary vasodilators in the rat. *Peptides* **7**, 231–5.

Holzer, P. (1991). Capsaicin: cellular targets, mechanisms of action and selectivity for thin sensory neurons. *Pharmacol. Rev.* **43**, 143–201.

Holzer, P. (1993). Capsaicin-sensitive nerves in the control of vascular effector mechanisms. In pain (ed. J.N. Wood), pp.191–218. Academic Press, London.

Hua, X-Y. and Lundberg, J.M. (1986). Dual capsaicin effects on ureteric motility: low dose inhibition mediated by calcitonin gene-related peptide and high dose stimulation by tachykinins? *Acta physiol. scand.* **128**, 453.

Hua, X-Y., Saria, A., Gamse, R., Theodorsson-Norheim, E., Brodin, E., and Lundberg, J.M. (1986). Capsaicin induced release of multiple tachykinins (substance P, neurokinin A and eledoisin-like material) from guinea-pig spinal cord and ureter. *Neuroscience* **19**, 313–19.

Hughes, S.R. and Brain, S.D. (1991). A calcitonin gene-related peptide (CGRP) antagonist (CGRP8-37) inhibits microvascular responses induced by CGRP and capsaicin in skin. *Br. J. Pharmacol.* **104**, 738–42.

Hughes, S.R. and Brain, S.D. (1994). Nitric oxide-dependent release of vasodilator quantities of calcitonin gene-related peptide from capsaicin-sensitive nerves in rabbit skin. *Br. J. Pharmacol.* **111**, 425–30.

Jamieson, A., Russell, N.J.W., and Rance, M.J. (1986). An assessment of the neurogenic component in models of inflammation. *Br. J. Pharmacol.* **86**, 787.

Jancsó, G., Kiraly, E., and Jancsó-Gabor, A. (1980*a*). Chemosensitive pain fibres and inflammation. *Int. J. Tissue Reactions* **2**, 57–66.

Jancsó, G., Kiraly, E., and Jancsó-Gabor, A. (1980*b*). Direct evidence for an axonal site of action of capsaicin. *Arch. Pharmacol.* **313**, 91–4.

Jancsó, G., Kiraly, E., Joo, F., Such, G. and Nagy, A. (1985). Selective degeneration by capsaicin of a subpopulation of primary sensory neurons in the adult rat. *Neurosci. Lett.* **59**, 209–14.

Jancsó, N. (1960). Role of nerve terminals in the mechanism of inflammatory reactions. *Bull. Millard Filmore Hosp.* **7**, 53–7.

Jancsó, N. (1968). Desensitization with capsaicin and related acylamides as a tool for studying the function of pain receptors. *Proc. 3rd Int. Pharmacol. Meeting*, Vol. 9 (ed. R.K.S. Lim, D. Armstrong, and E.G. Pardo), pp. 33–55. Pergamon Press, Oxford.

Jancsó, N., Jancsó-Gabor, A., and Szolcsányi, J. (1967). Direct evidence for neurogenic inflammation and its prevention by denervation and by pretreatment with capsaicin. *Br. J. Pharmacol.* **31**, 138–51.

Jancsó, N., Jancsó-Gabor, A., and Szolcsányi, J. (1968). The role of nerve endings in neurogenic inflammation induced in human skin and in the eye and paw of the rat. *Br. J. Pharmacol.* **33**, 32–41.

Jänig, W. and Lisney S.J.W. (1989). Small diameter myelinated afferents produce vasodilatation but not plasma extravasation in rat skin. *J. Physiol.* **415**, 477–86.

Jessell, T.M., Iversen, L.L., and Cuello, A.C. (1978). Capsaicin-induced depletion of substance P from primary sensory neurones. *Brain Res.* **152**, 183–8.

Kawasaki, H., Nuki, C., Saito, A., and Takasai, K. (1991). NPY modulates neurotransmission of CGRP-containing vasodilator nerves in rat mesenteric arteries. *Am. J. Physiol.—Heart circulatory Physiol.* **261** (3,30–3), H683–H690.

Kenins, P. (1981). Identification of the unmyelinated sensory nerves which evoke plasma extravasation in response to antidromic stimulation. *Neurosci. Lett.* **25**, 137–41.

Kenins, P. (1984). Electrophysiological and histological studies of vascular permeability after antidromic sensory nerve stimulation. In *Antidromic vasodilatation and neurogenic inflammation* (ed. L.A. Chahl, J. Szolcsányi, and F. Lembeck), pp. 175–88. Akademiai Kiado, Budapest.

Kenins, P. Hurley, J.V., and Bell, C. (1984). The role of substance P in the axon reflex in the rat. *Br. J. Dermatol.* **111**, 551–9.

Kidd, B.L., Mapp, P.I., Blake, D.R., Gibson, S.J., and Polak, J.M. (1990). Neurogenic influences in arthritis. *Ann. rheum. Dis.* **49**, 649–52.

Kolston, J. and Lisney, S.J.W. (1993). A study of vasodilator responses evoked by antidromic stimulation of A delta afferent nerve fibers supplying normal and reinnervated rat skin. *Microvasc. Res.* **46**, 143–7.

Koltzenburg, M. and McMahon, S.B. (1986). Plasma extravasation in the rat urinary bladder following mechanical, electrical and chemical stimuli: evidence for a new population of chemosensitive primary sensory afferents. *Neurosci. Lett.* **72**, 353–6.

Kowalski, M.L., Sliwinska-Kowalska, M., and Kaliner, M.A. (1990). Neurogenic inflammation, vascular permeability, and mast cells. II. Additional evidence indicating that mast cells are not involved in neurogenic inflammation. *J. Immunol.* **145**, 1214–21.

Laird, J.M.A., Chang, B., Hoey, R., and Cervero, F. (1991). Capsaicin-sensitive vagal afferent fibers and gastric motility: evidence for an 'axon reflex' mechanism. *J. gastrointest. Motility* **3**, 138–43.

Lam, F.Y. and Ferrell, W.R. (1993). Acute inflammation in the rat knee joint attenuates sympathetic vasoconstriction but enhances neuropeptide-mediated vasodilatation assessed by laser–Doppler perfusion imaging. *Neuroscience* **52**, 443–9.

LaMotte, R.H. (1992). Subpopulations of 'nocifensor neurons' contributing to pain and allodynia, itch and alloknesis. *Am. Pain Soc. J.* **1**, 115–26.

Lee, T.J., Saito, A., and Berezin, I. (1984). Vasoactive intestinal polypeptide-like substance: the potential transmitter for cerebral vasodilation. *Science* **224**, 898–901.

Lembeck, F., Donnerer, J., Tsuchiya, M., and Nagahisa, A. (1992). The non-peptide tachykinin antagonist, CP-96,345, is a potent inhibitor of neurogenic inflammation. *Br. J. Pharmacol.* **105**, 527–30.

Levine, J.D., Moskowitz, M.A., and Basbaum, A.I. (1985). The contribution of neurogenic inflammation in experimental arthritis. *J. Immunol.* **135**, 843–7.

Levine, J.D., Dardick, S.J., Roizen, M.F., Helms, C., and Basbaum, A.I. (1986). The contribution of sensory afferents and sympathetic efferents to joint injury in experimental arthritis. *J. Neurosci.* **6**, 3923.

Lewis, T. (1927). *The blood vessels of the human skin and their responses.* Shaw & Sons, London.

Lewis, T. (1937a). The nocifensor system of nerves and its reactions. I. *Br. med. J.* **1**, 431–5.

Lewis, T. (1937b). The nocifensor system of nerves and its reactions. II. *Br. med. J.* **1**, 491–4.

Lewis, T. and Grant, R.T. (1924). Vascular reactions of the skin to injury. Part II. The liberation of a histamine-like substance in injured skin; the underlying cause of factitious urticaria and of wheals produced by burning; and observations upon the nervous control of certain skin reactions. *Heart* **11**, 209–65.

Li, D.S., Raybould, H.E., Quintero, E., and Guth, P.H. (1992). Calcitonin gene-related peptide mediates the gastric hyperemic response to acid back-diffusion. *Gastroenterology* **102** (4 Pt 1), 1124–8.

Lou, Y.P., Franco-Cereceda, A., and Lundberg, J.M. (1992). Different ion channel mechanisms between low concentrations of capsaicin and high concentrations of capsaicin and nicotine regarding peptide release from pulmonary afferents. *Acta physiol. scand.* **146**, 119–27.

Lundberg, J.M. (1993). Capsaicin-sensitive nerves in the airways — implications for protective reflexes and disease. In *Neuroscience perspectives: capsaicin in the study of pain* (ed. J.N. Wood), pp. 219–27. Academic Press, London.

Lundberg, J.M., Brodin, E., Hua, X-Y., and Saria, A. (1984). Vascular permeability changes and smooth muscle contraction in relation to capsaicin-sensitive substance P afferents in the guinea-pig. *Acta physiol. scand.* **120**, 217–27.

Lundberg, J.M., Franco-Cereceda, A., Alving, K., Delay-Goyet, P., and Lou, Y.P. (1992). Release of calcitonin gene-related peptide from sensory neurons. *Ann. NY Acad. Sci.* **657**, 187–93.

Lynn, B. (1984). Effect of neonatal treatment with capsaicin on the numbers and properties of cutaneous afferent units from the hairy skin of the rat. *Brain Res.* **322**, 255–60.

Lynn, B. (1988). Neurogenic inflammation. *Skin Pharmacol.* **1**, 217–24.

Lynn, B. and Carpenter, S.E. (1982). Primary afferent units from the hairy sin of the rat hind limb. *Brain Res.* **238**, 29–43.

Lynn, B. and Cotsell, B. (1992). Blood flow increases in the skin of the anaesthetized rat that follow antidromic sensory nerve stimulation and strong mechanical stimulation. *Neurosci. Lett.* **137**, 249–52.

Lynn, B. and Shakhanbeh, J. (1988a). Neurogenic inflammation in the skin of the rabbit. *Agents Actions* **25**, 228–30.

Lynn, B. and Shakhanbeh, J. (1988b). Substance P content of the skin, neurogenic inflammation and numbers of C-fibres following capsaicin application to a cutaneous nerve in the rabbit. *Neuroscience* **24**, 769–75.

Lynn, B., Ye, W., and Cotsell, B. (1992). The actions of capsaicin applied topically to the skin of the rat on C-fibre afferents, antodromic vasodilatation and substance P levels. *Br. J. Pharmacol.* **107**, 400–6.

McCulloch, J., Uddman, R., Kingman, T.A., and Edvinsson, L. (1986). Calcitonin gene-related peptide: functional role in cerebrovascular regulation. *Proc. natl Acad. Sci., USA* **83**, 5731–5.

McDonald, D.M. (1988). Neurogenic inflammation in the rat trachea. I. Changes in venules, leucocytes and epithelial cells. *J. Neurocytol.* **17**, 583–603.

Maggi, C.A. (1991). Capsaicin and primary afferent neurons: from basic science to human therapy. *J. autonom. nerv. Syst.* **33**, 1–14.

Maggi, C.A. (193). The pharmacological modulation of neurotransmitter release. In *Capsaicin in the study of pain* (ed. J.N. Wood), pp.161–89. Academic Press, London.

Maggi, C.A. and Meli, A. (1986). The role of neuropeptides in the regulation of the micturition reflex. *J. autonom. pharmacol.* **6**, 133–62.

Maggi, C.A. and Meli, A. (1988). The sensory-efferent function of capsaicin-sensitive sensory neurons. *Gen. Pharmacol.* **19**, 1–43.

Maggi, C.A., Manzini, S., Giuliani, S., Santicioli, S., and Meli, A. (1986*a*). Extrinsic origin of the capsaicin-sensitive innervation of the rat duodenum: possible involvement of calcitonin gene-related peptide (CGRP) in the capsaicin-induced activation of intramural non-adrenergic non-cholinergic ('purinergic') neurones. *Naunyn-Schmiedebergs Arch. Pharmacol.* **334**, 172–80.

Maggi, C.A., Santicioli, S., Giuliani, S., Abelli, L., and Meli, A. (1986*b*). The motor effect of the capsaicin-sensitive inhibitory innervation of the rat ureter. *Eur. J. Pharmacol.* **126**, 333–6.

Maggi, C.A., Patacchini, R., Giuliani, S., Santicioli, P., and Meli, A. (1988). Evidence for two independent modes of activation of the 'efferent' function of capsaicin-sensitive nerves. *Eur. J. Pharmacol.* **156**, 367–73.

Maggi, C.A., Patacchini, R., Rovero, P., and Giachetti, A. (1993). Tachykinin receptors and tachykinin receptor antagonists. *J. autonom. Pharmacol.* **1993**, 23–93.

Malm, L. and Petersson, G. (1985). Tachykinins and nasal secretion. In *Tachykinin antagonists* (ed. R. Hakanson and F. Sundler), pp.199–202. Elsevier, Amsterdam.

Mandahl, A. and Bill, A. (1981). Ocular responses to antidromic trigeminal stimulation, intracameral prostaglandin E1 and E2, capsaicin and substance P. *Acta physiol. scand.* **112**, 331–8.

Mandahl, A. and Bill, A. (1984). Effects of the substance P antagonist, (D-Argl, D-Pro2, D-Trp7,9, Leu11)-SP on the miotic response to substance P, antidromic trigeminal nerve stimulation, capsaicin, prostaglandin E1, compound 48/80 and histamine. *Acta physiol. scand.* **120**, 27–35.

Marshall, I., Al-Kazwini, S.J., Holman, J.J., and Craig, R.K. (1986). Human and rat alpha-CGRP but not calcitonin cause mesenteric vasodilatation in rats. *Eur. J. Pharmacol.* **123**, 217–22.

Miyauchi, T., Ishikawa, T., Sugishita, Y., Saito, A., and Goto, K. (1987). Effects of capsaicin on nonadrenergic noncholinergic nerves in the guinea pig atria: role of calcitonin gene-related peptide as cardiac neurotransmitter. *J. cardiovasc. Pharmacol.* **10**, 675–82.

Moskowitz, M.A. and Buzzi, M.G. (1991). Neuroeffector functions of sensory fibres: implications for headache mechanisms and drug actions. *J. Neurol.* **238**, S18–S22.

Moskowitz, M.A., Brody, M., and Liu-Chen, L-Y. (1983). In vitro release of immunoreactive substance P from putative afferent nerve endings in bovine pia arachnoid. *Neuroscience* **9**, 809–14.

Nagy, J.I., Vincent, S.R., Staines, W.M.A., Fibiger, H.C., Reisine, T.D., and Yamamura, H.I. (1980). Neurotoxic action of capsaicin on spinal substance P neurons. *Brain Res.* **186**, 435–44.

Nagy, J.I., Iversen, L.L., Goedert, M., Chapman, D., and Hunt, S.P. (1983). Dose-dependent effects of capsaicin on primary sensory neurons in the neonatal rat. *J. Neurosci.* **3**, 399–406.

Nawa, H., Hirose, T., Takashima, H., Inayama, S., and Nakanishi, S. (1983). Nucleotide sequences of cloned cDNAs for two types of bovine substance P precursor. *Nature* **306**, 32–6.

Newbold, P. and Brain, S.D. (1993). The modulation of inflammatory oedema by calcitonin gene-related peptide. *Br. J. Pharmacol.* **108**, 705–10.

Nuki, C., Kawasaki, H., Takasaki, K., and Wada, A. (1994). Pharmacological characterization of presynpatic calcitonin gene-related peptide (CGRP) receptors on CGRP-containing vasodilator nerves in rat mesenteric resistance vessels. *J. Pharmacol. exp. Ther.* **268**, 59–64.

Ohkubo, T., Shibata, M., and Takahashi, H. (1990). [Participation of the sensory nerves in the inflammatory response induced by irritants.] *Nippon Yakurigaku Zasshi* **96**, 243–53.

Ohlen, A., Lindbom, L., Staines, W., Hökfelt, T., Cuello, A.C., Fischer, J.A., *et al.* (1987). Substance P and calcitonin gene-related peptide: immunohistochemical localisation and microvascular effects in rabbit skeletal muscle. *Naunyn-Schmiedebergs Arch. Pharmacol.* **336**, 87–93.

Olgart, L., Gazelius, B., Brodin, E., and Nilsson, G. (1977). Release of substance P-like immunoreactivity from the dental pulp. *Acta physiol. scand.* **101**, 510–12.

Pierau, F.-K., Lynn, B., Schütterle, S., and Basile, S. (1995). Heat-sensitive nociceptors induce flare-like antidromic vasodilation in the pig skin. *Soc. Neurosci. Abstr.* **21**, 262.3, p.648.

Pini, A. and Lynn, B. (1991). C-fibre function during the 6 weeks following brief application of capsaicin to a cutaneous nerve in the rat. *Eur. J. Neurosci.* **3**, 274–84.

Pini, A., Baranowski, R., and Lynn, B. (1990). Long-term reduction in the number of C-fibre nociceptors following capsaicin treatment of a cutaneous nerve in adult rats. *Eur. J. Neurosci.* **2**, 89–97.

Post, C., Butterworth, J.W., Strichartz, G.R., Karlsson, J.-A., and Persson, C.G.A. (1985). Tachykinin antagonists have potent local anaesthetic actions. *Eur. J. Pharmacol.* **117**, 347–54.

Ramnarine, S.I. and Rogers, D.F. (1994). Non-adrenergic, non-cholinergic neural control of mucus secretion in the airways. *Pulmonary Pharmacol.* **7**, 19–33.

Ramnarine, S.I., Harayama, Y., Barnes, P.J., and Rogers, D.F. (1994). 'Sensory-efferent' neural control of mucus secretion: characterization using tachykinin receptor antagonists in ferret trachea in vitro. *Br. J. Pharmacol.* **113**, 1183–90.

Rogers, D.F., Aursudkij, B., and Barnes, P.J. (1989). Effects of tachykinins on mucus secretion in human bronchi in vitro. *Eur. J. Pharmacol.* **174**, 283–6.

Rosell, S., Olgart, L., Gazelius, B., Panopoulos, P., Folkers, K., and Hörig, J. (1981). Inhibition of antidromic and substance P-induced vasodilatation by a substance P antagonist. *Acta physiol. scand.* **111**, 381–2.

Rosenfeld, M.G., Mermod, J.J., Amara, S.G., Swanson, L.W., Sawchenko, P.E., Rivier, J., Vale, W.W., and Evans, R.M. (1983). Production of a novel neuropeptide encoded by the calcitonin gene via tissue-specific RNA processing. *Nature* **304**, 129–35.

Saria, A. (1984). Substance P in sensory nerve fibres contributes to the development of oedema in rat hind paw after thermal injury. *Br. J. Pharmacol.* **82**, 217–22.

Saria, A., Lundberg, J.M., Skofitsch, G., and Lembeck, F. (1983). Vascular protein leakage in various tissues induced by substance P, capsaicin, bradykinin, serotonin, histamine and by antigen challenge. *Naunyn-Schmiedebergs Arch. Pharmacol.* **324**, 212–18.

Saria, A., Theodorsson-Norheim, E., Gamse, R., and Lundberg, J.M. (1985). Release of substance P- and substance K-like immunoreactivities from the isolated perfused guinea-pig lung. *Eur. J. Pharmacol.* **106**, 207–8.

Saria, A., Martling, C.R., Yan, Z., Theodorsson-Norheim, E., Gamse, R., and Lundberg, J.M. (1988). Release of multiple tachykinins from capsaicin sensitive sensory nerves in the lung by bradykinin, histamine, dimethylphenyl piperazinium, and vagal nerve stimulation. *Am. Rev. resp. Dis.* **137**, 1330–5.

Schmidt, A.W., McLean, S., and Heym, J. (1992). The substance P receptor antagonist CP-96, 345 interacts with calcium channels. *Eur. J. Pharmacol.* **215**, 351–2.

Sestini, P., Dolovich, M., Vancheri, C., Stead, R.H., Marshall, J.S., Perdue, M., *et al.* (1989). Antigen-induced lung solute clearance in rats is dependent on capsaicin-sensitive nerves. *Am. Rev. resp. Dis.* **139**, 401–6.

Skofitsch, G. and Jacobowitz, D.M. (1985). Calcitonin gene-related peptide coexists with substance P in capsaicin sensitive neurons and sensory ganglia of the rat. *Peptides* **6**, 747–54.

Smith, C.H., Barker, J., Morris, R.W, Macdonald, D.M., and Lee, T.H. (1993). Neuropeptides induce rapid expression of endothelial cell adhesion molecules and elicit infiltration in human skin. *J. Immunol.* **151**, 3274–82.

Stricker, S. (1876). Untersuchung über die Geffässerwurzeln des Ischiadus. *Sitz Kaiserl. Akad. Wiss. (Wien)* **3**, 173.

Szolcsányi, J. (1987). Selective responsiveness of polymodal nociceptors of the rabbit ear to capsaicin, bradykinin and ultra-violet radiation. *J. Physiol.* **388**, 9–23.

Szolcsányi, J. (1988). Antidromic vasodilatation and neurogenic inflammation. *Agents Actions* **23**, 4–11.

Szolcsányi, J., Sann, H., and Pierau, F.K., (1986). Nociception in pigeons is not impaired by capsaicin. *Pain* **27**, 247–60.

Szolcsányi, J., Anton, F., Reeh, P.W., and Handwerker, H.O. (1988). Selective excitation by capsaicin of mechano-heat sensitive nociceptors in rat skin. *Brain Res.* **446**, 262–8.

Tokuyama, K., Kuo, H.P., Rohde, J.A., Barnes, P.J., and Rogers, D.F. (1990). Neural control of goblet cell secretion in guinea pig airways. *Am. J. Physiol.* **259**, (2 Pt 1), L108–L115.

Tornebrandt, K., Nobin, A., and Owman, C. (1987). Contractile and dilatory action of neuropeptides on isolated human mesenteric blood vessels. *Peptides* **8**, 251–6.

Uddman, R., Edvinsson, L., Ekblad, E., Hakanson, R., and Sundler, F. (1986). Calcitonin gene-related peptide (CGRP): perivascular distribution and vasodilatory effects. *Regulat. Peptides* **15**, 1–23.

Wahlestedt, C., Beding, B., Ekman, R., Oksala, O., Stjernschantz, J., and Hákansen, R. (1986). Calcitonin gene-related peptide in the eye: release by sensory nerve stimulation and effects associated with neurogenic inflammation. *Regulat. Peptides* **16**, 107–15.

Webber, S.E., Lim, J.C., and Widdicombe, J.G. (1991). The effects of calcitonin gene-related peptide on submucosal gland secretion and epithelial albumin transport in the ferret trachea in vitro. *Br. J. Pharmacol.* **102**, 79–84.

Welk, E., Fleischer, E., Petsche, U., and Handwerker, H.O. (1984). Afferent C-fibres in rats after neonatal capsaicin treatment. *Pflügers Arch.* **400**, 66–71.

White, D.M. and Helme, R.D. (1985). Release of substance P from peripheral nerve terminals following electrical stimulation of the sciatic nerve. *Brain Res.* **336**, 27–31.

Williams, T.J. (1982). Vasoactive intestinal polypeptide is more potent than prostaglandin E2 as a vasodilator and oedema potentiator in rabbit skin. *Br. J. Pharmacol.* **77**, 505–9.

Xu, X.J., Hao, J.X., Wiesenfeld-Hallin, Z. Hakanson, R., Folkers, K., and Hokfelt, T. (1991). Spantide II, a novel tachykinin antagonist, and galanin inhibit plasma extravasation induced by antidromic C-fiber stimulation in rat hindpaw. *Neuroscience* **42**, 731–7.

Yamamato, T., Shimoyama, N., and Mizuguchi, T. (1993). Effects of FK224, a novel cyclopeptide NK_1 and NK_2 antagonist, and CP-96,345, a nonpeptide NK_1 antagonist, on development and maintenance of thermal hyperesthesia evoked by carrageenan injection in the rat paw. *Anesthesiology* **79**, 1042–50.

18 Nociceptors and neuroimmune interactions

CHRISTOPH STEIN

Introduction

Neuroimmune interactions have been described extensively in the central nervous system. Commonly, such interactions refer to the effects of compounds released from immune-competent cells upon central neurones or vice versa. The concept of an interrelation between peripheral sensory nerves and immune cells is relatively novel. This has been proposed by a number of authors, based mostly on microanatomical findings in inflammatory processes (reviewed in Weihe *et al.* 1990). Similarly to the situation in the central nervous system, mutual interactions may take place, that is, substances released from peripheral nerves may act on immune cells or vice versa. Effects resulting therefrom include immunomodulation and pro- or antiinflammatory, hyperalgesic or analgesic phenomena. This chapter is divided into two main parts, the first part covering substances released from peripheral neurones and the second part covering substances derived from immune cells. The focus will be on functional studies examining the crosstalk between cells of the immune system and peripheral sensory nerves. Auto- or paracrine actions of the respective compounds will not be discussed in detail.

Neurone-derived substances

Substance P

The most extensively studied compound is substance P (SP). SP is contained in dorsal root ganglion (DRG) neurones and is released from their peripheral and central terminals (see Lawson, Chapter 3, this volume). Receptors for SP have been demonstrated on T and B lymphocytes by cell-sorter and radioligand-binding techniques (McGillis *et al.* 1987, 1990; Bost and Pascual 1992). Moreover, messenger ribonucleic acid (mRNA) encoding SP receptor is constitutively expressed in mast cell lines (Ansel *et al.* 1993), in lymphocytes (Bost and Pascual 1992), and in macrophages (Bost *et al.* 1992). Apparently, the SP receptors expressed by immune cells are very similar to those expressed by neurones, as evidenced by radioreceptor binding assays and determination of the gene encoding the SP receptor (Bost and Pascual 1992; Bost *et al.* 1992).

So far, the majority of studies indicate that the effects of SP on cell-mediated immunity are stimulatory. SP has been shown to modulate immediate hypersensitivity responses by stimulating the generation of arachidonic acid-derived mediators from mast cells (McGillis *et al.* 1987). Furthermore, SP may influence mast-cell-mediated late inflammatory events by modulating the production and secretion of several cytokines. Thus, SP can induce mRNA for tumour necrosis factor α (TNFα) and stimulate TNF secretion in a murine mast-cell line or in freshly isolated mast cells (Ansel *et al.* 1993). Chemotaxis, lysosomal enzyme release, and phagocytosis by mononuclear and polymorphonuclear leucocytes are altered by SP (McGillis *et al.* 1987). SP enhances the synthesis of DNA, protein and immunoglobulin by T and B lymphocytes, respectively (McGillis *et al.* 1987). Furthermore, treatments that increase SP concentrations in the periphery increase the number of immunoglobulin-secreting B cells, and SP antagonists or depletion of SP-containing neurones reduce the organism's ability to synthesize immunoglobulins (Bost and Pascual 1992). In cultures of purified B lymphocytes or B-cell clones, SP augments immunoglobulin secretion (Bost and Pascual 1992). Mechanisms involved in these responses may include mobilization of intracellular Ca^{2+}, stimulation of Cl^- currents, and changes in the cell surface expression of cell adhesion molecules and cytokine receptors (Sudduth-Klinger *et al.* 1992; Kavelaars *et al.* 1993). Finally, some studies have suggested that these modulatory effects of SP are of importance in human diseases such as rheumatoid arthritis (McGillis *et al.* 1990) and inflammatory bowel disease (Mantyh *et al.* 1991).

Calcitonin-gene-related peptide (CGRP)

Similarly to SP, CGRP is contained and released from primary afferent nerves (see Lawson, Chapter 3, this volume). Anatomical studies have shown a close relationship between mast cells and CGRP-containing enteric nerves (Stead *et al.* 1987) and between various immunocytes and CGRP-immunoreactive cutaneous nerves under inflammatory conditions (Weihe *et al.* 1988; Hassan *et al.* 1992; Przewlocki *et al.* 1992). CGRP binding sites have been shown in germinal centres of lymph nodes (Popper *et al.* 1988; Gates *et al.* 1989) and on a macrophage-like cell line (Abello *et al.* 1991). CGRP can modulate mitogenic responses in human peripheral blood mononuclear cells (Casini *et al.* 1989), inhibit the production of H_2O_2 (Nong *et al.* 1989), and stimulate adenylate cyclase (Abello *et al.* 1991) in macrophages. In T cells CGRP induces cyclic adenosine monophosphate (cAMP) accumulation and inhibits the production of interleukin-2 (IL-2), TNFα, and interferon-gamma (IFN-γ) (Wang *et al.* 1992). In human epidermis, CGRP-containing nerve fibres are intimately associated with Langerhans cells and can inhibit their antigen-presenting functions (Hosoi *et al.* 1993). Taken together, these findings suggest an inhibitory role of CGRP on cellular immune functions.

Opioids

Several studies have detected opioid peptides in sensory ganglia (Botticelli *et al.* 1981; Przewlocki *et al.* 1983; Sweetnam *et al.* 1986; Quartu and Del Fiacco 1994) and in peripheral terminals of sensory nerves (Weihe *et al* 1985; Gibbins *et al.* 1987; Hassan *et al.* 1992; Hardebo *et al.* 1994). The expression of opioid peptides in sensory neurones seems to be somewhat selective in that only prodynorphin (and proenkephalin) but no proopiomelanocortin-derived peptides have been found so far (see also below). Opioid receptors have been demonstrated on immune cells, and opioid-mediated modulation of their proliferation and several of their functions (for example, chemotaxis, superoxide production, mast cell degranulation) has been reported (Sibinga and Goldstein 1988; Roy *et al.* 1991; Bryant and Holaday 1993; Hassan *et al.* 1993; Loh *et al.* 1993). Although these findings signal the potential for interactions between nociceptor-derived opioid peptides and their receptors on immune cells, direct functional evidence is lacking to date.

Immune-cell-derived substances

Opioids

Interactions between immune-derived opioid peptides and sensory nerves can result in the inhibition of pain. This notion has emerged during studies concerned with the local antinociceptive actions of opioids, which are particularly prominent in painful (hyper-algesic) inflammatory conditions (Barber and Gottschlich 1992; Stein 1993). Opioid receptors are present on peripheral sensory nerves and their endogenous ligands, opioid peptides, are found in resident immune cells within peripheral inflamed tissue. This concept will be outlined in detail.

Peripheral opioid receptors

Early studies have produced evidence for opioid binding on central processes of primary afferent neurones (LaMotte *et al* 1976; Fields *et al.* 1980; Ninkovic *et al.* 1982) and in the DRG (Ninkovic *et al.* 1982). More recently, opioid receptors have been demonstrated on the peripheral terminals, namely, on thinly myelinated and unmyelinated cutaneous nerves, by immunocytochemistry (Fig. 18.1; Stein *et al.* 1990*b*) and by autoradiography (Hassan *et al.* 1993). The advent of opioid receptor cloning has made it possible to generate more specific antisera to identify opioid receptors on small-diameter CGRP-containing neurones in the DRG and dorsal spinal cord by immunofluorescence (Dado *et al.* 1993) and to demonstrate opioid receptor mRNA in the DRG (Maekawa *et al.* 1994; M.K.H. Schäfer *et al.* 1994; M. Schäfer *et al.* 1995*a*). These findings are in line with functional studies indicating that capsaicin-sensitive C-fibre neurones mediate the peripheral antinociceptive effects of morphine (Bartho *et. al.* 1990). Following the occupation of neuronal opioid receptors by an opioid agonist, the excitability of the nociceptive input terminal or the propagation of action potentials is attenuated, possibly via inhibitory G proteins (Werz and MacDonald 1982; Frank 1985; Russell *et al.* 1987; Levine and Taiwo 1989; Andreev *et al.* 1994). In addition, the release of excitatory neuropeptides (for example, SP) from central and/or peripheral endings of primary afferents is inhibited (Mudge *et al.* 1979; Yaksh 1988; Yonehara *et al.* 1992). These mechanisms may account not only for the antinociceptive but also for the anti-inflammatory actions of opioids in peripheral tissues (Lembeck and Donnerer 1985; Barber and Gottschlich 1992).

After the induction of peripheral inflammation, the axonal transport of opioid receptors in fibres of the sciatic nerve is greatly enhanced (Hassan *et al.* 1993). Saturation and competition experiments indicate that the pharmacological character-istics of these receptors are very similar to those in the brain. Subsequently, the density of opioid receptors on cutaneous nerve fibres in the inflamed tissue increases and this increase is abolished by ligating the sciatic nerve (Hassan *et al.* 1993). These findings demonstrate that inflammation enhances the peripherally directed axonal transport of opioid receptors, which leads to an increase in their number (upregulation) on peripheral nerve terminals. This may partly explain why peripheral antinociceptive effects of exogenous opioids are enhanced under inflammatory conditions (Stein 1993). All three types (μ, δ, κ) of opioid receptors are apparently present in the periphery. This has been demonstrated using labels recognizing μ and δ receptors *in vitro* (Stein *et al.* 1990*b*; Hassan *et al.* 1993) and using selective ligands for all three receptor types *in vivo* (reviewed in Barber and Gottschlich 1992; Stein 1993).

A

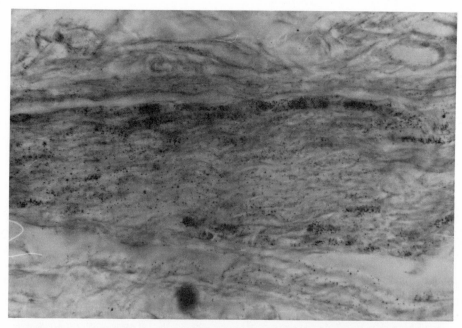

B

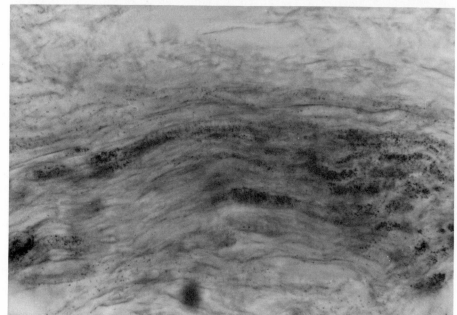

Fig. 18.1   Immunostaining of opioid receptors in subcutaneous (A) non-inflamed and (B) inflamed tissue of the rat paw. ImmunoGold silver-stained opioid receptors appear as black granules on small-diameter unmyelinated fibres in the longitudinal section of cutaneous sensory nerves. Reprinted from Stein *et al.* (1990*b*).

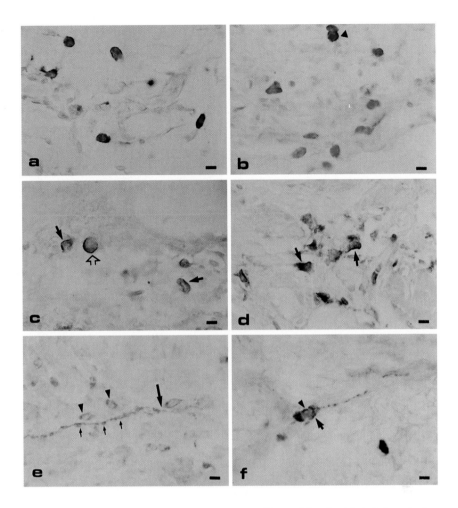

Fig. 18.2 Double staining of immunocytes, sensory neuropeptides, and β-endorphin in inflamed subcutaneous tissue of the rat paw. (a) T-lymphocytes; (b) B lymphocytes; (c) monocyte/macrophages; (d) macrophages contain β endorphin (brown staining). Panels (e) and (f) show β endorphin-containing cells (large arrows) in the vicinity of a sensory nerve (small arrows, brown staining). Reprinted with permission from Przewlocki *et al.* (1992).

Opioid peptides in cells of the immune system

Three families of opioid peptides have been characterized in the central nervous and neuroendocrine systems, each deriving from a distinct gene and precursor protein, namely proopiomelanocortin (POMC), proenkephalin (PENK), and prodynorphin. Appropriate processing yields their respective major representative opioid peptides beta-endorphin (END), Met-enkephalin (ME), and dynorphin (DYN). Each exhibits different affinities for the three opioid receptor types, μ, δ, and κ (Höllt 1986).

The issue of whether immune cells are capable of synthesizing opioid peptides, that is, whether the genes of precursor peptides are expressed and appropriately translated, has been a subject of controversy (reviewed in Sibinga and Goldstein 1988). Blalock and Smith (1980) were the first to demonstrate POMC-derived peptides in immunocytes. mRNA encoding POMC has been found in mouse splenocytes (Westly *et al.* 1986), lymphocytes (Buzzetti *et al.* 1989; Smith *et al.* 1990), and spleen macrophages (Lolait *et al.* 1986). Some of those cells express POMC mRNA similar to that found in the pituitary and in the hypothalamus, the classical loci for production of POMC-derived peptides (Lolait *et al.* 1986; Smith *et al.* 1990). Peripheral blood leucocytes (Buzzetti *et al.* 1989) and human thymus cells (Lacaze-Masmonteil *et al.* 1987) appear to contain POMC mRNA molecules that are about 200 nucleotides shorter than pituitary mRNA, raising doubts as to whether this shortened mRNA species gets translated into functional POMC protein. PENK mRNA has been demonstrated in normal lymphocytes (Rosen *et al.* 1989), in activated T lymphocytes, and in macrophages (Zurawski *et al.* 1986; Martin *et al.* 1987). This mRNA is highly homologous to rat brain PENK mRNA, abundant and apparently translated, since immunoreactive ME is released from these cells (Zurawski *et al.* 1986). In most of these early studies, cells were obtained from healthy human subjects or animals and were then stimulated *in vitro*.

More recent investigations have studied models that, due to the presence of inflammation, represent a persistent pathophysiological stimulation of the immune system *in vivo* (Stein *et al.* 1988). This may represent a condition that is closer to the clinical setting than some of the early *in vitro* studies. These studies have demonstrated mRNAs encoding POMC and PENK and their respective opioid peptide products END and ME within inflamed tissue. These peptides are found in resident T and B lymphocytes as well as in monocytes and macrophages (Fig. 18.2; Stein *et al.* 1990*b*; Przewlocki *et al.* 1992). Small amounts of DYN are also detectable by immunocytochemistry (Hassan *et al.* 1992). These findings indicate the presence and synthesis of opioid peptides in different types of inflammatory cells at the site of tissue injury. Thus, a growing body of evidence indicates that both POMC- and PENK-derived opioid peptides are produced by immune cells, but that the specific conditions of stimulation in the microenvironment are crucial (see also Heijnen *et al.* 1991; Sacerdote *et al.* 1991; van Woudenberg *et al.* 1992; Sharp and Linner 1993).

Release of opioid peptides from inflammatory cells

In order to interact with nociceptors and to produce analgesic effects, the opioid peptides must be released (Fig. 18.3). Although environmental stress is an effective stimulus (Stein *et al.* 1990*a,b*; Przewlocki *et al.* 1992), the exact mechanisms of opioid secretion within inflamed tissue are only beginning to be unravelled. Corticotrophin-releasing factor (CRF) is a major physiological secretagogue for opioid peptides in the pituitary. Its releasing effects are potentiated by IL-1 (Fagarasan *et al.* 1989), and IL-1 (and other cytokines) can stimulate END release directly (Bernton *et al.* 1987). Receptors for each of these agents are present on immune cells (Webster *et al.* 1990; Dinarello and Thompson 1991; Mousa *et al.* 1994). In the periphery, the local application of small, systemically inactive doses of CRF, IL-1, and other cytokines produces potent antinociceptive effects in inflamed, but not in non-inflamed tissue (Czlonkowski *et al.* 1993; Schäfer *et al.* 1994). These effects are reversible by immunosuppression with cyclosporin A, by passive immunization with antibodies against END, and by opioid antagonists. Furthermore, short-term (5–10 min) incubation with CRF or IL-1 can release END *in vitro* in immune cell suspensions prepared from lymph nodes (Schäfer *et al.* 1994). These findings are consistent with the notion that exogenous CRF and cytokines cause secretion of END from immune cells, which subsequently activates opioid receptors on sensory nerves to inhibit nociception.

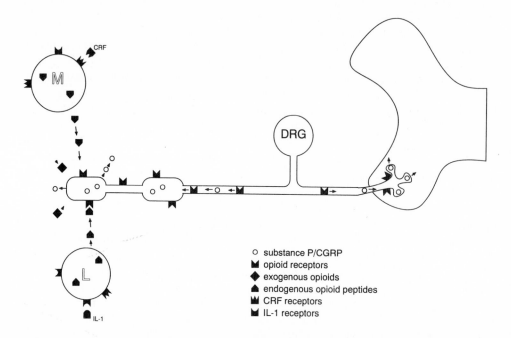

○ substance P/CGRP
opioid receptors
◆ exogenous opioids
▲ endogenous opioid peptides
CRF receptors
IL-1 receptors

Fig. 18.3 Schematic diagram of a primary afferent neurone. Its cell body is located in the dorsal root ganglion (DRG); opioid receptors (Hassan *et al.* 1993) and neuropeptides (Donnerer *et al.* 1992) are transported towards its central and peripheral terminals. Upon stimulation with cytokines (IL-1) or corticotrophin-releasing factor (CRF), opioid peptides are released from monocytes/macrophages (M) and/or from lymphocytes (L). Occupation of opioid receptors by exogenous or endogenous ligands can result in a decreased release of excitatory (proinflammatory) neuropeptides (for example, substance P/CGRP) and/or in a decreased excitability of the primary afferent neurone. For additional references see text.

Recent studies have examined the endogenous activation of this mechanism of pain control by stress. Consistent with previous reports (Karalis *et al.* 1991), CRF was found to be produced within the inflammatory site (Schäfer *et al.* 1995*b*). Both the inhibition of local CRF synthesis by antisense oligonucleotides and the *in vivo* antagonism of peripherally derived CRF abolished stress-induced peripheral opioid analgesia (Schäfer *et al.* 1995*b*). Apparently, locally expressed CRF triggers the release of opioid peptides from immune cells and thus, plays a crucial role in the local opioid inhibition of inflammatory pain.

Clinical studies

Local opioid interactions with nociceptors are of clinical relevance. A sizeable body of literature demonstrates the analgesic efficacy of exogenous opioids outside the central nervous system (reviewed in Stein 1993, 1995). To test opioid analgesic actions in the vicinity of peripheral sensory nerve terminals, several controlled studies have examined the intraarticular application of small, systemically inactive doses of morphine during knee surgery (reviewed in Stein 1995). The majority of these trials have reported significant analgesic effects. The fact that intraarticular naloxone antagonizes the effect of locally applied morphine (Stein *et al.* 1991) and anecdotal evidence for opioid binding in human synovial tissue (Lawrence *et al.* 1992) indicate that intraarticular opioid receptors are present and capable of mediating analgesia in human beings.

Opioid peptides are found in synovial tissue from patients undergoing arthroscopic knee surgery (Stein *et al.* 1993). These patients had acute traumata or chronic articular lesions and displayed histological signs of synovitis, that is, leucocytic infiltration. The opioid peptides are localized in synovial lining cells and in immune cells such as lymphocytes, macrophages, and mast cells. The prevailing peptides are END and ME, while only minor amounts of DYN are detectable (Stein *et al.* 1993). Consistent with these findings, there is an anecdotal report of opioid peptide release from human synovia *in vitro* (Yoshino *et al.* 1992). Opioids in synovial tissue are capable of interacting with intraarticular opioid receptors to produce clinically appreciable, local inhibition of pain. This has been demonstrated by the local administration of small, systemically inactive doses of the opioid antagonist naloxone, which causes increased postoperative pain in patients undergoing arthroscopic knee surgery (Stein *et al.* 1993). This suggests that opioid peptides are tonically released from inflamed synovial tissue and activate intraarticular opioid receptors to produce intrinsic inhibition of pain.

Pharmacokinetic aspects

How do immune-cell-derived opioid peptides reach their receptors on sensory neurones? This is not a trivial question since, under normal circumstances, tight intercellular contacts at the innermost layer of the perineurium act as a diffusion barrier for high-molecular-weight or hydrophilic substances such as peptides (Rechthand and Rapoport 1987; Olsson 1990). This barrier preserves homeostasis in the endoneurial tissue embedding peripheral neurones and continues up to the peripheral endings of afferent somatic and autonomic nerve fibres (Olsson 1990). An exception are non-corpuscular nerve endings, a subgroup of somatic afferents, which terminate either within the perineurium or lack it at their very tips (Burkel 1967; Heppelmann *et al.* 1990). Opioid receptors are located not only at the very tips of afferent nerve terminals but also within a considerable distance therefrom along axons (Frank 1985; Stein *et al.* 1990*a*; Hassan *et al.* 1993). These loci are clearly ensheathed by perineurium (Olsson 1990) and are potential sites of action for opioids.

Inflammatory conditions entail a deficiency of the perineurial barrier and/or an enhanced permeability of endoneurial capillaries (Rechthand and Rapoport 1987; Olsson 1990). A similar leakage can be produced experimentally by the extraneural application of hyperosmolar solutions (Rechthand and Rapoport 1987). Similarly to the situation at the blood–brain barrier (Rapoport and Robinson 1986), the effects of hyperosmolar solutions have been ascribed to a transient shrinkage of perineurial cells with subsequent widening of the zonulae occludentes (Rechthand and Rapoport 1987). Recent studies have shown that peripheral opioid analgesia and perineurial disruption coincide during the very early stages of an inflammatory reaction and that both can be mimicked by hyperosmolar solutions in normal tissue (Antonijevic *et al.* 1995). More-over, these investigations have demonstrated that either inflammatory or artificial disruption of the perineurium facilitates the passage of opioid peptides and of macro-molecules (such as horseradish peroxidase) to sensory neurones (Antonijevic *et al.* 1995). These findings have several interesting implications. Although initially discovered under inflammatory conditions, peripheral opioid analgesic effects can be brought about in normal tissue as well. The hitherto enigmatic observation that such effects are difficult to detect in non-inflamed tissue is thus explainable. Furthermore, these observations indicate an unrestricted transperineurial passage for peptides in inflammation and, thus, add a further integral component to the concept of a direct communication between immune cell-derived endogenous opioid peptides and sensory nerves.

Nerve growth factor (NGF)

NGF is the prototype of target-derived neurotrophic factors critical for the development and maintenance of specific peripheral and central neuronal populations (Eide *et al.* 1993). NGF accumulates in inflammatory sites or exudates caused by various noxious stimuli (Weskamp and Otten 1987; Aloe *et al.* 1992). Recently, T cells and mast cells have been shown to synthesize, store, and release NGF (Ehrhard *et al.* 1993; Leon *et al.* 1994). Receptors for NGF are expressed by DRG neurones (Carroll *et al.* 1992; Meakin and Shooter 1992). NGF is thought to bind to its receptor on nerve terminals and to be transported retrogradely together with its receptor to the cell body. Neurochemical studies have suggested an interaction of NGF with primary afferent neurones innervat-ing inflamed tissue. NGF increases in peripheral nerves (Donnerer *et al.* 1992) and it upregulates the synthesis of SP and CGRP in the DRG (Lindsay and Harmar 1989; Donaldson *et al.* 1992). Moreover, the axonal transport of both peptides towards the periphery is induced by NGF (Donnerer *et al.* 1992). The elevated levels of neuropep-tides probably result in their increased release from peripheral (Donnerer *et al.* 1992) and/or central (Garry and Hargreaves 1992) terminals. Since SP and CGRP are commonly considered excitatory and/or proinflammatory neuropeptides, these inves-tigations suggest that NGF plays a role in sustaining pain and inflammation (see also Mendell, Chapter 19, this volume).

Cytokines

A few studies have suggested an indirect interaction of cytokines and nociceptors. The injection of exogenous IL-1 into non-inflamed tissue has been shown to cause hyper-algesia, which was presumed to result from prostaglandin release (Ferreira *et al.* 1988). Macrophage-derived IL-1 enhances NGF synthesis in Schwann cells and other non-neuronal cells of the sciatic nerve after nerve lesion (Lindholm *et al.* 1987), and IL-1 may be produced and released from non-neuronal cells residing in the damaged nerve (Rotshenker *et al.* 1992). None of these studies has shown direct interactions between immune-cell-derived IL-1 and nociceptors.

Conclusions

At this time, the most extensively studied compounds mediating direct interactions between nociceptors and immunocytes are SP and opioids. SP is the prototype of a neuropeptide released from sensory neurones and its actions upon immune cells appear to be largely stimulatory. Some studies have suggested that these effects of SP are of importance in human diseases such as rheumatoid arthritis and inflammatory bowel disease. A large number of experimental and clinical trials have demonstrated interactions of exogenous and immune-cell-derived endogenous opioids with nociceptors, resulting in the inhibition of inflammatory pain. These findings have stimulated research into novel routes of opioid administration and into production, release, and pharmacokinetics of opioids in inflamed tissue. Clinical studies have already shown promising results, suggesting that peripheral opioid neuroimmune interactions provide a novel perspective for pain management and for the treatment of chronic inflammatory conditions.

Acknowledgements

This work was supported by NIH/NINDS grant RO1 NS32466.

References

Abello, J., Kaiserlian, D., Cuber, J.C., Revillard, J.P., and Chayvialle, J.A. (1991). Characterization of calcitonin gene-related peptide receptors and adenylate cyclase response in the murine macrophage cell line P388 D1. *Neuropeptides* **19**, 43–9.

Aloe, L., Tuveri, M.A., Carcassi, U., and Levi-Montalcini, R. (1992). Nerve growth factor in the synovial fluid of patients with chronic arthritis. *Arthritis Rheumatism* **35**, 351–5.

Andreev, N., Urban, L., and Dray, A. (1994). Opioids suppress spontaneous activity of polymodal nociceptors in rat paw skin induced by ultraviolet irradiation. *Neuroscience* **58**, 793–8.

Ansel, J.C., Brown, J.R., Payan, D.G., and Brown, M.A. (1993). Substance P selectively activates TNF-alpha gene expression in murine mastcells. *J. Immunol.* **150**, 4478–85.

Antonijevic, I., Mousa, S.A., Schäfer, M., and Stein, C. (1995). Perineurial defect and peripheral opioid analgesia in inflammation. *J. Neurosci.* **15**(1), 165–72.

Barber, A. and Gottschlich, R. (1992). Opioid agonists and antagonists: an evaluation of their peripheral actions in inflammation. *Med. Res. Rev.* **12**, 525–62.

Bartho, L., Stein, C., and Herz, A. (1990). Involvement of capsaicin-sensitive neurones in hyperalgesia and enhanced opioid antinociception in inflammation. *Naunyn-Schmiedebergs Arch. Pharmacol.* **342**, 666–70.

Bernton, E.W., Beach, J.E., Holaday, J.W., Smallridge, R.C., and Fein, H.G. (1987). Release of multiple hormones by a diret action of interleukin-1 on pituitary cells. *Science* **238**, 519–21.

Blalock, J.E. and Smith, E.M. (1980). Human leukocyte interferon: structural and biological relatedness to adrenocortical hormone and endorphins. *Proc. natl Acad. Sci., USA* **77**, 5972–4.

Bost, K.L. and Pascual, D.W. (1992). Substance P: a late acting B lymphocyte differentiation cofactor. *Am. J. Physiol.* **262**, C537–45.

Bost, K.L., Breeding, S.A., and Pascual, D.W. (1992). Modulation of the mRNAs encoding substance P and its receptor in rat macrophages by LPS. *Regional Immunol.* **4**, 105–12.

Botticelli, L.J., Cox, B.M., and Goldstein, A. (1981). Immunoreactive dynorphin in mammalian spinal cord and dorsal root ganglia. *Proc. natl Acad. Sci., USA* **78**, 7783–6.

Bryant, H.U. and Holaday, J.W. (1993). Opioids in immunologic processes. In *Opioids II. Handbook of experimental pharmacology*, Vol. 104 (ed. A. Herz, H. Akil, and E.J. Simon), pp. 361–92. Springer, Berlin.

Burkel, W.E. (1967). The histological fine structure of perineurium. *Anat. Rec.* **158**, 177–90.

Buzzetti, R., McLoughlin, L., Lavender, P.M., Clark, A.J.L., and Rees, L.H. (1989). Expression of pro-opiomelanocortin gene and quantification of adrenocorticotropic hormone-like immuno-reactivity in human normal peripheral mononuclear cells and lymphoid and myeloid malignancies. *J. clin. Invest.* **83**, 733–7.

Carroll, S.L., Silos-Santiago, I., Frese, S.E., Ruit, K.G., Milbrandt, J., and Snider, W.D. (1992). Dorsal root ganglion neurons expressing trk are selectively sensitive to NGF deprivation in utero. *Neuron* **9**, 779–88.

Casini, A., Geppetti, P., Maggi, C.A., and Surrenti, C. (1989). Effects of calcitonin gene-related peptide (CGRP), neurokinin A and neurokinin A (4–10) on the mitogenic response of human peripheral blood mononuclear cells. *Naunyn-Schmiedebergs Arch. Pharmacol.* **339**, 354–8.

Czlonkowski, A., Stein, C., and Herz, A. (1993). Peripheral mechanisms of opioid antinociception in inflammation: involvement of cytokines. *Eur. J. Pharmacol.* **242**, 229–35.

Dado, R.J., Law, P.Y., Loh, H.H., and Elde, R. (1993). Immunofluorescent identification of a delta-opioid receptor on primary afferent nerve terminals. *NeuroReport* **5**, 341–4.

Dinarello, C.A. and Thompson, R.C. (1991). Blocking IL-1: interleukin 1 receptor antagonist in vivo and in vitro. *Immunol. Today* **12**, 404–10.

Donaldson, L.F., Harmar, A.J., McQueen, D.S., and Seckl, J.R. (1992). Increased expression of preprotachykinin, calcitonin gene-related peptide, but not vasoactive intestinal peptide messenger RNA in dorsal root ganglia during the development of adjuvant monoarthritis in the rat. *Mol. Brain Res.* **16**, 143–9.

Donnerer, J., Schuligoi, R., and Stein, C. (1992). Increased content and transport of substance P and calcitonin gene-related peptide in sensory nerves innervating inflamed tissue: evidence for a regulatory function of nerve growth factor in vivo. *Neuroscience* **49**, 693–8.

Ehrhard, P.B., Erb, P., Graumann, U., and Otten, U. (1993). Expression of nerve growth factor and nerve growth factor receptor tyrosine kinase Trk in activated CD4-positive T-cell clones. *Proc. natl Acad. Sci., USA* **90**, 10984–8.

Eide, F.F., Lowenstein, D.H., and Reichardt, L.F. (1993). Neurotrophins and their receptors—current concepts and implications for neurologic disease. *Exp. Neurol.* **121**, 200–14.

Fagarasan, M.O., Eskay, R., and Axelrod, J. (1989). Interleukin-1 potentiates the secretion of β-endorphin induced by secretagogues in a mouse pituitary cell line (AtT-20). *Proc. natl Acad. Sci., USA* **86**, 2070–5.

Ferreira, S.H., Lorenzetti, B.B., Bristow, A.F., and Poole, S. (1988). Interleukin-1 beta as a potent hyperalgesic agent antagonized by a tripeptide analogue. *Nature* **334**, 698–700.

Fields, H.L., Emson, P.C., Leigh, B.K., Gilbert, R.F.T., and Iversen, L.L. (1980). Multiple opiate receptor sites on primary afferent fibres. *Nature* **284**, 351–3.

Frank, G.B. (1985). Stereospecific opioid receptors on excitable cell membranes. *Can. J. Physiol. Pharmacol.* **63**, 1023–32.

Garry, M.G. and Hargreaves, K.M. (1992). Enhanced release of immunoreactive CGRP and substance P from spinal dorsal horn slices occurs during carrageenan inflammation. *Brain Res.* **582**, 139–42.

Gates, T.S., Zimmerman, R.P., Mantyh, C.R., Vigna, S.R., and Mantyh, P.W. (1989). Calcitonin gene-related peptide-alpha receptor binding sites in the gastrointestinal tract. *Neuroscience* **31**, 757–70.

Gibbins, I.L., Furness, J.B., and Costa, M. (1987). Pathway-specific patterns of the co-existence of substance P, calcitonin gene-related peptide, cholecystokinin and dynorphin in neurons of the dorsal root ganglia of the guinea pig. *Cell Tissue Res.* **248**, 417–37.

Hardebo, J.E., Suzuki, N., and Owman, C. (1994). Dynorphin B is present in sensory and parasympathetic nerves innervating pial arteries. *J. autonom. nerv. Syst.* **47**, 171–6.

Hassan, A.H.S., Przewlocki, R., Herz, A., and Stein, C. (1992). Dynorphin, a preferential ligand for kappa-opioid receptors, is present in nerve fibers and immune cells within inflamed tissue of the rat. *Neurosci. Lett.* **140**, 85–8.

Hassan, A.H.S., Ableitner, A., Stein, C., and Herz, A. (1993). Inflammation of the rat paw enhances axonal transport of opioid receptors in the sciatic nerve and increases their density in the inflamed tissue. *Neuroscience* **55**, 185–95.

Heijnen, C.J., Kavelaars, A., and Ballieux, R.E. (1991). β-endorphin: cytokine and neuropeptide. *Immunol. Rev.* **119**, 41–63.

Heppelmann, B., Messlinger, K., Neiss, W.F., and Schmidt, R.F. (1990). Ultrastructural three-dimensional reconstruction of group III and group IV sensory nerve ending ('free nerve endings') in the knee joint capsule of the cat: evidence for multiple receptive sites. *J. comp. Neurol.* **292**, 103–16.

Höllt, V. (1986). Opioid peptide processing and receptor selectivity. *Ann. Rev. Pharmacol. Toxicol.* **26**, 59–77.

Hosoi, J., Murphy, G.F., Egan, C.L., Lerner, E.A., Grabbe, S., Asahina, A., and Granstein, R.D. (1993). Regulation of Langerhans cell function by nerves containing calcitonin gene-related peptide. *Nature* **363**, 159–63.

Karalis, K., Sano, H., Redwine, J., Listwak, S., Wilder, R.L., and Chrousos, G.P. (1991). Autocrine or paracrine inflammatory actions of corticotropin-releasing hormone in vivo. *Science* **254**, 421–3.

Kavelaars, A., Jeurissen, F., Von Frijtag Drabbe Kunzel, J., Herman Van Roijen, J., Rijkers, G.T., and Heijnen, C.J. (1993). Substance P induces a rise in intracellular calcium concentration in human T lymphocytes in vitro: evidence of a receptor-independent mechanism. *J. Neuroimmunol.* **42**, 61–70.

Lacaze-Masmonteil, T., De Keyzer, Y., Luton, J.P., and Bertagna, X. (1987). Characterization of proopiomelanocortin transcripts in human non-pituitary tissues. *Proc. natl Acad. Sci., USA* **84**, 7261–5.

LaMotte, C., Pert, C.B., and Snyder, S.H. (1976). Opiate receptor binding in primate spinal cord: distribution and changes after dorsal root section. *Brain Res.* **112**, 407–12.

Lawrence, A.J., Joshi, G.P., Michalkiewicz, A., Blunnie, W.P., and Moriarty, D.C. (1992). Evidence for analgesia mediated by peripheral opioid receptors in inflamed synovial tissue. *Eur. J. clin. Pharmacol.* **43**, 351–5.

Lembeck, F. and Donnerer, J. (1985). Opioid control of the function of primary afferent substance P fibres. *Eur. J. Pharmacol.* **114**, 241–6.

Leon, A., Buriani, A., Dal Toso, R., Fabris, M., Romanello, S., Aloe, L., and Levi-Montalcini, R. (1994). Mast cells synthesize, store, and release nerve growth factor. *Proc. natl Acad. Sci., USA* **91**, 3739–43.

Levine, J.D. and Taiwo, Y.O. (1989). Involvement of the mu-opiate receptor in peripheral analgesia. *Neuroscience* **32**, 571–5.

Lindholm, D., Heumann, R., Meyer, M., and Thoenen, H. (1987). Interleukin-1 regulates synthesis of nerve growth factor in non-neuronal cells of rat sciatic nerve. *Nature* **330**, 658–9.

Lindsay, R.M. and Harmar, A.J. (1989). Nerve growth factor regulates expression of neuropeptide genes in adult sensory neurons. *Nature* **337**, 362–4.

Loh, H.H., Smith, A.P., and Lee, N.M. (1993). Effects of opioids on proliferation of mature and immature immune cells. *Advan. exp. Med. Biol.* **335**, 29–33.

Lolait, S.J., Clements, J.A., Markwick, A.J., Cheng, C., McNally, M., Smith, I.A., and Funder, J.W. (1986). Pro-opiomelanocortin messenger ribonucleic acid and posttranslational processing of beta-endorphin in spleen macrophages. *J. clin. Invest.* **77**, 1776–9.

McGillis, J.P., Organist, M.L., and Payan, D.G. (1987). Substance P and immunoregulation. *Fed. Proc.* **46**, 196–9.

McGillis, J.P., Mitsuhashi, M., and Payan, D.G. (1990). Immunomodulation by tachykinin neuropeptides. *Ann. NY Acad. Sci.* **594**, 85–94.

Maekawa, K., Minami, M., Yabuuchi, K., Toya, T., Katao, Y., Hosoi, Y., Onogi, T., and Satoh, M. (1994). In situ hybridization study of mu- and kappa-opioid receptor mRNAs in the rat spinal cord and dorsal root ganglia. *Neurosci. Lett.* **168**, 97–100.

Mantyh, P.W., Catton, M., Maggio, J.E., and Vigna, S.R. (1991). Alterations in receptors for sensory neuropeptides in human inflammatory bowel disease. *Advan. exp. Med. Biol.* **298**, 253–83.

Martin, J., Prystowsky, M.B., and Angeletti, R.H. (1987). Preproenkephalin mRNA in T-cells, macrophages and mast cells. *J. Neurosci. Res.* **18**, 82–7.

Meakin, S.O. and Shooter, E.M. (1992). The nerve growth family of receptors. *Trends Neurosci.* **15**, 323–31.

Mousa, S.A., Mitchell, W.M., Hassan, A.H.S., Carter, L., and Stein, C. (1994). Corticotropin releasing factor receptors in inflamed tissue: autoradiographic identification. *Regulat. Peptides* **54**, 203–4.

Mudge, A.W., Leeman, S.E., and Fischbach, G.D. (1979). Enkephalin inhibits release of substance P from sensory neurons in culture and decreases action potential duration. *Proc. natl Acad. Sci., USA* **76**, 526–30.

Ninkovic, M., Hunt, S.P., and Gleave, J.R.W. (1982). Localization of opiate and histamine H1-receptors in the primary sensory ganglia and spinal cord. *Brain Res.* **241**, 197–206.

Nong, Y.H., Titus, R.G., Ribeiro, J.M., and Remold, H.G. (1989). Peptides encoded by the calcitonin gene inhibit macrophage function. *J. Immunol.* **143**, 45–9.

Olsson, Y. (1990). Microenvironment of the peripheral nervous system under normal and pathological conditions. *Crit. Rev. Neurobiol.* **5**, 265–311.

Popper, P., Mantyh, C.R., Vigna, S.R., Maggio, J.E., and Mantyh, P.W. (1988). The localization of sensory nerve fibers and receptor binding sites for sensory neuropeptides in canine mesenteric lymph nodes. *Peptides* **9**, 257–67.

Przewlocki, R., Gramsch, C., Pasi, A., and Herz, A. (1983). Characterization and localization of immunoreactive dynorphin, alpha-neoendorphin, metenkephalin and substance P in human spinal cord. *Brain Res.* **280**, 95–103.

Przewlocki, R., Hassan, A.H.S., Lason, W., Epplen, C., Herz, A., and Stein, C. (1992). Gene expression and localization of opioid peptides in immune cells of inflamed tissue. Functional role in antinociception. *Neuroscience* **48**, 491–500.

Quartu, M. and Del Fiacco, M. (1994). Enkephalins occur and colocalize with substance P in human trigeminal ganglion neurones. *NeuroReport* **5**, 465–8.

Rapoport, S.I. and Robinson, P.J. (1986). Tight-junctional modification as the basis of osmotic opening of the blood–brain barrier. *Ann. NY Acad. Sci.* **481**, 250–67.

Rechthand, E. and Rapoport, S.I. (1987). Regulation of the microenvironment of peripheral nerve: role of the blood–nerve barrier. *Progr. Neurobiol.* **28**, 303–43.

Rosen, H., Behar, O., Abramsky, O., and Ovadia, H. (1989). Regulated expression of proenkephalin A in normal lymphocytes. *J. Immunol.* **143**, 3703–7.

Rotshenker, S., Aamar, S., and Barak, V. (1992). Interleukin-1 activity in lesioned peripheral nerve. *J. Neuroimmunol.* **39**, 75–80.

Roy, S., Ge, B.L., Ramakrishnan, S., Lee, N.M., and Loh, H.H. (1991). [3H]Morphine binding is enhanced by IL-1-stimulated thymocyte proliferation. *FEBS Lett.* **287**, 93–6.

Russell, N.J.W., Schaible, H.G., and Schmidt, R.F. (1987). Opiates inhibit the discharges of fine afferent units from inflamed knee joint of the cat. *Neurosci. Lett.* **76**, 107–12.

Sacerdote, P., Rubboli, F., Locatelli, L., Ciciliato, I., Mantegazza, P., and Panerai, A.E. (1991). Pharmacological modulation of neuropeptides in peripheral mononuclear cells. *J. Neuroimmunol.* **32**, 35–41.

Schäfer, M., Carter, L., and Stein, C. (1994). Interleukin 1β and corticotropin-releasing factor inhibit pain by releasing opioids from immune cells in inflamed tissue. *Proc. natl Acad. Sci., USA* **91**, 4219–23.

Schäfer, M., Imai, Y., Uhl, G.R., and Stein, C. (1995a). Inflammation enhances peripheral μ-opioid receptor-mediated analgesia, but not μ-opioid receptor transcription in dorsal root ganglia. *Eur. J. Pharmacol.* **279**, 165–9.

Schäfer, M., Mousa, S.A., and Stein, C. (1995b). Corticotropin releasing factor present in inflamed tissue is crucial for intrinsic mechanisms of peripheral opioid antinociception. *Soc. Neurosci. Abstr.* **21**(1), 649.

Schäfer, M.K.H., Bette, M., Romeo, H., Schwaeble, W., and Weihe, E. (1994). Localization of kappa-opioid receptor mRNA in neuronal subpopulations of rat sensory ganglia and spinal cord. *Neurosci. Lett.* **167**, 137–40.

Sharp, B. and Linner, K. (1993). Editorial: What do we know about the expression of proopiomelanocortin transcripts and related peptides in lymphoid tissue? *Endocrinology* **133**, 1921A–1921B.

Sibinga, N.E.S. and Goldstein, A. (1988). Opioid peptides and opioid receptors in cells of the immune system. *Ann. Rev. Immunol.* **6**, 219–49.

Smith, E.M., Galin, F.S., Le Boeuf, R.D., Coppenhaver, D.H., Harbour, D.V., and Blalock, J.E. (1990). Nucleotide and amino acid sequence of lymphocyte-derived corticotropin: endotoxin induction of a truncated peptide. *Proc. natl Acad. Sci., USA* **87**, 1057–60.

Stead, R.H., Tomioka, M., Quinonez, G., Simon, G.T., Felten, S.Y., and Bienenstock, J. (1987). Intestinal mucosal mast cells in normal and nematode-infected rat intestines are in intimate contact with peptidergic nerves. *Proc. natl Acad. Sci., USA* **84**, 2975–9.

Stein, C. (1993). Peripheral mechanisms of opioid analgesia. *Anesthes. Analges.* **76**, 182–91.

Stein, C. (1995). The control of pain in peripheral tissue by opioids. *New Engl. J. Med.* **332**(25), 1685–90.

Stein, C., Millan, M.J., and Herz, A. (1988). Unilateral inflammation of the hindpaw in rats as a model of prolonged noxious stimulation: alterations in behavior and nociceptive thresholds. *Pharmacol. Biochem. Behav.* **31**, 445–51.

Stein, C., Gramsch, C., and Herz, A. (1990a). Intrinsic mechanisms of antinociception in inflammation. Local opioid receptors and β-endorphin. *J. Neurosci.* **10**, 1292–8.

Stein, C., Hassan, A.H.S., Przewlocki, R., Gramsch, C., Peter, K., and Herz, A. (1990b). Opioids from immunocytes interact with receptors on sensory nerves to inhibit nociception in inflammation. *Proc. natl Acad. Sci., USA* **87**, 5935–9.

Stein, C., Comisel, K., Haimerl, E., Lehrberger, K., Yassouridis, A., Herz, A., and Peter, K. (1991). Analgesic effect of intraarticular morphine after arthroscopic knee surgery. *New Engl. J. Med.* **325**, 1123–6. Comment in *New Engl. J. Med.* **325**, 1168–9.

Stein, C., Hassan, A.H.S., Lehrberger, K., Giefing, J., and Yassouridis, A. (1993). Local analgesic effect of endogenous opioid peptides. *Lancet* **342**, 321–4. Comment in *Lancet* **342**, 320.

Sudduth-Klinger, J., Schumann, M., Gardner, P., and Payan, D.G. (1992). Functional and immunological responses of Jurkat lymphocytes transfected with the substance P receptor. *Cell. mol. Neurobiol.* **12**, 379–95.

Sweetnam, P.M., Wrathall, J.R., and Neale, J.H. (1986). Localization of dynorphin gene product-immunoreactivity in neurons from spinal cord and dorsal root ganglia. *Neuroscience* **18**, 947–55.

Van Woudenberg, A.D., Hol, E.M., and Wiegant, V.M. (1992). Endorphin-like immunoreactivities in uncultured and cultured human peripheral blood mononuclear cells. *Life Sci.* **50**, 705–14.

Wang, F., Millet, I., Bottomly, K., and Vignery, A. (1992). Calcitonin gene-related peptide inhibits interleukin 2 production by murine T lymphocytes. *J. biol. Chem.* **267**, 21052–7.

Webster, E.L., Tracey, D.E., Jutila, M.A., Wolfe, S.A., and De Souza, E.B. (1990). Corticotropin-releasing factor receptors in mouse spleen: identification of receptor-bearing cells as resident macrophages. *Endocrinology* **127**, 440–52.

Weihe, E., Hartschuh, W., and Weber, E. (1985). Prodynorphin opioid peptides in small somatosensory primary afferents of guinea pig. *Neurosci. Lett.* **58**, 347–52.

Weihe, E., Nohr, D., Millan, M.J., Stein, C., Müller, S., Gramsch, C., and Herz, A. (1988). Peptide neuroanatomy of adjuvant-induced arthritic inflammation in rat. *Agents Actions* **25**, 255–9.

Weihe, E., Büchler, M., Müller, S., Friess, H., Zentel, H.J., and Yanaihara, N. (1990). Peptidergic innervation in chronic pancreatitis. In *Chronic pancreatitis* (ed. H.G. Beger, M. Büchler, H. Ditschuneit, and P. Malfertheiner), pp. 83–105. Springer, Berlin.

Weskamp, G., and Otten, U. (1987). An enzyme-linked immunoassay for nerve-growth factor (NGF): a tool for studying regulatory mechanisms involved in NGF production in brain and peripheral tissues. *J. Neurochem.* **48**, 1779–86.

Westly, H.J., Kleiss, A.J., Kelley, K.W., Wong, P.K.Y., and Yuen, P.H. (1986). Newcastle disease virus-infected splenocytes express the proopiomelanocortin gene. *J. exp. Med.* **163**, 1589–93.

Werz, M.A. and MacDonald, R.L. (1982). Heterogeneous sensitivity of cultured dorsal root ganglion neurones to opioid peptides selective for mu- and delta-opiate receptors. *Nature* **299**, 730–3.

Yaksh, T.L. (1988). Substance P release from knee joint afferent terminals: modulation by opioids. *Brain Res.* **458**, 319–24.

Yonehara, N., Imai, Y., Chen, J.-Q., Takiuchi, S., and Inoki, R. (1992). Influence of opioids on substance P release evoked by antidromic stimulation of primary afferent fibers in the hind instep of rats. *Regulat. Peptides* **38**, 13–22.

Yoshino, S.I., Koiwa, M., Shiga, H., Nakamura, H., Higaki, M., and Miyasaka, N. (1992). Detection of opioid peptides in synovial tissues of patients with rheumatoid arthritis [letter]. *J. Rheumatol.* **19**, 660.

Zurawski, G., Benedik, M., Kamp, B.J., Abrams, J.S., Zurawski, S.M., and Lee, F.D. (1986). Activation of mouse T-helper cells induces abundant preproenkephalin mRNA synthesis. *Science* **232**, 772–5.

PART 5
Nociceptor plasticity

19 Development of the nociceptor phenotype: role of nerve growth factor

LORNE M. MENDELL

Introduction

The notion that specialized nociceptors exist among the afferent fibre population is a relatively recent one. Although indirect evidence for the existence of these fibres had been available for many years (reviewed in Perl 1984; see also Perl, Chapter 1, this volume), it was not until much later that definitive single-unit studies revealed the presence of neurones selectively activated by stimuli that are potentially damaging to the skin. These studies in the cat (Burgess and Perl 1967; Bessou and Perl 1969) clarified that there are two major groups of nociceptive afferents, one of which conducts in the Aδ conduction velocity range and the other of which conducts in the C-fibre range. The former innervate receptors that are high-threshold mechanoreceptors (HTMs), whereas the latter are more diverse in their properties with many being sensitive to multiple modalities of stimulation (mechanical, thermal, chemical) giving rise to the name *polymodal nociceptor*. More recently, these two groups of fibres have been identified in the rat (Lynn and Carpenter 1982). This chapter focuses on the development of nociceptors, and particularly on the role of nerve growth factor (NGF) in determining the development of these sensory receptors.

Since the nociceptive afferent population is a constituent of the dorsal root ganglion, its development can be evaluated from the perspective of the development of sensory neurones. More specifically, it can be examined in terms of the different structures such as the axon or cell body, or functions such as the somatic action potential or peripheral receptor properties. Finally, the role of trophic factors in promoting development of nociceptors has become an area of intensive investigation that is deserving of comment in any such discussion.

Non-uniformity in the development of sensory ganglion cells and their projections

The heterogeneity of cells in the dorsal root ganglion (DRG) extends over many different dimensions that are useful in charting their development. They vary substantially in size (both soma and axon), in peptide content (reviewed in Lawson 1992 and Lawson, Chapter 3, this volume), and in electrophysiological properties (reviewed in Koerber and Mendell 1992). Historically, a very useful classification scheme, based on appearance in histological section with a Nissl stain, is the large-light/small-dark division. Large light cells are destined to become large, myelinated afferents, whereas small, dark cells are destined to become small myelinated or unmyelinated afferents (reviewed in Lawson 1992).

The birth dates of neurones in the DRG (that is, the time at which the last mitosis takes place as studied with thymidine autoradiography) are not uniform (Fig. 19.1). DRG cells are born on gestational days 12–14 in the rat (Lawson *et al.* 1974) and on days 10–13 in the mouse (Lawson and Biscoe 1979). The staining and size differences between large light and small dark cells can be distinguished at this time. In both rat (Lawson *et al.* 1974) and chick (Carr and Simpson 1978), the small dark cells are born later than the large light cells. This indicates that cells destined to be nociceptors are born later than those destined to respond to innocuous stimulation of the skin.

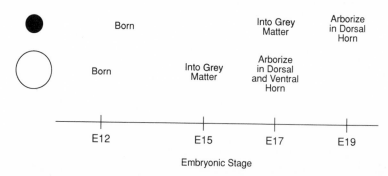

Fig. 19.1 The development of large light cells (open circles) as well as the arborization of their projections in the spinal cord occurs earlier than that of small dark cells (filled circles). Although specific stages are given, these are meant to be only approximate since the development of neurones supplying the forelimb occurs somewhat before the similar events for neurones innervating the hindlimb.

Studies with 1,1′-dioctadecyl-3,3,3′,3′-tetramethylindocarbocyanine perchlorate (diI) indicate that sensory cells project into the spinal cord in the order in which they are born (Fig. 19.1). Snider *et al.* (1992) demonstrated in rat cervical spinal cord that the large-diameter afferents destined to project to the motoneurone pool first penetrate in the grey matter at embryonic day 15 (E15), and arborize in the ventral horn by E17. Large-diameter cutaneous afferents have also arborized in laminae III and IV by E17 (see also Smith 1983). In contrast, afferents projecting to superficial layers, that is, prospective nociceptive afferents, enter the grey matter only at E17 and arborize in their terminal region by E19 (Ruit *et al.* 1992).

Another dimension along which sensory neurone development can be measured is the configuration of the somatic spike (Fig. 19.2). Early studies of Rohon–Beard cells in *Xenopus laevis*, which are sensory neurones that fail to survive the developmental period, revealed that spike properties change substantially during their brief lifetime (Baccaglini and Spitzer 1977; O'Dowd *et al.* 1988). Similar findings were made in *Xenopus* DRG cells (Baccaglini 1978). Initially, the inward current is carried primarily by Ca^{2+} with some contribution from Na^+; at this time the spike is tetrododoxin (TTX)-insensitive. As the cells mature, the contribution of Na^+ to the inward current increases. At a still later stage these cells develop spikes whose inward current is largely TTX-sensitive. This apparent change in ion channels associated with inward currents is in large part the result of changes in the expression of the K^+ channels, both the delayed rectifier as well as the Ca^{2+}-dependent K^+ current, which undergo significant increase both in strength (that is, current density) and in speed at this time. Similar studies of prenatal sensory neurones have been carried out in newly differentiated DRG neurones of chick

(Gottmann *et al.* 1988) and quail (Bader *et al.* 1985) maintained in culture. Under these conditions, the first currents to be expressed are carried by K$^+$ ions with Na$^+$ and Ca^{2+} currents becoming evident only later. Although the development of these currents is not uniform in this population of cells, after 2 days in culture virtually all cells express the entire array of currents (low- and high-voltage-activated Ca^{2+} currents as well as TTX-sensitive Na$^+$ currents). Thus there appears to be no obligatory pattern of development of expression of ion channels in DRG neurones, although culturing these cells may affect the expression of ion channels (Scott and Edwards 1980).

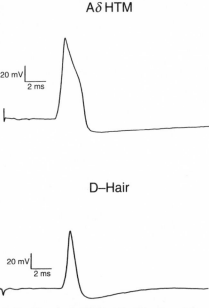

Aδ HTM

20 mV
2 ms

D–Hair

20 mV
2 ms

Fig. 19.2 Examples of somatic spikes from cat DRG cells. The top picture is from an Aδ HTM and demonstrates the characteristic inflection on the descending limb of the spike. Note also the long afterhyperpolarization. The bottom spike is from a low-threshold D-hair afferent with an axonal conduction velocity similar to that of the HTM. Note the briefer spike with the lack of an inflection on the descending limb. Adapted with permission from Fig. 2 of Traub and Mendell (1988).

Studies of the somatic spike in the rat DRG have revealed that these cells are differentiated at birth. Up to the very latest embryonic period (E19; Mirnics *et al.* 1993) or to postnatal day 0 (P0; Fulton 1987) all neurones in the DRG exhibit relatively broad spikes with an inflection on the falling phase that is generally attributed to a Ca^{2+} current (reviewed by Koerber and Mendell 1992) and have relatively long afterhyperpolarizations (AHP). Despite these general similarities, some correlated differences exist among the cells that provide some inkling concerning their eventual fate (Fulton 1987). Thus cells whose axons conduct relatively slowly are identified as prospective C fibres. Their somatic spikes tend to be broader with a clear inflection on the descending limb. They are associated with longer values of AHP, and are completely resistant to blockade by TTX. Fibres with slightly larger values of axonal conduction velocity, identified as prospective A fibres, tend to have somewhat narrower somatic spikes with a faster rising and a faster falling (but still with an inflection) phase and to exhibit partial sensitivity to TTX.

During the first 2 weeks of postnatal life all cells, but particularly prospective A fibres, increase their axonal conduction velocity, as anticipated from increased axonal diameter and the myelination that occurs during this period (Friede and Samorajski 1968). One group of neurones with the smallest values of axonal conduction velocity continues to exhibit the broadest somatic spikes (Fig. 19.3). Two types of somatic spikes can be distinguished among the more rapidly conducting A fibres. One group, restricted largely to the slowest axonal conduction velocities, displays relatively broad, TTX-insensitive spikes with an inflection on the descending limb; the other group whose conduction velocities cover the entire A-fibre spectrum has TTX-sensitive spikes with no evidence of any inflection on the descending limb (Harper and Lawson 1985; reviewed in Koerber and Mendell 1992).

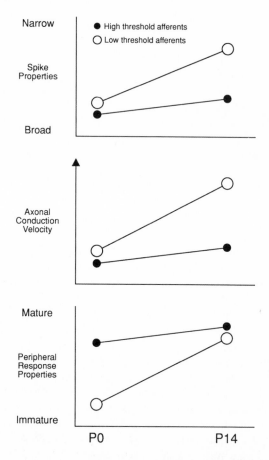

Fig. 19.3 Postnatal development of properties of sensory ganglion cells. The properties of somatic spikes change substantially between postnatal days 0 (P0) and 14 (P14) for low-threshold mechanoreceptors, presumably the large light cells (open circle) in that they change from broad to narrow, whereas the broad spikes of high-threshold neurones (presumably small dark cells, filled circles) remain broad although with some decrease in width. The axonal conduction velocity (a continuous variable denoted by arrowhead on ordinate) and peripheral response properties of large light cells (low-threshold afferents) change substantially, whereas for small dark cells the postnatal changes are relatively small.

Parallel evidence is now accumulating that DRG neurones systematically express different Na^+ and K^+ channels depending on their size and thus presumably their spike shape. Large cells tend to have a preponderance of rapid, TTX-sensitive Na^+-channels and rapid K^+-channels (I_A), whereas in small cells slower TTX-insensitive Na^+ channels and slower K^+ channels (delayed rectifier) tend to predominate (Campbell 1992; Caffrey *et al.* 1992).

The importance of this maturational scheme in the context of studies of development of nociceptors becomes clear when it is recognized that somatic action potentials display systematic differences in the mature animal according to the receptor type innervated in the periphery (Fig. 19.2). It has been shown in several species that afferents whose adequate stimulus is best described as mechanical nociception tend to have relatively broad somatic action potentials with inflections on their descending limb (Nicholls and Baylor 1968; Rose *et al.* 1986; Koerber *et al.* 1988; Traub and Mendell 1988; Ritter and Mendell 1992). From this perspective, mechanical nociceptors with myelinated (Aδ) axons resemble relatively immature neurones. The situation with regard to cells with unmyelinated axons is similar in that the somatic spikes of all these neurones are broad with prominent inflections on the descending limb regardless of whether they supply low- or high-threshold mechanoreceptors (Traub and Mendell 1988). Cells with myelinated axons activated by non-nociceptive stimuli exhibit brief somatic spikes without inflections. Thus, spikes in cells that are born later during development resemble those in immature neurones. One interpretation would be that cells born earlier would have access to more of some factor permitting maturation. However, since these cells are differentiated into large light and small dark from the very beginning (see above), it seems more likely that the spike phenotype is also specified very early.

Functional differentiation of the somatic spike is unlikely to determine the extent of impulse conduction through the ganglion since the cell body is electrically distant from where the axon gives off the side branch going to the cell body. Experimental evidence suggests that this branch point rather than the cell body itself is principally responsible for frequency sensitivity of conduction through the ganglion (Ito and Saiga 1959; Gallego and Eyzaguirre 1978; Stoney 1990).

The adequate stimulus of individual sensory neurones also exhibits changes during the perinatal period (M. Fitzgerald 1987). By E17 individual fibres can be classified as slowly or rapidly adapting although their firing frequencies are much lower than those of the adult pattern, presumably at least in part as a result of the lack of myelination. Some of these neurones are sensitive to noxious heating or mechanical stimulation. At slightly later stages (E18) mechanoreceptors sensitive to light touch or brushing and insensitive to thermal stimulation can be identified. These persist during the initial 2 weeks of postnatal life but gradually disappear, either maturing into the mechanoreceptors seen in adults, or becoming insensitive as the innervation of the skin changes during this period. Although all afferent fibre types can be detected at birth, low-threshold mechanoreceptors (LTMs) are much more immature in their sensory response properties than nociceptors, both the C-fibre polymodal nociceptors and the Aδ HTMs (Fig. 19.3). Maturation of sensory receptor properties thus occurs in the inverse order of cell birth, and this could reflect the additional step that the large, low-threshold afferents must go through in order to be fully mature, namely, myelination of the axon making possible the high-frequency conduction required to display mature receptor properties.

An important difference between cells innervating nociceptors and low-threshold afferents is that the former release peptides such as calcitonin gene-related peptide (CGRP) (Morton and Hutchison 1989) and substance P (Duggan *et al.* 1987) in addition to excitatory amino acids. There is evidence in other systems that the release of peptides requires Ca^{2+} channels of the L-type (Lemos and Nowycky 1989), so it is possible that the broad somatic spike of nociceptors is a reflection of channels that are necessary in the presynaptic terminals. Thus, the differentiation of somatic spikes may very well reflect physiological imperatives rather than being a consequence of the developmental time-table. In addition, since all sensory neurones have broad spikes during their early development, it may be that a period of peptide release is necessary during ontogeny. One possibility is that the peptides released during development are not transmitters such as CGRP or substance P, but rather growth factors such as NGF, brain-derived neurotrophic factor (BDNF), or neurotrophin 3 (NT-3) whose release from neurones would enable them to serve as trophic factors (Schecterson and Bothwell 1992).

It is interesting that, despite the presence of substance P in the somata of rat sensory neurones at birth, one anticipated result of its release peripherally, namely, neurogenic extravasation (Kenins 1981; Jänig and Lisney 1989), does not develop until about 10 days after birth (M. Fitzgerald and Gibson 1984). This indicates that the axon reflex is not present at birth despite the apparent availability of the appropriate peptide transmitter, although perhaps in lower than adult concentrations (M. Fitzgerald and Gibson 1984; Marti *et al.* 1987). Thus, further maturation in the function of C fibres occurs despite the adult pattern of receptive field and peptide transmitter. In this regard it is interesting that, although the central projections of C fibres into the superficial laminae of the spinal cord are well developed anatomically at birth (M. Fitzgerald and Swett 1983) and although their activation via mustard oil is capable of causing subthreshold depolarization and central sensitization (M. Fitzgerald 1991), they only become able to elicit impulse activity in dorsal horn neurones (M. Fitzgerald 1985) and in motor neurones (M. Fitzgerald and Gibson 1984; Hori and Watanabe 1987) after P8. Complete maturation of C-fibre central physiology may be delayed to some extent by the relatively late development of the neurones of the substantia gelatinosa to which they project (Altman and Bayer 1984). The fact that motorneurones are depolarized by C-fibre volleys from birth (see M. Fitzgerald 1991) would also argue that the deficit in the response of neonatal dorsal horn neurones is postsynaptic rather than presynaptic.

NGF is required for the survival of nociceptive neurones

The development of sensory neurones has long been known to be dependent on the action of growth factors. The most extensively characterized and studied growth factor, NGF, was shown originally to exert its action primarily on cells derived from neural crest, specifically cells of the autonomic ganglia and sensory ganglia (Levi-Montalcini and Hamburger 1953). Many of the early studies were carried out on these cells in culture where it was shown that NGF promoted their survival and was a required constituent of defined media for these neuronal types. It was also demonstrated that NGF would promote neurite elongation of these neurones, determining not only the extent of process outgrowth but also its direction. These studies are reviewed elsewhere (Purves 1988) and are not the focus of this chapter.

The role of NGF in the development of the sensory neurone population has been established by eliminating NGF from the developing animal using antibodies acting against NGF. In early studies the effects of such anti-NGF treatments (administered systemically) in neonatal animals was found to be more profound on the population of autonomic neurones than on sensory neurones (Levi-Montalcini and Cohen 1956; reviewed in Purves 1988). Typically, cell counts of autonomic ganglia revealed cell losses of 70 or 80 per cent after neonatal anti-NGF (with reciprocal effects, that is, increases in cell number after administration of NGF; Schafer *et al.* 1983), whereas the cell loss in the DRG was rarely greater than 40 per cent (Hulsebosch *et al.* 1987; E.M. Johnson *et al.* 1989). The apparent insensitivity of DRG neurones compared to sympathetic neurones turned out to be the result of timing differences in NGF requirement. When anti-NGF was administered to the pregnant mother, a much larger fraction of DRG neurones failed to survive in the neonate (Gorin and Johnson 1979). More recent experiments have revealed that anti-NGF treatments beginning 2 days after birth are much less effective in reducing the number of cells in the DRG (Lewin *et al.* 1992*b*; see below), although such treatments reduce the size of the sympathetic ganglia.

Further studies have indicated that neonatal sensory neurones undergo changes interpreted as sprouting in response to treatment with anti-NGF (Hulsebosch *et al.* 1987). This seems paradoxical in view of the reported effects of NGF in stimulating sprouting (Diamond *et al.* 1992). However, Hulsebosch *et al.* (1987) have suggested that this sprouting represents a response to the loss of cells induced by the anti-NGF treatment, that is, the stimulus for sprouting induced by denervation more than compensates for the loss of NGF.

In these early studies it was clear that sensory neurones were not equally affected by treatments with anti-NGF, with the small cells in the ganglion being affected to the greatest extent (Goedert *et al.* 1984; Hulsebosch *et al.* 1987). Although it is difficult to correlate soma size with axon size except in the most general terms (for reviews, see Willis and Coggeshall 1991; Lawson 1992), the findings were that C fibres and thinly myelinated Aδ fibres required NGF for survival to a much greater extent than did large-diameter Aβ fibres. Consistent with these findings it was also reported that anti-NGF treatments selectively deplete the DRG of cells containing peptides such as CGRP and substance P (Otten *et al.* 1980; Goedert *et al.* 1984). More recently, it was demonstrated that cells requiring NGF for survival project to the superficial layers of the dorsal horn (Ruit *et al.* 1992). All of these findings suggest that the development of nociceptive neurones in the DRG requires NGF, although one could not conclude that this requirement for NGF for survival is limited to nociceptive afferents.

Neurones requiring NGF for survival would be anticipated to express receptors for this trophic factor. A number of experimental data are consistent with this. Richardson and collaborators demonstrated that the high-affinity NGF receptor is located preferentially on small-diameter DRG neurones expressing some (CGRP, substance P) but not all (fluoride-resistant acid phosphatase (FRAP)) markers used to characterize these neurones (Verge *et al.* 1989). The availability of antibodies to the high-affinity NGF receptor, tyrosine kinase A (*trk*A), has permitted confirmation of their preferential location on small-diameter afferents, again with a subpopulation of such cells not expressing this receptor and thus presumably not being regulated by NGF (McMahon *et al.* 1994).

NGF is required for maintenance of the HTM phenotype

Recent physiological studies have confirmed the selective effects of NGF on the development of nociceptive neurones (Ritter *et al.* 1991; Lewin *et al.* 1992*b*). Recordings were made from the axons of sensory ganglion cells in the dorsal root in 5–6 week old anaesthetized rats treated neonatally with anti-NGF. The search stimulus was an electrical shock delivered to the sural nerve dissected free of surrounding tissue but left in continuity with the periphery. Units were characterized according to their axonal conduction velocity, adequate stimulus, and receptive field location. The properties of myelinated Aβ fibres were found to be unaffected by anti-NGF treatment (Fig. 19.4). However, Aδ fibres exhibited considerable changes in their distribution of receptor types. In control age-matched animals 40 per cent of the Aδ units responding to electrical stimulation of the sural nerve were characterized as HTMs, 30 per cent were low-threshold hair afferents (D-hairs), and 30 per cent were innervated subcutaneous receptors (referred to as 'Deep' receptors). In rats treated from birth with anti-NGF for 5 weeks (Ritter *et al.* 1991), the proportion of HTMs dropped precipitously with an increase in the proportion of LTMs, specifically the D-hairs (see below) (Fig. 19.4).

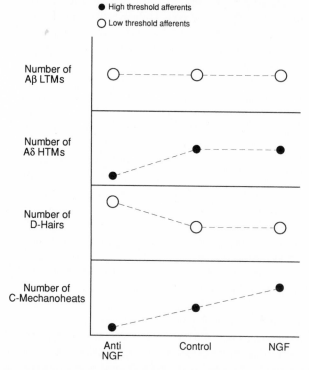

Fig. 19.4 Effects of manipulation of postnatal NGF levels on the number of receptors for different types. Aβ afferents exhibit no change after increase or decrease of NGF levels. Aδ HTMs exhibit decreased numbers after anti-NGF but no change when excess NGF is given. Aδ D-hairs exhibit reciprocal changes after anti-NGF and no change after excess NGF. C-fibre mechanoheat receptors are diminished in number after anti-NGF and increased in number after NGF.

Restricting the time of administration of anti-NGF led to the conclusion that there is a critical period for these effects of anti-NGF; this critical period encompassed the period from 4 days to 11 days postnatally (Lewin *et al.* 1992*b*).

One possible contributor to the critical period might be the timing of access of anti-NGF to the skin which is critical in this process (see below). This has been assessed by examining the distribution of IgG molecules in neonatal rats after systemic administration (Tonra and Mendell 1995). Access to the epidermis was always restricted compared to the dermis, but no differences were seen over the initial 2-week postnatal period.

The depletion of Aδ HTMs is consistent with previous findings that NGF is required for the survival of nociceptors. However, the experimental results were not completely consistent with this interpretation because *both* other receptors types in the Aδ conduction velocity range did not increase by the same proportion as might have been expected had the anti-NGF simply prevented survival of most of the HTMs. Additional studies have shown that the depletion of HTMs by anti-NGF can occur without detectable DRG cell death. This was demonstrated by administering anti-NGF from 2–14 days postnatally, beyond the time during which NGF is required for DRG neurone survival (Lewin *et al.* 1992*b*). This dissociation confirms that cell death is not required for the anti-NGF-induced depletion of HTMs.

If HTMs are depleted in the absence of cell death, it follows that they must be converted into some other type of afferent fibre. Since the D-hair population was found to exhibit an increase corresponding to the loss of HTMs (Lewin *et al.* 1992*b*), it was concluded that depriving the animal of NGF at a critical period (4–11 days postnatally) prevents the maintenance of the HTM phenotype and that these neurones 'switch' their phenotype to that of D-hairs. This change persists into the adult, when these recordings were made.

The axonal conduction velocity of HTMs surviving anti-NGF treatment during the critical period was lower on average than normal (Lewin *et al.* 1992*b*). Axons are growing during this period as evidenced by increases in conduction velocity from 0–2 weeks (Fulton 1987; Fig. 19.2) and increasing further by 5–6 weeks (Lewin *et al.* 1992*b*). Anatomically, the increase in diameter of the growing axons would be expected to increase the proportion of axons with myelination (Friede 1972; Voyvodic 1989). Conversely, a decrease in diameter due to anti-NGF might reduce the proportion of myelinated axons. This raises the possibility that anti-NGF administered in the neonatal period prevents growth of axons destined to become Aδ nociceptors rather than causing their conversion to D-hairs. These neurones might remain unmyelinated and thus not be counted as Aδ fibres.

There are several reasons to suggest that the failure for afferents to grow after anti-NGF is not the correct explanation. If afferents were not counted because they were C-fibres, in effect, this would be the equivalent of cell death in terms of evaluating the proportions of Aδ fibres of the different types for which evidence to the contrary has been obtained (see above). The shrinkage hypothesis is also not supported by the finding that the afferent-fibre diameter spectrum remained unchanged after anti-NGF (Ritter *et al.* 1991). Furthermore, mechanically sensitive unmyelinated afferents in these animals exhibit thresholds lower than normal Aδ HTMs (Lewin and Mendell 1994), not higher as is noted for surviving Aδ afferents in animals treated with anti-NGF (Lewin *et al.* 1992*b*; see below). Therefore, the mechanoreceptive unmyelinated afferents that emerge after anti-NGF treatment do not appear to represent Aδ afferents that have shrunk.

Taken together, these results suggest that NGF is required for normal development of HTMs and that in its absence these neurones develop into D-hairs. The interpretation of these findings requires examination of the normal development of skin sensory innervation. In a previous section the maturation of somatic membrane properties during the first 2 postnatal weeks was described. In addition the axons of these fibres are increasing in diameter and are becoming myelinated (Friede and Samorajski 1968) as evidenced by the dramatic increase in axonal conduction velocity that occurs over this period (Fulton 1987; M. Fitzgerald and Fulton 1992). The innervation of the skin begins during fetal life reaching the proximal hindlimb (in the rat) by E14 and the toes by E19. Although the skin is innervated at birth, the adult organization is not achieved for at least 2 postnatal weeks (M.J.T. Fitzgerald 1967; Reynolds *et al.* 1991). Innervation of the skin is initially rather diffuse consisting of an undifferentiated plexus of nerve processes reaching the epidermal surface. The switch to the adult pattern (Kruger *et al.* 1989) occurs during the first 2 postnatal weeks, and involves a withdrawal of nerve processes from the outer layers of the epidermis to the dermis (M.J.T. Fitzgerald 1967; Reynolds *et al.* 1991).

It may seem paradoxical that afferent fibres, particularly nociceptors, have recognizable, relatively well defined receptive field properties at birth (see above) despite the immature pattern of skin innervation existing at that time. This mismatch suggests that the adequate stimulus of sensory fibres may be determined by the properties of the fibre itself as well as of its receptor in the skin. Similar conclusions have been reached from studies of receptive field properties of regenerating afferents (R.D. Johnson and Munson 1991; Lewin and McMahon 1991*a,b*; R.D. Johnson *et al.* 1995; Koerber *et al.* 1995). In this regard it is interesting that afferents exhibiting the most mature receptive field properties at birth are nociceptive afferents, and these are the afferents whose membrane properties, as determined from measurements of the somatic spike, are closest to those observed in the adult.

This pattern of normal development provides a backdrop against which the changes after anti-NGF treatment can be viewed. Since mechanical nociceptors can be recognized before the critical period for the NGF's action on the HTM phenotype, we can infer that the role of NGF during the critical period is not to determine the phenotype, but rather to maintain it. From an anatomical point of view, the critical period for the action of NGF occurs at a time during which substantial rearrangement of skin innervation is taking place (see above). It has been demonstrated that NGF levels are relatively high in the skin during the perinatal period (Constantinou *et al.* 1994), particularly in the epidermal layers (Davies *et al.* 1987; Schechterson and Bothwell 1992). Lewin *et al.* (1992*b*) have suggested that these NGF levels are required during the critical period to maintain the HTM terminals in the epidermal layers where they reside in the adult (Kruger *et al.* 1981, 1985). If NGF levels are reduced by administering anti-NGF, the HTM terminals would migrate into the dermis, a shift that is taking place in parallel for many other cutaneous terminals during this period. Thus, the role of NGF would be to promote the maintenance of the HTM terminals in the epidermal layers, and, in the absence of this factor, these fibres could innervate different receptors in the dermal layer.

Additional evidence for physiological changes in HTMs after treatment with anti-NGF emerge from the finding that the mechanical threshold of HTMs that survive after anti-NGF treatment during the critical period, that is, are not converted to D-hairs, increases significantly (Lewin *et al.* 1992*b*). Anti-NGF treatments outside the critical period are ineffective in changing the mechanical threshold. A potential conflict arises in assessing the effects of anti-NGF administered during the critical period on mechanical threshold: on the one hand, anti-NGF causes cells destined to be HTMs to develop into ultrasensitive D-hairs and, on the other, it raises the threshold of the surviving HTMs. It would appear that the latter action is attributable directly to the action of anti-NGF since, when NGF is administered during the same time period, reciprocal changes occur, that is, HTM threshold decreases (Lewin *et al.* 1993) and HTM spike width increases (Ritter and Mendell 1992) (see below). Thus, the correlation between membrane properties and mechanical threshold appears to hold for HTMs, and the conversion to D-hairs presumably is triggered by the anti-NGF, but the phenotypic switch itself involves additional mechanisms (Ritter *et al.* 1991).

Other evidence indicating disruption of HTMs by anti-NGF comes from studies of antidromic vasodilatation induced by stimulation of the peripheral branch of cut peripheral nerves. After administration of anti-NGF from 2–14 days postnatally the vasodilatation induced in 5- to 6-week-old animals either by Aδ or by C fibres is significantly reduced in amplitude compared to that induced in control animals of the same age (Lewin *et al.* 1992*a*). Since these treatments are not accompanied by decreased numbers of Aδ or C fibres, it follows that the neurones have undergone changes in their peripheral effector function. This disruption has been attributed to depletion of CGRP terminals in the epidermis (Tonra *et al.* 1992). In contrast, neurogenic extravasation is not altered in anti-NGF treated animals; this action is thought to be mediated by substance P release from terminals in the skin (see discussion in Lewin *et al.* 1992*a*), which suggests that substance P-containing fibres are affected to a much lesser extent by anti-NGF than CGRP-containing fibres.

Administration of anti-NGF in the immediate postnatal period (2–14 days) also has considerable effects on the development of C-fibre receptive field types (Lewin and Mendell 1994). The clearest result is that the proportion of fibres sensitive to noxious heat, whether alone or in combination with noxious mechanical stimulation (C-mechanoheat fibres), falls dramatically (Fig. 19.3). These units are replaced by a novel group of mechanoreceptors with a much lower threshold than that of C fibres in control animals. However, the sensitivity of the other mechanically sensitive receptors, that is, the remaining C-mechanoheat fibres, C-mechanocold fibres, etc., is not altered. This selectivity rules out changes in skin properties, for example, thickness, in accounting for the increased sensitivity of the C-fibre mechanoreceptors. Relating the loss of C-mechanoheat afferents to the decrease in C-fibre evoked antidromic vasodilatation seen under the anti-NGF treatments (see above) suggests that at least most of these afferents use CGRP as a transmitter.

Behavioural changes after anti-NGF

It is striking that no changes in responsiveness to nociceptive stimulation have been noted after anti-NGF despite the dramatic alterations in nociceptor phenotypes (Lewin *et al.* 1993). The threshold for mechanical stimulation remains the same. If D-hairs converted from Aδ HTMs maintained their original central connections, one would anticipate that nociceptive pathways would be activated by extremely gentle stimuli. However, recent data (Lewin and Mendell, in press) indicate that cells in lamina I are not activated to any greater extent by Aδ LTMs after anti-NGF treatment over the critical period. This suggests that the central connectivity of these converted fibres has switched so that these afferents no longer activate central nociceptive pathways. It is important to contrast these findings with those of Urschel *et al.* (1991) who demonstrated hypoalgesia in response to anti-NGF treatments of neonatal rats. However, in these cases the rats were treated from birth, after which it is known that there is considerable loss in the number of sensory neurones (see above). Since the cells that are depleted are restricted largely to peptide-containing, small neurones, it seems likely that the hypoalgesia after these anti-NGF treatments is the result of the survival of fewer nociceptive afferents.

The studies with anti-NGF suggest that NGF is required for the survival and differentiation of nociceptors and for the maintenance of the nociceptor phenotype. For Aδ neurones, NGF appears to be responsible for the maintenance of the HTM phenotype; among C fibres the major action of NGF appears to be in maintaining the noxious heat sensitivity of these afferents. These actions are highly selective and additional experiments have confirmed that anti-NGF has no influence on the development of Aβ mechanoreceptors (Lewin *et al.* 1992*b*).

Developmental effects of NGF

A similar series of experiments has revealed that systemic administration of NGF can have substantial effects on the development of nociceptors. Unlike anti-NGF, it does not alter the relative proportions of Aδ mechanoreceptors, suggesting that NGF is normally present to excess as far as the maintenance of the Aδ HTM phenotype is concerned.

Although the proportion of Aδ HTMs is not altered by excess NGF in the neonate, their mechanical threshold is decreased if the NGF is administered in the immediate postnatal period (0–2 weeks; Lewin *et al.* 1993). This decrease in threshold is not permanent, lasting up to about 9 weeks of age. The proportion of Aδ HTMs that are rapidly adapting, normally about 20 per cent of the total, falls to virtually 0 per cent in these preparations. Furthermore, the population of mechanically insensitive Aδ afferents (identified in response to electrical stimulation of the sural nerve and the skin (Meyer and Campbell 1988) but insensitive to high-intensity mechanical stimulation of the electrically determined receptive field) also falls precipitously after administration of NGF. In conjunction with the reciprocal findings after anti-NGF, these results suggest that NGF regulates the mechanical sensitivity of Aδ HTMs in the neonate, and that the mechanically insensitive units require more NGF in order to become mechanically sensitive. It is interesting that a similar decrease in mechanically insensitive units is observed in the inflamed joint (Schaible and Schmidt 1985). This analogy between the effects of inflammation and administration of NGF has led to suggestions that NGF upregulation after injury may play a pivotal role in inducing the resultant hyperalgesia (Lewin and Mendell 1993*a*; Lewin *et al.* 1994; Woolf *et al.* 1994).

Reciprocity in the actions of NGF and anti-NGF is also observed in the changes in the C-fibre population after neonatal administration. Systemic administration of NGF in the neonate results in an increase in the proportion of units sensitive to noxious heat (Lewin and Mendell 1994), precisely the reverse of what occurs after anti-NGF administration in the neonate. The mechanism by which NGF alters the peripheral responsiveness to noxious heat is not known although behavioural studies in adults suggest that NGF might act peripherally via degranulation of mast cells (Lewin *et al.* 1994).

The mechanism by which NGF might influence the mechanosensitivity of sensory neurones is not known. One possibility is that the terminals in the skin might undergo sprouting (Diamond *et al.* 1992), thus providing additional transduction sites contributing to the production of the generator potential. Such sprouting is almost certainly highly localized since the receptive field areas of individual mechanoreceptors do not increase after NGF administration (Lewin *et al.* 1993).

The action of NGF on developing nociceptors is not restricted to peripheral changes. The hyperalgesia resulting from NGF administration may have a central component (Lewin *et al.* 1993), perhaps as a result of the upregulation of substance P and neurokinin A that has been noted in sensory ganglia of neonatal rats exposed to NGF (Vedder *et al.* 1993). The ability for NGF to upregulate tachykinins may correlate with the developmental expression of *trk* receptors in those neurones (Ehrhard and Otten 1994).

Genetic analysis of trophic factors and sensory neurone development.

Recent experiments have made use of transgenic mice over- or underexpressing NGF in the skin. This was accomplished by attaching sense or antisense NGF complementary DNA to the keratin promoter, which restricted the alterations in NGF levels to the skin. These animals were found to have altered nociceptive function, the NGF-overexpressing ones being mechanically hyperalgesic and the underexpressing ones being mechanically hypoalgesic (Davis *et al.* 1993). Knockouts of the high-affinity receptor for NGF (*trk*A) also result in hypoalgesia (Smeyne *et al.* 1994). Since these changes occur from the earliest developmental stages and last throughout the life of the animal, they cannot be specifically localized to the developmental or to any other period. Nonetheless, they are consistent with the view that the altered levels of NGF produced by systemic administration of NGF or its antibody are acting at the skin.

This genetic approach will prove to be more and more useful. For example, knockouts of various *trk* receptors that are the high-affinity receptors for the various neurotrophins (*trk*A for NGF; *trk*B for BDNF; *trk*C for NT-3) have revealed that these trophic factors may be affecting different populations of DRG neurones since different neurone types are eliminated in the knockout mice (reviewed in Mendell 1995). The findings are in agreement with the localization of *trk* receptors, suggesting that BDNF and the *trk*B receptor may be specific for large-diameter cutaneous afferents (Klein *et al.* 1993; Ernfors *et al.* 1994) and the NT-3/*trk*C receptor system may be specific for large-diameter muscle afferents (Klein *et al.* 1994).

Conclusion

The plasticity of nociceptors during development must be viewed in the context of changes that are occurring during the development of the organism. It is now clear from numerous studies that the birth of a neurone is no guarantee of its survival and that neurones must compete for the limited amount of appropriate trophic substance available in their target and possibly elsewhere in their environment. Survival does not mean that the neurone's fate is determined, since the absence of the appropriate trophic factor during and beyond the period at which it is required for survival can cause the neurone to stray from its normal developmental programme and develop into some other type of neurone. Although much remains to be discovered concerning the mechanisms of action of trophic factors, the studies on NGF and nociceptors indicate that they interact continuously to affect development as well as function once the developmental period is over.

Acknowledgements

I thank Alain Rueff and James Tonra for helpful comments. LMM's work was supported by NIH: PO1 NS 14899, RO1 NS 32264, and RO1 NS 16996 (Javits Neuroscience Award).

References

Altman, J. and Bayer, S.A. (1984). The development of the rat spinal cord. *Advan. Anat. Embryol. Cell Biol.* **85**, 1–166.

Baccaglini, P.I. (1978). Action potentials of embryonic dorsal root ganglion neurones in Xenopus tadpoles. *J. Physiol.* **283**, 585–604.

Baccaglini, P.I. and Spitzer, N.C. (1977). Developmental changes in the inward current of the action potential of Rohon–Beard neurones. *J. Physiol.* **271**, 93–117.

Bader, C.R., Bertrand, D., and Dupin, E. (1985). Voltage-dependent potassium currents in developing neurones from quail mesencephalic neural crest. *J. Physiol.* **366**, 129–51.

Bessou, P. and Perl, E.R. (1969). Response of cutaneous sensory units with unmyelinated fibers to noxious stimuli. *J. Neurophysiol.* **34**, 116–31.

Burgess, P.R. and Perl, E.R. (1967). Myelinated afferent fibres responding specifically to noxious stimulation of the skin. *J. Physiol.* **190**, 541–62.

Caffrey, J.M., Eng, D.L., Black, J.A., Waxman, S.G., and Kocsis, J.D. (1992). Three types of sodium channels in adult rat dorsal root ganglion neurons. *Brain Res.* **592**, 283–97.

Campbell, D.T. (1992). Large and small vertebrate sensory neurons express different Na and K channel subtypes. *Proc. natl Acad. Sci., USA* **89**, 9569–73.

Carr, V.M. and Simpson, S.B., Jr. (1978). Proliferative and degenerative events in the early development of chick dorsal root ganglia. I. Normal development. *J. comp. Neurol.* **182**, 727–40.

Constantinou, J., Reynolds, M.L., Woolf, C.J., Safieh-Garabedian, B., and Fitzgerald, M. (1994). Nerve growth factor levels in developing rat skin: upregulation following skin wounding. *NeuroReport* **5**, 2281–4.

Davies, A.M., Bandtlow, C., Heumann, R., Korsching, S., Rohrer, H., and Thoenen, H. (1987). Timing and site of nerve growth factor synthesis in developing skin in relation to innervation and expression of the receptor. *Nature* **326**, 353–8.

Davis, B.M., Lewin, G.R., Mendell, L.M., Jones, M.E., and Albers, K.M. (1993). Altered expression of nerve growth factor in the skin of transgenic mice leads to changes in response to mechanical stimuli. *Neuroscience* **56**, 789–92.

Diamond, J., Holmes, M., and Coughlin, M. (1992). Endogenous NGF and nerve impulses regulate the collateral sprouting of sensory axons in the skin of the adult rat. *J. Neurosci.* **12**, 1454–66.

Duggan, A.W., Morton, C.R., Zhao, Z.Q., and Hendry, I.A. (1987). Noxious heating of the skin releases immunoreactive substance P in the substantia gelatinosa of the cat: a study with antibody microprobes. *Brain Res.* **403**, 345–9.

Ehrhard, P.B. and Otten, U. (1994). Postnatal ontogeny of the neurotrophin receptors trk and trkB mRNA in rat sensory and sympathetic ganglia. *Neurosci. Lett.* **166**, 207–10.

Ernfors, P., Lee, K.-F., and Jaenisch, R. (1994). Mice lacking brain-derived neurotrophic factor develop with sensory deficits. *Nature* **368**, 147–50.

Fitzgerald, M. (1985). The postnatal development of cutaneous afferent fibre input and receptive field organization in the rat dorsal horn. *J. Physiol.* **364**, 1–18.

Fitzgerald, M. (1987). Cutaneous primary afferent properties in the hind limb of the neonatal rat. *J. Physiol.* **383**, 79–92.

Fitzgerald, M. (1991). The developmental neurobiology of pain. In *Proceedings of the 6th World Congress on Pain* (ed. M.R. Bond, J.E. Charlton, and C.J. Woolf), pp. 253–61. Elsevier, Amsterdam.

Fitzgerald, M. and Fulton, B.P. (1992). The physiological properties of developing sensory neurons. In *Sensory neurons: diversity, development and plasticity* (ed. S.A. Scott), pp. 287–306. Oxford University Press, Oxford.

Fitzgerald, M. and Gibson, S. (1984). The postnatal physiological and neurochemical development of peripheral sensory C fibres. *Neuroscience* **13**, 933–44.

Fitzgerald, M. and Swett, J. (1983). The termination pattern of sciatic nerve afferents in the substantia gelatinosa of neonatal rats. *Neurosci. Lett.* **43**, 149–54.

Fitzgerald, M.J.T. (1967). Perinatal changes in epidermal innervation in rat and mouse. *J. comp. Neurol.* **126**, 37–42.

Friede, R.L. (1972). Control of myelin formation by axon caliber (with a model of the control mechanism) *J. comp. Neurol.* **144**, 233–52.

Friede, R.L. and Samorajski, T. (1968). Myelin formation in the sciatic nerve of the rat. *J. Neuropathol. exp. Neurol.* **27**, 546–71.

Fulton, B.P. (1987). Postnatal changes in conduction velocity and soma action potential parameters of rat dorsal root ganglion neurones. *Neurosci. Lett.* **73**, 125–30.

Gallego, R. and Eyzaguirre, C. (1978). Membrane and action potential characteristics of A- and C nodose ganglion cells studied in whole ganglia and in tissue slices. *J. Neurophysiol.* **41**, 1217–32.

Goedert, M., Otten, U., Hunt, S.P., Chapman, D., Schlumpf, M., and Lichtensteiger, W. (1984). Biochemical and anatomical effects of antibodies against nerve growth factor on developing rat sensory ganglia. *Proc. natl Acad. Sci., USA* **81**, 1580–4.

Gorin, P.D. and Johnson, E.M. (1979). Experimental autoimmune model of nerve growth factor deprivation: effects on developmental peripheral sympathetic and sensory neurons. *Proc. natl Acad. Sci., USA* **76**, 5382–6.

Gottmann, K., Dietzel, I.D., Lux, H.D., Huck, S., and Rohrer, H. (1988). Development of inward currents in chick sensory and autonomic precursor cells in culture. *J. Neurosci.* **8**, 3722–32.

Harper, A.A. and Lawson, S.N. (1985). Electrical properties of rat dorsal root ganglion neurones with different peripheral nerve conduction velocities. *J. Physiol.* **359**, 47–63.

Hori, Y. and Watanabe, S. (1987). Morphine-sensitive components of the flexion reflex in the neonatal rat. *Neurosci. Lett.* **78**, 91–6.

Hulsebosch, C.E., Perez Polo, J.R., and Coggeshall, R.E. (1987). In vivo ANTI-NGF induces sprouting of sensory axons in dorsal roots. *J. comp. Neurol.* **259**, 445–51.

Ito, M. and Saiga, M. (1959). The mode of impulse conduction through the spinal ganglion. *Jap. J. Physiol.* **9**, 33–42.

Jänig, W. and Lisney, S.J. (1989). Small diameter myelinated afferents produce vasodilatation but no plasma extravasation in rat skin. *J. Physiol.* **415**, 477–86.

Johnson, E.M., Jr, Osborne, P.A., and Taniuchi, M. (1989). Destruction of sympathetic and sensory neurons in the developing rat by a monoclonal antibody against the nerve growth factor (NGF) receptor. *Brain Res.* **478**, 166–70.

Johnson, R.D. and Munson, J.B. (1991). Regenerating sprouts of axotomized cat muscle afferents express characteristic firing patterns to mechanical stimulation. *J. Neurophysiol.* **66**, 2155–8.

Johnson, R.D., Taylor, J.S., Mendell, L.M. and Munson, J.B. (1995). Rescue of motoneuron and muscle afferent functions in cats by regeneration into skin. I. Properties of afferents. *J. Neurophysiol.* **73**, 651–61.

Kenins, P. (1981). Identification of the unmyelinated sensory nerves which evoke plasma extravasation in response to antidromic stimulation. *Neurosci. Lett.* **25**, 137–41.

Klein, R., Smeyne, R.J., Wurst, W., Long, L.K., Auerbach, B.A., Joyner, A.L., and Barbacid, M. (1993). Targeted disruption of the *trk*B neurotrophin receptor gene results in nervous system lesions and neonatal death. *Cell* **75**, 113–22.

Klein, R., Silos- Santiago, I., Smeyne, R.J., Lira, S.A., Brambilla, R., Bryant, S., Zhang, L., Snider, W.D., and Barbacid, M. (1994). Disruption of *trk*C, the neurotrophin-3 receptor gene, eliminates Ia muscle afferents and results in movement abnormalities consistent with the loss of proprioception. *Nnature* **368**, 249–51.

Koerber, H.R. and Mendell, L.M. (1992). Functional heterogeneity of dorsal root ganglion cells. In *Sensory neurons:' diversity, development and plasticity* (ed. S.A. Scott), pp. 77–96. Oxford University Press, Oxford.

Koerber, H.R., Druzinsky, R.E., and Mendell, L.M. (1988). Properties of somata of spinal dorsal root ganglion cells differ according to peripheral receptor innervated. *J. Neurophysiol.* **60**, 1584–96.

Koerber, H.R., Mirnics, K., and Mendell, L.M. (1995). Properties of regenerated primary afferents and their central connections. *J. Neurophysiol.* **73**, 693–702.

Kruger, L., Perl, E.R., and Sedivec, M.J. (1981). Fine structure of myelinated mechanical nociceptor endings in cat hairy skin. *J. comp. Neurol.* **198**, 137–54.

Kruger, L., Sampogna, S.L., Rodin, B.E., Clague, J., Brecha, N., and Yeh, Y. (1985). Thin-fiber cutaneous innervation and its intraepidermal contribution studied by labeling methods and neurotoxin treatment in rats. *Somatosens. Res.* **2**, 335–56.

Kruger, L., Silverman, J.D., Mantyph, P.W., Sternini, C., and Brecha, N.C. (1989). Peripheral patterns of calcitonin-gene-related peptide general somatic sensory innervation: cutaneous and deep terminations. *J. comp. Neurol.* **280**, 291–302.

Lawson, S.N. (1992). Morphological and biochemical cell types of sensory neurons. In *Sensory neurons: diversity, development and plasticity* (ed. S.A. Scott), pp. 27–60. Oxford University Press, Oxford.

Lawson, S.N. and Biscoe, T.J. (1979). Development of mouse dorsal root ganglia: an autoradiographic and quantitative study. *J. Neurocytol.* **8**, 265–74.

Lawson, S.N., Caddy, K.W.T., and Biscoe, T.J. (1974). Development of rat dorsal root ganglion neurones. Studies of cell birthdays and changes in mean diameter. *Cell Tissue Res.* **153**, 399–413.

Lemos, J. and Nowycky, M.C. (1989). Two types of calcium channels coexist in peptide-releasing vertebrate nerve terminals. *Neuron* **2**, 1419–26.

Levi-Montalcini, R. and Cohen, S. (1956). In vitro and in vivo effects of a nerve growth-stimulating agent isolated from snake venom. *Proc. natl Acad. Sci., USA* **42**, 695–9.

Levi-Montalcini, R. and Hamburger, V. (1953). A diffusible agent of mouse sarcoma producing hyperplasia of sympathetic ganglia and hyperneurotization of viscera in the chick embryo. *J. exp. Zool.* **123**, 233–87.

Lewin, G.R. and McMahon, S.B. (1991*a*). Physiological properties of primary sensory neurons appropriately and inappropriately innervating the skin in adult rats. *J. Neurophysiol.* **66**, 1205–17.

Lewin, G.R. and McMahon, S.B. (1991*b*). Physiological properties of primary sensory neurons appropriately and inappropriately innervating skeletal muscle in adult rats. *J. Neurophysiol.* **66**, 1218–31.

Lewin, G.R. and Mendell, L.M. (1993*a*). Nerve growth factor and nociception. *Trends Neurosci.* **16**, 353–9.

Lewin, G.R. and Mendell, L.M. (1994). Regulation of cutaneous C-fiber heat nociceptors by nerve growth factor in the developing rat. *J. Neurophysiol.* **71**, 941–9.

Lewin, G.R. and Mendell, L.M. Maintenance of modality specific connections in the spinal cord after neonatal NGF deprivation. *Eur. J. Neurosci.* (in press).

Lewin, G.R., Lisney, S.J.W., and Mendell, L.M. (1992*a*). Neonatal anti-NFG treatment reduces the A and C-fiber evoked vasodilator responses in rat skin: evidence that nociceptor afferents mediate antidromic vasodilatation. *Eur. J. Neurosci.* **4**, 1213–18.

Lewin, G.R., Ritter, A.M., and Mendell, L.M. (1992*b*). On the role of nerve growth factor in the development of myelinated nociceptors. *J. Neurosci.* **12**, 1896–905.

Lewin, G.R., Ritter, A.M., and Mendell, L.M. (1993). Nerve growth factor induced hyperalgesia in the neonatal and adult rat. *J. Neurosci.* **13**, 2136–49.

Lewin, G.R., Rueff, A., and Mendell, L.M. (1994). Peripheral and central mechanisms of NGF-induced hyperalgesia. *Eur. J. Neurosci.* **6**, 1903–12.

Lynn, B. and Carpenter, S.E. (1982). Primary afferent units from the hairy skin of the rat hind limb. *Brain Res.* **238**, 29–43.

McMahon, S.B., Armanini, M.P., Ling, L.H., and Phillips, H.S. (1994). Expression and co-expression of *trk* receptors in subpopulations of adult primary sensory neurons projecting to identified peripheral targets. *Neuron* **12**, 1161–71.

Marti, E., Gibson, S.J., Polak, J.M., Facer, P., Springall, D.R., Van Aswega, G., Aitchison, M., and Koltzenberg, M. (1987). Ontogeny of peptide and amino-containing neurons in motor, sensory and autonomic regions of rat and human spinal cord. *J. comp. Neurol.* **266**, 332–59.

Mendell, L.M. (1995). Neurotrophic factors and the specification of neural function. *Neuroscientist* **1**, 26–34.

Meyer, R.A. and Campbell, J.N. (1988). A novel electrophysiological technique for locating cutaneous nociceptive and chemospecific receptors. *Brain Res.* **441**, 81–6.

Mirnics, K., Glickstein, S.B., and Koerber, H.R. (1993). Membrane properties of single primary afferents and their projections in the embryonic rat spinal cord. *Soc. Neurosci. Abstr.* **19**, 48.

Morton, C.R. and Hutchison, W.D. (1989). Release of sensory neuropeptides in the spinal cord: studies with calcitonin gene-related peptide and galanin. *Neuroscience* **31**, 807–15.

Nicholls, J.G. and Baylor, D.A. (1968). Specific modalities and receptive fields of sensory neurons in the CNS of the leech. *J. Neurophysiol.* **31**, 740–56.

O'Dowd, D.K., Ribera, A.B., and Spitzer, N.C. (1988). Development of voltage-sensitive calcium, sodium and potassium currents in Xenopus spinal neurons. *J. Neurosci.* **8**, 792–805.

Otten, U., Goedert, M., Mayer, N., and Lembeck, F. (1980). Requirement of nerve growth factor for the development of substance P containing neurones. *Nature* **287**, 158–9.

Perl, E.R. (1984). Pain and nociception. In *Handbook of physiology* Section I. *The nervous system.* Vol. III. *Sensory processes,* Part 2 (ed. I Darian-Smith), pp. 915–75. American Physiological Society, Bethesda, Maryland.

Purves, D. (1988). *Body and brain. A trophic theory of neuronal connections.* Harvard University Press, Cambridge, Massachusetts.

Reynolds, M.L., Fitzgerald, M., and Benowitz, L.I. (1991). GAP-43 expression in developing cutaneous and muscle nerves in the rat hindlimb. *Neuroscience* **41**, 201–11.

Ritter, A.M. and Mendell, L.M. (1992). The somal membrane properties of physiologically identified sensory neurons in the rat: effects of nerve growth factor. *J. Neurophysiol.* **68**, 2033–41.

Ritter, A.M., Lewin, G.R., Kremer, N.E., and Mendell, L.M. (1991). Requirement for nerve growth factor in the development of myelinated nociceptors in vivo. *Nature* **350**, 500–2.

Rose, R.D., Koerber, H.R., Sedivec, M.J., and Mendell, L.M. (1986). Somal action potential duration differs in identified primary afferents. *Neurosci. Lett.* **63**, 259–64.

Ruit, K.C., Elliot, J.L., Osborne, P.A., Yan, Q., and Snider, W.D. (1992). Selective dependence of mammalian dorsal root ganglion neurons on nerve growth factor during embryonic development. *Neuron* **8**, 573–87.

Schafer, T., Schwab, M.E., and Thoenen, H. (1983). Increased formation of preganglionic synapses and axons due to a retrograde trans-synaptic action of nerve growth factor in the rat sympathetic nervous system. *J. Neurosci.* **3**, 1501–10.

Schaible, H.G. and Schmidt, R.F. (1985). Effects of an experimental arthritis on the sensory properties of fine articular afferent units. *J. Neurophysiol.* **54**, 1109–26.

Schecterson, L.C. and Bothwell, M. (1992). Novel roles for neurotrophins are suggested by BDNF and NT-3 mRNA expression in developing neurons. *Neuron* **9** 449–63.

Scott, B.S. and Edwards, B.A.V. (1980). Electric membrane properties of adult mouse DRG neurons and the effect of culture duration. *J. Neurobiol.* **11**, 291–301.

Smeyne, R.J., Klein, R., Schnapp, A., Long, L.K., Bryant, S., Lewin, A., Lira, S., and Barbacid, M. (1994). Severe sensory and sympathetic neuropathies in mice carrying a disrupted *Trk*/NGF receptor gene. *Nature* **368**, 246–9.

Smith, C.L. (1983). The development and postnatal organization of primary afferent projections to the rat thoracic spinal cord. *J. comp. Neurol.* **220**, 29–43.

Snider, W.D., Zhang, L., Yusoof, S., Gorukanti, N., and Tsering, C. (1992). Interaction between dorsal root axons and their target motor neurons in developing mammalian spinal cord. *J. Neurosci.* **12**, 3494–3508.

Stoney, S.D. Jr (1990). Limitations on impulse conduction at the branch point of afferent axons in frog dorsal root ganglion. *Exp. Brain Res.* **80**, 512–24.

Tonra, J.R. and Mendell, L.M. (1995). Immunoglobulin localization in rat skin, DRG and spinal cord after rabbit sera injections. *Soc. Neurosci. Abstr.* **21**; 605.17.

Tonra, J.R., Lewin, G.R., McMahon, S.B., and Mendell, L.M. (1992). Rearrangement of CGRP-IR fibers in skin following neonatal anti-NGF treatment. *Soc. Neurosci. Abstr.* **18**, 60.10.

Traub, R.J. and Mendell, L.M. (1988). The spinal projection of individual identified A-delta—and C-fibers. *J. Neurophysiol.* **59**, 41–55.

Urschel, B.A., Brown, P.B., and Hulsebosch, C.E. (1991). Differential effects on sensory processes and behavioral alterations in the rat after treatment with anti-bodies to nerve growth factor. *Exp. Neurol.* **114**, 44–52.

Vedder, H., Affolter, H.U., and Otten, U. (1993). Nerve growth factor (NGF) regulates tachykinin gene expression and biosynthesis in rat sensory neurons during early postnatal development. *Neuropeptides* **24**, 351–7.

Verge, V.M.K., Richardson, P.M., Benoit, R., and Riopelle, R.J. (1989). Histochemical characterization of sensory neurons with high-affinity receptors for nerve growth factor. *J. Neurocytol.* **18**, 583–91.

Voyvodic, J.T. (1989). Target size regulates calibre and myelination of sympathetic axons. *Nature* **342**, 430–3.

Willis, W.D. and Coggeshall, R.E. (1991). *Sensory mechanisms of the spinal cord* (2nd edn). Plenum Press, New York.

Woolf, C.J., Safieh-Garabedian, B., Ma, Q.-P, Crilly, P., and Winter, J. (1994). Nerve growth factor contributes to the generation of inflammatory sensory hypersensitivity. *Neuroscience* **62**, 327–31.

20 Properties of regenerated nociceptor afferents

S.J.W. LISNEY

Introduction

The preceding chapters of this book have provided a persuasive justification for considering nociceptors and their associated afferents separately from other types of peripheral sensory unit. For example, in skin nerves nociceptor afferents outnumber all the other kinds of afferent taken together (Lynn and Carpenter 1982; Leem *et al.* 1993), and on these grounds alone some special significance can be inferred. As well as this, nociceptive afferents are involved in much more than simply transmitting information about noxious events occurring in the periphery to the central nervous system (CNS). Neuropeptides released from their central terminals as conventional transmitters/ neuromodulators (principally substance P, calcitonin gene-related peptide, and neuro-kinin A) are also released from their peripheral terminals, where they are involved in bringing about a range of local actions that together contribute to the initial stages of inflammation (see Lynn, Chapter 17, this volume). These actions include vasodilatation, increased vascular permeability, and direct and/or indirect effects on leucocyte mobility and activation. This dual afferent/efferent action of nociceptive fibres does not seem to be shared by other types of sensory unit. Levine *et al.* (1993) and Otsuka and Yoshioka (1993) have recently reviewed these functional aspects of the tachykinins in nociceptive afferents and their articles can be consulted in conjunction with the chapters by Lynn and Stein in this book. The main interest in nociceptive afferents, however, lies with their role in signalling tissue damage, and in the relationship between this activity and the triggering of nocifensive reflex responses, and also the initiation and maintenance of painful sensations. This connection between nociceptor afferent activity and pain is also the reason for the interest in nociceptor properties after peripheral nerve injury and regeneration.

The extent to which general sensibility returns to anything approaching normal after peripheral nerve injury depends on a host of factors, and, broadly speaking, these fall into two categories. The first includes factors that are local to the injury site, for example, the extent of the damage caused, whether or not the nerve is repaired and how immediately this is done, and whether there is secondary infection, and the main effect of these is in influencing the number of fibres that survive the injury and eventually re-establish a functional ending with an appropriate peripheral target. These factors also influence the degree to which surviving fibres show abnormal properties. The second category covers events occurring at sites distant from the injury, and includes changes such as alterations in the distribution and synaptic efficacy of the central terminals of the injured/regenerated fibres. These contribute to alterations in the central processing of the incoming information carried by the injured/regenerated fibres. The sum of all these changes together determines the quality of recovery after nerve injury. At one end of the spectrum the recovery might be very good—with no detectable sensory deficits or abnormalities (as is usually the case after crush injury, for example)—to being disturbingly poor—with clear deficiencies and abnormalities of sensation, including inappropriate, abnormal patterns of pain.

The association between major nerve injuries and an ongoing experience of abnormal pains has long been recognized (see, for example, Mitchell *et al.* 1864), but there are still many aspects of these pains that are poorly understood and that continue to puzzle (for recent books containing appropriate articles see Fields 1990; Jänig and Schmidt 1992; Wall and Melzack 1994; see also Chapter 21 by Ochoa *et al.* in this book). This is why there is still a continuing effort to find out what happens to nociceptive afferents after injury and regeneration. This chapter will deal with what happens to the injured fibres themselves but, as mentioned just previously, the changes that peripheral nerve damage triggers in the central nervous system must be remembered as these are likely to be equally, or possibly even more, important in determining the overall outcome as far as pain sensibility is concerned (for review articles see McMahon 1992; Wolff 1992).

Studies in man

Efforts to describe the time course and quality of the return of sensations after nerve injury in man began in the early part of this century, initially with the work of Head and his associates, Sherren and Rivers. Head arranged for the nerves supplying the back of one of his hands to be cut and then, with the help of Sherren and Rivers, he followed the progress of the reinnervation process (Head and Sherren 1905; Head *et al.* 1905; Rivers and Head 1908). The testing protocols included application of both mechanical and thermal noxious stimuli, so the findings of this extended study should have given indications on the regeneration of nociceptor afferents. From their testing of skin sensibility, Head, Sherren, and Rivers concluded that the ability to perceive pain and to detect extreme temperatures reappeared before the ability to detect light touch, pressure, and temperatures in the low-to-middle range. They explained this apparent difference in the rate of recovery of different sensibilities by proposing there were two distinct sensory systems, the so-called 'protopathic' one subserving pain and extreme temperature sensibility and the 'epicritic' one involved in touch and pressure sensation and in moderate temperature discrimination. The implication was that the nociceptive and certain temperature sensitive afferents, making up the protopathic system, regenerated more quickly than did the other classes of afferent fibres. Subsequent studies were unable to offer support for these ideas (for example, Trotter and Davies 1909; Boring 1916; Sharpey-Schafer 1929), finding that after nerve injury the submodalities of sensation return at more or less the same rate, with perhaps the ability to sense warmth being delayed. This pattern of recovery has recently been confirmed by Van Boven and Johnson (1994) in a carefully conducted study of a series of patients who had had unavoidable nerve damage as a consequence of corrective surgery of the jaw.

These kinds of study give general insights into the recovery from nerve injury but many things will have contributed to the overall picture obtained, including the extent of regeneration of the various groups of afferent fibres and the adaptive changes that will have taken place in the central nervous system in response to the altered input received from the regenerated fibres. It follows that other kinds of investigation are needed to obtain detailed information on what has happened to the nociceptive afferents. Those working in the clinical setting seem to have few tests for assessing the function of small fibres on their own, the main two being a test based on the ability of these fibres to initiate neurogenic inflammatory responses (see, for example, Parkhouse and Le Quesne 1988; Walmsley and Wiles 1991) and microneurography (see, for example, Nystrom and Hagbarth 1981; Ochoa et al. 1987; Ochs et al. 1989). Of these two, microneurography is the more precise, but up to now there have been few full reports of studies using the technique to investigate nociceptor afferent function after peripheral nerve injury (see, for example, Nystrom and Hagbarth 1981; Ochoa et al. 1987; Ochs et al. 1989) and, by the nature of the method, the results are likely to be just a snapshot of what is happening across the population of nociceptor afferents. To get a broader view of the properties of these afferents after injury it has been necessary to turn to experimental work involving laboratory animals.

Experiments on laboratory animals

Survival of injured afferent fibres

Investigations into the effects of cutting limb nerves in experimental animals and allowing them to regenerate or, alternatively, deliberately causing a stump neuroma to form have shown that 20–40 per cent of the sensory neurones supporting axons in the nerve die (for reviews see Aldskogius et al. 1985; Lisney 1989). This loss seems to be entirely of neurones supporting unmyelinated axons: if any cells supporting myelinated axons die after injury they are very few indeed. It is generally held that the closer the injury is to the cell body, that is, the more proximal it is, then the greater the loss is likely to be (Glover 1967; Ygge 1989; also see Lisney 1989 for a discussion). In most studies the degree of sensory neurone loss was estimated by making cell body counts of the appropriate dorsal root ganglia. Others have adopted a different approach and counted the numbers of axons present in the peripheral nerves themselves. Both strategies have their drawbacks, the main one so far as the present discussion is concerned being that neither has given any information about the relative survival of different types of sensory neurone. This shortcoming does not matter for the myelinated afferents because, if none is lost, then it is reasonable to assume that all the types originally present in the nerve survive and in the same proportions. It is feasible that the injury and regeneration process could cause some surviving axons to change their phenotype, but the electro-physiological evidence to date suggests this does not happen, at least not to any measurable degree (see below). Thus, it seems that the full complement of Aδ-nociceptor afferents survives in the proximal stump of any injured nerve and is therefore available for regeneration.

The lack of detailed information is more of a problem in assessing what happens among the sensory neurones with unmyelinated axons. The work involving cell body counts does not help because there are no reliable markers/indicators that enable cells to be assigned to particular afferent types. Knowing that the cell is large or small is not enough because of the possibility of size changes—particularly shrinkage—in the surviving ones. Thus, these studies have not been able to give any indication about whether C-fibre polymodal nociceptor afferent neurones survive better than the other C-fibre afferent types. The same identification problem applies to the axon-counting studies, where the picture is made more complicated still by the presence of the unmyelinated axons of postganglionic sympathetic neurones. The picture gained from electrophysiological studies of those C-fibre neurones that have survived injury and regenerated back to skin, however, is that all the afferent types found in normal nerves are still present and in about their normal proportions (Shea and Perl 1985): this suggests that the loss of different kinds of C-fibre sensory neurones is on a *pro rata* basis. Thus, in the proximal stump of an injured nerve there are likely to be 20–40 per cent fewer C-fibre nociceptor units available for regeneration than were originally present.

Regeneration across the injury site

Not all the myelinated and unmyelinated axons that survive injury manage to grow across the injury site and enter the distal stump (for a review see Lisney 1989). A much higher proportion of the surviving axons manage to negotiate an injury site if their basement membrane tubes remain intact, for example, after crushing or freezing, than when their continuity is interrupted. This is certainly true for myelinated sensory axons supplying skin (Horch and Lisney 1981). After a simple transection injury—without any form of repair—75–85 per cent of myelinated and unmyelinated axons manage to regenerate into the distal stump (see Lisney 1989 for references), a figure that is only slightly improved if a repair procedure is carried out.

While this is the picture after experimental injury in small cutaneous nerves in animals, where it was possible to exercise a measure of control over the surgical procedures, it is unlikely to be that seen in the clinical setting. Here few injuries are as simple as a clean cutting through of the nerve and there will be the possibility of other complicating factors such as additional soft tissue injury, damage to the ends of the nerve stumps, foreign body contamination, and wound infection.

Since only 70 per cent or so of the original population of fibres survive injury (see above), and then at best only 70–80 per cent of those manage to regenerate into the distal stump, it follows that no more than half to two-thirds of the original population of nociceptor afferents will be present in the distal stump to resupply peripheral targets with sensory endings. It therefore becomes crucially important to know the extent to which the nociceptive neurones that do re-establish an ending in an appropriate target tissue exhibit what might be called 'normal properties'. There have been few studies that have specifically addressed this question and again they have been carried out using small cutaneous nerves in the common laboratory species.

Properties of regenerated nociceptor afferents with myelinated axons

Burgess and Horch (1973) recorded from populations of myelinated afferent fibres in normal cat sural nerves and in ones that had regenerated after transection or crush injury 10 to 25 months before. They compared the proportions, axonal conduction velocities proximal to the injury, and receptor characteristics of the various types of afferent present and found that the units sampled from the regenerated nerves resembled those of the normal nerves in all respects. Aδ afferents in the cat sural nerve, whether associated with nociceptor or hair receptor endings, do not have direct spinal projections via the dorsal columns and Burgess and Horch found this was also the case after injury and regeneration (Burgess and Horch 1973; see also Horch 1976), indicating that injury does not trigger any sort of extensive reorganization of the central collaterals of these fibres.

This general picture of an eventual return to normal properties after simple cut or crush injuries has been confirmed in subsequent studies (see, for example, Horch and Lisney 1981; Sanders and Zimmermann 1986; Lewin and McMahon 1991), although, as a minor point, Horch and Lisney (1981) found changes in conduction velocity distal to the injury site.

There is evidence that Aδ afferent fibres supplying skin in rats have an effector function as well as their expected afferent one. A brief volley of impulses in Aδ fibres results in a transient increase in skin blood flow (Jänig and Lisney 1989; Kolston and Lisney 1993) and an argument has been presented that it is the Aδ nociceptive afferents that are involved (Lewin et al. 1992). These responses are still present after peripheral nerve injury and regeneration, but with a tendency to be smaller (Kolston and Lisney 1993). Given that not all the injured fibres will have regenerated into the distal stump and then that not all of those that did will have managed to reform a peripheral ending, it is reasonable to suggest that the reduction in the size of the responses is due to a decrease in the number of Aδ nociceptor units supplying the skin rather than a reduction in the effector capability of the fibres themselves. If this is the correct reading of the situation, it adds to the argument that the properties of Aδ nociceptor afferents are not greatly altered after injury and regeneration.

A problem with the interpretation of these findings remains, and it concerns the 'silent', or unresponsive, nociceptor afferents described in previous chapters. The first units in this group to be reported fell in the C-fibre category, but it is now clear that Aδ-fibre units have to be included as well (Handwerker et al. 1991; Meyer et al. 1991). These units would not have been considered in the earlier experimental work on regeneration and so they went overlooked. They have to be brought into the picture, however, because it is possible that nerve injury and/or regeneration can act as a trigger—like inflammation in the vicinity of the receptor ending—that switches the change from being unresponsive, or 'silent', to being responsive. Thus, a unit that was originally unresponsive could become one of the 'normally' responsive units in a regenerated nerve. The same argument should be kept in mind when thinking about the regeneration of neurones with unmyelinated axons.

Properties of regenerated nociceptor afferents with unmyelinated axons

Shea and Perl (1985) surveyed the receptive properties of unmyelinated afferent units supplying the rabbit ear at various times after nerve injury. By 5 to 8 months a stable situation had been reached in which all the unmyelinated afferent types found in normal preparations were present and in the same proportions: thus nociceptor afferent units—of which most were of the polymodal kind—still made up 80 per cent of the population. There was no evidence that any specific afferent type regenerated faster than any of the others. By this time the regenerated C-fibre nociceptor afferents showed response characteristics that were virtually the same as those of units from normal nerves, with the one exception that about 20 per cent of the regenerated polymodal ones had lower thresholds to heat stimuli. A similar finding has been reported for regenerated C-fibre noxious heat receptor afferents supplying the cat's foot pad (Dickhaus et al. 1976), but here it was felt that the threshold was reduced across all the units in the sample rather than in just a fraction of them. Both groups of investigators proposed that this change in threshold could contribute to an increased sensitivity of reinnervated skin to thermal stimuli.

Shea and Perl's (1985) study focused on the receptive properties of the regenerated units, but C polymodal nociceptor afferents have an 'effector' action as well, initiating neurogenic inflammation. The ability of these units to engage in this response after regeneration has been demonstrated at a gross level using whole-nerve antidromic stimulation or application of irritants to the skin in the presence of Evans's blue dye as a marker of plasma extravasation (see, for example, Janscó and Király 1983; Lisney 1987; Brenan *et al.* 1988), but this approach says nothing about the ability of individual units to contribute to the response. Bearing in mind the evidence for profound changes in neuropeptide synthesis by injured sensory neurones (see the following section), it is quite possible that the impression of reasonably successful regeneration given by these experiments is false. It could be that a few regenerated units were releasing much greater than normal amounts of neuropeptides and in doing so giving an impression of a greater degree of reinnervation than was the case: alternatively, many fibres could each have been releasing smaller than normal quantities and therefore giving the opposite impression. Bharali and Lisney (1992) attempted to tackle this aspect of the issue by looking at the ability of single C-fibre units in normal and regenerated rat saphenous nerves to evoke plasma extravasation. They found that not every polymodal nociceptor unit studied gave detectable signs of plasma extravasation after antidromic stimulation, in both normal and regenerated nerves, and there seemed to be no difference in properties (conduction velocity, receptive thresholds) for those that did and those that did not. As far as it was possible to tell, there was no difference in the sizes of the area of plasma extravasation in the two conditions.

As with the Aδ nociceptor units, the amount of information available is scant but what there is suggests that the majority of C-fibre nociceptor afferent units that manage to resupply their target tissue and reform a receptor ending show few, if any, abnormal features. A comparison of some aspects of the time course of the reinnervation of skin by C-fibre polymodal nociceptor afferents after nerve transection is shown in Fig. 20.1.

Changes in neuropeptides

Whilst electrophysiological experiments carried out to date have not shown up any striking changes in receptive properties of regenerated afferents, including the nociceptor afferents, there is a wealth of evidence showing widespread alterations in the expression of neuropeptides and membrane receptors by injured sensory neurones. These changes have recently been reviewed elsewhere (see Hökfelt *et al.* 1994) and the details will not be covered again here. Essentially, the changes occurring after axotomy that have been observed so far are as follows: for *small dorsal root ganglion (DRG) neurones* (generally associated with unmyelinated afferents), *downregulation* of substance P, calcitonin gene-related peptide (CGRP), somatostatin, neuropeptide Y receptor mRNA and *upregulation* of vasoactive intestinal polypeptide (VIP), galanin and its mRNA, cholecystokinin (CCK), neuropeptide Y, CCK_B receptor mRNA; for *large DRG neurones* (generally associated with myelinated afferents), *downregulation* of CGRP and *upregulation* of VIP, neuropeptide Y, galanin, neuropeptide Y mRNA, CCK mRNA. These changes are not all of equal magnitude. There are other findings that could be taken to indicate further changes in biochemical activity of injured sensory neurones. For example, there is evidence pointing to increased production of α adrenergic receptors (McMahon 1991) and of Na$^+$ channels (Devor *et al.* 1993). With all these changes, however, there is no certainty as to which ones are occurring in nociceptor afferents. This is because it has not yet been possible to establish definitive links between the neuropeptide profile of a sensory neurone and its normal adequate stimulus (for a discussion of this see Lawson, Chapter 3, this volume). It seems there may be a better correlation between neuropeptide profile and the type of tissue supplied, that is, whether skin, muscle, or a visceral structure, and, what is more, the profile can change if the afferents are rerouted to reinnervate a different kind of target (see, for example, McMahon *et al.* 1991; Horgan and Van der Kooy 1992).

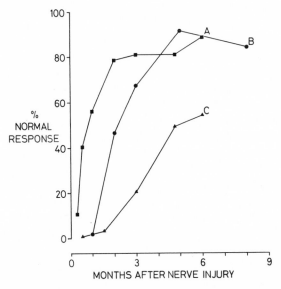

Fig. 20.1 Graph illustrating aspects of the time course of reinnervation of skin by C-fibre polymodal nociceptor afferents after peripheral nerve transection. Trace A (filled squares) shows the time course of regeneration of C fibres from the proximal to the distal stump of transected rat saphenous nerves. From Lisney (1987). Trace B (filled circles) shows the time course with which C-fibre polymodal nociceptor units reinnervate the rabbit ear with readily identifiable receptor endings. From Shea and Perl (1985). Trace C (filled triangles) shows the time course of the return in the ability of C-fibre polymodal nociceptor units to produce plasma extravasation following antidromic nerve stimulation. From Lisney (1987). Results from several animals contributed to each point in each set of data.

The delay between regeneration into the distal stump and functional reinnervation of skin (trace A compared with trace B) can probably be accounted for simply in terms of the time it would have taken for the axons to regrow over the necessary distance. Although there would have been differences in regeneration distance between animals in the two series, these would only have been in the order of a few 10s of mm, and with an average regeneration rate of 2 mm/day, this alone would not be enough to account for all of the delay.

The delay between reinnervation of the skin with functionally identifiable endings and the ability to evoke neurogenic plasma extravasation (traces B and C, respectively) cannot, however, be explained away in terms of regeneration time. It seems that regenerated C-fibre polymodal nociceptor afferent endings regain their receptive capabilities much more quickly than their ability to contribute to neurogenic inflammation. Substance P and CGRP synthesis are both downregulated following injury (see main text), so the delay might occur because it takes longer for the normal synthesis and/or transport of these neuropeptides to be re-established than it does for other aspects of the biochemical activity of these C-fibre polymodal nociceptor afferent neurones.

Undoubtedly, these alterations in neuropeptide expression will be better described by future work and additional substances added to the lists, but at the same time it is important to ask what mechanism(s) trigger(s) the changes and do the changes have any significance? There are few clues at present to the answer to the first of these questions, although retrograde transport of nerve growth factor (NGF) seems to have a role to play (Fitzgerald *et al.* 1985). Fitzgerald and colleagues found that delivery of excess amounts of NGF to the cut end of damaged rat sciatic nerves prevented the expected changes in substance P levels from taking place. Experiments to see whether the same happens with other neuropeptides have yet to be carried out.

Several lines of argument can be used to make a case for attributing significance to these altered patterns of neuropeptide synthesis. When sensory neurones are injured, the emphasis of their functional activity switches from one in which acting as lines of communication between the periphery and the CNS was to the fore to one in which survival and regeneration dominate. Thus, the pattern of ongoing biochemical reactions in the cell body would be expected to change from a situation in which structural integrity has to be maintained and in which activities such as stimulus transduction, impulse propagation, and transmitter synthesis and release are supported to one in which the activity is directed towards supporting outward growth of the regenerating axon process. If this is so, one could expect a temporary decrease in transmitter synthesis and an increased production of materials associated with axonal growth, and, generally speaking, this is what has been observed. For example, there is a decreased synthesis of substance P, the presumed excitatory transmitter at the central terminals of nociceptor afferents (see Hökfelt *et al.* 1994 for references), and an increased expression of growth-related molecules such as GTPase-activating protein, GAP-43 (Strittmatter *et al.* 1992; Booth and Brown 1993). The possible increase in synthesis of α-adrenergic receptors and Na^+ channels mentioned earlier would also be appropriate if axonal elongation were taking place. As well as being part of an overall response in which injured neurones redirect their resources to regeneration, the downregulation of transmitter production may have the extra benefit of reducing the likelihood of effective transmission from afferents to dorsal horn neurones at a time when these fibres are regenerating and when they might be activated inappropriately.

The changes described may also have pathophysiological significance, especially if regeneration and reinnervation of appropriate peripheral targets is incomplete across a population of fibres, or if the changes induced by injury are not reversed if regeneration is successful. The neuropeptides associated with nociceptor afferents, particularly substance P and CGRP, have peripheral actions that are important in initiating inflammatory responses. Weihe and Nohr (1992) have proposed that any sort of disturbance in their release after injury could contribute to the abnormalities found in some chronic pain states by exacerbating inflammatory processes. Devor (see, for example, Devor and Rappaport 1990; Devor 1991, 1994) has suggested that increased production of Na^+ channels and other membrane components that can influence its excitability, and their incorporation into the nerve membrane, could cause an abnormally raised excitability. The consequence of this could be inappropriate impulse initiation, particularly at sites where these molecules might accumulate such as the endings of nerves trapped in a neuroma.

Although there is not a clear picture as to which neuropeptides are present in Aδ- and C-fibre nociceptor afferents and, hence, as to what changes occur in the biochemistry of these neurones when they are injured and are regenerating, this must be an important area for investigation. It is likely that there are more neuropeptides to be identified: some may prove to be reliable markers of sensory neurone subgroups, whereas others might provide the key to understanding events that follow injury, such as the changes in central synaptic activity that underlie injury-induced plasticity.

Changes in properties of nociceptive afferents after injury of neighbouring or distant fibres

Two experiments have been reported in which injury to a group of nerve fibres has altered the properties of unmyelinated nociceptor afferent units not directly involved in the original injury. The first instance is where transection and regeneration of a peripheral nerve of one side of a rat caused a reduction in the ability of impulse activity in the same nerve on the other side of the animal to evoke plasma extravasation (Allnatt *et al.* 1990; Kolston *et al.* 1991). In recent work it has been shown that this reduction in the magnitude of the evoked plasma extravasation response is matched by a decrease in the substance P content of the nerves (Perry *et al.* 1994). The implication of these observations is that at least one property of polymodal nociceptor afferents in the unoperated nerve, their ability to evoke plasma extravasation, has been changed. It has been proposed that this change is brought about by a transneuronal signal, this being a signal that passes from injured neurones on one side of the body to intact ones on the other side via the spinal cord. There is other evidence for contralateral effects involving transneuronal signals from experiments in which peripheral nerve activity has been altered, either as a result of injury (see, for example, Rotshenker and Tal 1985; Souyri and Bourre 1989; Menéndez and Cubas 1990; Booth and Brown 1993; McLachlan *et al.* 1993) or following experimental induction of arthritis (see, for example, Bileviciute *et al.* 1993; Donaldson *et al.* 1993; Mapp *et al.* 1993). In both these models, injury and arthritis, the reason for the changes is uncertain but it may be that alterations in the biochemical activity in a group of peripheral neurones on one side of the body (see above), however they are brought about, are mirrored on the other side but possibly in an attenuated form. The changes may be of some benefit, for example, by initiating or facilitating a compensatory change on the uninjured side that might help the animal to adapt to loss of function on the injured side, but in other instances the change might be inappropriate—as seems to be the case in the experimental arthritis models. The nature of the signal and how it is conveyed are also unknown but, in some instances at least, it seems that capsaicin-sensitive afferents are involved. Topical application of capsaicin to peripheral nerve results in a selective loss of C-fibre polymodal nociceptor afferents, while other afferent populations are left virtually untouched (Pini *et al.* 1990; Pini and Lynn 1991). Donaldson *et al.* (1995), working with one of the experimental arthritis models, have found that capsaicin pretreatment of the nerve supplying the joint in which arthritis is induced prevents the spread of the condition to the other side. We have obtained the same sort of result in recent nerve injury experiments (Scott, Perry, and Lisney, unpublished observations). We have found that, when rat saphenous nerves which have been pretreated with capsaicin are cut and allowed to regenerate, there is no evidence of the contralateral changes expected on the basis of our previous work: there is no change in the contralateral plasma extravasation response and no change in the substance P content of the nerves. Thus, in these two experimental situations, C-fibre polymodal nociceptor afferents appear to be part of the signalling pathway. As for the signal itself, the first stage could be the same as that involved in triggering the changes in neuropeptide synthesis in injured neurones discussed earlier, that is, it may be related to changes in the levels of retrogradely transported NGF. Another aspect of these transneuronal responses that is unclear is how the signal—or a derivative of it—makes its way to the other side.

Another form of novel interaction between damaged nerve fibres and undamaged nociceptor afferents has been described by Sato and Perl (1991). In experiments with several types of nerve injury they found that C polymodal nociceptor units that were not damaged directly by the original injury developed an increased α-adrenergic excitability and increased responsiveness to noxious thermal stimuli. Thus, injury of some fibres in a nerve can alter the responsiveness of uninjured polymodal nociceptor afferents in the same nerve, presumably through a change in the gene expression regulating α-adrenergic receptors or their actions in these afferents. The signal for this change in gene expression has not yet been determined, but again it could be linked with a change in the profile of material carried in the retrograde transport to the cell body of the uninjured neurones. This increased responsiveness of nociceptor afferents not directly involved in an injury could contribute to the pain that sometimes follows major nerve trauma, for example, the pain of reflex sympathetic dystrophy, and these results—taken together with those on transneuronal effects—clearly indicate that the repercussions of nerve injury are more widespread than has been imagined up to now.

Properties of fibres in animal models of peripheral neuropathy

As well as the work already described on the properties of sensory nerve fibres that have regenerated and resupplied peripheral targets, several research groups have studied what happens to these fibres when regeneration has deliberately been hindered to some degree. The extreme example is the stump neuroma model, in which regeneration is stopped by ligating the proximal stump of the cut nerve and/or capping it with a short length of polythene tube. This model is particularly aimed at reproducing what might happen after limb amputation. In other models, attempts have been made to produce a graded degree of damage to a nerve trunk. In one of these, first introduced by Bennett and his colleagues (Bennett and Xie 1988; Sugimoto *et al.* 1990; Munger *et al.* 1992) and subsequently used by Guilbaud's group (see, for example, Attal *et al.* 1990; Guilbaud *et al.* 1993) and Carlton and Coggeshall's group (see, for example, Carlton *et al.* 1991; Coggeshall *et al.* 1993), several loosely tied ligatures are placed around the sciatic nerve of rats. The ligatures are tied tightly enough to stop them from moving but slackly enough to cause only a slight constriction of the nerve when it is viewed by eye. A second model has been introduced by Seltzer and co-workers (1990). In this case a suture is passed through the sciatic nerve so that when it is tightened the dorsal one-third to one-half of the nerve is tied off. Again, the rat is the animal that has been used. Finally, DeLeo *et al.* (1994) have described a peripheral neuropathy model in which the sciatic nerve of rats is damaged by freezing. Animals operated upon in any one of these ways are likely to show abnormal behaviours indicative of a painful, neuropathic condition. For the purposes of the present discussion the question is, to what extent could abnormal properties of nociceptor afferents in the affected nerves contribute to these conditions?

Sensory nerve fibres caught up in a neuroma exhibit a range of abnormal features and these have been reviewed extensively by Devor (Devor and Rappaport 1990; Devor 1991, 1994). These features include the following: spontaneous discharge (originating from both the nerve endings trapped in the neuroma and from neuronal cell bodies in the

DRG); increased sensitivity of these ectopic impulse generator sites to mechanical and thermal stimuli, ischaemia, and catecholamines; and abnormal interactions between fibres. Three types of interaction have been reported: (1) a tightly linked, one-to-one coupling between axons, which is likely to have an ephaptic basis; (2) an activation of afferent fibres by impulse traffic in sympathetic postganglionic fibres caught up in the same neuroma, which is not by an ephaptic mechanism; and (3) a modulation of activity in spontaneously discharging neuroma fibres brought about by trains of impulses in neighbouring fibres other than postganglionic sympathetic ones.

Most of the information about these abnormal properties has come from recordings of myelinated fibre activity in teased-fibre preparations. The law of averages predicts that at least some of the recordings would have been made from Aδ-nociceptor afferent units, but the nature of the experiments was such that there can be no certainty of this. What is clear is that much of the abnormal barrage of impulses is carried by myelinated fibres that were not originally of a nociceptive kind. Some of these abnormal features have been shown to be shared by unmyelinated fibres ending in neuromata. For example, a proportion of them show spontaneous activity, the neuroma endings can be excited in the same way as can those of myelinated fibres, and they are capable of taking part in fibre-to-fibre interactions (see Lisney 1989; Devor and Rappaport, 1990; Amir and Devor 1992; Devor 1994, for references). By no means are all the unmyelinated afferents involved but, given the high proportion of unmyelinated afferents that are nociceptive, it is reasonable to expect some of the fibres showing these features to be nociceptive ones.

Very much less is known about changes in properties of afferent fibres in the other peripheral neuropathy models. There is general agreement that the nerve constriction model produces a fibre loss that affects the large-diameter myelinated fibres the most severely, with there being a less extensive loss of smaller myelinated and unmyelinated fibres (Gautron *et al.* 1990; Basbaum *et al.* 1991; Carlton *et al.* 1991; Munger *et al.* 1992; Nuylten *et al.* 1992; Coggeshall *et al.* 1993), but there is only one full paper on the effects of this kind of injury on the functional characteristics of the afferent fibres, namely, that of Kajander and Bennett (1992). They found that within the first 3 days of causing the injury spontaneous discharges developed in Aβ- and Aδ-afferent fibres, but only rarely in C fibres. There were no results on the properties of afferent fibres that still conducted through the area of constriction. Sato and Perl (1991) have reported on the properties of C-fibre nociceptor afferents not directly injured in the nerve hemiligation model and their main findings have been mentioned already (see previous section).

If the underlying mechanisms producing abnormal behaviour and signs of pain in these animal models are to be properly understood, it will be essential for very much more information than this to be obtained. At the moment it is unclear whether nociceptor afferents make a major and specific contribution to the development of these changes or whether theirs is a minor role.

Concluding remarks

The results available to date show that regenerated myelinated and unmyelinated nociceptor afferents will, given time, reassume normal properties if they manage to resupply an appropriate peripheral target. This applies to both their afferent and efferent functions. On the other hand, when successful regeneration is not achieved and possibly also when there is injury to neighbouring and possibly even distant nerve fibres, these afferents can show a range of abnormal properties. Although it is tempting to take these abnormalities and use them as the basis of explanations for disturbed sensation and pain after nerve injury, the fact is that a large number of non-nociceptive afferents show the same abnormal properties, so that it is difficult to know how much significance to attribute to the altered nociceptor afferents, how much to alterations in the afferent fibre population as a whole, and how much to changes elsewhere in the nervous system.

Important keys to a better understanding of events that follow nerve injury are likely to come with increased knowledge of the changes in the pattern of cell metabolism triggered by injury. Already there are clear pointers that changes in what is happening in terms of the cells' biochemistry are important: for example, changes in levels of α-adrenergic receptor and Na^+ channel synthesis and/or changes in their distribution in neurones in which regeneration has been thwarted provide an explanation for the increased excitability observed in damaged neurones. Further characterization of such changes in cell activity is needed, as are details of the mechanisms bringing about the changes. The new, recently developed models of neuropathic pain are likely to be important, but efforts now need to be directed to finding out what changes in afferent fibre properties are triggered by the injuries and what happens in other parts of the nervous system in these animals.

References

Aldskogius, H., Arvidsson, J., and Grant, G. (1985). The reaction of primary sensory neurons to peripheral nerve injury with particular emphasis on transganglionic changes. *Brain Res. Rev.* **10**, 27–46.

Allnatt, J.P., Dickson, K.E., and Lisney, S.J.W. (1990). Saphenous nerve injury and regeneration on one side of a rat suppresses the ability of the contralateral nerve to evoke plasma extravasation. *Neurosci. Lett.* **118**, 219–22.

Amir, R. and Devor, D. (1992). Axonal cross-excitation in nerve-end neuromas: comparison of A- and C-fibers. *J. Neurophysiol.* **68**, 1160–6.

Attal, N., Jazat, F., Kayser, V., and Guilbaud, G. (1990). Further evidence for 'pain-related' behaviours in a model of unilateral peripheral neuropathy. *Pain* **41**, 235–51.

Basbaum, A.I., Gautron, M., Jazat, F., Mayes, M., and Guilbaud, G. (1991). The spectrum of fiber loss in a model of neuropathic pain in the rat: an electron microscopic study. *Pain* **45**, 359–67.

Bennett, G.J. and Xie, Y.-K. (1988). A peripheral mononeuropathy in rat that produces disorders of pain sensation like those seen in man. *Pain* **33**, 87–107.

Bharali, L.A.M. and Lisney, S.J.W. (1992). The relationship between unmyelinated afferent type and neurogenic plasma extravasation in normal and reinnervated rat skin. *Neuroscience* **47**, 703–12.

Bileviciute, I., Lundeberg, T., Ekblom, A., and Theodorsson, E. (1993). Bilateral changes of substance P-, neurokinin A-, calcitonin gene-related peptide- and neuropeptide Y-like immunoreactivity in rat knee joint synovial fluid during monoarthritis. *Neurosci. Lett.* **153**, 37–40.

Booth, C.M. and Brown, M.C. (1993). Expression of GAP-43 mRNA in mouse spinal cord following unilateral peripheral nerve damage: is there a contralateral effect? *Eur. J. Neurosci.* **5**, 1663–76.

Boring, E.G. (1916). Cutaneous sensation after nerve division. *Quart. J. Exp. Psychol.* **10**, 1–95.

Brenan, A., Jones, L., and Owain, N.R. (1988). The demonstration of the cutaneous distribution of saphenous nerve C-fibres using a plasma extravasation technique in the normal rat and following nerve injury. *J. Anat.* **157**, 57–66.

Burgess, P.R. and Horch, K.W. (1973). Specific regeneration of cutaneous fibers in the cat. *J. Neurophysiol.* **36**, 101–14.

Carlton, S.M., Dougherty, P.M., Pover, C.M., and Coggeshall, R.E. (1991). Neuroma formation and numbers of axons in an experimental peripheral neuropathy. *Neurosci. Lett.* **131**, 88–92.

Coggeshall, R.E., Dougherty, P.M., Pover, C.M., and Carlton, S.M. (1993). Is large myelinated fiber loss associated with hyperalgesia in a model of experimental peripheral neuropathy in the rat? *Pain* **52**, 233–42.

DeLeo, J.A., Coombs, D.W., Willenbring, S., Colborn, R.W., Fromm, C., Wagner, R., and Twitchell, B.B. (1994). Characterization of a neuropathic pain model: sciatic cryoneurolysis in the rat. *Pain* **56**, 4–16.

Devor, M. (1991). Neuropathic pain and injured nerve: peripheral mechanisms. *Br. Med. Bull.* **47**, 619–30.

Devor, M. (1994). Pathophysiology of injured nerve. In *Textbook of pain* (ed. P.D. Wall and R. Melzack), pp. 79–100. Churchill-Livingstone, London.

Devor, M. and Rappaport, H.Z. (1990). Pain and the pathophysiology of damaged nerve. In *Pain syndromes in neurology* (ed. H.L. Fields), pp. 47–83. Butterworths, London.

Devor, M., Govrin-Lippmann, R., and Angelides, K. (1993). Na$^+$ channel immunolocalization in peripheral mammalian axons and changes following nerve injury and neuroma formation. *Neurosci.* **13**, 1976–92.

Dickhaus, H., Zimmerman, M., and Zotterman, Y. (1976). The development in regenerating cutaneous nerves of C-fibre receptors responding to noxious heating of the skin. In *Sensory functions of the skin in primates* (ed. Y. Zotterman), pp. 415–23. Pergamon Press, Oxford.

Donaldson, L.F., Seckl, J.R. and McQueen, D.S. (1993). A discrete adjuvant-induced mono-arthritis in the rat; effects of adjuvant dose. *J. Neurosci. Meth.* **49**, 5–10.

Donaldson, L.F., McQueen, D.S., and Seckl, J.R. (1995). Neuropeptide gene expression and capsaicin-sensitive primary afferents: maintenance and spread of adjuvant arthritis in the rat. *J. Physiol.* **486**, 473–82.

Fields, H.L. (1990). *Pain syndromes in neurology.* Butterworths, London.

Fitzgerald, M., Wall, P.D., Goedert, M., and Emson, P.C. (1985). Nerve growth factor counter-acts the neurophysiological and neurochemical effects of chronic sciatic nerve section. *Brain Res.* **332**, 131–41.

Gautron, M., Jazat, F., Ratinahirana, H., Hauw, J.J., and Guilbaud, G. (1990). Alterations in myelinated fibres in the sciatic nerve of rats after constriction: possible relationships between the presence of abnormal small myelinated fibres and pain related behaviour. *Neurosci. Lett.* **111**, 62–7.

Glover, R.A. (1967). Sequential cellular changes in the nodosal ganglion following section of the vagus nerve at two levels. *Anat. Rec.* **157**, 248.

Guilbaud, G., Gautron, M., Jazat, F., Ratinahirana, H., Hassig, R., and Hauw, J.J. (1993). Time course of degeneration and regeneration of myelinated nerve fibres following chronic loose ligatures of the rat sciatic nerve: can nerve lesions be linked to the abnormal pain-related behaviours? *Pain* **53**, 147–58.

Handwerker, H.O., Kilo, S., and Reeh, P.W. (1991). Unresponsive afferent nerve fibres in the sural nerve of the rat. *J. Physiol.* **435**, 229–42.

Head, H. and Sherren, J. (1905). The consequences of injury to the peripheral nerves in man. *Brain* **28**, 116–338.

Head, H., Rivers, W.H.R., and Sherren, J. (1905). The afferent nervous system from a new aspect. *Brain* **28**, 99–115.

Hökfelt, T., Zhang, X., and Wiesenfeld-Hallin, Z. (1994). Messenger plasticity in primary sensory neurons following axotomy and its functional implications. *Trends Neurosci.* **17**, 22–30.

Horch, K.W. (1976). Ascending collaterals of cutaneous neurons in the fasciculus gracilis of the cat during peripheral nerve regeneration. *Brain Res.* **117**, 19–32.

Horch, K.W. and Lisney, S.J.W. (1981). On the number and nature of regenerating myelinated axons after lesions of cutaneous nerves in the cat. *J. Physiol.* **313**, 275–86.

Horgan, K. and Van der Kooy, D. (1992). Visceral targets specify calcitonin gene-related peptide and substance P enrichment in trigeminal afferent projections. *J. Neurosci.* **12**, 1135–43.

Jänig, W. and Lisney, S.J.W. (1989). Small diameter myelinated afferents produce vasodilatation but not plasma extravasation in rat skin. *J. Physiol.* **415**, 477–86.

Jänig, W. and Schmidt, R.F. (1992). *Reflex sympathetic dystrophy*. VCH, Weinheim.

Janscó, G. and Király, E. (1983). Cutaneous nerve regeneration in the rat: reinnervation of the denervated skin by regenerative but not by collateral sprouting. *Neurosci. Lett.* **36**, 133–7.

Kajander, K.C. and Bennett, G.J. (1992). Onset of a painful peripheral neuropathy in rat: a partial and differential deafferentation and spontaneous discharge in A beta and A delta primary sensory afferent neurons. *J. Neurophysiol.* **68**, 734–44.

Kolston, J. and Lisney, S.J.W. (1993). A study of vasodilator responses evoked by antidromic stimulation of Aδ afferent nerve fibers supplying normal and reinnervated rat skin. *Microvasc. Res.* **46**, 143–57.

Kolston, J., Lisney, S.J.W., Mulholland, M.N.C., and Passant, C.D. (1991). Transneuronal effects triggered by saphenous nerve injury on one side of a rat are restricted to neurones of the contralateral, homologous nerve. *Neurosci. Lett.* **130**, 187–9.

Leem, J.W., Willis, W.D., and Chung, J.M. (1993). Cutaneous sensory receptors in the rat foot. *J. Neurophysiol.* **69**, 1684–99.

Levine, J.D., Fields, H.L., and Basbaum, A.L. (1993). Peptides and the primary afferent nociceptor. *J. Neurosci.* **13**, 2273–86.

Lewin, G.R. and McMahon, S.B. (1991). Physiological properties of primary sensory neurons appropriately and inappropriately innervating skin in the adult rat. *J. Neurophysiol.* **66**, 1205–17.

Lewin, G.R., Lisney, S.J.W., and Mendell, L.M. (1992). Neonatal anti-NGF treatment reduces the Aδ- and C-fibre evoked vasodilator responses in rat skin: evidence that nociceptor afferents mediate antidromic vasodilatation. *Eur. J. Neurosci.* **4**, 1213–18.

Lisney, S.J.W. (1987). Functional aspects of the regeneration of unmyelinated axons in the rat saphenous nerve. *J. Neurol. Sci.* **80**, 289–98.

Lisney, S.J.W. (1989). Regeneration of unmyelinated axons after injury of mammalian peripheral nerve. *Quart. J. Exp. Physiol.* **74**, 757–84.

Lynn, B. and Carpenter, S.E. (1982). Primary afferent units from the hairy skin of the rat hind limb. *Brain Res.* **238**, 29–43.

McLachlan, E.M., Jänig, J., Devor, M., and Michaelis, M. (1993). Peripheral nerve injury triggers noradrenergic sprouting within dorsal root ganglia. *Nature* **363**, 543–6.

McMahon, S.B. (1991). Mechanisms of sympathetic pain. *Br. med. Bull.* **47**, 584–600.

McMahon, S.B. (1992). Dorsal horn plasticity and RSD. In *Reflex sympathetic dystrophy* (ed. W. Jänig and R.F. Schmidt), pp. 143–61. VCH, Weinheim.

McMahon, S.B., Lewin, G.R., Anand, P., Ghatei, M.A., and Bloom, S.R. (1991). Quantitative analysis of peptide levels and neurogenic extravasation following regeneration of afferents to appropriate and inappropriate targets. *Neuroscience* **33**, 67–75.

Mapp, P.I., Terenghi, G., Walsh, D.A., Chen, S.I., Cruwys, S.C., Garrett, N., Kidd, B.L., Polak, J.M., and Blake, D.R. (1993). Monoarthritis in the rat knee induces bilateral and time-dependent changes in substance P and calcitonin gene-related peptide immunoreactivity in the spinal cord. *Neuroscience* **57**, 1091–6.

Menéndez, J.A. and Cubas, S.C. (1990). Changes in contralateral protein metabolism following unilateral sciatic nerve section. *J. Neurobiol.* **21**, 303–12.

Meyer, R.A., Davis, K.D., Cohen, R.H., Treede, R.-D., and Campbell, J.N. (1991). Mechanically insensitive afferents (MIAs) in cutaneous nerves of the monkey. *Brain Res.* **561**, 252–61.

Mitchell, S.W., Morehouse, G.R., and Keen, W.W. (1864). *Gunshot wounds and other injuries of nerves*. Lippincott, Philadelphia.

Munger, B.L., Bennett, G.J., and Kajanader, K.C. (1992). An experimental painful neuropathy due to nerve constriction. I. Axonal pathology in the sciatic nerve. *Exp. Neurol.* **118**, 204–14.

Nuylten, D., Kuper, R., Lammens, M., Dorn, R., Van Hees, J., and Gybels, J. (1992). Further evidence for myelinated as well unmyelinated fibre damage in a rat model of neuropathic pain. *Exp. Brain Res.* **91**, 73–8.

Nystrom, B. and Hagbarth, K.E. (1981). Microelectrode recordings from transected nerves in amputess with phantom limb pain. *Neurosci. Lett.* **27**, 211–16.

Ochoa, J., Cline, M., Dotson, R., and Marchettini, P. (1987). Pain and paresthesias provoked mechanically in human cervical root entrapment (sign of Spurling). Single sensory unit antidromic recording of ectopic, bursting, propagated nerve impulse activity. In *Effects of injury on trigeminal and spinal somatosensory systems* (ed. L.M. Pubols and B.J. Sessle), pp. 389–97. Alan R. Liss, New York.

Ochs, G., Schenk, M., and Struppler, A. (1989). Painful dysaesthesias following peripheral nerve injury: a clinical and electrophysiological study. *Brain Res.* **496**, 228–40.

Otsuka, M. and Yoshioka, K. (1993). Neurotransmitter functions of mammalian tachykinins. *Physiol. Rev.* **73**, 229–308.

Parkhouse, N. and Le Quesne, P.M. (1988). Quantitative objective assessment of peripheral nociceptive C-fibre function. *J. Neurol., Neurosurg., Psychiat.* **51**, 28–34.

Perry, M.J.M., Scott, C., Keen, P., and Lisney, S.J.W. (1994). Substance P content of normal and regenerated rat saphenous nerves. *J. Physiol.* **476**, 49–50P.

Pini, A. and Lynn, B. (1991). C-fibre function during the 6 weeks following a brief application of capsaicin to a cutaneous nerve in the rat. *Eur. J. Neurosci.* **3**, 274–84.

Pini, A., Baranowski, R., and Lynn, B. (1990). Long term reduction in the number of C-fibre nociceptors following capsaicin treatment of a cutaneous nerve in adult rats. *Eur. J. Neurosci.* **2**, 89–97.

Rivers, W.H.R. and Head, H. (1908). A human experiment in nerve division. *Brain* **31**, 323–40.

Rotshenker, S. and Tal. M. (1985). The transneuronal induction of sprouting and synapse formation in intact mouse muscles. *J. Physiol.* **360**, 387–96.

Sanders, K.H. and Zimmermann, M. (1986). Mechanoreceptors in rat glabrous skin: redevelopment after nerve crush. *J. Neurophysiol.* **55**, 644–59.

Sato, J. and Perl, E.R. (1991). Adrenergic excitation of cutaneous pain receptors induced by peripheral nerve injury. *Science* **251**, 1608–10.

Seltzer, Z., Dubner, R., and Shir, Y. (1990). A novel behavioral model of neuropathic pain disorders produced in rats by partial sciatic nerve injury. *Pain* **43**, 205–18.

Sharpey-Schafer, E. (1929). The effects of denervation of a cutaneous area. *Quart. J. Exp. Physiol.* **19**, 85–107.

Shea, V.K. and Perl, E.R. (1985). Regeneration of cutaneous afferent unmyelinated (C) fibers after transection. *J. Neurophysiol.* **54**, 502–12.

Souyri, F. and Bourre, J.M. (1989). Altered metabolism of rat contralateral sciatic nerve after microinjection into the endoneurium of the ipsilateral sciatic nerve. *Neurosci. Lett.* **96**, 351–5.

Strittmatter, S.M., Vartanian, T., and Fishman, M.C. (1992). GAP-43 as a plasticity protein in neuronal form and repair. *J. Neurobiol.* **23**, 507–20.

Sugimoto, T., Bennett, G.J. and Kajander, K.C. (1990). Transsynaptic degeneration in the superficial dorsal horn after sciatic nerve injury: effects of a chronic constriction injury, transection, and strychnine. *Pain* **42**, 205–13.

Trotter, W. and Davies, H.M. (1909). Experimental studies in the innervation of the skin. *J. Physiol.* **38**, 134–246.

Van Boven, R.W. and Johnson, K.O. (1994). A psychophysical study of the mechanisms of sensory recovery following nerve injury in humans. *Brain* **117**, 149–67.

Wall, P.D. and Melzack, R. (ed.) (1994). *Textbook of pain* (3rd edn). Churchill-Livingstone, London.

Walmsley, D. and Wiles, P.G. (1991). Early loss of neurogenic inflammation in the human diabetic foot. *Clin. Sci.* **80**, 605–10.

Weihe, E. and Nohr, D. (1992). A neuroimmune sensory-sympathetic link in the pathophysiology and chronic pain cycle of reflex sympathetic dystrophy (RSD)? In *Reflex sympathetic dystrophy* (ed. W. Jänig and R.F. Schmidt), pp. 281–300. VCH, Weinheim.

Wolff, C.J. (1992). Maladaptive neuronal plasticity and reflex sympathetic dystrophy. In *Reflex sympathetic dystrophy* (ed. W. Jänig and R.F. Schmidt), pp. 125–41. VCH, Weinheim.

Ygge, J. (1989). Neuronal loss in lumbar dorsal root ganglia after proximal compared to distal sciatic nerve resection: a quantitative study in the rat. *Brain Res.* **478**, 193–5.

21 Pathophysiology of human nociceptor function

JOSÉ L. OCHOA, JORDI SERRA, AND
MARIO CAMPERO

This chapter deals with aspects of the pathophysiology of nociceptors, mostly C nociceptors, and in the human context. It will be assumed that the pathophysiology of nociceptors in experimental animals has been studied primarily in order to contribute to the understanding of health-related issues in humans. Therefore any sizeable departures idiosyncratic to the animal condition that do not match descriptions in humans are probably of lesser relevance. The present review is not intended to be all-inclusive; emphasis will be laid on themes that have been investigated by, or have interested the authors. Subjects to be covered include those listed below, but normal and abnormal phenomena will not be dissociated in separate sections.

1. *Normal background data:*

(a) brief description of the fine anatomy of human cutaneous nociceptors;

(b) brief description of receptor characteristics of human C polymodal and Aδ nociceptors, innervating skin and skeletal muscle;

(c) description of the elementary cognitive attributes of somatic sensations (pain and itch) evoked by selective activation of C polymodal and Aδ nociceptors supplying skin and muscle in humans;

(d) vascular reactions of the human skin induced by antidromic excitation of C nociceptors, and their interactions with sympathetic vasomotor responses;

(e) afferent and vascular responses of the human skin induced by local administration of substances that sensitize common C nociceptors and also 'silent' C-nociceptor afferents.

2. *Abnormal biological states affecting structure and function of human nociceptors, or the central processing of their afferent input:*

(a) brief description of the fine structural pathology of human unmyelinated fibres;

(b) sensitization of human C nociceptors;

(c) abnormal release of low-temperature co-activated, centrally gated, human C-nociceptor input;

(d) secondary hyperalgesia: a critique;

(e) 'sympathetically maintained pain' and the C nociceptor: a critique.

Fine structure of nociceptors: order and disorder

Unmyelinated axons innervating human skin were classically studied through the use of vital stains such as methylene blue (Woollard *et al.* 1940). It is possible that some of the strands stained vitally were conglomerates of multiple unmyelinated axons. The same is probably true for the 'fibrae organicae' first dissected out by Remak (1838) from human sympathetic nerves (Fig. 21.1). The unmyelinated axons that normally penetrate the epidermis are clearly discernible by electron microscopy (Fig. 21.2). In terms of their functional submodality it is not definitely established whether intraepidermal C axons are warm-specific or nociceptor-specific receptors. Woollard (1936, p. 56), who was aware of intraepidermal axons in human skin, doubted that the epidermis was 'in any way the special site of pain'. It is very unlikely that these intraepithelial C fibres are sympathetic efferent terminals. It is also unlikely that they represent the naked endings of myelinated axons.

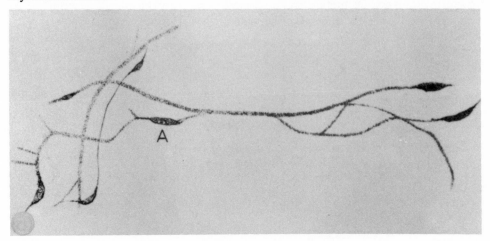

Fig. 21.1   Fibrae organicae from the sympathetic nerve of a man, enlarged about 150 times. A, Nodule with a nucleolus. Reproduced from Remak (1838).

The innervation of the human epidermis has been reassessed recently taking advantage of immunohistochemical stains using labelled antibodies to the neuropeptide protein gene product (PGP 9.5; Kennedy and Wendelschafer-Crabb 1993). Through confocal light microscopy and electron microscopy, immunostained unmyelinated axons were found by those authors in all cell layers of the human epidermis, and may reach quite close to the surface.

Within nerve trunks serving human skin, the unmyelinated fibre population is organized in typical cellular strands containing multiple axons, well separated from one another by intervening membrane-bound Schwann cell processes (Fig. 21.3). In the sural nerve those axons are three to four times more numerous than myelinated axons. Their calibre spectrum is unimodal, peaking at about 1.6 μm in our preparations of sural nerves (Ochoa and Mair 1969a; Ochoa 1970). With ageing, and in neuropathies, unmyelinated axons drop out. Survivor axons issue tiny sprouts that make their calibre spectrum bimodal, and their Schwann cell processes budd into typical profiles. The

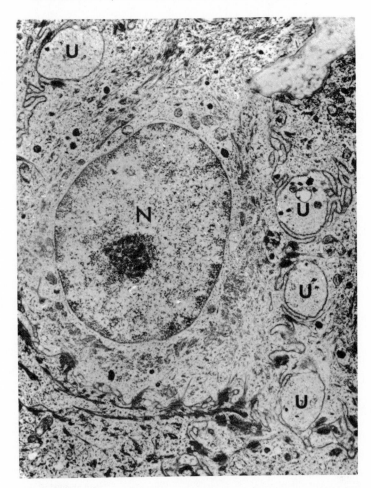

Fig. 21.2 Electron micrograph of tangential section through human non-hairy epidermis. Four profiles (U), presumably axons, are lodged extracellularly in between basal layer cells. A keratinocyte is cut through its nucleus (N). The specimen was fixed by immersion in 4 per cent buffered glutaraldehyde, post-osmicated and embedded in Epon. Uranyl acetate and lead citrate stain; 8250 ×. Reproduced with permission from Ochoa (1984).

remaining 'denervated' Schwann cell bands also have typical fine structural features (Ochoa and Mair 1969b; Ochoa 1970; Fig. 21.4). Until recently there was no way to distinguish somatic from sympathetic unmyelinated axons through light or electron microscopy of somatic nerves. The utilization of specific lectins has made it possible to differentially label with surface markers the axolemma of sensory axons, even in humans (Mori 1986; Kusunoki *et al.* 1991; Shimizu *et al.* 1994).

The fine structure and pathology of Aδ nociceptors in human skin remain to be described (see Kruger and Halata, Chapter 2, this volume). The fine structural pathology of nociceptors from human muscle also awaits description (see Mense, Chapter 7, this volume), but it would be surprising if it differed from the pathology of nociceptor fibres in cutaneous nerves.

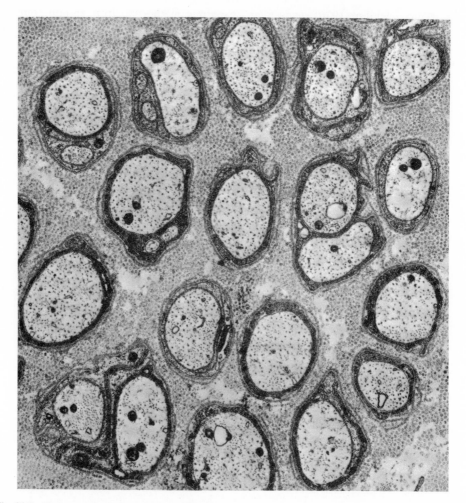

Fig. 21.3 Electron micrograph of normal human unmyelinated fibres from cross-section of cutaneous nerve fascicle. In contrast to autonomic and muscle nerves, most axons here are individualized in separate Schwann cell processes. The specimen was fixed by immersion in 4 per cent buffered glutaraldehyde, post-osmicated, and embedded in Epon. Uranyl acetate and lead citrate stain; 9750×. Reproduced with permission from Ochoa (1984).

Some electrophysiological receptor characteristics of human nociceptors

Nociceptors from various species generally display the high receptor threshold described originally by Zotterman (1933, 1936) in animal nerves. When C-nociceptor afferents were shown to respond to strong mechanical, thermal, and chemical stimuli in mammals, they were eventually termed *polymodal nociceptors* (Iggo 1959; 1960; Bessou and Perl 1969; see reviews by Burgess and Perl 1973; Perl 1984, Perl, Chapter 1, this volume). Torebjörk and Hallin (1970), Hallin and Torebjörk (1970), and Van Hees and Gybels (1972) pioneered intraneural microrecordings of human C nociceptors, having described their adequate stimuli, receptor thresholds, adaptation rates, and conduction velocities.

Torebjörk and Hallin (1976) devised an ingenious method to differentiate somatic afferent from sympathetic efferent C units in human cutaneous nerves. They took advantage of the use-determined latency delay observed when natural excitation of recorded C-nociceptor afferents is superimposed upon their rhythmic stimulation by electrical pulses.

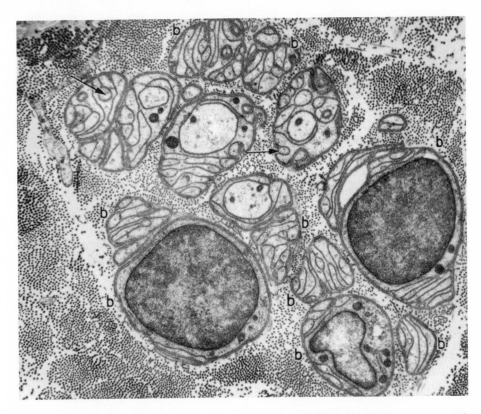

Fig. 21.4 A conglomerate of unmyelinated fibres exhibit all the changes due to age: budding of Schwann cells; denervated bands (b) three of them nucleated; and ultrathin axons (arrowed). Man aged 59 years; 8000 ×. Reproduced with permission from Ochoa and Mair (1969*b*).

In a study of 71 C nociceptors supplying glabrous and hairy skin in human volunteers, it was found that the units were polymodal in the sense that they all responded to noxious mechanical and heat stimuli. The few units tested for chemical responsiveness became spontaneously active following histamine injection. Conduction velocities ranged from 0.5 to 1.5 m/s. The receptive fields of these cutaneous human C polymodal nociceptors were small, usually 2 × 2 to 3 × 3 mm. In most instances two or three C-nociceptor units that had receptive fields closely clustered in the glabrous skin of the hand were recorded from the same intraneural site (Ochoa and Torebjörk 1989). Evidence to support the claim that individual human C-nociceptor axons that can be recorded through an intraneural microelectrode can also be stimulated through the same electrode was obtained by 'marking' the particular C unit through repetitive intraneural microstimulation; immediate recording under those circumstances displays a sudden reversible shift in latency, as shown in figure 2 of Ochoa and Torebjörk (1989).

Whereas well deserved attention has been given to the receptor behaviour of cutaneous C polymodal nociceptors in response to low-temperature stimuli in several animal species (Bessou and Perl 1969; Iggo and Ogawa 1971; Georgopoulos 1976, 1977; Saumet *et al.* 1985), responses of human polymodal nociceptors to low temperature have been reported succinctly (Torebjörk 1974; Torebjörk and Hallin 1976). Recent observations on 55 human cutaneous C polymodal nociceptors have revealed that a substantial subpopulation (40 per cent) responds consistently to low-temperature stimuli with a low mean firing rate (Campero *et al.* 1994). The low discharge frequency of C polymodal nociceptors in response to noxious low temperature may be due to impaired impulse transmission of unmyelinated fibres at temperatures of 3–4°C (Paintal 1967). It is likely that these units are, at least in part, responsible for low-temperature-induced pain and, therefore, also for low-temperature-induced hyperalgesia (Campero *et al.* 1994). Preliminary animal studies show that cutaneous polymodal nociceptors may become sensitized to low temperature after transient challenge to their receptors with noxious low temperature (P. Reeh, personal communication). Possible sensitization of nociceptors to low temperature remains to be investigated in neuropathic patients.

For reasons that remain to be determined, afferent units with thin myelinated Aδ fibres are much less likely to be recorded through microneurography than are larger myelinated (Aβ) fibres, or even C fibres. Obviously, the calibre of Aδ fibres must be just critically small enough for the Vallbo–Hagbarth electrode to pierce or hook, a feature that would not apply to the larger multiaxonal unmyelinated fibre complexes. The receptor characteristics of human myelinated nociceptors were briefly described by Torebjörk and Ochoa (1990) who found that in the glabrous skin these units are usually not polymodal. Their receptor thresholds are high, they have fast adaptation rate, and their conduction velocities are in the Aδ range (see Torebjörk and Ochoa 1990, Fig. 2).

Cognitive attributes of somatic sensations (pain and itch) evoked by selective activation of C polymodal nociceptors and Aδ nociceptors from skin and muscle in human volunteers

Elementary sensations evoked by selective activation of identifiable cutaneous C-nociceptor units are specific in terms of their subjective quality (Torebjörk and Ochoa 1980; Ochoa and Torebjörk 1983). Furthermore, they conform to the Stevens law in terms of subjective magnitude (Ochoa and Torebjörk, unreported) and predict the anatomical site of the pertinent cutaneous receptor through surprisingly precise locognosis (Ochoa and Torebjörk 1989). The same general cognitive characteristics apply to Aδ nociceptors from skin (Torebjörk and Ochoa 1980, 1990).

In the combined method of intraneural microstimulation and microrecording as used for investigation of cognitive attributes of somatic sensations (Torebjörk and Ochoa 1980), the intrafascicular electrode is primarily used to deliver trains of weak electrical stimuli while the experimenter gently adjusts its position and attends to the evoked sensations that the subject reports. Once an intrafascicular site is reached where intraneural microstimulation evokes a weak monofocally projected painful sensation, the psychophysical studies are initiated. The apparatus is eventually switched to the recording mode and the search then starts for sensory units recordable from the site of intraneural microstimulation. The unit search relies on administration of natural stimuli to the cutaneous territory of the nerve with emphasis on the field of projected sensation (PF). Alternatively, the intrafascicular electrode may be used primarily in the recording mode to search for units through a conventional natural stimulus–nerve impulse response strategy. In either case the cognitive sensory data accrued from microstimulation is matched against the electrophysiological data obtained from recording classified units (Ochoa and Torebjörk 1983, 1989; Torebjörk and Ochoa 1990). For intraneural microstimulation, square-wave pulses of 0.25 ms duration are used in trains of 3, 5, or 30 Hz, lasting usually 2 to 5 s to allow sufficient time for sensory detection. The amplitude of the stimulating pulses is gradually raised from 0 to a level at which the subject first feels a sensation at threshold. The subjects are given no cues as to when intraneural stimuli are given or what parameters are used during the stimulation. They describe in their own words the qualities and temporal profiles of sensations evoked by intraneural microstimulation and map on a real-size picture of their limb the locations and sizes of the cutaneous areas where sensations were projected (PF).

The quality of pain evoked as a threshold sensation during weak intraneural microstimulation of C nociceptors is typically described as dull or burning. The first quality tends to predominate in glabrous skin, whereas the second is more typical of hairy skin. The painful sensation thus evoked by repetitive electrical pulses is sustained rather than intermittent. Intermittency characterizes tactile sensations evoked by intraneural microstimulation of rapidly adapting low-threshold mechanoreceptors. The duller burning pain evoked by intraneural microstimulation of C nociceptors persists during selective block of myelinated fibres, as achieved by compression ischaemia of the tested limb. The monofocal cutaneous site of projection (PF) of the painful sensation evoked during intraneural microstimulation at C-nociceptor recording sites most commonly matches the physical location of the receptor of the recorded fibre. The spatial correspondence is particularly good for units in the glabrous skin of the hand; here, the closeness between receptive and projected fields is within 10 mm in the vast majority of cases (Ochoa and Torebjörk 1989). The psychophysical threshold for pain evoked by natural stimuli not only depends on stimulus intensity but also, importantly, on the rate at which stimulus energy increases (Yarnitsky *et al.* 1992). The mean firing frequency of C polymodal nociceptors increases significantly with increasing rates of stimulus temperature rise, whereas the receptor threshold does not change. However, in keeping with psychophysical studies (Yarnitsky and Ochoa 1990*a*), steeper slopes of temperature rise, by producing increased frequency response of nociceptors, cause the minimum afferent input required for psychophysical detection of pain to be attained earlier, thus decreasing the threshold for pain detection.

For Aδ nociceptors supplying the skin of the human hand, the cognitive outcome of their selective microstimulation is *sui generis*. The evoked sensation is characteristically sharp pricking pain rather than dull or burning pain. Sharp cutaneous pain cannot be evoked during selective blockade of myelinated fibres by means of compression ischaemia, at a time when only unmyelinated fibres continue to conduct. The locus of projected sensation of sharp pricking pain evoked by activation of Aδ nociceptors supplying human skin predicts the physical locus of the pertinent receptor at least as accurately as in the case of C nociceptors (Torebjörk and Ochoa, unpublished (1980) 1990; Fig. 21.2). These joint studies have been adjudicated before (Torebjörk 1992, p. 136, referring to Torebjörk 1985, p. 231). Plate 1 illustrates the psychophysical and microneurographic characteristics of an Aδ nociceptor from the glabrous skin of the middle finger of one of the present authors.

Selective activation of certain cutaneous units wired through C polymodal nociceptors evokes itch rather than pain (Torebjörk and Ochoa 1981; Schmidt *et al.* 1993). The itch submodality is confined to skin afferents; muscle nociceptors only evoke pain. Unlike cutaneous nociceptors, one single quality of sensation; that is, cramp-like pain, can be evoked through intraneural microstimulation of human muscle nociceptors (Torebjörk and Ochoa 1980; Ochoa and Torebjörk 1981; Marchettini 1993; Simone *et al.* 1994).

Vascular reactions induced by antidromic excitation of C nociceptors and their interactions with sympathetic vasomotor responses

Antidromically triggered vasodilatation is a well known event (Stricker 1876; Bayliss 1901; Langley 1923; Hinsey and Gasser 1930; Lewis 1937; Chapman *et al.* 1961; see Lynn, Chapter 17, this volume). Not surprisingly, electrical stimulation of the peripheral end of freshly divided nerve roots in man elicits rubor in dermatomal distribution (Foerster 1933). This chemically based vasodilator reaction, eventually attributed to neurosecretion of substance P, is believed today to be largely mediated by calcitonin gene-related peptide (CGRP; Brain and Escott 1994). Prolonged repetitive electrical microstimulation at painful intensities of nerve fascicles projecting to the hand consistently elicits warming of coherent districts of the skin. This is precisely and sensitively detected by thermography (Comstock *et al.* 1986; Ochoa *et al.* 1987*a*; Plate 2).

This regional warming is not abolished after postganglionic sympathetic denervation of human skin, which rules out the possibility that it might be due to temporary use-dependent blockade of sympathetic efferent vasoconstrictor fibres (Comstock *et al.* 1986; Ochoa *et al.* 1987*a*). Another reason to rule out sympathetic efferent phenomena as a determinant of such regional vasodilatation is the observation that the effect becomes prominent only after stimulation is discontinued (Ochoa *et al.* 1993). Thus, the phenomenon is most probably antidromic. The cutaneous receptive field for the nerve fascicle being stimulated matches well the discrete territory of skin that displays the antidromic vasodilator phenomenon. This provides neuroanatomical evidence that C-nociceptor units contained in individual nerve fascicles are distributed into well defined partial somatotopic domains within the total nerve territory. Furthermore, as argued (by Ochoa *et al.* (1987*a*), this proves that the matching fields of projected sensation evoked by intraneural stimulation of skin nerve fascicles legitimately represent the anatomical receptive field of those fascicles, rather than being 'condensed abstractions of the brain' (Wall and McMahon 1985).

Striking interactions occur between orthodromic sympathetic vasoconstrictor and antidromic vasodilator effects of C-fibre stimulation. They carry potential clinical relevance. During high-intensity intraneural stimulation, when both sympathetic and somatic systems are co-activated, skin temperature becomes decreased diffusely in the tested limb. This is because reflex sympathetic vasoconstriction overrides the co-activated antidromic vasodilator effect induced by stimulation of C nociceptors. After termination of the stimulus the skin temperature increases regionally, within the territory of the stimulated fascicle. Upon renewed stimulation the regional warming induced by antidromic neurosecretion from C nociceptors is again rapidly erased (Ochoa *et al.* 1993). The fact that both sympathetic vasomotor and antidromic sensory mechanisms may determine changes in the colour and temperature of the skin is clinically relevant. There exist interesting medical conditions of neuropathic origin, to be described further below, that feature prominent deviations of skin temperature, such as erythralgia (Lewis 1933, 1942) or the ABC syndrome (Ochoa 1986), the triple cold syndrome [Ochoa and Yarnitsky 1990, 1994] and the heterogeneous 'reflex sympathetic dystrophy' (RSD) (Bonica 1979). Thus it is useful from the diagnostic point of view to remain aware that 'neuropathic' painful syndromes associated with vascular phenomena need not necessarily imply sympathetic pathophysiology.

It has been assumed that the neurovascular apparatus and the operant mechanism responsible for antidromically induced vasodilatation of human skin are identical to those responsible for local vasodilatation in response to substances that cause neurogenic inflammation and sensitization of nociceptors. Recent evidence supports the concept that flare and antidromic vasodilatation may have different mechanisms (Serra *et al.* 1994*b*). Langley (1921) suggested that the neural system responsible for the flare response that follows noxious stimulation of the skin is the same as the system responsible for the antidromic vasodilatation. However, Lewis (1937) cautioned: 'When both posterior root vasodilatation and flare were thought to depend on sensory nerves, one system for the two reactions was a natural conception; but the identity of the nerves underlying these two reactions has not been proved'. It is known that the skin flush that follows antidromic stimulation is due to capillary dilatation with no intervention of deeper arterioles, as it persists after clamping the aorta (Langley 1923). Recent histophysiological experiments also suggest that antidromic vasodilatation is a vascular effect primarily at the 'minute' vessel level (Kenins 1984; Bharali and Lisney 1992). On the other hand, the flare response is entirely an arteriolar phenomenon (Lewis 1927; Serra *et al.* 1994*c*). Antidromic stimulation would activate unmyelinated nociceptor axons and would trigger antidromic release of substances capable of inducing plasma extravasation and visible capillary flushing. In contrast, activation of the neural system mediating the flare response would trigger arteriolar vasodilatation and secondary flushing in a wide area surrounding the injury site.

In the clinical context, antidromic vasodilatation is defective or absent in patients who have lost peripheral unmyelinated axons (Plate 3). This is probably the reason that the flare response becomes sluggish with age (Helme *et al.* 1985).

Vascular and sensory reactions of the skin induced by local administration of substances that excite or sensitize nociceptors

Following intradermal injection of the irritant capsaicin, flare and hyperalgesia may develop in a broad surrounding area. The neurogenic flare mechanism is resolved locally in the skin (Lewis 1927) and it has been proposed that it spreads through local axon reflexes involving C polymodal nociceptors (Szolcsányi *et al.* 1992). However, the hypothetical existence of a distinct subset of 'nocifensor' nerve fibres specifically arranged for the flare reaction remains viable (Lewis 1937; see LaMotte, Chapter 16, this volume). In addition to the flare, cutaneous hyperalgesia develops surrounding the injection site (Simone et al. 1989; LaMotte et al. 1991; Torebjörk et al. 1992). A distinction has been made between the hyperalgesia that appears at the site of cutaneous injury, 'erythralgia' (Lewis 1942) or primary hyperalgesia (Hardy et al. 1952, pp. 123–33), and the hyperalgesia beyond it, 'nocifensor tenderness' (Lewis 1936, 1942) or secondary hyperalgesia (Hardy et al. 1952, pp. 123–33). Secondary hyperalgesia has been characterized as occurring only in response to mechanical stimuli, without associated heat hyperalgesia (Raja et al. 1984; LaMotte et al. 1991). There is general agreement that primary hyperalgesia is due to the sensitization of cutaneous nociceptor terminals (LaMotte et al. 1982, 1983, 1992; Campbell and Meyer 1983; Torebjörk et al. 1984).

Failure to detect sensitization in common polymodal C nociceptors in the area of secondary hyperalgesia during capsaicin experiments in animals or humans (Baumann et al. 1991; LaMotte et al. 1992) has led to the proposition that secondary hyperalgesia might be mediated by dorsal horn neurones previously sensitized by a C-nociceptor afferent barrage (LaMotte et al. 1991; Simone et al. 1991; Torebjörk et al. 1992). However, recent experiments (Serra et al. 1993, 1994a–c) using dynamic telethermography show that, following capsaicin injection, the flare response occurs over an area much larger than that usually detected by visual inspection or by laser Doppler blood flow measurement. Such flare reflects underlying arteriolar dilatation and extends into the area commonly considered to be that in which secondary hyperalgesia occurs (Serra et al. 1993; (Plate 4). In this area, pain thresholds are lowered and pain magnitude estimates are increased for punctuate mechanical stimuli. For heat hyperalgesia, threshold values are little changed, but there is definite heat hyperalgesia for suprathreshold stimuli. The broad area of heat hyperalgesia can be delineated only by delivering stimuli well above pain threshold, which may explain the differences between this and previous studies. Increased pain response to heat stimuli in the area of secondary hyperalgesia was unambiguously described by Hardy et al. (1952, pp. 123–33).

The most striking finding of these experiments (Serra et al. 1993, 1994a,b) is that the area of punctate mechanical hyperalgesia precisely matches the area of heat hyperalgesia, and both match the very large area of flare. Such matching was well described by Lewis (1935–6) and has significant implications. Even if nociceptive input to the dorsal horn follows somatotopic order (Bullit 1991), such input, if pathogenetic, could not be so accurate as to result in sensitization of precisely those dorsal horn neurones whose receptive fields match a remote local vascular process of the skin. It is reasonable to envisage this vascular-sensory matching as the consequence of related mechanisms resolved at peripheral level (see LaMotte, Chapter 16, this volume). However, it remains to be established how flare and hyperalgesia are linked.

Although the common polymodal C nociceptor does not change its properties in the area of secondary hyperalgesia (Campbell et al. 1988; Baumann et al. 1991; LaMotte et al. 1992), this need not imply that secondary hyperalgesia cannot be due to sensitizaton of peripheral units. Recently discovered 'silent' C or Aδ nociceptor units that become active during inflammation (Davis et al. 1993; Handwerker et al. 1993) appeal as likely subsets of peripheral nociceptors responsible for signalling secondary hyperalgesia. To the best of our knowledge the behaviour of these units has not been

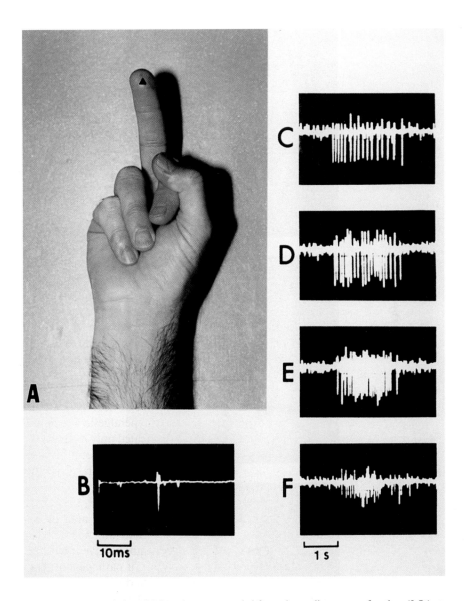

Plate 1 Receptor characteristics of Aδ nociceptor recorded from the median nerve of author (J.O.) at upper arm level. (A) The receptive field in the tip of the middle finger was small, about 2 × 2 mm (triangle). (B) The conduction velocity was 31.9 m/s. (C) The unit's response was slowly adapting to von Frey stimulation at 51 g. (D) Von Frey 100-g stimulus induced a more vivid response. (E) The most intense response was evoked by painful needle prick. (F) Sympathetic reflex activity but no response from the Aδ nociceptor was observed when the receptive skin region was briefly touched by a glowing match evoking pain.

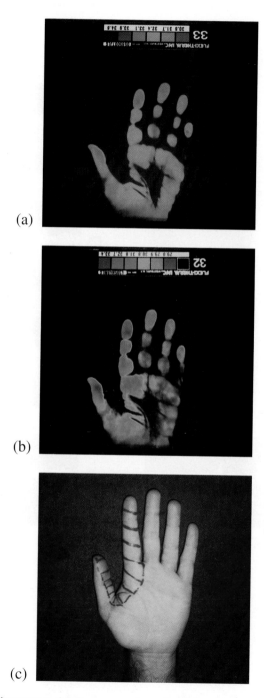

(a)

(b)

(c)

Plate 2 (a) Baseline thermogram showing an even thermal emission profile in the palm and fingers. Note relative hyperthermia of fingertips. (b) Regional hyperthermia mostly affecting index and thumb (2 min after discontinuation of painful intraneural microstimulation). (c) Area of projection of paraesthesiae induced by painful intraneural microstimulation matches the area of antidromic vasodilatation.

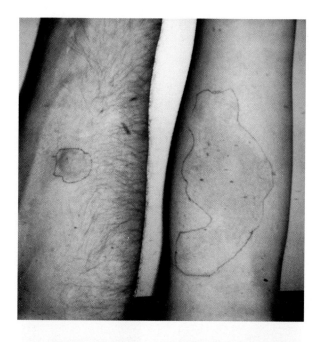

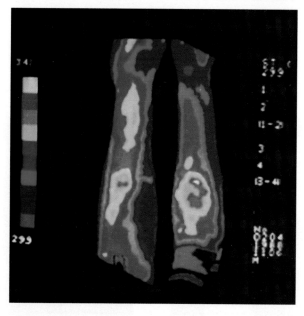

Plate 3 (Top panel) Absence of surrounding flare in response to intradermal histamine test in patient with small fibre neuropathy (left) compared to broad response in normal volunteer (right). (Lower panel) Corresponding thermograms.

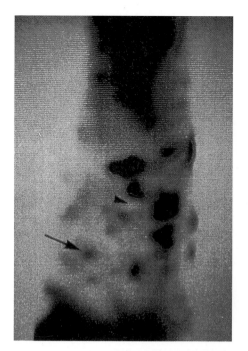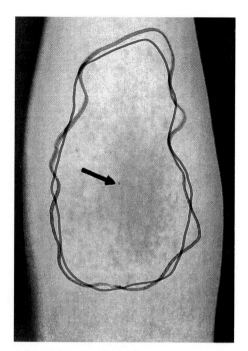

Plate 4 (Left) Early thermographic image (30 s postinjection) of the flare response following intradermal capsaicin injection (100 mg in 10 ml) in the anterior aspect of the forearm of a volunteer subject. (Right) There is spatial matching between the areas of mechanical hyperalgesia to punctate stimulation (green) and of heat hyperalgesia (red) and the area of both visual and thermographic flare.

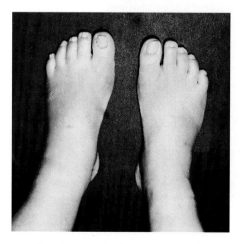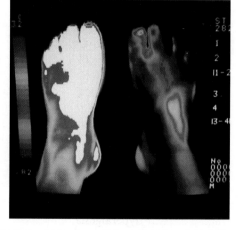

Plate 5 (Left) Episode of spontaneous cooling of the right foot, which appears less swollen than the left. In parallel, pains and hyperalgesias were spontaneously relieved on the right foot. (Right) Infrared thermography showing hypothermia of the transiently asymptomatic right foot and hyperthermia of the persistently symptomatic left foot.

reported in areas of secondary hyperalgesia. A recent study in human volunteers (Serra *et al.* 1995) identified peripheral units fulfilling the criteria for 'silent' nociceptors whose receptors become sensitized in the area of secondary hyperalgesia. They display significant reduction of receptor threshold or enhanced firing in response to mechanical or heat stimuli. This type of 'silent' nociceptor that becomes sensitized during inflammation probably contributes to the pathophysiology of secondary hyperalgesia.

Injection of capsaicin aimed at the receptive field of primary nociceptor endings within human skeletal muscle may also sensitize those nociceptors (Simone *et al.* 1992).

Some hyperexcitable states of nociceptors in human disease

The observations that follow apply to common C polymodal nociceptors and, in our experience, also to 'mechanically insensitive' or 'silent' C nociceptors. Data on the hyperexcitability of Aδ human nociceptors is unavailable in published form. Once C nociceptors are in the sensitized hyperexcitable state it becomes impossible, under available criteria, to determine retrospectively whether the unit was a common C polymodal nociceptor or a silent C nociceptor. Microneurography combined with psychophysical and thermographic studies has provided evidence that sensitizaton of primary nociceptors may explain a spectrum of positive sensory and antidromic vasomotor symptoms (Cline and Ochoa 1986; Ochoa *et al.* 1987*b*; Cline *et al.* 1989). The criteria for sensitization under these circumstances include abnormal reduction of the receptor threshold and abnormal spontaneous or stimulus-induced afferent discharge. In the case of the patient reported in detail by Cline *et al.* (1989), spontaneous discharge of C nociceptors was not a feature. In that patient the striking abnormalities were reduction of receptor threshold to normally non-noxious levels, and prolonged afterdischarges evoked by brief mechanical stimuli.

Hyperexcitability of primary C nociceptors carries predictable clinical cognitive correlates. The pathologically prolonged aftersensation of pain is obviously determined by the abnormally prolonged nociceptor afterdischarge. The duration of the afterdischarges matches the duration of the hyperalgesic pain, as delineated through the use of a manual analogue device (Cline *et al.* 1989). Another obvious clinical correlate of C-nociceptor hyperexcitability obtains for mechanical hyperalgesia: gentle natural mechanical stimuli can now effectively activate nociceptors and evoke pain at abnormally low thresholds. The mechanical hyperalgesia determined by sensitized C nociceptors is of the 'static' subtype (Ochoa *et al.* 1989; Ochoa and Yarnitsky 1993; Koltzenburg *et al.* 1993). This kind of hyperalgesia has a typical dull or burning painful quality and resists selective A-fibre blockade. The clinical pathophysiological profile of this kind of hyperalgesia is quite distinct from the 'dynamic', 'allodynic' subtype of mechanical hyperalgesia (Ochoa *et al.* 1989; Ochoa and Yarnitsky 1993; Koltzenburg *et al.* 1993).

It is logically anticipated that sensitizaton of polymodal nociceptors should determine not only static mechanical hyperalgesia but also hyperalgesia to heat and to low temperature. Heat hyperalgesia is indeed a key feature of the human syndrome determined by sensitization of C nociceptors. It is for that reason that such a hyperalgesic state was termed *polymodal hyperalgesia* (Ochoa 1986; Ochoa *et al.* 1987*b*; Cline *et al.* 1989; Culp *et al.* 1989). Cold hyperalgesia does not come up as an issue in the context of sensitized C nociceptors for the simple reason that application of low temperature to the symptomatic parts of these patients actually soothes the painful symptoms. This is what has been called *cross-modality receptor threshold modulation* (XTM). This term describes the relief of both pain and mechanical hyperalgesia by passive cooling of the symptomatic parts (during differential block of tactile and cold-specific input). Increasing the temperature of those parts worsens pain and mechanical hyperalgesia. Such a striking influence of temperature has been construed as a clinical sign of nociceptor sensitization (Ochoa 1986; Ochoa *et al*. 1987*b*; Cline *et al*. 1989) and is taken to reflect modulation of the biophysical properties of the excitable membrane of polymodal nociceptors (Culp *et al*. 1989). We have also observed that, through a cooling effect, sympathetically mediated vasoconstriction also relieves polymodal hyperalgesia. However, by virtue of the theoretical principle of cross-modality threshold modulation, there would exist a critical level below which low temperature no longer soothes but evokes pain in patients with sensitized C polymodal nociceptors. Lewis (1936) actually wrote: 'cooling abolishes the pain unless a low temperature is reached . . . ice gives pain, indistinguishable from that induced by heat.' The issue of sensitization of C nociceptors to *low temperature* will be further discussed below.

Clinical and experimental observations on polymodal hyperalgesia and XTM in patients and volunteers allowed us to conceptualize a clinical condition caused by sensitization of primary peripheral nociceptors—the ABC syndrome (Ochoa 1986, 1993*b*; Ochoa *et al*. 1987*b*; Cline *et al*. 1989). This syndrome is seen, albeit not commonly, in a subgroup of patients with neuropathy. Its prevalence remains to be established. One key clinical feature of sensitization of C polymodal nociceptors is the rubor or erythema of the symptomatic parts. This is what led Lewis to term this condition 'erythralgia' (Lewis 1936). The underlying vasodilatation is active, rather than the expression of sympathetic vasoparalysis (see fig. 4 in Ochoa 1986). Sensitization of primary nociceptors has been recorded as the cause of a combined neurosensory and neurovascular painful ABC syndrome in a subgroup of patients with diabetic neuropathy. The case of the patient to be described briefly below (Mrs K) displays the whole clinical spectrum of manifestations of the ABC syndrome. The case illustrates another striking feature of C-nociceptor hyperexcitability, which also carries a straight clinical cognitive correlate. That is *multiplication of afferent nerve impulses* in response to finite receptor stimulation. This feature partially fits not only the concept of hyperalgesia but also the concept of 'hyperpathia' (Merskey and Bogduk 1994). Such a receptor–response anomaly is not necessarily associated with a reduced receptor threshold of the C nociceptor.

Case report

Mrs K, a 30-year-old patient with long-standing insulin-dependent diabetes mellitus, carried a chronic polyneuropathy with prominent sensory symptoms and trophic dysfunction. She complained of severe spontaneous pains involving mostly the lower extremities, in stocking distribution. She also complained of distal cutaneous hyperalgesia and her symptomatic skin was red, hot, and moderately swollen. She also expressed clear heat hyperalgesia. She had become aware of the beneficial effect of passive cooling upon her spontaneous pain and mechanical hyperalgesia (XTM). Although the patient expressed typical symptomatology of the ABC syndrome, a consultant had recommended sympathectomy as therapy for 'reflex sympathetic dystrophy'. Thermography revealed marked hyperthermia of the symptomatic parts, and quantitative sensory testing marked heat hyperalgesia. Autonomic testing documented ability to engage reflex vasoconstriction, indicating that the erythema was not due to sympathetic vasoconstrictor paralysis. Microneurographic recordings at ankle level (Serra, Campero, and Ochoa, unreported) from cutaneous nerve fascicles supplying symptomatic skin revealed spontaneous bursting discharges in single units, probably low-threshold mechanoreceptors, that were observed to be ongoing for prolonged periods of time. Such discharges were of distal nerve origin as they persisted during an effective local anaesthetic nerve block given proximal to the site of recording. These spontaneous discharges are the likely substrate for the ongoing tingling paraesthesiae described by the patient. In addition, there were abnormal afferent responses in C polymodal nociceptors: after single electrical impulses delivered to the receptive field their axons fired consistently with an abnormal repetitive discharge (Fig. 21.5). Effective activation of sympathetic outflow failed to modify the receptor threshold or to induce the discharge of sensitized nociceptors.

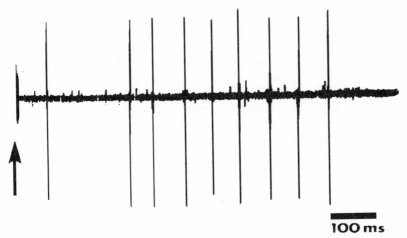

100 ms

Fig. 21.5 Painful diabetic neuropathy. An abnormal repetitive discharge in a single C nociceptor unit of the superficial peroneal nerve in response to a brief (0.25-ms) square-wave electrical stimulus applied to the unitary receptive field in the dorsum of the foot.

A significant incidental observation was recorded during one clinical visit. The patient arrived volunteering the information that her left foot was relatively painless and was not tender to gentle mechanical stimulation. The temporarily asymptomatic foot was neither red nor hot when tested (Plate 5). After a few hours the left foot went back to its typically symptomatic, hyperalgesic and hyperthermic state. This episode is best explained through circumstantial interjection of a strong sympathetic vasoconstrictor output to that foot. It would exemplify the capacity of the sympathetic vasoconstrictor system to override neurogenic antidromic vasodilatation, as shown experimentally in humans (Ochoa *et al.* 1993). In keeping with the concept of XTM of polymodal nociceptors, the active cooling induced by sympathetic vasoconstrictor activity probably rectified the excitability of the nociceptor membrane in the patient. This would prevent it from firing spontaneously and from responding to adequate stimulus energies with an abnormally low receptor threshold, or with a multiplied afferent response.

This evidence reinforces the concept that primary peripheral mechanisms may by themselves explain crippling hyperalgesia in neuropathic patients. Furthermore, this and other evidence indicate that multiplication of stimulus-induced afferent discharge in primary *low-threshold mechanoreceptors* may by itself explain unpleasant but not necessarily painful 'dysaesthetic' dynamic hyperalgesia or 'allodynia' (Campero *et al.* 1994, and unpublished observations).

Conceptualizing a neuropathic syndrome caused by central release of cold pain

Application of a painless low-temperature stimulus to the skin activates cold-specific channels subserved by small-calibre myelinated fibres (MacKenzie *et al.* 1975; Adriaensen *et al.* 1983). For low-temperature stimuli of noxious intensity, simultaneous co-activation of nociceptor channels subserved by unmyelinated C polymodal nociceptors is believed to mediate the characteristic painful cold sensation (Torebjörk 1974; LaMotte *et al.* 1982; Saumet *et al.* 1985). For high-temperature stimuli of noxious intensity, the activation of unmyelinated C polymodal nociceptors mediates the familiar burning pain sensation (Van Hees and Gybels 1981; Hallin *et al.* 1982; Ochoa and Torebjörk 1989; Torebjörk and Ochoa 1990; Yarnitsky *et al.* 1992). In turn, noxious mechanical stimuli to skin normally evoke typical sharp or dull burning pain devoid of any thermal quality. However, noxious mechanical stimulation of skin during a differential nerve block that selectively spares C-fibre input in normal volunteers evokes delayed burning pain without a mechanical sharp or dull component (Hallin and Torebjörk 1976; Ochoa and Torebjörk 1989). Correspondingly, intraneural microstimulation of identified C nociceptors typically evokes burning pain after a relatively long reaction time; such pain is resistant to selective unmyelinated fibre block (Ochoa and Torebjörk 1989). Nevertheless, during noxious low-temperature stimulation of human skin, the normal subjective experience is one of cold pain rather than of burning pain. What became of the burning component (Yarnitsky and Ocoa 1990*b*)?

Selective experimental blockade of cold-specific cutaneous input releases the magnitude of pain induced by noxious low temperature and changes its subjective quality into 'a burn' (Yarnitsky and Ochoa 1990*b*). This paradoxical phenomenon, like the thermal grill illusion of Thunberg (Craig and Bushnell 1994), is interpreted as being due to central disinhibition or unmasking. The modulation normally exerted by cold-specific Aδ neural input upon the quality and magnitude of C-fibre mediated pain (induced by low temperature) is found to be defective in certain patients with small-calibre fibre neuropathy. The abnormal condition is not aetiology-related, it is pathophysiology-related. These patients typically express a combination of cold hyperalgesia (featuring paradoxical burning quality), cold hypoaethesia, and cold skin (the triple cold syndrome: Ochoa and Yarnitsky 1990, 1994). The cutaneous hypothermia prevailing in symptomatic parts in these patients is due to vasospasm caused by partial sympathetic denervation supersensitivity secondary to unmyelinted fibre loss. The minimal requirement for spatial summation of the polymodal nociceptor painful input explains the prominence of the nociceptor-mediated cold hyperalgesia even in the presence of substantial loss of small-calibre fibres. The triple cold syndrome is the mirror image of the erythralgia or ABC syndrome, both syndromes emerging as independent clinical entities with definable abnormal mechanisms.

In patents with triple cold syndrome related to chronic progressive axonal poly-neuropathy, the failing neural function follows a dynamic gradient along the limbs, in keeping with the 'dying-back' process (Cavanagh 1964; Fig. 21.6). Indeed, proximally in the symptomatic limb, these patients display normal thresholds for cold pain and cold sensation, whereas in the symptomatic area there is cold hypoaesthesia associated with cold hyperalgesia. Occasionally, further distal to the hyperalgesic region there is global hypoaesthesia and hypoalgesia. It cannot be overemphasized that, together with a careful clinical history and neurological examination, tests such as thermography and quantitiative sensory testing, provide highly suggestive profiles both for the ABC syndrome and the triple cold syndrome (Verdugo and Ochoa 1992; Fig. 21.7).

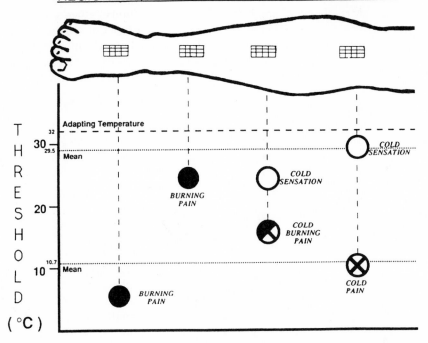

Fig. 21.6 Schematic representation of the regional gradient of thresholds for cold sensation and pain induced by low-temperature stimuli, measured at four points along the symptomatic limb by means of a quantitative thermotest. The ramps of low-temperature stimuli start from an adapting skin temperature of 32°C. Just below knee level, cold sensations and cold pain are felt at normal threshold values, with normal subjective qualities. At proximal leg level, cold sensation is detected at elevated threshold and pain induced by low temperature is detected at a moderately reduced threshold; it has an abnormal cold-burning quality. At distal leg level, pain is perceived at a hyperalgesic low threshold with burning quality; there is no cold sensation nor cold pain in response to low-temperature stimuli. Distally, on the foot, there is global hypoaesthesia and hypoalgesia; noxious low-temperature stimuli evoke burning pain at abnormally elevated thresholds. Reproduced with permission from Ochoa and Yarnitsky (1994).

Secondary sensitization of central neurones as a hypothetical pathogenetic mechanism of neuropathic pains and hyperalgesias

It has been proposed that certain forms of hyperalgesia following peripheral nerve injury result from secondary central nervous system (CNS) dysfunction (Lindblom and Verrillo 1979; Ochoa 1982; Fruhstorfer 1984; Wall 1984; Meyer et al. 1987). Tissue injury or inflammation may actually cause hyperexcitability of wide-dynamic-range convergent CNS neurones: they display an exaggerated response and expand their receptive fields to peripheral input (see Dubner 1991). This pathophysiological profile might explain some clinical observations described in patients thought to have 'centralized' neuropathic pains. They complain of pains that by far outlast the primary peripheral damage and that progressively worsen and expand in area. However, the theory is questioned by a clear-cut clinical dichotomy: expansion of spontaneous pain and hyperalgesia rarely occur following organic nerve injury; when gross expansion occurs, there is almost invariably absence of underlying organic nerve injury (Campero *et al.* 1992). In our opinion, the history of ideas behind the concept of 'centralization' of neuropathic pains is full of contradictions (Ochoa 1994; Ochoa and Verdugo 1995).

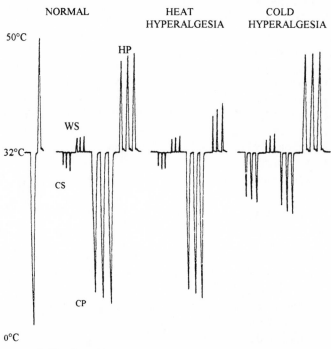

Fig. 21.7 (Centre panel): Heat hyperalgesia as seen in the ABC syndrome. (Right panel): Profile of the triple cold syndrome—cold hypoaesthesia associated with cold hyperalgesia.

It is possible to assess hypothetical 'centralization' in patients with chronic pains and hyperalgesias of organic neuropathic origin (Cline *et al.* 1989). This goal can be addressed by directly questioning the brain about the comparative quality and magnitude of pain evoked from the peripheral sensory apparatus projecting to symptomatic and control skin. Pain is evoked by means of intraneural stimulation, after bypassing potentially sensitized nerve endings. The method has been applied recently to assess central versus peripheral mechanisms of hyperalgesia in volunteers with capsaicin-induced secondary hyperalgesia (Torebjörk *et al.* 1992). Torebjörk (1993) has proposed that this experimental method be applied to the future study of clinical hyperalgesia. We have combined microneurography and microstimulation to excite identified low-threshold mechanoreceptors supplying hyperalgesic skin in patients, while measuring psychophysically the quality, localization, and, especially, the magnitude of evoked sensations. In patients with chronic regional 'neuropathic' pains, either with or without demonstrable organic mononeuropathy, selective stimulation of low-threshold mechanoreceptors has thus far failed to evoke pain (Dotson *et al.* 1992; Campero and Ochoa, unpublished). In other words, excitation of such units in patients evokes sensations similar to those experienced by normal volunteers (Ochoa and Torebjörk 1983). These findings fail to support secondary sensitization of central neurones as the cause of pain induced by weak excitation of tactile afferent units in these types of 'neuropathic' pain patients.

The recent human experiments on skin injury described above reveal that the area of secondary hyperalgesia that has been attributed to 'centralization' contains sensitized 'silent' or mechanically insensitive afferents (MIAs) (Serra *et al.* 1995). These results again question the concept that experimentally induced secondary hyperalgesia is necessarily due to transynaptic hyperexcitability of central neurones.

It remains possible, but unlikely in our opinion, that some individuals with painful neuropathy might harbour secondary centralized hyperexcitability and might benefit from administration of *N*-methyl-D-aspartate (NMDA) receptor antagonists. On the other hand, we believe that these powerful compounds (and their unwanted side-effects) should not be administered to patients whose painful neuropathic mechanisms are clearly peripheral (Ochoa 1993*a*). Establishing the viability of the 'centralized' neuropathic pain mechanism is a goal of major practical importance to be undertaken through rigorous scientific experiments in patients.

Reassessment of possible roles of the sympathetic system in generating vasomotor signs, neuropathic pains, and hyperalgesias

There exist defined criteria for the assessment of neuropathic anomalies of skin temperature, which traditionally tend to be attributed to imbalance of sympathetic outflow. Four patterns with pathophysiological significance emerge from thermographic recording of cutaneous responses to sympathetic reflex provocation, somatic local anaesthetic nerve block, sympathetic ganglion block, or blood vessel adrenoceptor block. One cold pattern is due to exaggerated sympathetic vasoconstrictor tone; the other implies chronic postganglionic sympathetic denervation and adrenoceptor supersensitivity. One warm pattern reflects acute suppression of the sympathetic vasoconstrictor tone; the other is unrelated to sympathetic activity, being caused by antidromic somatosensory (nociceptor) release of vasodilator substances (Ochoa *et al.* 1987*a*; Thomas and Ochoa 1993; see chapter 10 of Rosenbaum and Ochoa 1993). Thermographic recognition of these patterns is a prerequisite for proper interpretation of the meaning of temperature anomalies in neuropathic pain patients.

Pathophysiological interactions may occur between sympathetic efferent and sensory antidromic neurovascular functions in humans (Ochoa *et al.* 1993) and in an animal model of painful peripheral neuropathy (Bennett and Ochoa 1991). This issue becomes relevant to neuropathic pains because blood flow is a key determinant of skin temperature, an energy which in turn may critically activate or deactivate the excitable membrane of cutaneous nociceptor afferents (XTM). In the clinical realm this hierarchical predominance of sympathetically induced vasoconstriction over antidromic vasodilatation may mask the clinical profile of naturally 'hot' neuropathic syndromes (Plate 5). In addition, the sympathetically determined cooling effect opportunistically soothes heat-dependent nociceptor-mediated pains and hyperalgesias (Ochoa 1986; Ochoa *et al.* 1987*b*; Cline *et al.* 1989). This interaction might carry potential therapeutic value. Rather than assuming that sympatholysis is the only way to control painful syndromes associated with vasomotor imbalance, the opposite possibility should be assessed individually. Indeed, sympathomimetic drugs might be useful to treat patients with painful neuropathy caused by sensitization of nociceptors to heat.

Patients with 'neuropathic' pains who display vasomotor signs qualify for the diagnostic term 'reflex sympathetic dystrophy' (RSD) and after sympathetic block become suspect for 'sympathetically maintained pains'. However, testing for pain without proper control of placebo effect (both inert and active) is misleading (see Turner *et al.* 1994). Certain subpopulations of 'neuropatic pain' patients express a very high incidence of placebo response (Verdugo and Ochoa 1991, 1994*a*). The significance of subjective symptom relief in response to diagnostic sympathetic blocks has been re-examined and attributed to placebo effect in patients with posttraumatic causalgia, with RSD, and with painful polyneuropathy (McGlone *et al.* 1993; Verdugo and Ochoa 1994*b*; Verdugo *et al.* 1994; Jadad *et al.* 1995; Fig. 21.8). Doubts about the prevalence of the sympathetically maintained pain status (Blumberg 1993; Schott 1995) have been increased by the results of controlled studies in neuropathic monkeys (Carlton *et al.* 1993).

The human nociceptor and sympathetic pains

After dismissal of the early suggestion that the sympathetic system contributes to clinical pain states by conveying somatosensory afferent messages, it was for a long time hypothesized that, within peripheral nerves, sympathetic fibres pathologically activate 'pain' fibres ('artificial synapse': Doupe *et al.* 1944; Nathan 1947). This idea was subsequently abandoned (see historical analysis in Ochoa and Verdugo 1993), but the concept of pain caused by sympathetic actions was still maintained by the observation that patents with 'causalgia–RSD', even in the absence of demonstrable nerve lesion, often report improvement following sympathetic blocks (see Bonica 1979). This clinical evidence called for scientific endorsement as did the origin of certain clinical phenomena that could not be explained by the anatomical and functional organization

---

Fig. 21.8 (Top) Spontaneous pain outcome in response to phentolamine sympathetic block (protocol A: baseline (bas.), saline, and phentolamine (phentol.) phases). Note the pure placebo effect expressed within 30 min during the saline phase in 22 of 76 patients, and the slow, steady response during the saline and phentolamine phases in seven patients. In the 47 patients in whom saline did not induce a placebo response, the active blocker did not induce any effect. (Centre) Outcome for dynamic mechanical hyperalgesia (DMH) in response to phentolamine sympathetic block (protocol A) in 32 patients. The individual (* :intermediate profile) whose symptom was eventually abolished during phentolamine had initially expressed substantial placebo response followed by intervening reversal. Otherwise, the overall profile for dynamic mechanical hyperalgesia relief is similar to that for the spontaneous pain response: either placebo response or no response. (Bottom) Outcome for static mechanical hyperalgesia (SMH) in response to phentolamine sympathetic block (protocol A) in 51 patients. The overall profile is similar to those for spontaneous pain and DMH responses: most patients failed to respond and patients who responded did so through a placebo effect. Reproduced with permission from Verdugo and Ochoa (1994*b*).

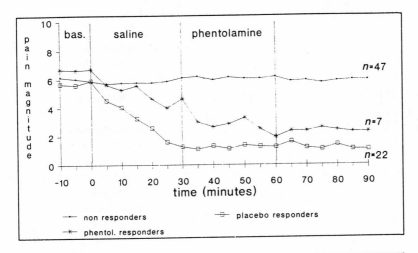

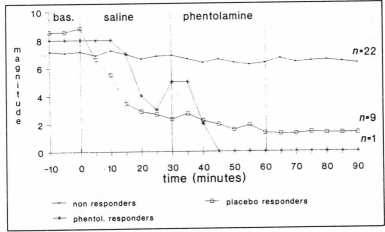

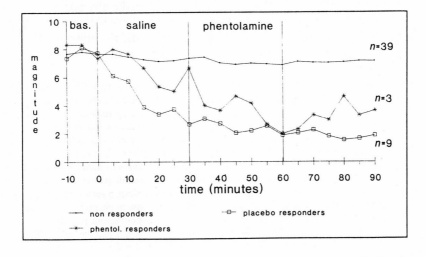

of the peripheral nervous system, such as non-dermatomal sensory loss and muscle weakness with normal tendon reflexes. But the worst hurdle at the periphery was the fact that, in many RSD patents, gentle touch hurts. Those needs were felt to be satisfied by including a sympathetic clause in the secondary 'centralization' theory of pain (Evans 1946*a,b*; Livingston 1947, pp. 209–23). For Loh and Nathan (1978) the whole profile was reconciled as follows: the sympathetic system did act, but indirectly, upon sensitized central cells.

It is unlikely that the output of *noradrenaline* could change the characteristics of peripheral endings of types I and II mechanoreceptors and hair receptors so that activation of these receptors causes pain, or that it could lower the threshold of delta or nonmyelinated nociceptors so that they would be excited by minimal mechanical stimuli. It is more likely that constant firing has caused a change in *central* activity. This might be a relaxation of tonic inhibition or increased facilitation, Either or both of these, or other mechanisms, could affect neurones of lamina 5 on which mechanoreceptor and nociceptor fibres converge; in this case these neurones might be fired by slight tactile stimulation.

The sympathetic imperative, as imposed by the observed relief of pain during sympatholysis, called for a more comprehensive 'centralized' hypothesis than that proposed by Loh and Nathan. This was provided by the sympathetically maintained pain (SMP) theory of Roberts (1986). A primary injury would trigger a nociceptive barrage that would sensitize dorsal horn neurones. Under those circumstances touch would cause pain because the sensitized central cells are pain-signalling and anatomically convergent. Sympathetic blocks would relieve pain by preventing sympathetic activity from activating tonically tactile corpuscles whose triggered input would excite those sensitized second-order cells. While Roberts' theory remains intellectually satisfying, when indirectly tested by us and others in patients with causalgia–RSD it does not hold. The use of microneurography has thus far failed to gather supporting evidence, in either normal human volunteers or mononeuropathic pain patients, that the sympathetic system, through activation of low-threshold mechanoreceptor units, might trigger unwanted afferent input (Dotson *et al.* 1990, 1992; Campero and Ochoa, unpublished observations). The theory of Roberts is also at odds with the clinical observation that causalgia–RSD patients not only do not worsen but may actually improve subjectively when their large-calibre fibres are stimulated with TENS units (Wall and Sweet 1967). Nevertheless, the theory remains popular and has been re-examined and re-appraised (see Campbell *et al.* 1988, 1992, 1993; Gracely *et al.* 1991, 1992; Koltzenburg *et al.* 1994). Those authors have considered the primary nociceptor to be an important player in the sympathetic–afferent equation. In patients, discrete foci of previously sensitized nociceptors would maintain in a chronic state the otherwise transient secondary central cell hyperexcitability (see Woolf and Thompson 1991 for experimental data). Sympathetic activity would determine spontaneous pain and hyperalgesia for as long as nociceptors maintain central ells hyperexcitable. The scientific strength of this interpretation is very difficult to assess as it relies entirely on subjective patient reports prompted by ceremonial clinical interventions such as a local anaesthetic block.

The recycled scientific ideas behind RSD–SMP have also taken into account a concept that originally goes back half a century (Jung 1941; Lewis 1942) and was then restated in the 1970s (Hanington-Kiff 1977) 'Superficial pain and hyperpathia in Sudeck's atrophy are due to the influence of noradrenaline on sensory nerve endings. This would explain why guanethidine first exacerbates, and then relieves these features of Sudeck's atrophy. Possibly the sensory nerve endings have been rendered susceptible in the injured limb.' The peripheral nociceptor itself would be primarily sensitized by physical trauma. The hyperexcitable behaviour of those units would be responsible for the subjective sensory symptomatology and their newly developed adrenergic chemosensitivity would explain the 'sympathetically maintained' clinical status, that is, the subjective pain relief by sympathetic blocks (see Sato and Perl 1991; Perl 1992*a,b*; and Lisney, Chapter 20, this volume). It should be emphasized that the model of sensitization of C nociceptors to adrenergic stimulation in the rabbit ear has not been shown to be associated with pain behaviour. On the other hand, does this interpretation still require an added central mechanism whereby convergent pain signalling cells are also sensitized? In any case, if this peripheral mechanism were responsible for all RSD–SMP syndromes, sympathectomy should always relieve these pain conditions and we know that this is not the case. The observation by Sato and Perl (1991) that 'after nerve damage, but not in its absence, sympathetic stimulation and norepinephrine [noradrenaline] were excitatory for a subset of skin C nociceptors . . .' is at variance with a prior report by Wallin *et al.* (1976) based on Swedish human microneurographic recordings. In patients with 'causalgia' whose spontaneous pain and allodynia were reactivated by topical application of noradrenaline (see Swedish results reissued by Torebjörk 1990), the responses of C nociceptors to mechanical and electrical stimulation in the symptomatic skin were normal. In attempting to reconcile this conflict it is useful to bear in mind that a large percentage of 'causalgia–RSD' patients do not have an organic nerve injury (Ochoa 1993*a*, 1994, 1996; Ochoa *et al.* 1994; Schott 1995).

Our limited testing of responsiveness to sympathetic stimulation of sensitized C polymodal nociceptors from patients with painful 'causalgic' polyneuropathy has been negative thus far (see Case report for Mrs K.).

References

Adriaensen, H., Gybels, J., Handwerker, H.O., and Van Hees, J. (1983). Response properties of thin myelinated fibers in human skin nerves. *J. Neurophysiol.* **49**, 111–22.

Baumann, T.K., Simone, D.A., Shain, C.N., and LaMotte, R.H. (1991). Neurogenic hyperalgesia: the search for the primary cutaneous afferent fibers that contribute to capsaicin-induced pain and hyperalgesia. *J. Neurophysiol.* **66**, 212–27.

Bayliss, W.M. (1901). On the origin from the spinal cord of the vasodilator fibres of the hind limb, and on the nature of these fibres. *J. Physiol., London,* **26**, 173–209.

Bennett, G. and Ochoa, J. (1991). Thermographic observations on rats with experimental neuropathic pain. *Pain* **45**, 61–7.

Bessou, P. and Perl, E.R. Response of cutaneous sensory units with unmyelinated fibers to noxious stimuli. *J. Neurophysiol.* **32**, 1025–43.

Bharali, L.A., and Lisney, S.J. (1992). The relationship between unmyelinated afferent type and neurogenic plasma extravasation in normal and reinnervated rat skin. *Neuroscience* **47**, 703–12.

Blumberg, H. (1993). Mechanisms of reflex sympathetic dystrophy and sympathetically maintained pain syndrome (Abstract). 7th World Congress on Pain, Paris, France, 1993.

Bonica, J.J. (1979). Causalgia and other reflex sympathetic dystrophies. In *Advances in pain research and therapy*, Vol. 3, (ed. J.J. Bonica, J.C. Liebeskind, and D.J. Albe-Fessard), pp. 141–66. Raven Press, New York.

Brain, S.D. and Escott, K.J. (1994). Calcitonin gene-related peptide. *Agents Actions* **41** (suppl. C), C262–263.

Bullit, E. (1991). Somatotopy of spinal nociceptive processing. *J. comp. Neurol.* **321**, 279–90.

Burgess, P.R., and Perl, E.R. (1973) Cutaneous mechanoreceptors and nociceptors. In *Handbook of sensory physiology*. Vol. II, *Somatosensory system*, (ed. A. Iggo), pp. 29–78. Springer-Verlag, Berlin.

Campbell, J.N., and Meyer, R.A. (1983). Sensitization of unmyelinated nociceptive afferents in monkey varies with skin type. *J. Neurophysiol.* **49**, 98–110.

Campbell, J.N., Raja, S.N., and Meyer, R.A. (1988). Painful sequelae of nerve injury. In *Proceedings of the 5th World Congress on Pain* (ed. R. Dubner, G.F. Gebhart, and M.R. Bond), pp. 135–43.. Elsevier Science Publishers, Amsterdam.

Campbell, J.N., Meyer, R.A., Davis, K.D., and Raja, S.N. (1992). Sympathetically maintained pain. A unifying hypothesis. In *Hyperalgesia and allodynia* (ed. W.D. Willis), pp. 141–9. Raven Press, New York.

Campbell, J.N., Raja, S.N., and Meyer, R.A. (1993). Pain and the sympathetic nervous system: connecting the loop. In *New trends in referred pain and hyperalgesia* (ed. L. Vecchiet, D. Albe-Fessard, and U. Lindblom, pp. 99–108. Elsevier Science Publishers, Amsterdam.

Campero, M., Ochoa, J., and Pubols, L. (1992). Receptive fields of hyperalgesia confine to districts of injured nerves; fields 'expand' in 'RSD' without nerve injury. *Soc. Neurosci. Abstr.* **18**, 287.

Campero, M., Serra, J., and Ochoa, J.L. (1994). Response of human cutaneous C-polymodal nociceptors elicited by low temperature stimulation. *J. Neurol.* **241**, (Suppl. 1), S61 (abstract).

Carlton, S.M., Gondesen, K., Palecek, J., Rees, H., Dougherty, P.J., and Willis, W.D. (1993). Behavioral and electrophysiological consequences of phentolamine administration in neuropathic primates. *Soc. Neurosci. Abstr.* **19**, 520.

Cavanagh, J.B. (1964). The significance of the 'dying back' process in experimental and human neurological disease. *Int. Rev. exp. Pathol.* **3**, 219–67.

Chapman, L.F., Ramos, A.O., and Goodell, H. (1961). Neurohumoral features of afferent fibers in man. *Arch. Neurol.* **4**, 617–50.

Cline, M., and Ochoa, J.L. (1986). Chronically sensitized C nociceptors in skin. Patient with hyperalgesia, hyperpathia, and spontaneous pain. *Soc. Neurosci. Abstr.* **12**, 331.

Cline, M.A., Ochoa, J.L., and Torebjörk, E. (1989). Chronic hyperalgesia and skin warming caused by sensitized C nociceptors. *Brain* **12**, 621–47.

Comstock, W., Ochoa, J., and Marchettini, P. (1986). Neurogenic warming of human hand provinces by activation of the unmyelinated population of single skin nerve fascicles. *Soc. Neurosci. Abstr.* **12**, 331.

Craig, A.D., and Bushnell, M.C. (1994). The thermal grill illusion: unmasking the burn of cold pain. *Science* **265**, 252–5.

Culp, W.J., Ochoa, J.L., Cline, M.A., and Dotson, R. (1989). Heat and mechanical hyperalgesia induced by capsaicin: cross modality threshold modulaton in human C nociceptors. *Brain* **112**, 1317–31.

Davis, K.D., Meyer, R.A., and Campbell, J.N. (1993). Chemosensitivity and sensitization of nociceptive afferents that innervate the hairy skin of monkey. *J. Neurophysiol.* **69**, 1071–81.

Dotson, R., Ochoa, J., Cline, M., Roberts, W.J., Yarnitsky, D., Simone, D., and Marchettini, P. (1990). Sympathetic effects on human low threshold mechanoreceptors. *Soc. Neurosci. Abstr.* **16**, 1280.

Dotson, R., Ochoa, J.L., Cline, M., Marchettini, P., and Yarnitsky, D. (1992). Intraneural microstimulation of low threshold mechanoreceptors in patients with causalgia/RSD/SMP. *Soc. Neurosci. Abstr.* **18**, 290.

Doupe, J., Cullen, C.H., and Chance, G.O. (1944. Post traumatic pain and the causalgic syndrome. *J. Neurol. Neurosurg. Psychiat.* **7**, 33–48.

Dubner, R. (1991) Pain and hyperalgesia following tissue injury: new mechanisms and new treatment. (Editorial comment). *Pain* **44**, 213–14.

Evans, J.A. (1946a). Reflex sympathetic dystrophy. *Surg. Clin. North America* **26**, 780–90.

Evans, J.A. (1946b). Reflex sympathetic dystrophy. *Surg. Gynecol. Obstet.* **82**, 36–43.

Foerster, O. (1933). The dermatomes in man. *Brain* **56**, 1–39.

Fruhstorfer, H. (1984). Thermal sensibility changes during ischemic nerve block. *Pain* **20**, 355–61.

Georgopoulos, A.P. (1976). Functional properties of primary afferent units probably related to pain mechanisms in primate glabrous skin. *J. Neurophysiol.* **39**, 71–83.

Georgopoulos, A.P. (1977). Stimulus–response relations in high-threshold mechanothermal fibers innervating primate glabrous skin. *Brain Res.* **128**, 547–52.

Gracely, R.H., Lynch, S., and Bennett, G.J. (1991). The central process responsible for AβLTM-mediated allodynia in some patients with RSD is sensitive to perfusion of the microenvironment of nociceptor terminals. *Soc. Neurosci. Abstr.* **17**, 439.

Gracely, R.H., Lynch S., and Bennett, G.J. (1992). Painful neuropathy: altered central processing maintained dynamically by peripheral input. *Pain* **51**, 175–94.

Hallin, R.G., and Torebjörk, H.E. (1970), C-fibre components in electrically evoked compound potentials recorded from human median nerve fascicles in situ. *Acta soc. med. upsaliensis* **75**, 77–80.

Hallin, R.G., and Torebjörk, H.E. (1976). Studies on cutaneous A and C fibre afferents, skin nerve blocks and perception. In *Sensory functions of the skin in primates, with special reference to man*, Wenner-Gren International Symposium, Vol. 27 (ed. Y. Zottermann), pp. 137–49). Pergamon Press, Oxford.

Hallin, R.G., Torebjörk, H.E., and Wiesenfeld, Z. (1982). Nociceptors and warm receptors innervated by C fibres in human skin. *J. Neurol. Neurosurg. Psychiat.* **45**, 313–19.

Handwerker, H.O., Schmidt, R., Forster, C., Schmelz, M., Traversa, R., and Torebjörk, H.E. (1993). Microneurographic assessment of sensitive and insensitive C-fibers in human skin nerve. *Soc. Neurosci. Abstr.* **19**, 1404.

Hannington-Kiff, J.G. (1977). Relief of Sudeck's atrophy by regional intravenous guanethidine. *Lancet* **1**, 1132–3.

Hardy, J.D., Wolff, H.G., and Goodell, H. (1952). *Pain sensations and reactions.* Williams & Wilkins, Baltimore.

Helme, R.D., and McKernan, S. (1985). Neurogenic flare responses following topical application of capsaicin in humans. *Ann. Neurol.* **18**, 505–9.

Hinsey, J.C., and Gasser, H.S. (1930). The component of the dorsal root mediating vasodilatation and the Sherrington contracture. *Am. J. Physiol.* **92**, 679–89.

Iggo, A. (1959). Cutaneous heat and cold receptors with slowy conducting (C) afferent fibres. *Quart. J. exp. Physiol.* **44**, 362–70.

Iggo, A. (1960). Cutaneous mechanoreceptors with afferent C fibres. *J. Physiol., London* **152**, 337–53.

Iggo, A., and Ogawa, H. (1971). Primate cutaneous thermal nociceptors. *J. Physiol., London*, **216**, 77P–8P (abstract).

Jadad, A.R., Carroll, D., Glynn, C.J., and McQuay, H.J. (1995). Intravenous regional sympathetic blockade for pain in reflex sympathetic dystrophy: a systematic review and a randomized, double-blind crossover study. *J. Pain Symptom Management.* **10**, 13–20.

Jung, V.R. (1941). Die allgemeine Symptomatologie der Nervenverletzungen und ihre physiologischen Grundlangen. *Enarzt* **14**, 493–516.

Kenins, P. (1984). Electrophysiological and histological studies of vascular permeability after antidromic sensory nerve stimulation. In *Antidromic vasodilatation and neurogenic inflammation* (ed. L.A. Chahl, J. Szolcsányi, and F. Lembeck), pp.175–91. Akadémiai Kiadó, Budapest.

Kennedy, W.R., and Wendelschafer-Crabb, G. (1993). The innervation of human epidermis. *J. neurol. Sci.* **115**, 184–90.

Koltzenburg, M., Lundberg, L.E.R., and Torebjörk, E. (1993). Dynamic and static components of mechanical hyperalgesia in human hairy skin. Significant addendum. *Pain* **53**, 363.

Koltzenburg, M., Torebjörk, H.E., and Wahrén, L.K. (1994). Nociceptor modulated central sensitization causes mechanical hypralgesia in acute chemoenic and chronic neuropathic pain. *Brain* **117**, 579–91.

Kusunoki, S., Inoue, K., Iwamori, M., Nagai, Y., and Mannen, T. (1991). Fucosylated glycoconjugates in human dorsal root ganglion cells with unmyelinated axons. *Neurosci. Lett.* **126**, 159–62.

LaMotte, R.H., Thalhammer, J.G., Torebjörk, H.E., and Robinson, C.J. (1982). Peripheral neural mechanisms of cutaneous hyperalgesia following mild injury by heat. *J. Neurosci.* **2**, 765–81.

LaMotte, R.H., Thalhammer, J.G., and Robinson, C.J. (1983). Peripheral neural correlates of magnitude of cutaneous pain and hyperalgesia: a comparison of neural events in monkey with sensory judgments in human. *J. Neurophysiol.* **50**, 1–26.

LaMotte, R.H., Shain, C.N., Simone, D.A., and Tsai, E.E.P. (1991). Neurogenic hyperalgesia: psychophysical studies of unerlying mecanisms. *J. Neurophysiol.* **66**, 190–211.

LaMotte, R.H., Lundberg, L.E.R., and Torebjörk, E. (1992). Pain, hyperalgesia and activity in nociceptive C units in humans after intradermal injection of capsaicin. *J. Neurophysiol.* **448**, 749–64.

Langley, J.N. (1921). *The autonomic nervous system.* Cambridge University Press, London.

Langley, J.N. (1923). Antidromic action. Part I. *J. Physiol.* **LVII**, 428–46.

Lewis, T. (1927). *The blood vessels of the human skin and their responses.* Shaw & Sons, London.

Lewis, T. (1933. Clinical observations and experiments relating to burning pain in the extremities, and to so-called 'Erythromelalgia' in particular. *Clin. Sci.* **1**, 175–211.

Lewis, R. (1935–6). Experiments relating to cutaneous hyperalgesia and its spread through somatic nerves. *Clin. Sci.* **2**, 373–421.

Lewis, T. (1936). *Vascular disorders of the limbs, described for practitioners and students.* Macmillan, London.

Lewis, T. (1937). The nocifensor system of nerves and its reactions. *Br. Med. J.* March, 491–4.

Lewis, T. (1942). *Pain.* Macmillan, London.

Lindblom, U., and Verrillo, R.T. (1979). Sensory functions in chronic neuralgia. *J. Neurol. Neurosurg. Psychiat.* **42**, 422–35.

Livingston, W.K. (1947). *Pain mechanisms.* Macmillan, New York.

Loh, L., and Nathan, P.W. (1978). Painful peripheral states and sympathetic blocks. *J. Neurol. Neurosurg. Psychiat.* **41**, 664–71.

McGlone, F., Dean, J., and Dhar, S. (1993). A sympathetic response to sympathetic block in RSD? *Abstracts 7th World Congress on Pain, Paris, France, 1993*, p. 350. IASP Press, Seattle.

MacKenzie, R.A., Burke, D., Skuse, N.F., and Lethlean, K. (1975). Fibre function and perception during cutaneous nerve block. *J. Neurol. Neurosurg. Psychiat.* **38**, 865–73.

Marchettini, P. (1993). Muscle pain: animal and human experimental and clinical studies. *Muscle Nerve* **16**, 1033–9.

Merskey, H. and Bogduk, N. (ed.) (1994). *Classification of chronic pain: description of chronic pain syndromes and definition of pain terms.* IASP (International Association for the Study of Pain) Press, Seattle.

Meyer, R.A., Campbell, J.N., and Raja, S.N. (1987). Hyperalgesia following peripheral nerve injury. In *Effects of injury on trigeminal and spinal somatosensory systems* (ed. L.M. Pubols and B.J. Sessle), pp. 383–8. Alan R. Liss, New York.

Mori, K. (1986). Lectin *Ulex europaeus* agglutinin I specifically labels a subset of primary afferent fibers which project selectively to the superficial dorsal horn of the spinal cord. *Brain Res.* **365**, 404–8.

Nathan, P.W. (1947). On the pathogenesis of causalgia in perpheral nerve injuries. *Brain* **70**, 145–70.

Ochoa, J.L. (1970). The structure of developing and adult sural nerve in man and the changes which occur in some diseases. A light and electron miroscopic study. Unpublished PhD thesis, University of London.

Ochoa, J.L. (1982). Pain in local nerve lesions. In *Abnormal nerves and muscles as impulse generators* (ed. W. Culp and J.L. Ochoa), pp. 568–87. Oxford University Press, New York.

Ochoa, J.L. (1984). peripheral unmyelinated units in man: structure, function, disorder, and role in sensation. In *Advances in pain research and therapy*, Vol. 6 (ed. L. Kruger and J.C. Liebeskind). Raven Press, New York.

Ochoa, J.L. (1986). The newly recognized painful ABC syndrome: thermographic aspects. *Thermology* **2**, 65–107.

Ochoa, J.L. (1993*a*). Guest Editorial: Essence, investigation, and management of 'Neuropathic' pains: hopes from acknowledgment of chaos. *Muscle Nerve* **16**, 997–1008.

Ochoa, J.L. (1993*b*). The human sensory unit and pain. New concepts, syndromes and tests. *Muscle & Nerve* **16**, 1009–16.

Ochoa, J.L. (1994). Pain mechanisms in neuropathy. Current Science ISMN 1–85922–678–7 ISSN 1350–7540. *Curr. Opin. Neurol.* **7**, 407–14.

Ochoa, J.L. (1996). Chronic pains associated with positive and negative sensory, motor and vasomotor manifestations. Clinical entities and differential diagnosis of their physiopathological and psychopathological substrates. In *Behavioral and brain sciences*, (ed. S. Harnard, W. Roberts, and P.J. Cordo). Cambridge University Press, New York. (In press.)

Ochoa, J.L., and Mair, W.G.P. (1969*a*). The normal sural nerve in man. I. Ultrastructure and numbers of fibres and cells. *Acta neuropathol.* **13**, 197–216.

Ochoa, J.L., and Mair, W.G.P. (1969*b*). The normal sural nerve in man. II. Changes in axons and Schwann cells due to age. *Acta neuropathol.* **13**, 217–39.

Ochoa, J.L., and Torebjörk, H.E. (1981). Pain from skin and muscle. *Pain* **11**, S87 (Abstract).

Ochoa, J.L., and Torebjörk, H.E. (1983). Sensations evoked y intraneural microstimulation of single mechano-receptor units innervating the human hand. *J. Physiol.* **342**, 633–54.

Ochoa, J.L., and Torebjörk, H.E. (1989). Sensations evoked by selective intraneural microstimulation of identified C nociceptor fibres in human skin nerves. *J. Physiol.* **415**, 583–99.

Ochoa, J.L., and Verdugo, R.J. (1993). Reflex sympathetic dystrophy. Definitions and history of the ideas. A critical review of human studies. In *The evaluation and management of cloinical autonomic disorders* (ed. P.A. Low), pp. 473–92. Little, Brown & Co, Boston.

Ochoa, J.L., and Verdugo, R.J. (1995). Reflex sympathetic dystrophy: a common clinical avenue for somatoform expression. *Neurol. Clin.* **13**, 351–63.

Ochoa, J.L., and Yarnitsky, D. (1990). Triple cold ['CCC'] painful syndrome. *Pain Suppl.* **5**, S278 (abstract).

Ochoa, J.L., and Yarnitsky, D. (1993). Mechanical hyperalgesias in neuropathic pain patients: dynamic and static subtypes. *Ann. Neurol.* **33**, 465–72.

Ochoa, J.L., and Yarnitsky, D. (1994). The triple cold ('CCC') syndrome: cold hyperalgesia, cold hypoesthesia and cold skin in peripheral nerve disease. *Brain* **117**, 185–97.

Ochoa, J.L., Comstock, W.J., Marchettini, P., and Nizamuddin, S. (1987*a*). Intrafascicular nerve stimulation elicits regional skin warming that matches the projected field of evoked pain. In *Fine afferent nerve fibers and pain* (ed. R.F. Schmidt, H.G. Schaible, and C. Vahle-Hinz), pp. 475–9. VCH, Weinheim.

Ochoa, J.L., Cline, M., Comstock, W., Culp, W.J., Dotson, R., Marchettini, P., and Torebjörk, H.E. (1987*b*). Painful syndrome newly recogniz4ed: polymodal hyperalgesia with cross modality threshold modulaton and rubor. Its basis: sensitized nociceptors plus antidromic vasodilatation. *Soc. Neurosci. Abstr.* **57**, 12.

Ochoa, J.L., Roberts, W.J., Cline, M.A., Dotson, R., and Yarnitsky, D. (1989). Two mechanical hyperalgesias in human neuropathy. *Soc. Neurosci. Abstr.* **15** (1), 472.

Ochoa, J., Yarnitsky, D., Marchettini, P., Dotson, R., and Cline, M. (1993). Interactions between sympathetic vasoconstrictor outflow and C nociceptor-induced antidromic vasodilatation in man. *Pain* **54**, 191–6.

Ochoa, J.L., Verdugo, R.J., and Campero, M. (1994). Pathophysiological spectrum of organic and psychogenic disorders in 270 'neuropathic' pain patients fitting the description of 'Causalgia' or 'RSD'. In *Proceedings of the 7th World Congress on Pain*. Vol. 2, *Progress in pain research management* (ed. G.F. Gebhart, D.L. Hammond, and T.S. Jensen), pp.483–94. IASP Press, Seattle.

514   *Pathophysiology of human nociceptor function*

Paintal, A.S. (1967). A comparison of the nerve impulses of mammalian non-medullated nerve fibres with those of the smallest diameter medullated fibres.l *J. Physiol.* **193**, 523–33.

Perl, E.R. (1984). Characterization of nociceptors and their activation of neurons in the superficial dorsal horn: first steps for the sensation of pain. In *Advances in pain research and therapy* (ed. L. Kruger and J.C. Liebeskind), pp. 23–51. Raven Press, New York.

Perl, E.R. (1992*a*). Alterations in the responsiveness of cutaneous nociceptors: sensitization by noxius stimuli and the induction of adrenergic responsiveness by nerve injury. In *Hyperalgesia and allodynia*, (ed. W.D. Willis), pp. 59–80. Raven Press, New York.

Perl, E.R. (1992*b*). Nociceptors and primary hyperalgesia (discussion). In *Hyperalgesia and allodynia* (ed. W.D. Willis), pp. 167–71. Raven Press, New York.

Raja, S.N., Campbell, J.N., and Meyer, R.A. (1984). Evidence for different mechanisms of primary and secondary hyperalgesia following heat injury to the glabrous skin. *Brain* **107**, 1179–88.

Remak, R. (1838). *Observationes anatomicae et microscopicae de systematis nervosi structura.* Berlin.

Roberts, W.J. (1986). A hypothesis on the physiological basis for causalgia and related pains. *Pain* **24**, 297–311.

Rosenbaum, R.B., and Ochoa, J.L. (1993). *Carpal tunnel syndrome and other disorders of the median nerve.* Butterworth-Heinemann, Boston.

Sato, J., and Perl, E.R. (1991). Adrenergic excitation of cutaeous pain receptors induced by peripheral nerve injury. *Science* **251**, 1608–10.

Saumet, J.L., Chery-croze, S., and Duclaux, R. (1985). Response of cat skin mechanothermal nociceptors to cold stimulation. *Brain Res. Bull.* **15**, 529–32.

Schmidt, R., Torebjörk, H.E., and Jørum, E. (1993). Pain and itch from intraneural micro-stimulation. *Abstracts: 7th World Congress in Pain*, p. 143. IASP Press, Seattle.

Schott, G.D. (1995). An unsympathetic view of pain. *Lancet* **345**, 634–5.

Serra, J., Campero, M., and Ochoa, J. (1993). 'Secondary' hyperalgesia (capsaicin) mediated by C-nociceptors. *Soc. Neurosci. Abstr.* **19**, 965.

Serra, J., Campero, M., and Ochoa, J.L. (1994*a*). Mechanisms of neurogenic flare in human skin. *J. Neurol.* **241**, S34 (abstract).

Serra, J., Campero, M., and Ochoa, J.L. (1994*b*). Common peripheral mechanism for neurogenic flare and hyperalgesia (capsaicin) in human skin. *Muscle Nerve* Suppl. 1, S250 (abstract).

Serra, J., Campero, M., and Ochoa, J. (1995). Sensitization of 'silent' C-nociceptors in areas of secondary hyperalgesia (SH) in humans. *Neurology* **Suppl. 4**, A365 (abstract).

Shimizu, J., Murayama, S., Kusonoki, S., Inoue, K., and Kanazawa, I. (1994). Selective labeling of somatic afferent C fibers in human sural nerve by UEA-I Lectin. *Muscle Nerve* **Suppl. 1**, S217 (abstract).

Simone, D.A., Baumann, T.K., and LaMotte, R.H. (1989). Dose-depedent pain and mechanical hyperalgesia in humans after intradermal injection of capsaicin. *Pain* **38**, 99–107.

Simone, D.A., Sorkin, L.S., Oh, U., Chun, J.M., Owens, C., LaMotte, R.H., and Willis, W.D. (1991). Neurogenic hyperalgesia: central neural correlates in responses of spinothalamic tract neurons. *J. Neurophysiol.* **66**, 228–45.

Simone, D., Caputi, G., Marchettini, P., and Ochoa, J. (1992). Cramping pain and deep hyperalgesia following intramuscular injection of capsaicin. *Soc. Neurosci. Abstr.* **18**, 134.

Simone, D.A., Marchettini, P., Caputi, G., and Ochoa, J.L. (1994). Identification of muscle afferents subserving sensation of deep pain in humans. *J. Neurophysiol.* (1876). **72**, 883–9.

Stricker, S. (1876). Untersuchung über die geffässerwurzein des Ischiadicus. *Sitz Kaiserl. Akad. Wissenschr (Wien)* **3**, 173.

Szolcsányi, J., Pintér, E., and Pethö, G. (1992). Role of unmyelinated afferents in regulation of microstimulation and its chronic distortion after trauma and change. In *Reflex sympathetic dystrophy, pathophysiological mechanisms and clinical implications* (ed. W. Jänig and R.F. Schmidt), pp. 245–61. VCH, Weinheim.

Thomas, P.K., and Ochoa, J.L. (1993). Clinical features and differential diagnosis. In *Peripheral neurpathy* (3rd edn), (ed. P. Dyck, P.K. Thomas, J.W. Griffin, P.A. Low, and J.F. Podulso), pp. 749–74. W.B. Saunders, Philadelphia.

Torebjörk, H.E. (1974). Afferent C units responding to mechanical, thermal and chemical stimuli in human non-glabrous skin. *Acta physiol. scand.* **94**, 374–90.

Torebjörk, H.E. (1985). Nociceptor activation and pain. *Phil. Trans. R. Soc., London* **308**, 227–34.

Torebjörk, H.E. (1990). Clinical and neurophysiological observations relating to pathophysiological mechanisms in reflex sympathetic dystrphy. In *Reflex sympathetic dystrphy* (ed. M. Stanton-Hicks, W. Jänig, and R.A. Boas), pp. 71–80. Kluwer Academic Publishers, Boston.

Torebjörk, H.E. (1992). Nociceptive and non-nociceptive afferents contributing to pain and hyperalgesia in humans. In *Hyperalgesia and allodynia* (ed. W.D.J. Willis), pp. 135–90. Raven Press, New York.

Torebjörk, H.E. (1993). Human microneurography and intraneural microstimulation in the study of neuropathic pain. *Muscle Nerve* **16**, 1056–62.

Torebjörk, H.E. and Hallin, R.G. (1970). C-fibre units recorded from human sensory nerve fascicles in situ. *Acta soc. med. upsaliensis* **75**, 81–4.

Torebjörk, H.E., and Hallin, R.G. (1976). Skin receptors supplied by unmyelinated (C) fibres in man. In *Sensory functions of the skin in primates with special reference to man* (ed. Y. Zotterman), pp. 475–85. Pergamon Press, Oxford.

Torebjörk, H.E. and Ochoa, J.L. (1980). Specific sensations evoked by activity in single identified sensory units in man. *Acta physiol. scand.* **18**, 1445–7.

Torebjörk, H.E. and Ochoa, J.L. (1981). Pain and itch from C-fibers stimulation. *Soc. Neurosci. Abstr.* **7**, 228.

Torebjörk, H.E. and Ochoa, J.L. (1990). New method to identify nociceptor units innervating glabrous skin of the human hand. *Exp. Brain Res.* **81**, 509–14.

Torebjörk, H.E., LaMotte, R.H., and Robinson, C.J. (1984). Peripheral neural correlates of magnitude of cutaneous pain and hyperalgesia: simultaneous recordings in humans of sensory judgments of pain and evoked responses in nociceptors with C-fibers. *J. Neurophysiol.* **51**, 325–39.

Torebjörk, H.E., Lundberg, L.E.R., and LaMotte, R.H. (1992). Central changes in processing of mechanoreceptive input in capsaicin-induced secondary hypralgesia. *J. Physiol.* **448**, 765–80.

Turner, J.A., Deyo, R.A., Loeser, J.D., Von Koff, M., and Fordyce, W.E. (1994). The importance of placebo-effects in pain treatment and research. *J. Am. med. Soc.* **271**, 1609–14.

Verdugo, R.J., and Ochoa, J.L. (1991). High incidence of placebo responders among chronic neuropathic pain patients. *Ann. Neurol.* **30**, 229 (abstract).

Verdugo, R., and Ochoa, J.L. (1992). Quantitative somatosensory thermotest. A key method for functional evaluation of small caliber afferent channels. *Brain* **115**, 893–913.

Verdugo, R.J., and Ochoa, J.L. (1994a). Placebo response in chronic, causalgiform, 'neuropathic' pain patients. Study and Review. *Pain Rev.* **1**, 33–46.

Verdugo, R.J., and Ochoa, J.L. (1994b). 'Sympathetically maintained pain.' I. Phentolamine block questions the concept. *Neurology* **44**, 1079–82.

Verdugo, R.J., Campero, M., and Ochoa, J.L. (1994). Phentolamine sympathetic block in painful polyneuropathies. II. Further questioning of the concept of 'sympathetically maintained pain'. *Neurology* **44**, 1083–5.

Van Hees, J., and Gybels, J. (1972). Pain related to single afferent C fibres from human skin. *Brain Res.* **67**, 387–402.

Van Hees, J., and Gybels, J. (1981). C nociceptor activity in human nerve during painful and non painful skin stimulation. *J. Neurol. Neurosurg. Psychiat.* **44**, 600–7.

Wall, P.D. (1984). The hyperpathic syndrome: a challenge to specificity theory. In *Somatosensory mechanisms,* Wenner-Gren International Symposium, Vol. 41 (ed. C. Von Euler, O. Franzén, U. Lindblom, and D. Ottoson), pp. 327–37. Macmillan, London.

Wall, P.D., and McMahon, S.B. (1985). Microneurography and its relation to perceived sensation. A critical review. *Pain* **21**, 209–29.

Wall, P.D. and Sweet, W.H. (1967). Temporary abolition of pain in man. *Sci. Abstr.* **155**, 108–9.

Wallin, G., Torebjörk, E., and Hallin, R. (1976). Preliminary observations on the pathophysiology of hyperalgesia in the causalgic pain syndrome. In *Sensory functions of the skin in primates* (ed. Y. Zotterman), pp. 489–502. Pergamon Press, Oxford.

Woolf, C.J., and Thompson, S.W.N. (1991). The induction and maintenance of central sensitization is dependent on N-methyl-D-aspartic receptor activaton; implications for the treatment of post-injury pain hypersensitivity states. *Pain* **44**, 293–300.

Woolward, H.H. (1936). Intra-epidermal nerve endings. *J. Anat.* **71**, 54–9.

Woollard, H.H., Weddell, G., and Harpman, J.A. (1940). Observations on the neurohistological basis of cutaneous pain. *J. nat.* **74**, 413–40.

Yarnitsky, D., and Ochoa, J.L. (1990a). Study of heat pain sensation in man. I: Perception thresholds, rate of stimulus rise and reaction time. *Pain* **40**, 85–91.

Yarnitsky, D., and Ochoa, J.L. (1990b). Release of cold-induced burning pain by block of cold-specific afferent input. *Brain* **113**, 893–902.

Yarnitsky, D., Simone, D., Dotson, R., Cline, M., and Ocoa, J. (1992). Single C nociceptor responses and psychophysical parameters of evoked pain: effect of rate of rise of heat stimuli in humans. *J. Physiol., London* **450**, 581–92.

Zotterman, Y. (1933). Studies in the peripheral nervous mechanism of pain. *Acta med. scand.* **80**, 186–242.

Zotterman, Y. (1936). Specific action potentials in the lingual nerve of cat. *Skand. Arch. Physiol.* **75**, 105–20.

Index

A-fibres (fastest conducting fibres)
 β-type, cutaneous mechanoreceptive, pain and
  406
 δ-type, see Aδ-fibres
 discovery/historical studies 13
 mechanoheat sensitive, see A mechanoheat
  nociceptors
 polymodal 328
 see also myelinated fibres
Aδ-fibres
 coding of information about peripheral injury 97
 corneal 97
 cutaneous afferent 22–3, 97, 357–9, 494, 495–6
  cognitive attributes of somatic sensations
   evoked by selective activation of 495–6
 DRG somata of 84
 intraepidermal 45
 mechanically-insensitive 373, 374
 nociceptive types 85, 357–9
 non-nociceptive types 85
 development 462–3
 discovery/historical studies 13, 14, 17, 22–3
 effector function 477
 injury and regeneration 476–7
A mechanoheat nociceptors (AMH)
 corneal 159–60
 skin 119–20, 128–30, 358
  heat hyperalgesia 370, 371
  heat pain signalling 131–3
  heat responses 121, 128–30, 358
  mechanical responses 121, 133–6
  type I 120, 121, 128, 358
  type II 120, 121, 128, 358
A mechanoreceptors (AM), cutaneous 358, 359
ABC syndrome/erythralgia 500–1, 503, 504
 triple cold syndrome mirroring 502
acetic acid, corneal, polymodal unit responses 157,
  158
acetylcholine 270–1
N-acetylgalactosamine-binding lectins, labelling
  with 42
acid, dilute 274–6
 cornea 274–5
  polymodal unit responses 157, 158
 skin 275–6
  C-fibre responses 26
acid phosphatase, see fluoride-sensitive acid
  phosphatase
ACTH (corticotrophin)-releasing factor, opioids
  and 443–5
action potentials
 coupling, see coupling
 thin fibre 18
 see also discharge; impulse

activation of nociceptors, spreading sensitisation in
  response to 381–2
adenosine effects 311
adenylate cyclase-linked G-protein-coupled
  receptors 304–6
adrenaline effects 268–9
 in skeletal muscle 188
α2-adrenoceptors
 hyperalgesia and 382
 noradrenaline and 269, 305–6
adrenocorticotrophic hormone (corticotrophin)-
  releasing factor, opioids and 443–5
aesthesiometers, corneal 171
age-related changes in fine structure 490, 493
AH6809 336, 337
airways/respiratory tract
 efferent actions of nociceptors 422, 426, 427, 428
 high-threshold receptors 222–3
 neuropeptide effects 426
algogen, see pain
alimentary tract, see gastrointestinal tract
allodynia 364–5, 370–1, 390–404 passim
 hyperalgesia vs. 370–1
 mechano- 406
alloknesis 391, 396
allyl-isothiocyanate (mustard oil) on skin 284–5,
  359–61
alpha-2 adrenoceptors, see adrenoceptors
amino acids
 excitatory 271, 380
  cutaneous hyperalgesia and 380
  long-term potentiation and 102, 103
 markers, DRG 75
γ-aminobutyric acid 271
cAMP 309–11
 bradykinin responses and 268, 336
 prostaglandin responses and 268, 336, 337
 sensitization role 309–11
 long-term, in Aplysia 105
AMPA, cutaneous dysaesthesiae and 404
Amphioxus spp., coiling-reflex 325
amplification of signal (in signal transduction) 245,
  247–53
anaesthetics, general, see general anaesthetics; local
  anaesthetics
analgesia, peripheral opioid 445–6
 stress-induced 444–5
anatomy, see structure
ankle joint afferents, mechanosensitivity 206
antidromic excitation of C nociceptors, vascular
  reactions induced by 496–7
antinociception, endogenous, articular afferents 212–13
antipruritic state, painful cutaneous stimulation
  setting up 393